Taste of Home

BEST OF

Comfort Food Diet

COOKBOOK

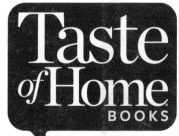

Taste of Home BOOKS

REIMAN MEDIA GROUP, INC.
GREENDALE, WI

Taste of Home | Reader's Digest

A TASTE OF HOME/READER'S DIGEST BOOK
© 2013 Reiman Media Group, Inc.
5400 S. 60th St., Greendale WI 53129
All rights reserved.

Taste of Home and Reader's Digest are registered trademarks
of The Reader's Digest Association, Inc.

EDITORIAL
Editor-in-Chief: **CATHERINE CASSIDY**
Creative Director: **HOWARD GREENBERG**
Editorial Operations Director: **KERRI BALLIET**

Managing Editor, Print and Digital Books: **MARK HAGEN**
Associate Creative Director: **EDWIN ROBLES JR.**

Editor: **CHRISTINE RUKAVENA**
Art Director: **JESSIE SHARON**
Layout Designer: **NANCY NOVAK**
Contributing Layout Designers: **MATT FUKUDA, MÉLANIE LÉVESQUE**
Editorial Production Manager: **DENA AHLERS**
Copy Chief: **DEB WARLAUMONT MULVEY**
Copy Editor: **MARY C. HANSON**
Content Operations Manager: **COLLEEN KING**
Executive Assistant: **MARIE BRANNON**
Editorial Intern: **DEVIN MULERTT**
Copy Desk Intern: **KAITLIN STAINBROOK**

Chief Food Editor: **KAREN BERNER**
Food Editor: **JAMES SCHEND; PEGGY WOODWARD, RD**
Associate Food Editor: **KRISTA LANPHIER**
Associate Editor/Food Content: **ANNIE RUNDLE**
Recipe Editors: **MARY KING; JENNI SHARP, RD; IRENE YEH**

Test Kitchen and Food Styling Manager: **SARAH THOMPSON**
Test Cooks: **MATTHEW HASS, LAUREN KNOELKE**
Food Stylists: **KATHRYN CONRAD (SENIOR), SHANNON ROUM, LEAH REKAU**
Prep Cooks: **MEGUMI GARCIA, NICOLE SPOHRLEDER, BETH VANOPDORP**

Photography Director: **STEPHANIE MARCHESE**
Photographers: **DAN ROBERTS, JIM WIELAND**
Photographer/Set Stylist: **GRACE NATOLI SHELDON**
Set Stylists: **STACEY GENAW, MELISSA HABERMAN, DEE DEE JACQ**

Business Analyst: **KRISTY MARTIN**
Billing Specialist: **MARY ANN KOEBERNIK**

BUSINESS
General Manager, Taste of Home Cooking Schools: **ERIN PUARIEA**

Vice President, Brand Marketing: **JENNIFER SMITH**
Vice President, Circulation and Continuity Marketing: **DAVE FIEGEL**

READER'S DIGEST NORTH AMERICA
Vice President, Business Development and Marketing: **ALAIN BEGUN**
President, Books and Home Entertainment: **HAROLD CLARKE**
General Manager, Canada: **PHILIPPE CLOUTIER**
Vice President, Operations: **MITCH COOPER**
Chief Operating Officer: **HOWARD HALLIGAN**
Vice President, Chief Sales Officer: **MARK JOSEPHSON**
Vice President, General Manager, Milwaukee: **FRANK QUIGLEY**
Vice President, Digital Sales: **STEVE SOTTILE**
Vice President, Chief Content Officer: **LIZ VACCARIELLO**
Vice President, Global Financial Planning & Analysis: **DEVIN WHITE**

THE READER'S DIGEST ASSOCIATION, INC.
President and Chief Executive Officer: **ROBERT E. GUTH**

For other **TASTE OF HOME BOOKS** and products,
visit us at **TASTEOFHOME.COM.**

For more **READER'S DIGEST PRODUCTS** and information, visit
RD.COM (in the United States) or see **RD.CA** (in Canada).

International Standard Book Number: **978-1-61765-234-9**
Library of Congress Control Number: **2013940211**

COVER PHOTOGRAPHY
Photographer: **DAN ROBERTS**
Food Stylist: **SHANNON ROUM**
Set Stylist: **DEE DEE JACQ**

PICTURED ON FRONT COVER:
Family-Favorite Cheeseburger Pasta, page 196.

PICTURED ON BACK COVER:
Seasoned Chicken Strips, page 156; Ice Cream Sandwich Dessert, page 428;
Tangy Pulled Pork Sandwiches, page 451.

PRINTED IN CHINA.
13579108642

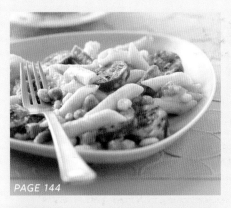
PAGE 144

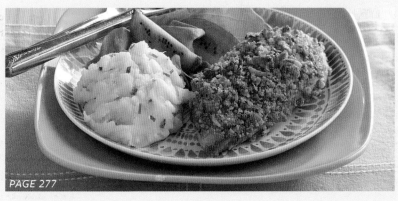
PAGE 277

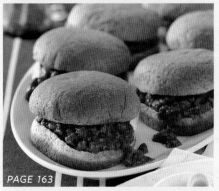
PAGE 163

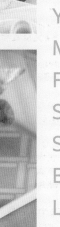
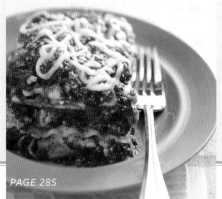
PAGE 402

PAGE 285

TABLE OF CONTENTS

This PROVEN PLAN is your key to a healthier lifestyle and trimmer figure—even if your days are busy!

Some other weight-loss plans expect you to spend lots of time in the kitchen or squeeze group meetings into your already busy schedule. The Taste of Home Comfort Food Diet, however, is simple, offering **commonsense tools that keep your weight-loss goals on track**...without serious commitments on your time.

In this best-of edition of Comfort Food Diet Cookbook, we've included prep and cook times with every recipe, so you can quickly match up your calorie needs with the amount of time you have available to spend in the kitchen.

You'll also see that **each chapter is arranged by calories** so you can quickly find the recipes that meet your goals. In addition, a special bonus chapter loaded with slow cooker favorites promises to have healthy dinners ready without much work on your part!

The basics behind the Comfort Food Diet are simple: **watch your portion sizes, record your calories and get moving** every day. But it's the idea that you can easily **enjoy the foods you and your family love and still lose weight** that makes this program a winner. Let's get started!

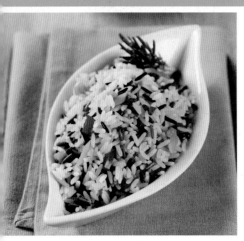

A NEW WAY TO EAT
PAGE 10

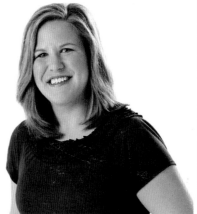

CHRISTY'S SUCCESS STORY
PAGE 38

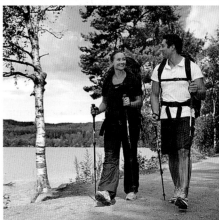

MOVE IT AND LOSE IT! PAGE 34

Comfort Food Diet Basics

Do the words "comfort food" and "diet" go together? Yes! With a little planning, the right recipes and reasonable portions you'll drop pounds and serve your family's favorite meals. Read on to discover how the Taste of Home Comfort Food Diet works and how readers like you have succeeded in their goals.

1 Eat three meals and two snacks a day for a total of 1,400 calories.

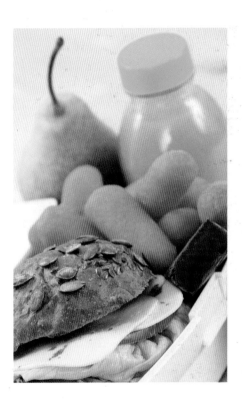

If you're a woman, shoot for a total calorie consumption of 1,400 calories per day. Men should consume 1,500 calories per day. Check with your doctor before you begin this plan to see if this calorie guideline is appropriate for you. Then consider the Six-Week Meal Plan on pages 42-63. There you'll find detailed menus that total roughly 1,400 calories per day.

Use the following guide to distribute calories through the day:

- 350 calories for breakfast

- 450 calories for lunch

- 500 calories for dinner

- Two 50-calorie or two 100-calorie snacks, depending on the total calories you're aiming for per day. You can consume more or less calories in a snack or meal than what is suggested here as long as your daily total is 1,400 or 1,500 calories.

2 | Start a food diary to keep track of everything you eat. See pages 470-471 for blank Do-It-Yourself Meal-Planning Worksheets.

Keeping a food diary is a key to success on the Comfort Food Diet. By writing down everything you eat, you can easily identify eating habits you hadn't noticed previously. You're also less likely to cheat if you know you'll have to jot down that sundae you had at lunch or the extra cookie you snuck in after dinner.

Use your food journal or the Meal-Planning Worksheets to help you plan menus in advance as well. Browse through this cookbook and decide which of the hearty dishes you plan to make. Map out menus and snacks for an entire day in advance, then go back and record what you actually ate.

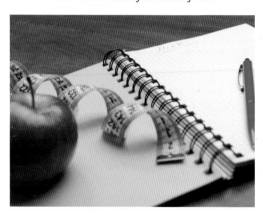

Always remember to watch portion sizes, and review the Nutrition Facts at the end of each recipe to learn what a serving size is. If you increase the serving size, the amount of calories (and nutrients) will obviously increase as well.

It's also important to understand that you can mix and match foods however you'd like as long as you stay within the 1,400 or 1,500 daily calorie limit.

For instance, let's say you prepare Asian Chicken with Pasta (p. 180) for lunch. Note that the recipe makes six servings, but the nutrition facts are based on one serving of 1½ cups. As such, you can enjoy one serving and serve the rest to family members or refrigerate the leftovers for a handy lunch or dinner tomorrow.

The guideline for lunch is 450 calories, and one serving of pasta weighs in at 320 calories. This means you can also enjoy ½ cup of 1% chocolate milk (85 calories) and carrots (free food) for a lunch that totals only 405 calories. You can add another food that is about 45 calories, or you can spend those calories later in the day. It's up to you—as long as your daily caloric intake meets the 1,400 or 1,500 goal.

3

See the Snacks Calorie List (pages 84-85), the Free Foods List (page 41) and the calorie breakdowns before each chapter when pairing foods with entrees.

The lunch example covered in Step 2 noted that ½ cup of 1% chocolate milk was 85 calories. How would you know that? Simply turn to pages 84-85 for the Snacks Calorie List. There you'll find dozens of ideas for low-calorie bites that don't require a recipe. These items are great for snacking, and they also make tasty additions to meals as demonstrated by the lunch example. While these items come in at 100 calories or less, you still need to write them down in your food diary.

Similarly, the Free Foods List offers many items you can enjoy without guilt. In fact, these foods are so light, there's no need to worry about their calorie content as long as you follow any portion restrictions they might offer.

The chapters in *Best of Comfort Food Diet Cookbook* are broken down into Snacks, Breakfasts, Lunches, Dinners, Side Dishes, Desserts and Slow Cooker Favorites. Most chapters begin with lower-calorie staples and end with higher-calorie specialties.

If you ate a lunch below the 450 calorie guideline, you may want to consider a higher-calorie dinner. If you enjoyed a high-calorie breakfast and morning snack, you may want to stick with a lunch that's a bit lighter.

Many of the chapters overlap a little, making meal planning easy! For example, some of the higher-calorie lunches would make wonderful low-calorie dinners. You could also look at the calorie breakdown at the beginning of the side dish chapter and choose one of those recipes for a meat-free lunch or substantial snack.

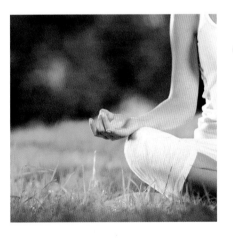

4

Add exercise to burn extra calories.

Find a form of exercise that you would enjoy doing every day or on a regular basis. Walking is a great way to start exercising. Walking with family or friends is a great motivator to keep you going.

Swimming, yoga, biking or a dance fitness program are fun ways to exercise. These activities can also be done alone or with family and friends. Choosing an activity that keeps you interested will make you want to exercise. You may have to change activities every few months to maintain that spark.

I Walked Away From My Sedentary Lifestyle!

By Pam Holmes
Lincoln, Nebraska

The Comfort Food Diet helped me lose more than half my body weight and got me moving again!

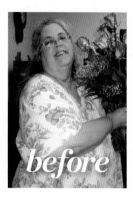

before

I remember being eight years old, wearing one of the many beautiful hand-sewn dresses my mother made for me and thinking that if I cinched the belt tighter, I wouldn't look so fat.

Things changed after I had been married for a few years. The pounds piled on after each of my three sons was born. I was no longer fat; I was morbidly obese. In July 2009, my doctor weighed me at 328 pounds. Before that visit, I had no idea how much I weighed. I didn't own a scale.

In my career, I had earned my bachelor's degree in elementary education. But I took a sedentary desk job as an administrative assistant at a university, so I got little exercise and brought a lot of unhealthy snacks to work with me. I snacked all day in front of my computer.

And for 30 years, I ate anything and everything I wanted. I love food, and I never limited myself, even though I was battling high blood pressure for the last 15 years. My doctor had me on five different medications, and it was still borderline high.

At home, I just wanted to sit in my chair and watch TV. My kitchen chair had wheels, and I would roll around in it while I prepared and cleaned up meals. It just hurt my legs too much to stand or walk.

Vacations and other fun activities were limited because I couldn't walk very far. Physical activity of any sort was completely out of the question.

I started half-heartedly to lose some weight after that eye-opening visit to the doctor in July 2009. Giving up my beloved carbonated full-sugar soft drinks helped me lose 24 pounds. But it was not enough.

Scary news

In December 2009, I went to the doctor complaining that my heart was pounding hard after even the slightest physical exertion. The doctor ordered an EKG and told me the test seemed to show that I had already had a heart attack. Even though subsequent tests with a cardiologist proved that my heart was fine, his words finally got my attention. It was now or never.

So I launched a "get healthy for life" campaign. If I wanted to maintain any serious weight loss, I knew I couldn't do a short-term "fix" but needed a lifestyle change.

To start, I simply cut back on my overall food intake by eliminating between-meal snacks and eating only one helping of the food I prepared for my family. As the pounds came off, I got more motivated and started cooking and eating healthier foods like fruits, vegetables, lean beef, chicken and fish.

I found many wonderful low-fat and low-calorie recipes in the *Comfort Food Diet Cookbook* and

after

loved that the nutritional facts were listed for each recipe. It was easy for me to monitor my calorie intake. My husband and son even enjoyed (and still enjoy) the recipes I prepare from the cookbook, too—and they're both real meat-and-potato guys.

I also started walking. Running was not a possibility for me since my knee and hip joints are bad. But I knew that if I didn't start moving, I would lose my ability to get around. I was almost 60 years old and afraid I was going to lose my mobility.

The end of my steep, quarter-mile-long driveway became my first walking goal. My husband, Duane, walked with me a few times. I was always huffing and puffing; he was not. That motivated me to walk a little farther down the road every night.

The first time I made it to the end of our road—1.25 miles—I felt like Rocky, and I did a little dance. I still tell people that spot is where I had my "Rocky moment."

I walk a lot farther now, and I also took up bicycling again. What a joy it is after not being on a bike in 30 years!

Losing weight and maintaining it!

Through my path to weight loss, I set interim goals as I shed pounds. I wanted to get into the 240s before a friend's wedding and to the 220s before my 40th wedding anniversary. I especially wanted to weigh less than 200 pounds by my 60th birthday. And two months before the big 6-0, I weighed in at 199.6 pounds. I was officially in ONE-derland!

A year and a half after beginning my "get healthy for life" campaign, I reached my ultimate goal of weighing

160 pounds. My total weight loss was 172 pounds, and I am now less than half the size I used to be!

Currently, I weigh 150 pounds. My blood pressure has returned to normal, and my doctor is slowly weaning me off all the medications. I went from a size 5X to an extra-large or large in blouses, and I now wear a size 10 in jeans. Never in my adult life have I been this small.

To maintain my weight, I eat breakfast again after skipping that meal for years. I eat a lot of salads for lunch. I love them with grilled chicken breast and a drizzle of low-fat dressing. Fruit is my favorite snack—I eat grapes like candy! For dinner, I usually eat whatever I prepare for my family, but I give myself a smaller portion. And fruit makes a great dessert!

I still love home-style comfort food, and I find that it's not too tricky to swap ingredients to make dishes healthier with little or no difference in taste. I still make recipes from the *Comfort Food Diet Cookbook*. And I still eat out sometimes, but I make healthier choices. I look on the restaurant's website beforehand so I can pick a wholesome dish to order and avoid less healthy options.

My active life

Now I can do anything! I can literally walk for miles. My house is cleaner, too, because I have more energy to do housework.

My grandchildren and I also have so much fun together now, because I can stay active for longer periods of time. I can't wait to go to the amusement park with them! (That was a great motivator to lose weight.)

Counted cross-stitch is something I enjoy again, too. It's a satisfying hobby and not just because of the lovely things I'm making. When my fingers and mind are busy, it keeps me out of the kitchen.

I can't even name all of the differences this weight loss has made in my life. I can get a regular-sized bath towel around me after a shower. I can cross my legs. I don't have to ask for a seat belt extender on an airplane, and I can sit in a lawn chair! I have confidence and self-esteem; I feel like a first-class citizen again.

There are no great secrets to weight loss. It's hard work, and it takes discipline. But you will never regret the day you decided to get healthy, and that turning point will ring in your memory as a great one. By losing half of myself—178 pounds—I regained my whole life.

A New Way To Eat

Counting calories may be the key to losing weight, but it's still important to make sure you're getting good nutrition so you can be more active—and have more fun! Here's how to bring balance and variety to your diet.

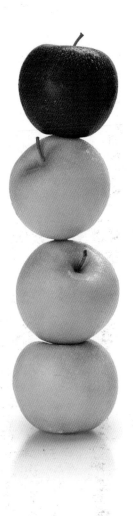

Fiber

Most Americans do not eat as much fiber as they should. Your daily fiber goal should be 20 to 30 grams, which includes soluble and insoluble fiber.

Insoluble fiber can be found in whole wheat and brown rice, while soluble fiber is a part of oatmeal, beans and barley. Soluble fiber helps to lower cholesterol, and insoluble fiber keeps your digestive tract healthy.

Along with aiding digestion, consuming the right amount of fiber each day can help lower your risk of heart disease and diabetes. The best part? Fiber helps keep you feeling full, which can help prevent you from overeating and keep you on track with your diet.

Tips to help boost your fiber

- Making soup? Add extra veggies.

- Add wheat germ or oat bran to yogurt and casseroles. You won't notice the difference.

- Add a tablespoon or two of ground flaxseed to your morning smoothie.

- Leave the skins on when you eat fruits and vegetables.

- Toss some garbanzo beans or kidney beans in your salad.

- Choose whole grain breads and crackers. Whole wheat or whole grain flour should be listed as the first ingredient on the food label.

Protein

The body needs a constant supply of protein to repair and rebuild cells that are worn or damaged. About half of the protein we consume creates enzymes, which help cells carry out necessary chemical reactions. Proteins also transport oxygen to cells, help muscles contract and produce antibodies. Men should consume about 55 grams of protein a day, while women should consume about 45 grams per day.

Carbohydrates

Moderation is key when consuming carbohydrates. Carbs shouldn't be feared when you're on a diet, because they energize your body, which is necessary for your daily exercise.

There are two types of carbohydrates: sugar and starch. Sugars are in fruit, milk and granulated sugar, and starches include grains and potatoes. Your body converts all sugars and starches to glucose—a source of energy.

Positive carbohydrate choices include whole grains, reduced-fat dairy products and a variety of fruits and vegetables. Want to eliminate empty calories? Cut out packaged cakes, pies and cookies. These choices are highly processed and don't contribute to a healthy diet.

Cholesterol

Although saturated and trans fats have a larger effect on blood cholesterol than eating foods high in cholesterol, you should still limit your daily intake of cholesterol to 300 mg. Cholesterol is found in foods from animals, such as eggs, meat and dairy products.

Fat

Believe it: There are some healthy fats! Monounsaturated and polyunsaturated fats, which are found in olive and canola oils and nuts and seeds, are all healthier options. Adults should limit fat to about 30% of their calories each day. This means you should be eating no more than 50 grams of fat daily if you are consuming 1,400 to 1,500 calories per day.

Saturated Fat

While saturated fat is found mostly in high-fat meats and dairy foods, it is also found in coconut oil, palm kernel oil and some processed foods. Consume only 17 grams of saturated fat per day, which is 10% of calories following a 1,400 to 1,500 calorie-a-day diet.

Trans Fat

LDL (bad) cholesterol increases with saturated fat and trans fat, increasing your risk of coronary artery disease. Trans fats can also decrease HDL (good) cholesterol. Limit trans fat as often as you can, and try to stay below 1.5 to 2.0 grams per day. Foods that commonly contain trans fat include vegetable shortening, stick margarine, fried foods, processed foods and store-bought baked goods.

Sodium

Restrict sodium to no more than 2,300 mg a day—equivalent to about one teaspoon of table salt. The best way to reduce salt is to cut back on restaurant and processed foods like canned vegetables, deli meat and condiments.

Generally, a food product that has been prepared for you to buy—such as frozen dinners and convenience products—will contain a high amount of sodium. Read food labels and purchase lower-sodium products when you can.

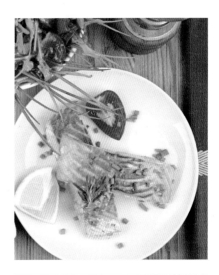
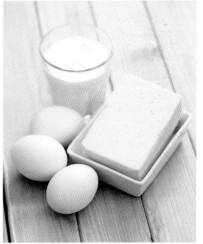
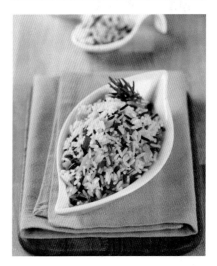

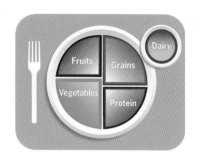

The Dish On MyPlate

Step up to the USDA's new plate (or MyPlate) and change your eating habits for the better.

IT'S EASIER TO EAT RIGHT, thanks to the U.S. Department of Agriculture (USDA). The government agency that built the long-standing Food Guide Pyramid has replaced it with a dinner plate in an effort to make following a healthy diet a no-brainer.

The aptly named MyPlate symbol (shown above) is divided into four sections—fruits, vegetables, grains and protein—with a "cup" on the side to represent dairy. What immediately catches your eye is that fruits and veggies fill half the plate, with protein making up the smallest portion.

If that isn't the way your plate looks during dinner time, prepare for an appetite adjustment.

How can the MyPlate symbol make healthy eating easier? Instead of encouraging you to figure out how many servings of this and that you should eat each day, as in the old pyramid, the plate helps you visualize the symbol when you dish up your meal. Figure out how to make your plate look more like MyPlate. Maybe it's trading the potato chips for cut-up fresh fruit or splitting that huge steak with your spouse. You can even apply the symbol to a fast-food meal!

The key messages of the USDA's revised dietary guidelines are:

- Enjoy food, but eat less

- Avoid oversized portions

- Make half your plate fruit and vegetables

- Make at least half your grains whole grains

- Drink water instead of sugary drinks

- Choose fat-free or 1% (low-fat) milk

- Check the sodium in foods—and aim low

More ways to save on calories and fat when eating out:

- Ask for condiments on the side

- Choose packets of light dressings

- Skip the salt and fat (like bacon and cheese)

- Avoid supersized portions and buffets

- Don't eat on the run

- Check out fast-food restaurants' nutritional information for their menu items on their websites before you go

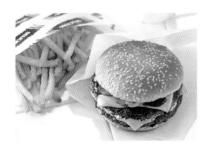

Say your typical drive-thru dinner consists of a hearty double cheeseburger, fries and a soda.

Instead of eating from the bag, assemble it on a dinner plate and see how it compares to MyPlate. The bun and burger (grains and protein) may fill one half of the plate, but the cheese adds extra fat and sodium. The fries spill over the entire other half, and though they're potatoes, they're loaded with fat, calories and sodium—hardly a nutritious choice.

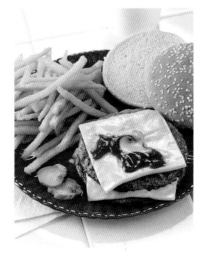

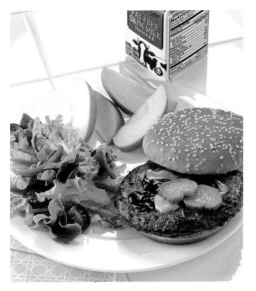

How do you make that fast-food meal look like MyPlate? You can still choose a burger and bun; just downsize to a single patty, skip the cheese and opt for a whole grain bun if it's available. For the other half of the plate, order a side salad. Some fast-food restaurants also offer fruit choices. Don't forget to swap out soda for milk. You'll cut the fat, calories and sodium, add nutrients and jumpstart a habit that will do your body good.

Want to learn more about the USDA's guidelines and how to make them work for you? Visit **choosemyplate.gov.**

Portion Size Chart

Large restaurant portions and super-sized fast-food meals make it hard to remember how big a standard healthy serving really is. Keep these visuals in mind when estimating a proper portion size.

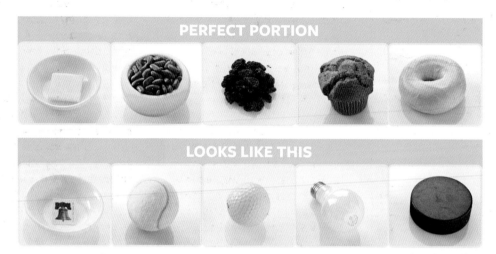

PERFECT PORTION

LOOKS LIKE THIS

- **1 teaspoon butter,** a postage stamp or the tip of your thumb

- **1 cup beans,** a tennis ball or a cupped handful

- **2 tablespoons dried fruit or nuts,** a golf ball or a small cupped handful

- **1 small muffin,** the round part of a light bulb

- **1 small bagel,** a hockey puck (3" diameter)

- **3 ounces meat,** a purse pack of tissues or your outstretched palm

- **1 dinner roll,** a bar of soap or half your palm

- **1 pancake,** a music CD

- **1 tablespoon salad dressing,** a silver dollar

- **1 cup chips,** a tennis ball or a cupped handful

- **1 3x3-inch piece of cake,** a tennis ball

Get Your (Nutrition) Facts Straight!

The nutrition information found on packaged foods makes it easy to buy the healthiest food for your family.

Nutrition Facts

Serving Size 1/4 Cup (30g)
Servings Per Container About 38

Amount Per Serving

Calories 200 Calories from Fat 150

	% Daily Value*
Total Fat 17g	**26%**
Saturated Fat 2.5g	**13%**
Trans Fat 0g	
Cholesterol 0mg	**0%**
Sodium 120mg	**5%**
Total Carbohydrate 7g	**2%**
Dietary Fiber 2g	**8%**
Sugars 1g	
Protein 5g	

Vitamin A 0%	•	Vitamin C 0%
Calcium 4%	•	Iron 8%

*Percent Daily Values are based on a 2,000 calorie diet.

Regulated by the Food Safety and Inspection Service and the Food and Drug Administration, Nutrition Facts panels are found on nearly every item in the grocery store. And while food labels can be a bit confusing, they're not impossible to translate once you understand them.

Serving Size

The top of the Nutrition Facts panel (see example) lists serving information. Food manufacturers follow guidelines that ensure the serving sizes of like products are comparable. This makes it a cinch for shoppers to determine which brand of orange juice offers the most vitamin C per serving, which spaghetti sauce has the least calories and so on.

CALORIES. The panel lists the number of calories each serving contains—and how many of those calories come from fat. In the example above, there are 200 calories in one serving, and 150 of them come from fat. Remember, however, that if you ate ½ cup (or 2 servings), you'd take in 400 calories, of which 300 would be fat.

FATS. Also listed is the total number of fat grams per serving and how many of those grams come from saturated and trans fats (the "bad" fats).

CARBOHYDRATES. The Total Carbohydrate figure lists all of the carbs contained in the item. Since dietary fiber and sugars are of special interest to consumers, their amounts are highlighted individually as well as being included in the total carb number.

The sugars listed include those that occur naturally in foods, such as lactose in milk, as well as sugars that are added during processing.

Percent Daily Value

The Percent Daily Value listed on the nutrition panel indicates how much each component in the product contributes to a 2,000-calorie-per-day eating plan. In the example at left, the total fat for a serving comprises 26% of the daily value, whereas the sodium comprises 5%.

Manufacturers must list the Percent Daily Value of vitamin A, vitamin C, calcium and iron on every food label, so consumers will know how the product fits into a well-balanced diet. Other vitamins and minerals may also be listed, depending on the space on the label and the manufacturer's preference.

If the Daily Value for calcium, iron, vitamin A, etc. is more than 10%, the product is generally considered to be a good source of that particular nutrient.

At the end of the nutrition label, you'll find an ingredients list—a requirement on all food products that contain more than one ingredient. Ingredients are listed in order, with the most major component (based on weight) of the product listed first and other ingredients following in decreasing order.

Rewriting My Own History as 'In Shape' not 'Overweight'

By Richelle Fry
Springdale, Arkansas

I lost 65 pounds in a year and gained better health and the confidence to take control of my life!

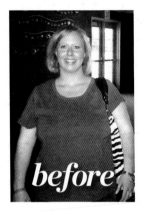

before

I have struggled with my weight all my life. When I was growing up, I was always a little bit bigger than the other kids. And I continued to gain weight into my 20s until 215 pounds were packed onto my 5-foot-1-inch frame. When I was 23, I had to have back surgery. At 26, I had back surgery again. The extra weight I was carrying continued to be a big problem.

A few years ago, I lost almost 70 pounds in a very short time and in a very unhealthy way. Around that time, I met my best friend and husband, Terry, and I gained all the weight back. I lost my job and I wasn't sure what my next step was going to be. Terry encouraged me to pursue my lifelong dream of earning my college degree in history, which I love.

For the first time, I felt happy. I had a happy home, a wonderful husband who found me beautiful and a great new direction in my life. I knew I weighed too much, but I wasn't inspired to do anything about it.

Baby steps toward success

When I returned to college, I was determined to succeed, so I worked really hard. But that left me with little time for eating. Each day, I ended up having one large, unhealthy meal late in the evening. That's when I realized that my habits had to stop. I wouldn't be able to do my best in any area of my life if I wasn't feeling my best. So I decided to make some healthy changes.

I started by incorporating more fruits, vegetables and yogurt into my diet. Rather than one huge meal a day, I tried to eat several small meals. I drank less diet soda—which was very difficult for me—and more water.

Exercise is not my favorite thing, but I made a conscious decision to walk more, especially around campus. Then Terry and I started walking through our neighborhood in the evenings; this is something

we still do. Our walks serve two great purposes: we get daily exercise, and we have a chance to reconnect after a busy day. Even when I'm tired or don't feel like walking, Terry encourages me to go with him since it's a great way to spend time together.

Terry's mother also lives with us. As I started losing weight and wanted to continue, we made the effort to eat better as a family. We shared big salads loaded with vegetables. We ate leaner meats. Now, chicken shows up on our menu at least four times a week. Terry makes the best meat loaf, so we switched out the ground beef for lean ground turkey. Now we have a lighter way to enjoy our favorite comfort food. We avoid fatty foods and all fast-food.

after

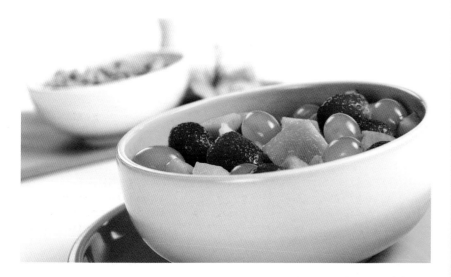

Richelle's Easy Changes

- Find someone to encourage you
- Drink less soda
- Drink more water
- Put flavor packets in your water to keep your taste buds interested
- Cook with lean meats
- Go for a walk—relax and exercise at the same time
- Indulge only a little bit
- Don't be hard on yourself

Even snacking got healthier. My current favorite snack is popcorn, especially when it's air-popped. I often put some fat-free butter and cheese seasonings on it, but it's also great plain. And I find that I really do love salads. I usually eat a small salad four times a day or whenever my stomach starts rumbling. And my top way to get going in the morning is with a serving of oatmeal sprinkled with a pinch of cinnamon.

Little indulgences

My sweet tooth has been an obstacle along the way, despite my newfound love for salads. I adore cookies and desserts, so it's hard for me to walk through our kitchen and not indulge in the sweets. I have to ask myself if I really want the cookie or if I just want it because I see it. It's kind of like going to the grocery store when you are hungry—you don't need all that junk food, but you see it and it looks good, so you buy it. Then you get home and instantly regret going overboard.

I strongly believe that you should not deprive yourself. When I want a cookie, I break off a small piece to satisfy my craving—and that's it. Having a small portion of what you are craving will not ruin your day or throw you off your healthy path. If you've watched your food choices and portion sizes the last few days, a little indulgence will not be the end of the world. If I have a weak moment and eat too many calories, I try not to beat myself up over it. I'm human and make mistakes. I just get back on my healthy path again the next day.

In one year, I have lost 65 pounds and know that I've done it gradually by watching what I eat and working exercise into my day. Now I have tons of confidence and higher self-esteem. My back feels better than ever. I'm happy to know that Terry and I can continue to have fun visiting many historical sites, since our healthy lifestyle will ensure a long life together.

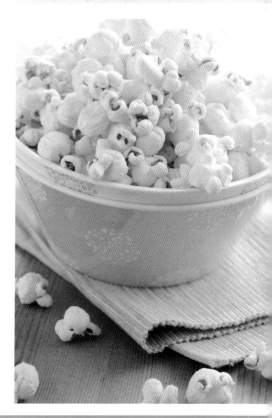

Shop Smart for Family Groceries

Making healthy decisions is a snap with these supermarket strategies.

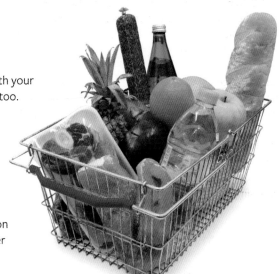

The grocery store can feel like a foreign country when you're trying to eat healthier.

You could probably find the soda, frozen pizza and packaged cookies with your eyes closed. But mapping out fresh and nutritious foods can be simple, too. Learning your way around the healthy options is easier than you think.

Spend less time in the middle of the store, looking through row upon row of processed foods. Instead, allocate most of your time and money on the outer aisles, where the gems like fresh fruits and vegetables are kept.

Yes, many of the foods that are the best choices for healthy eaters are on the perimeter of the store. That includes produce, dairy and the butcher section, with its array of fresh meat and fish.

Getting to know these parts of the store is beneficial because many of your meals can follow this formula: choose your protein, then add vegetables, fruit and a whole grain to make a meal. You'll still need to go to the middle of the store for pasta, rice, frozen foods and other items. But avoid the big sections of processed foods like chips, meals in a box or a can, cookies and candy that beckoned to you in the past.

It's tempting to blame your busy lifestyle for preventing you from having the time to shop for healthy foods. But it doesn't take any longer to shop for healthy foods than it does for unhealthy ones. Save yourself some time at the grocery store by planning your meals and writing out grocery lists. You'll save time in the kitchen, too, because you won't be staring into your refrigerator, wondering what to make for dinner.

Shopping healthy is all about choosing the right foods for your meal plan: lean, unprocessed meat and fish, high-quality fruits and vegetables, whole grains and low-fat dairy. Eating healthy means taking these basic starters and preparing them for your family without adding unnecessary fat and calories.

About Produce

When it comes to good-for-you staples, fresh produce is best, followed closely by frozen fruits or vegetables. Canned products are a distant third.

Spend a lot of time in the fresh produce section and get to know your naturally healthy foods. You recognize your old favorites—carrots, celery, potatoes...but what about jicama? Or kale? Your new favorite food could be right in front of you, and you don't even know it yet!

Trying new produce is one of the fun parts of healthy eating. Give yourself the goal of trying a new fruit or vegetable every week. Have your family members take turns at picking a new fresh food, and try it together. If you like it, find a way to incorporate it into your meals.

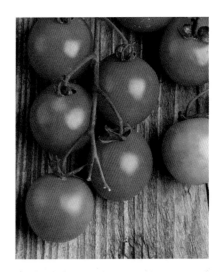

The produce manager can explain individual produce items and how they're best prepared. Ask questions; these folks like to share their knowledge—but make sure to ask for healthy ways to make your newfound favorites.

Fresh produce is even fresher at the farmers market. If there's one near you, get there early so you're guaranteed the best selection. Talk to the farmers who grow the produce you're buying. They are used to eating what they grow, so they often have simple recipes and healthy preparation tips to share.

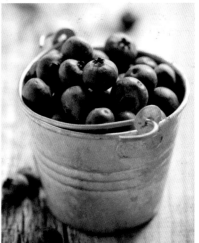

About Meat & Fish

When you're at the meat counter, avoid processed meats like sausage. They're often made with high-fat ingredients and a number of additives. Instead, look for fresh chicken and turkey with the occasional lean cuts of beef and pork.

When buying your chicken or turkey, either buy skinless or remove the skin and fat at home so your pieces are lean. The breast is leanest. When buying ground turkey, make sure it is ground breast, not turkey pieces; those "pieces" can include skin and have as much fat as regular ground beef!

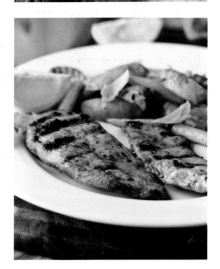

For red meat, cuts that include the word "round" or "loin" are generally leaner. Look for firm meat that smells and looks fresh with no off-color areas. Read the packages to make sure your meat wasn't injected with water, flavorings or preservatives.

And if you're buying fish, choose fresh, firm fish that doesn't smell fishy. It's OK to ask when it was delivered to the store. If the fresh fish looks or smells iffy, go for frozen seafood instead.

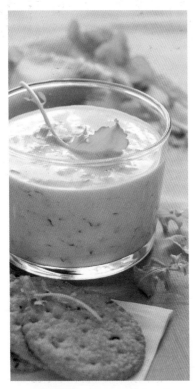

Knowing The Ins & Outs

While sticking to the perimeter of the store can help you pick healthy items, you will need to venture into the aisles for some packaged and canned foods. When choosing these foods, get into the habit of checking Nutrition Facts labels (see the guide on page 15).

Look for foods that don't get many of their calories from fat, and aim for items that are low in saturated fat. Select non-fat or low-fat options at the dairy case.

When the carbohydrate total on the label is more than twice the amount of sugar, the food is usually loaded with complex carbohydrates that are good for you. Consider making these items a part of your family's weekly menu plan.

Many items found in the deli or bakery, however, are not required to provide nutrition facts. Luckily, many of today's supermarkets make this information available upon request. When in doubt, ask. You'd be surprised at how often nutrition information is available.

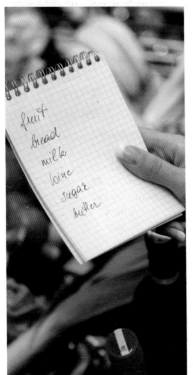

Here's another important tip for successful healthy shopping: Don't go to the grocery store when you're hungry. And if your kids are looking for a snack, this may not be the best time to bring them along. You'll be tempted to give in to instant gratification (junk food), and you won't stick to your healthy eating plan either. Eat something substantial and satisfying before you leave the house.

And finally, the best shopping advice: If it's not good for you, simply don't put it in your cart. That way you can't take it home and eat it!

Lighten Up Your Family Favorites!

Cut calories and keep your gang satisfied by tweaking your most popular recipes.

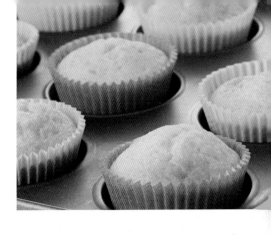

Dinner standbys:

- When serving pasta and rice, pay attention to portion sizes. A serving of cooked rice is ½ or ⅔ cup, while pasta is usually 1½ ounces, uncooked, per serving.

- A serving of meat is considered 4 ounces, uncooked.

- 10-inch flour tortillas have about 200 calories before any fillings are added. To go lighter, choose 6- or 8-inch tortillas instead.

- See the Portion Size Chart on page 14 for visual cues of common portion sizes.

- Until you get a feel for typical serving sizes, measure portions with measuring cups and spoons. It will help you keep on track.

- Choose lean meat when cooking. Look for skinless white-meat poultry, pork with "loin" in the name and beef with "loin" or "round" in the name.

- Consider low-sodium/no-sodium alternatives when cooking with packaged foods, boxed mixes, olives, cheese and savory seasoning mixes. Instead of canned products, choose fresh or frozen corn, sliced mushrooms, green beans and others.

- Cut back on adding high-calorie ingredients such as olives, cheese and avocado.

Dessert favorites:

- When adding chopped mix-ins such as nuts, chips, raisins or coconut to desserts, decrease the amount a bit. Try using mini chips. Toast nuts and coconut so smaller amounts have stronger flavor.

- Reduce the amount of frosting. You can usually cut the amount by ¼ or ⅓ without missing out.

- When making frosting, confectioners' sugar can almost always be decreased without losing any of the sweetness. One tablespoon of confectioners' sugar equals 29 calories.

- Using reduced-fat butter and reduced-fat cream cheese works well in homemade frosting. Since these lighter products tend to be soft-set, the recipe may need less liquid.

- When baking, replace ¼ or ½ of the butter or oil in a recipe with unsweetened applesauce. But keep in mind that applesauce is a better replacement for oil than it is for butter.

- If you're substituting a substantial amount (½ to 1 cup) of applesauce for fat, you can cut down on sugar a bit due to the natural sweetness of the applesauce.

- Oftentimes, sugar can be decreased slightly without making a difference in the recipe. This is especially true for recipes that are over 40 years old since they tend to be disproportionately high in sugar.

- One tablespoon of sugar equals 48 calories—so be careful when adding it to any of your baked goods.

- If your lightened-up cakes turn out tough with a dense texture, try substituting cake flour for all-purpose flour the next time you prepare them.

- It's rather difficult to lighten cookie recipes successfully and keep the original shape and texture. The best option is to prepare your little treats as usual and savor a single serving.

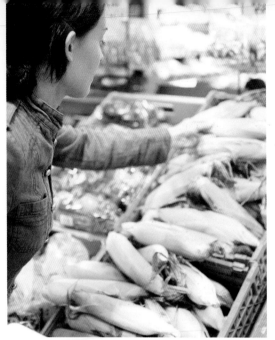

Supermarket Savvy

The next time you hit the grocery store, keep these slimmed-down substitutions in mind. Consider the foods pictured, and you'll cut back on calories and fat...and you might even trim a few dollars off your grocery bill.

buy this **instead of this**

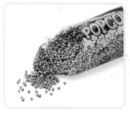 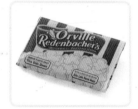

- How long has it been since you popped a big bowl of popcorn on the stove? Maybe you've forgotten just how easy it is or haven't noticed the cost of those microwave bags lately.

- Instead, with a heavy saucepan, a small amount of oil and a few minutes, you can have popcorn seasoned your way without all the salt, artificial flavor and coloring of some microwave versions.

buy this **instead of this**

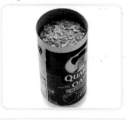 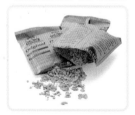

- Hot oatmeal can be a comforting start on a chilly morning, but the cost of those quick-and-easy "instant" packets adds up. They also contain additives and sugar.

- Instead, get the real thing. Add some fresh or dried fruit, honey or nuts to old-fashioned or quick-cooking oats for a more nutritious breakfast. Or try our Raisin Oatmeal Mix on page 104.

buy this **instead of this**

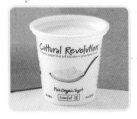 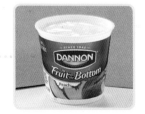

- Not only are you paying more for a few berries, but you're also paying for added sugar, high fructose corn syrup and food coloring.

- Instead, pick up some plain yogurt and add your own fresh fruit for sweetness and additional nutrients. It will also cost you less in calories.

buy this	instead of this	

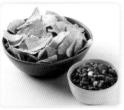 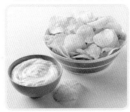

- When a crunchy craving hits, don't reach for a bag of salty chips and fatty dip.

- Instead, enjoy some salsa and baked chips. One ounce of chips and ¼ cup salsa contains fewer than 130 calories and has only 3 grams of fat. The same amounts of chips and dip packs on nearly 300 calories and a whopping 20 grams of fat.

buy this **instead of this**

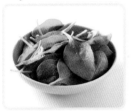 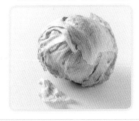

- Think all leafy greens are the same? While spinach and iceberg offer about the same calories and fiber cup for cup, you don't have to settle for a lackluster salad.

- Instead, enjoy a spinach salad that's loaded with far more vitamins and minerals. Spinach is a good source of vitamins K, A, C and folate and magnesium.

buy this **instead of this**

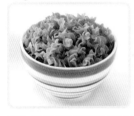 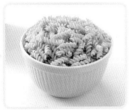

- Pasta is an all-time dinner staple in most homes. Don't feel you have to forget pasta just because you're trying to lose weight.

- Instead, make a smarter pick with whole wheat pasta and work more fiber into your diet. It has three times as much fiber per serving as plain pasta. Be sure to read the ingredient list on the box to check for 100% whole wheat flour.

buy this **instead of this**

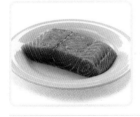 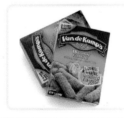

- Fish is high in protein, low in calories and can be a great source of heart-healthy omega-3 fatty acids. But those handy breaded or sauced frozen fish products can be high in calories and fat.

- Instead, buy fresh or plain frozen fish fillets and season them with your own breading or herbs.

buy this **instead of this**

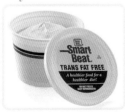 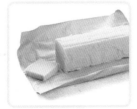

- If you're watching your cholesterol and intake of saturated fats, you might have given up butter and switched to stick margarine. Think you've made a change for the better?

- Instead, make a real difference and switch to margarine in tubs. It has ⅓ the trans fat of stick margarine! Compare labels to find the brands lowest in trans fat.

I Lost 110 Pounds...
And Gained a New Attitude!

By Jeffrey Jacobs
Minneapolis, Minnesota

After changing my eating habits, counting calories and cooking my own meals, I'm feeling healthier than ever!

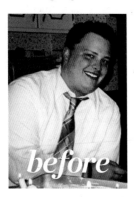

before

Even at my heaviest, I never thought I looked overweight. I still pictured myself as a teenager with broad shoulders and a great jawline. Unfortunately, that wasn't the case.

I have been obese since I began college. Most people gain the infamous "Freshman 15," but I think I gained the "Freshman 40." In fact, between the ages of 18 and 27, I think I gained almost 90 pounds.

I loved food. Eating made me happy in so many ways—the texture of the food, the satisfaction of being full and, of course, the flavor. If a plate of brownies was set before me, I shamelessly ate every last crumb. Give me a pie, and before the day was over, it was gone. Pizza? Hope you ordered your own because I alone could eat an entire one...effortlessly.

It wasn't until my body began shouting for help that I realized I had to do something about my weight. I was 27, yet I developed the problems of an unhealthy 55-year-old man. I was pre-diabetic and nearly hypertensive. I had both a high heart rate and high cholesterol, and I began experiencing sleep apnea. I realized that if I continued to gain weight, my health would be in serious trouble.

I didn't have much of a goal in mind, and I just thought I'd try to get healthy. I wanted to see my jawline again. I wanted to feel better. I wanted to lose weight.

My biggest challenge was cutting back the amount of unhealthy food I ate. Instead of eating excessively until I was uncomfortable, I began focusing on a few small meals and snacks until I was satisfied. Calorie counting and portion control were key. I looked at an item's calorie count, noted the portion size and then determined if eating the item was worth the calories involved.

Best of all, I got cooking! I realized that opening a can

after

of this and adding a jar of that doesn't constitute cooking... and those convenience products can pack on calories quickly. By staying away from processed foods, I instantly felt healthier.

Once I got the cooking bug, I quickly learned how to double, and sometimes even triple, recipes. This way I had plenty of leftovers, ensuring I'd eat right throughout the week.

I also began exercising. Since an expensive gym membership didn't fit my budget, I found ways to exercise for free. I ran outdoors and took advantage of a weight set collecting dust in my basement. I also followed an exercise DVD.

By changing my habits and staying consistent, I began losing weight. When I lost 80 pounds, and saw how close I

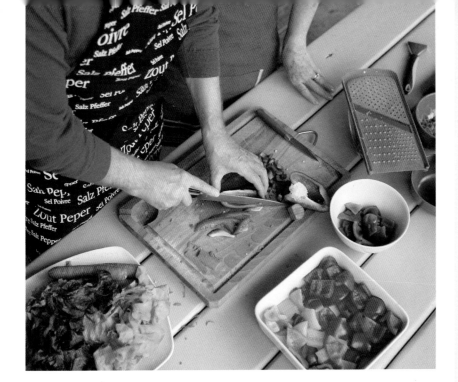

was to reaching the 100-pound mark, I found the motivation to keep going. Like everyone trying to lose weight, however, I eventually reached a plateau.

While it's a very discouraging feeling, I realized that I had to push through the plateau in order to start losing again. The best way I found to deal with the situation was to change my exercise habits and even my diet. I gave my metabolism a run for its money with a good offensive game plan.

I thought of this as a competition. If my opposing team, my metabolism, caught on to my tricks and tactics, I simply changed my strategy a little. I mixed up my workouts; I ate breakfast earlier or lunch later. I was surprised how well this worked!

I also allowed myself the chance to occasionally eat the foods I craved. When I convinced myself that I could no longer eat cookies, for instance, I ended up telling myself that I just "had to have those cookies one last time." I constantly found myself having a "one-last-time" experience.

Now I tell myself that I will, indeed, have those cookies...just not today, just not right now. I know that if I watch the calories I take in, then I'll be able to enjoy a cookie or two another day. Or, better yet, I can try to find a low-calorie recipe for those same cookies and work them into my menu plan. I'm able to enjoy my favorite comfort foods as long as I eat them in moderation, take portion size into consideration and account for their calories.

By pushing myself and making changes to the way I ate, I far surpassed my goal, changing my life for the better! I lost a total of 110 pounds, and I went from a size 40 waist to a size 30. Best of all, that jawline I missed so much? It's back for good, and I couldn't be happier.

1 **SHOP LOCALLY.** I purchase my meat from local butchers who don't use growth hormones, and I shop at public and farmers markets. I even go so far as to visit independent coffee shops and restaurants. These establishments are special because of the owner's capability to use fresh, organic and local foods. It is such a refreshing feeling to know where the foods you eat come from.

2 **DRINK UP!** Make water your new beverage of choice. Not only does drinking plenty of water help fill you up, but you'll be amazed at how it helps your skin, too. I've always had acne problems, and those issues decreased substantially once I started drinking more water. Best of all, water is an easy, healthy and economical choice.

3 **GO LEAN.** Health-conscious people tend to avoid meat as a protein source. While fat and cholesterol play a part in meat proteins, remember that meats aren't bad for you in moderation... and you need the protein. It's essential to think smart when choosing proteins. Fresh tuna, for instance, is a great way to work lean protein into your diet.

Out Of The Kitchen...
Not Out Of Control

Don't leave your diet goals at home when you go out.
Keep your healthy-eating momentum when you dine at...

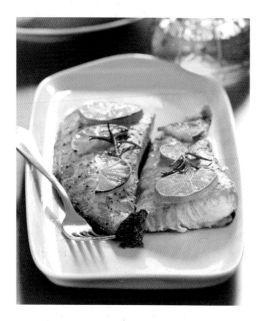

A Restaurant

Go fish! Most family restaurants have a number of fish and seafood options from which you can choose. Resist the urge to order fried shrimp or anything with a cream or butter sauce.

If seafood's not your thing, there are other smart options. Stir-fries, lean cuts of meat and baked chicken dishes are healthier than other menu items. Look for items that are baked, roasted, poached, broiled or steamed. Avoid those that are fried or come with a heavy sauce.

Check out the appetizers, and you might find something that makes an ideal low-calorie entree at a normal portion size. Grilled vegetable platters and side salads (with the dressing on the side) are great options. But if you order a normal entree, watch your portion size and try to save half for leftovers the next day.

The Vending Machine

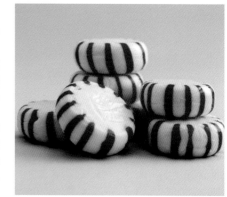

Vending machines seem like a great idea when hunger comes calling. Whether at work or cheering the kids on at an after-school activity, vending machines promise comforting nibbles—but deliver few rewards.

If you need to drop a few coins into a vending machine, spend them on baked chips or pretzels. Similarly, small bags of snack mix and plain animal crackers are decent snacks. Many machines offer an assortment of mints and low-sugar gum. Give these options a try, as the strong flavor of peppermint will often curb any cravings.

A Party

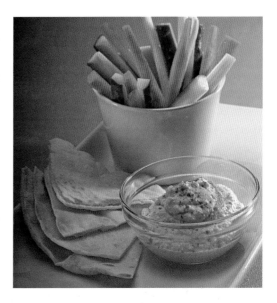

Family celebrations mean good people, good times and good food—that may not be good FOR you. That mile-long buffet is probably stocked with high-calorie foods that can easily tempt you.

Look for items such as veggie and fruit platters, boiled shrimp and whole wheat crackers. Decide which items you really have to try and which you can do without. Stay clear of fried foods and be leery of thick dips and spreads. Try a salsa or chutney instead.

The best way to avoid overindulging at a party is to eat something healthy before you arrive. If your stomach is full, you'll spend less time at the buffet and more time having fun!

The Office

Home cooks are often so busy packing lunches for the kids they forget to fill a brown bag for themselves. Bring your own lunch to work, and you can easily keep your caloric goals intact and avoid the vending machine.

Bring a few snacks to work, too. For many people, the lure of high-calorie snacks is greatest at the workplace. Keep a container of nuts or low-calorie snack mix in your office, or whip up a batch of Granola-to-Go Bars (p. 101) or Cafe Mocha Mini Muffins (p. 91) to keep on hand when you're on the job.

Thanks to the Comfort Food Diet, I'm an Active Mom Again!

By Tami Kuehl
Loup City, Nebraska

Being 56 pounds lighter, I'm enjoying more quality family time than ever.

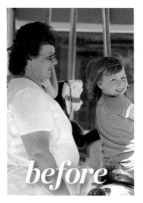

before

I have always grappled with my weight—even as a child. And like many newlywed women, once I walked down the aisle, I stopped worrying about managing my eating habits and let myself go. Then I gained even more weight while pregnant with my daughter, Bailey, as well as during the postpartum depression that followed. I had trouble keeping up with my active little girl.

One of the hobbies Bailey and I enjoyed together was scrapbooking. But something important was missing from our early projects: pictures of the two of us. Self-conscious about my weight, I shied away from cameras. I realized that not only was my lifestyle unfair to Bailey, I was cheating myself as well.

My daughter began to ask questions in the kitchen and take an interest in cooking and baking. I knew I had to change my bad habits so she would learn how to make healthier choices and avoid the struggles that I'd endured my entire life.

Changing My Life

In January 2011, my life changed when I started to follow the Comfort Food Diet. I quickly developed the tools I need to live more healthfully. It isn't like any other diet I've been on; I can eat real food, and it tastes good.

I like to plan my meals in advance and cook up a storm on weekends so I can reheat dishes during the week. Choosing recipes that include similar ingredients and ones that freeze or store well has helped me save time and money.

Keeping track of my calorie intake also hugely affected my weight loss. Now that I'm good at estimating calories, I realize I used to consume more than 5,000 on some days. To help with calorie counting, I have relied on the *Comfort Food Diet Cookbook* as well as a calorie guide. In fact, I have two copies: one in the house and one in the car so I can check nutrition facts at restaurants and make better food choices.

The more my weight drops, the more active I want to be. My best piece of workout equipment is Max, our West Highland terrier, because I cannot put him in the closet when I get tired of him. The two of us walk four times a day, totaling up to a mile each, weather permitting. And since I'm so much more energetic, Bailey and my husband, Shane, and I enjoy frequent bike rides and Nintendo Wii Fit competitions on family game nights.

Exercise is built into my work life, too. My family home is close to both of my seasonal part-time jobs, so I typically walk to and from work. During the day, I also walk to the post office and the bank as well as home for lunch with Shane. According to my pedometer, I average between 8,000 and 9,000 steps each day. I can hardly believe the impact this increased activity has had on both my body and lifestyle.

after

Overcoming Obstacles

Along with all these successes, I've had to navigate some challenges, too. For one, I needed to make a big effort to steer clear of those tempting, ooey-gooey sweets at the office, church events and family gatherings. I satisfy my sweet tooth with just a bite or two, or with 100-calorie snacks from the supermarket.

In the end, it's all about choices. I still have the occasional ice cream bar, a serving of dessert or a miniature candy bar, but I adjust my calories for that day to include them.

I've also worked hard to drink more water and consume the nutrients I need. Now, I take a water bottle everywhere. So I can have a larger supper, my days include many smaller, nutrient- and fiber-filled meals and snacks. Lately, I've been enjoying granola bars, fruit, popcorn, and green salads topped with ingredients like chicken, nuts, apples and chickpeas, plus a tasty low-calorie dressing.

Lastly, I've had to deal with some physical issues, including arthritis in my right ankle, which used to be an easy excuse for inactivity. Finding shoes that fit well was key. The right equipment and professional help when needed have allowed me to overcome my biggest physical challenge.

Looking Forward

I can honestly say it took me just three months to lose the "baby weight" I had been packing on during the seven years since Bailey was born. In the first 12 weeks of dieting, I lost 35 pounds, and now I'm down 56 pounds. I'm currently at 220 pounds and I'd like to lose about 45 more. The progress I've made toward my goal has built up so much energy that I'm practically bursting at the seams to move. My walking pace is nearly a jog, and Max has a hard time keeping up. I used to call that pace my "ticked-off strut," but since starting the Comfort Food Diet, it has become my normal gait.

It's clear that my new lifestyle is beginning to have an effect on Bailey, too, because she frequently asks about calories and makes comments about unhealthy foods. Sometimes she holds up her hands and says, "Mommy, you used to be this wide, but now you are only this wide."

My weight-loss journey has been made simple with a few small, complementary changes: reducing my calorie intake and increasing my activity. I don't feel like I'm on a "diet" or sacrificing, and the excitement of losing those pounds keeps me motivated. I am sleeping better, my joints don't ache as much as they used to, and I'm almost always smiling. Though I'm usually on the go, I do let myself slow down when I walk by a store window—just to catch a glimpse of my reflection.

Top 5 Restaurant Tricks

Eating away from home can be nerve-racking when you don't have control over every ingredient that goes into a meal. Here are five rules of thumb that help me stay on track.

1 **JUST BECAUSE IT'S CALLED A SALAD** doesn't mean it's good for you. Opt for lots of greens with grilled meat instead of the fried stuff. Ask for the dressing on the side, and, if it's available, go for light vinaigrette—you'll be glad you did.

2 **ORDER FROM THE KIDS' MENU.** These portions satisfy and keep me from returning to "super size." At many fast-food restaurants, the kids' meals also include a side of fresh fruit and smaller desserts.

3 **GET THE (NUTRITION) FACTS.** Most chain restaurants publish nutritional information, and many local ones do, too. Ask the cashier or your server for a copy; many are also available online.

4 **SKIP THE BREADS, ROLLS AND BUNS.** These pack in a lot of extra calories. If you're having a sandwich, go open-faced, or order without the bread so you can splurge on dessert.

5 **"SAVE" YOUR CALORIES.** If I know I'm eating supper at a restaurant, I'll fix a light breakfast and lunch. I may have fruit, granola and yogurt for breakfast and a green salad with apple at lunch. This leaves me with plenty of calories to enjoy at dinner!

What's Eating You?

Avoid emotional overeating with these tips.

If a bad day at work or home sends you straight to the refrigerator to cope, you already know something about emotional eating.

If you haven't ever downed a carton of ice cream, a bag of chips or a package of cookies in response to frustration in your life, you probably aren't an emotional eater. Consider yourself lucky.

There's nothing wrong with eating a modest amount of a favorite food because it makes you feel content. After all, comfort food is what this book is all about.

But when stress, anxiety or sadness drives you to eat more and more, or you're so preoccupied with negative feelings that you don't even notice what you're eating, it's time to confront the problem and deal with it.

Emotional eating can quickly sabotage a sensible eating plan. Here are the symptoms to help determine if you are an emotional eater.

- You eat to try to make yourself feel better rather than because you are hungry.

- It's hard to find food that is satisfying, so you don't stop eating when you're full. You keep looking for that one food that will "hit the spot."

- You eat while doing something routine such as watching TV, surfing the Internet or folding laundry. When the package suddenly hits empty, you can't believe you mindlessly ate it all.

- You get a craving for a specific food, and it seems to be related to feeling bored, lonely, angry, hopeless, underappreciated or some other negative emotion.

Finding out what makes you overeat is the key to stopping it. You cannot skip this step if you want long-term success in reaching and maintaining a healthy, comfortable body weight.

The emotional eating cycle starts with a brief period of pleasure while you're

eating, followed by a feeling of failure and a promise to eat healthy going forward.

Unfortunately, though, the whole loop usually starts again. Stepping off the roller coaster and onto stable ground requires determining the "why."

The trick is not to make yourself feel worse by trying to smother those emotions with food. There are better ways to process those feelings—without wrecking your weight-loss goals. Try one (or more) of these tips:

- **WRITE IT DOWN.** Keeping a food journal is a powerful way to track and control what you eat. Here's a way to make it even more effective: Don't just keep a food diary—keep a mood diary, too.

  When you write down what you're eating—and remember, you have to be honest and include the wayward

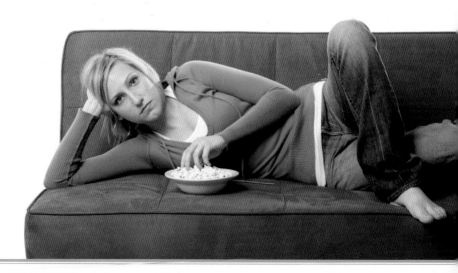

treats and binges—take a moment to note how you're feeling, too.

You may start to see patterns between your food choices and your emotional state. Spotting patterns is the first step to changing them.

- **BREAK THE CHAIN.** Once you identify your emotional-eating triggers, you can deal with them in more constructive ways.

This may mean asking yourself some tough questions: What needs aren't being met, or what feelings aren't being expressed? Can you vent them in a more constructive way than heading to the fridge? Breaking the chain of events or feelings that leads to emotional eating may be as simple as picking up the phone (instead of a bag of chips) and calling a friend. Or taking the dog for a walk. Or doing something fun until the craving passes.

- **STOP AND THINK.** Now that you're more mindful of your emotional state, you'll be able to assess your situation honestly.

When you catch yourself at the pantry door, stop and ask: Am I hungry? Is my body telling me it needs more fuel— or is my head saying there's some emotional need that isn't being met? Why do I really want to eat? What can I do instead of eating?

- **BE FOOD-CONSCIOUS.** As you become aware of your own food/mood connections, it's easy to overreact and cut yourself off from eating food you love. Don't.

Watching what you eat shouldn't be an exercise in deprivation. Shoot for moderation instead.

Eat slowly so you can hear your body telling you it's physically satisfied.

Don't eat in front of the TV or computer, or while you're doing something else. Focus on the food. Savor it.

Keep some favorite foods in the house, but in smaller quantities so that you're not tempted to overdo it.

GRAB A PEN:
- Make a list of all the things you'll do when you meet your weight-loss goal.

- Write a letter describing why you are sad, angry, frustrated—whatever the feeling is that you are trying to forget by eating. Tear the letter up or keep it to look at later. (Or deliver it, but not before at least 24 hours of thought.)

COUNT PLUSES:
- How many people told you how great you looked this week?

- How did you feel when you stepped on the scale and realized you had lost weight?

- How close are you to getting back into those jeans that used to fit?

DISTRACT YOURSELF:
- Fight boredom at all costs. Pick up a library book or even a trashy novel.

- Hone your mental sharpness by working your way through a crossword puzzle or something similar.

- If you hear the kitchen calling you when you know it shouldn't, head to the bathroom instead. A hot bath will relax you and get your mind off eating.

- Listen to relaxing music, your favorite CD or your iPod. Enjoy some "me" time.

BE GOOD TO YOUR BODY:
- Is the fridge calling? Go to bed early. Your body will appreciate extra sleep more than extra calories.

- Drink a glass of water or two. You might be thirsty rather than hungry, or the feeling of fullness from the water may take your mind off eating.

- Exercise boosts your mood. So walk up and down the steps at home or do other light exercise. Pull out your favorite CD and dance to the music. Get moving!

LOOK AHEAD:
- Plan your wardrobe. What can you pull from your closet that you haven't worn in years? What new piece of clothing should you buy yourself for losing 15 pounds? What's the first new thing you'll try on when you've reached your goal?

- Plan—and take—a vacation. Losing weight is hard work. Keeping it off is even harder. When you feel like you might actually consider wearing a swimsuit, start planning a vacation that lets you do it.

- To help fund your vacation or new wardrobe, reward yourself for each good choice. Put $1 in a money jar each time you avoid emotional eating. Start today!

Losing Weight For Real This Time!

By Kim Bennett
Jackson, Tennessee

Having a full, busy life distracted me from taking care of myself and losing weight—until I got serious.

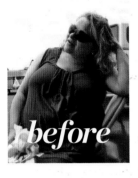

before

Following fad diet plans has never really worked out well for me. Having been plump since I was a toddler, I started my first "diet" before seventh grade. The weight came off quickly, but I gained it back just as fast. A year after my son was born, I weighed the same as I did the day I brought him home from the hospital. When I put on a bathing suit in the summer of 2010, I held 198 pounds on my 5-foot-3-inch frame and was totally disheartened. I was shocked when I looked at photos of myself—was I really that big?

During the year, my job as a sixth grade language arts teacher is stressful, and I work more than full time. I also have a 6-year-old daughter and a 2-year-old son, and my parents have both been ill. For a long time, I didn't have good coping skills to help me deal with feeling sad or stressed. So I ate. That overstuffed feeling became normal for me, and the pounds kept piling on.

I was tired of feeling this way—and so was my husband! He has always been supportive, and we decided that together, we were ready to make some serious changes for the better. I knew I could do it this time.

Three key elements

I said, "good-bye, diet mentality." This time, I approached weight loss as a new lifestyle instead of a short-term fix. I found that weight loss is basically a mathematical formula. I had to eat less and move more if I wanted to see any sort of change.

There were three integral elements to my weight-loss success. The first was nutrition. Instead of talking about a "diet," my daughter and I worked on healthy eating, and we learned how to make better choices. Fruit and vegetable portions increased, and our intake of simple carbohydrates decreased. I made sure we were eating enough protein, too. The recipes in the *Comfort Food Diet Cookbook* were really great, because they helped me modify our meals but were family-friendly, so everyone passed them around the table with pleasure.

The second element was movement. I created a caloric deficit by moving more. I didn't always need to exercise formally, since I am a middle school teacher and a mother of two. My days are always busy, so I'm not sitting much—but I still needed to move. I started to wear a pedometer and aim for 15,000 steps every day. It was easy to take a few extra steps, and the pedometer made it simple to see my progress.

The third element of my weight loss was the emotional component. I had to figure out what made me eat poorly. I identified my triggers and found ways to subvert them. If I knew I was going to be sad or stressed, such as when my husband was out of town for several weeks, I made sure to plan some relaxation for myself. Sometimes it was as simple as a hot bath after the kids were

after

asleep or finding a babysitter for a few hours to devote some time to myself. I started to listen to my body and not my emotions when it came to hunger. Then I could be smart and more deliberate about my actions.

Planning ahead and saving calories

Planning meals was another key to staying on track. Though it was a big challenge for me, I've integrated it into my daily life. Instead of not having a plan, I now make sure that we have two or three servings of fish each week and that we eat a rainbow of produce. Every week we have a family outing to the farmers market, so we eat lots of fresh produce and get our vitamins and nutrients.

And when I get up each day, I reach for a yogurt, my new staple breakfast food. Sometimes I make extra breakfast items on the weekend to heat up throughout the week, such as individual ham and cheese frittatas, a recipe I got from an earlier version of the *Comfort Food Diet Cookbook*.

As much as I try to plan each dinner, that time of day can quickly go awry. So I have a stash of quick-and-easy meal ideas that I can whip up if necessary. It's no trouble to keep meal-size portions of browned lean ground beef or turkey in the freezer. That way, I can pull it out and reheat it on really hectic evenings.

Another speedy idea: I mix the cooked ground meat with low-fat, low-sugar spaghetti sauce and serve it over shirataki noodles, thin Japanese noodles that are low in calories.

I also freeze casseroles or casserole ingredients for fast dinner prep. A deli rotisserie chicken weighed out in portions is easily paired with fresh or frozen vegetables as a dinner.

Slow cookers are my new friends, too! I put an entree in one, and two vegetable sides in other ones. When I get home, a hot meal is ready.

My snacks are also important, because I need to keep my energy level up and my hunger low. I love string cheese, nuts, seeds, vegetable sticks with Greek yogurt dip and hard-boiled eggs. I portion out items at home.

I keep healthy, individual desserts around the house for the whole family. When I make a dessert, I portion it and store it in containers right away. Then it's a conscious decision to get another whole dessert instead of scooping out "just a little more." When I'm tempted to eat more, I head to bed.

Every step counts

All of these changes in the last year have helped me lose 63 pounds. I now weigh in at 135 pounds, which is a healthy weight for my frame. My wonderful husband, who was enthusiastic as I implemented this new style of eating for our family, has lost 45 pounds, too!

I will maintain my weight loss by monitoring calories and keeping up my activity level. I take my kids outside to ride bikes and play, or we stay inside and compete in fun, active video games. I use my elliptical machine, and I try to take the stairs instead of the elevator. I walk to the store instead of driving.

But I do occasionally stray. I've even gained a few pounds here and there. When that happens, I am disappointed

Kim's Healthy Substitutes

1 Greek yogurt is a great substitute for sour cream. It works well in dip mixes.

2 Instead of using spray oil, I use a pastry brush to spread oil evenly. It's also easier to measure.

3 Being Southern, I drink a lot of iced tea. I sweeten it with sugar substitute.

4 Instead of flavored coffee creamer, I use unsweetened vanilla almond milk. It makes my coffee rich and creamy without added sugar.

but not discouraged. I just take a deep breath and dive right back into my healthy lifestyle.

Permanent changes

My family, neighbors and coworkers have been my cheering section. I get compliments daily and requests for weight loss advice. My husband has been so supportive, and I could not have achieved this goal without him.

I am now much healthier and happier and better equipped to keep up with my kids, my house and my job. The side benefits are greater confidence and self-esteem. I'm thrilled to be making positive, permanent changes that improve my life and the lives of everyone around me.

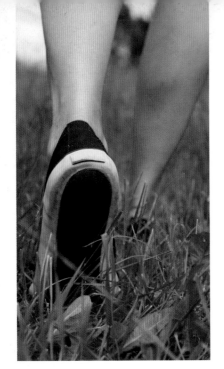

Move It and Lose It!

Combine exercise with healthy eating to burn more calories and lose more weight.

The Comfort Food Diet suggests adding exercise to your week for surefire calorie-burning success. And while it might seem intimidating at first, it's easier than you think to take that first step–literally.

Whatever activity you choose should be easy, affordable and, most of all, fun! Try to find a form of exercise that you'd enjoy doing every day...or at least on a very regular basis. Consider options that fit into your schedule and meet with your doctor's approval. Look for opportunities to work out with a spouse, family member or friend. Then grab your walking shoes and take that first step!

Walk It Off!

Walking is a perfect way to start an exercise routine. After all, you can burn roughly 100 calories by briskly walking a mile. In addition, walking lowers blood pressure and improves cholesterol.

If you're new to fitness walking, begin with a daily 10-minute stroll. Those 10 minutes will likely turn into 20 minutes or more in a matter of days. Set a goal for yourself to walk every day for one week. Get out there and enjoy a walk around the neighborhood!

During the next week, pay attention to the speed with which you move. The average walking speed is between 1½ and 2½ mph, but a good walking speed is 3 to 4 mph. Start using short strides with quick heel-to-toe movements. Long strides may cause your front foot to act like a brake, jarring your joints and slowing you down.

Using a pedometer, start increasing your steps by 10 to 20 percent per week. You are at a great level when you've reached 10,000 steps per day or 70,000 steps per week.

Your muscles need oxygen, so don't forget to inhale deeply and exhale fully, both to a count of three. When possible, walk on soft surfaces such as dirt, sand or grass—these areas are gentle on your joints. Always stretch before and after walking to prevent muscles from tightening or cramping.

One of the benefits of walking is that you can fit in a long walk once during the day, or you can walk for short bursts throughout the day and still burn calories. In other words, if you can't fit in a 45-minute walk, you can take three 15-minute walks instead.

Walking with a buddy can make the time fly, motivate you to stick with it and

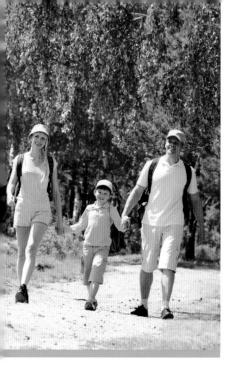

push you to increase your pace. Better yet, grab your family and take a relaxing walk together.

- Enjoy a family walk before dinner to discuss the day's events.

- Make walking a special event by taking the gang to the zoo, a museum or a shopping mall.

- When the kids are frustrated, walk around the block with them. They'll burn off the stress, and you'll all burn calories.

Regardless of how you work this activity into your day, be sure to carve out walking time in your schedule. Remember, the ultimate goal is to lose weight, feel good and become the best you can be. Commit to walking regularly, and with a little dedication and perseverance, you'll take a big step in the right direction.

Get Moving!

In a landmark Harvard study of some 40,000 women over the age of 45, those who walked as little as one hour a week—even at a stroll—were half as likely to have heart attacks or blocked coronary arteries as those who rarely walked for exercise. Walking is easier with good form, so follow these easy tips for proper posture to start your path to healthier tomorrows!

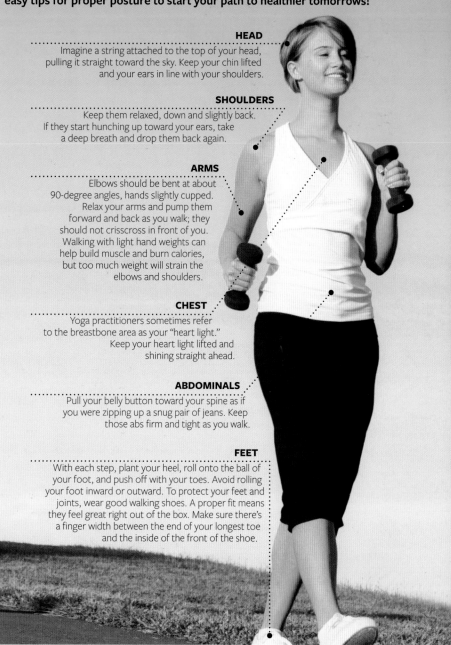

HEAD
Imagine a string attached to the top of your head, pulling it straight toward the sky. Keep your chin lifted and your ears in line with your shoulders.

SHOULDERS
Keep them relaxed, down and slightly back. If they start hunching up toward your ears, take a deep breath and drop them back again.

ARMS
Elbows should be bent at about 90-degree angles, hands slightly cupped. Relax your arms and pump them forward and back as you walk; they should not crisscross in front of you. Walking with light hand weights can help build muscle and burn calories, but too much weight will strain the elbows and shoulders.

CHEST
Yoga practitioners sometimes refer to the breastbone area as your "heart light." Keep your heart light lifted and shining straight ahead.

ABDOMINALS
Pull your belly button toward your spine as if you were zipping up a snug pair of jeans. Keep those abs firm and tight as you walk.

FEET
With each step, plant your heel, roll onto the ball of your foot, and push off with your toes. Avoid rolling your foot inward or outward. To protect your feet and joints, wear good walking shoes. A proper fit means they feel great right out of the box. Make sure there's a finger width between the end of your longest toe and the inside of the front of the shoe.

Before & After

Two of the most critical parts of a workout—the warm-up and cooldown—are also two of the most misunderstood.

Few things have evolved as dramatically in the field of exercise science as the understanding of proper warm-ups and cooldowns. Done correctly, they make exercise safer and more enjoyable. Are you doing them the right way? Here's what you need to know.

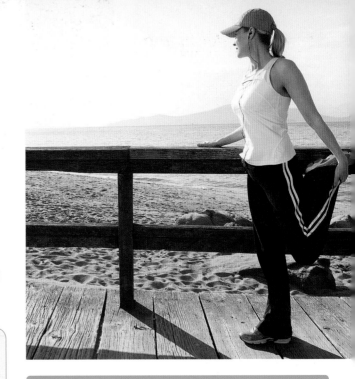

WARMING UP

Think back to high school gym class. The typical warm-up was probably a few bouncy stretches, and if you're still warming up that way, it's time to change. Research has repeatedly shown that stretching before you exercise does nothing to increase flexibility or prevent injuries.

Instead, the best warm-up is a slow, gentle version of the activity you're about to do. For example, if you're planning a run, start with a brisk walk. Before playing tennis, make some slow practice swings. Warming up this way slowly raises your heart rate, moves blood to your muscles and warms ligaments and tendons. These important physiological changes reduce your risk of injury and make your workout more comfortable, which means you'll be more likely to do it again.

COOLING DOWN

Cooling down is just as important as warming up because it gradually decreases your heart rate and body temperature and helps prevent muscle cramping and soreness. To cool down, simply follow the guidelines for a good warm-up and continue the same physical activity at a slower pace. After a 30- to 40-minute workout, spend 5 to 10 minutes cooling down.

Once you finish your cooldown, it's time to stretch. Warm muscles will stretch more easily, and frequent stretching increases your range of motion, reducing your chance of injury.

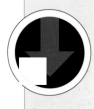

WORK OUT RIGHT

Warm-up and cooldown suggestions for popular activities:

PHYSICAL ACTIVITY	METHOD
AEROBICS	5-10 minutes at low intensity on a stair-climber
WEIGHT TRAINING	Walking on a treadmill for 5-10 minutes. Also, do a few repetitions with light weights before moving to your full load.
RUNNING	Walking or slow jogging
SWIMMING	Slow crawl
CYCLING	Flat terrain in lower gears
HIKING	Hike on flat terrain at minimal altitude
RACQUETBALL	Brisk walk or light jog and graduated-tempo volleying
ELLIPTICAL/ STAIR-CLIMBER	Light aerobic activity, such as walking, or low-tempo step exercise

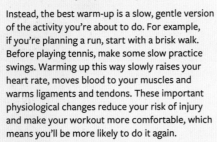

Hints for safer hiking

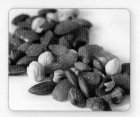

Prevent dehydration and fatigue by bringing water and nonperishable snacks, such as peanut butter and jelly sandwiches, granola and trail mix.

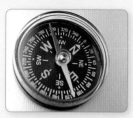

Bring a compass and cell phone as well as a clearly marked map of the area to keep you on track. Always tell someone who won't be with you where you are going.

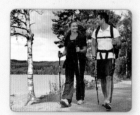

Add trekking poles to prevent injury. They help maintain balance and take strain off of your knees and ankles.

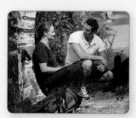

When you get tired take a break. Stumbles and falls happen more often when you've overdone it. Stretch a little, have a drink and snack, then get back to it.

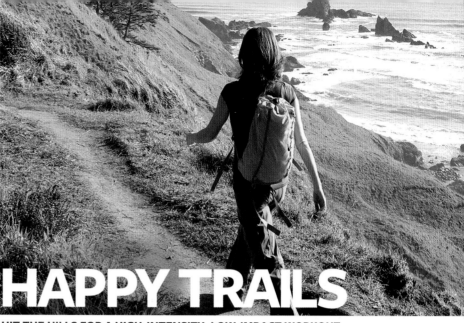

HAPPY TRAILS

HIT THE HILLS FOR A HIGH-INTENSITY, LOW-IMPACT WORKOUT

When you need a change of pace from the gym, look outdoors for a new way to tone up. Hiking burns calories, costs next to nothing and has a way of clearing your head. So read our tips and head outside, and make Mother Nature your workout partner!

WHY HIKE?

Compared to walking, hiking increases your workout's intensity. Your core abdominal and back muscles work harder as they stabilize you over uneven surfaces. And if you're hiking up a hill, all of your muscles—including your heart—get a better workout. Hiking on a steep grade and rough terrain also works hip flexors, quads, hamstrings, calves and glutes, so you get a firmer backside.

GET GOING

- Start out slowly and keep a consistent pace to help preserve your energy.

- Ask park rangers about trail elevation and layout to gauge your hike's intensity before you go. Search your state's Department of Natural Resources website for local trails.

- Consider your socks. The wrong pair can leave you blistered and miserable. Opt for two layers. Start with a thin polyester liner that wicks moisture, and top those with thicker, warmer socks. Bring a fresh pair of both types to change midway through long hikes.

- Make a smart shoe choice. If you'll be on a well-groomed trail, opt for light and comfortable cross-trainers. A rocky, off-the-beaten path area requires good-fitting boots with a sturdy toe.

- Layer up in colder months. Start with modern performance underwear made from moisture-wicking polyester or polypropylene. Top with polyester fleece to trap warmth without making clothes soggy from sweat. Add wind- and water-resistant pants, gloves, and a coat and hat, if needed.

I Was My Own Biggest Loser.

By Christy Sprotte
Kaukauna, Wisconsin

I shed 60 pounds and learned a lot about myself along the way.

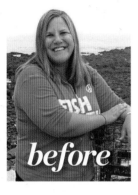

before

Like most women on their wedding day, I felt as though I was the most beautiful bride... despite the fact that I didn't reach my weight-loss goal prior to the big day.

During the flurry of wedding planning, I visited bridal boutiques and was shocked to discover that based on my measurements, I had to try on gowns from the plus-sized department.

I quickly began a fad diet and a few months later became ill. My doctor told me that I had developed a kidney stone that could very likely have been caused by the diet I was following. I decided to forgo the diet and concentrate on wedding plans.

Even though my weight wasn't where I wanted it to be on the big day, it was a glorious summer wedding nonetheless, and I couldn't have been happier.

As autumn quickly approached, and I settled into marital bliss, I decided it was time to revisit my goals and take off those extra pounds. I wanted to do this not only for me, but also for the family my husband and I planned to have.

I work as a psychologist at a middle school, and when a coworker proposed a weight-loss competition for the staff, I jumped onboard. I knew the friendly wager was the exact shove I needed to start shedding pounds.

Like the TV show, "The Biggest Loser," each participant was matched with a friend. Everyone weighed in with his or her partner weekly, and after 3 months the pair who lost the most pounds and percentage of weight won a monetary award.

I was motivated to win that prize, but knew the pounds weren't going to simply melt off. I recalled having some success in the past using food journals to track what I ate and count calories. By logging my food intake, I became much more aware of what I ate every day as well as the portion sizes.

I combined journaling with meal planning and drinking eight glasses of water daily. I also started walking 15 minutes a day, and it was much easier than I imagined. Eventually, I worked my way up to a minimum of 30 minutes of cardio activity every day in addition to strength-training exercises three times a week.

My attitude, however, was the most challenging obstacle I faced. You see, I am a perfectionist by nature, and because of this, I quickly became disappointed in myself when I overindulged or skipped a workout. Instead of pushing myself harder the next time, my self-criticism would set me back, and I would ignore my goals for several days.

Eventually, I realized that one of the most important factors in weight loss is consistency. It dawned on me that when I strayed too far from the path, I undid several weeks of weight-loss success. I quickly learned that humans make mistakes, and that I needed to let them go in order to move forward.

after

I began following an 80-20 rule. By this I mean that I ate healthy 80% of the time and indulged the remaining 20% of the time. This truly helped me as I became less flustered and found it easier to stick to my goals. I found that maintaining an overall healthy lifestyle isn't as challenging when you treat yourself occasionally, hold yourself accountable and forgive yourself for any mishaps that might occur.

Since I work in a school where tempting snacks, such as birthday cakes, muffins and other sweets, make regular appearances, I began taking healthy snacks to work. Low-fat string cheese, light yogurt, apples and bananas helped me avoid all of those enticing treats found in the teachers lounge. I also began eating every 3 to 4 hours in order to control my hunger and curb any cravings.

Whenever I felt like giving up, I reminded myself of the reasons I wanted to trim down in the first place.

Besides needing a healthy body to carry a child, I also wanted to be able to teach my family how to stay healthy.

I was determined to gain the skills and confidence I needed to maintain a healthy lifestyle before my husband and I had children and started our own family. And the best way to do that was to lose the weight and understand what it takes to eat right and live well.

Three months later the contest came to an end, and my partner and I were announced the winners...we lost the most weight! I was 50 pounds lighter and I was thrilled to win the award. I realized, however, that my greatest prize was gaining the skills I needed to maintain a healthy lifestyle for myself.

Currently, I am down 60 pounds, and I couldn't feel better. While my journey began as a plus-sized bride, today I am a happy, healthy wife, ready for anything that comes my way.

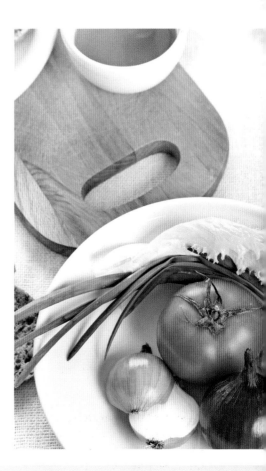

The secrets to my success

While on my weight-loss journey, I relied on a few secrets that helped me shed pounds and stay motivated.

- **PLAN, PLAN, PLAN.** Every weekend, my husband and I plan our meals for the upcoming week and then do our shopping. All of the recipes from the *Comfort Food Diet Cookbook* have been a huge help!

- **CHECK IN OR CHECK OUT.** Don't be afraid of the scale. Weekly weigh-ins are great. Losing 5 pounds gained over the holidays is significantly easier than losing 25

pounds gained carelessly by not keeping track of your weight.

- **DO SOME SURFING.** The Web is a great place for information and interactive tools on weight-loss. If you have plans to go out to dinner, you can even check the menu online and plan your order in advance.

- **DOWNSIZE DINNERWARE.** In order to keep myself from feeling deprived, I ate dinners off salad plates. This made me feel as though the portions were larger, and I felt fuller quickly.

- **TREAT YOURSELF.** I love desserts, so eliminating them from my diet was not realistic. Instead, I found low-calorie alternatives and allowed myself indulgences.

- **STIR IT UP.** Mixing up my exercise routine is motivating and keeps my body in fat-burning mode. My exercise routine includes hiking, biking, jogging, using an elliptical trainer and following a few exercise DVDs.

Free Foods List

Add these foods to your menu plan without worry.

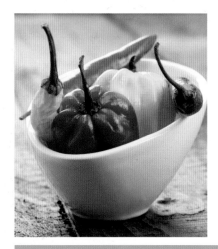 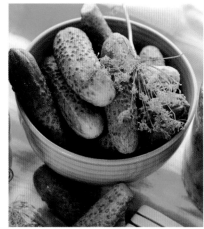 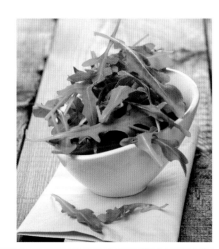

Listed at right are items considered "free foods" on the Comfort Food Diet. **A free food is an item that has fewer than 20 calories and 5 or less grams of carbohydrates per serving.** Whether you add these items to your meal plan, rely on them for snacks or simply use them to enhance the flavors of your favorite dishes, **feel free to enjoy as many free foods as you'd like.**

Free foods are an ideal way to fill you up because they are mostly non-starchy vegetables. When you make a low-calorie turkey sandwich, for instance, give it a bit of crunch with sliced cucumber, pickles or even radishes. Or **pump up the flavor** with fresh herbs, horseradish or hot pepper sauce...and don't worry about adding up any calories these items might contain.

On the far right, you'll find a section that offers more free foods with specific portion sizes. Feel free to enjoy a serving of these items and not count the calories— but **if you eat them in portions larger than what's noted in the list, the calories will have to count toward your daily goal.**

Eat All You Want

- Artichoke
- Artichoke hearts
- Asparagus
- Baby corn
- Bamboo shoots
- Bean sprouts
- Beans (green, wax, Italian)
- Beets
- Broccoli
- Broth or bouillon
- Brussels sprouts
- Cauliflower
- Carrots
- Celery
- Cucumber
- Eggplant
- Flavored sugar-free gelatin
- Garlic
- Green onions or scallions
- Greens (collard, kale, mustard, turnip)
- Hearts of palm
- Herbs (fresh or dried)
- Horseradish
- Hot pepper sauce
- Jicama
- Kohlrabi
- Leeks
- Lemon juice
- Mixed vegetables (without corn, peas or pasta)
- Mushrooms (fresh)
- Mustard
- Okra
- Onions
- Pea pods
- Pickles
- Radishes
- Rutabaga
- Salad greens (lettuce, romaine, chicory, endive, escarole, arugula, radicchio, watercress)
- Sauerkraut
- Spices
- Spinach
- Squash (summer, crookneck, zucchini)
- Sugar snap peas
- Swiss chard
- Tomato (fresh or canned)
- Turnips
- Vinegar
- Water chestnuts
- Worcestershire sauce

Free Foods and Beverages—Drink as Much as You Want

- Carbonated or mineral water
- Club soda
- Coffee (unsweetened or with sugar substitute)
- Diet soft drinks
- Drink mixes (sugar-free)
- Flavored water (20 calories or less)
- Tea (unsweetened or with sugar substitute)
- Tonic water (diet)
- Water

Free Foods with Restricted Portions

- Barbecue sauce, *2 teaspoons*
- Cream cheese (fat-free), *1 tablespoon ($\frac{1}{2}$ ounce)*
- Creamer:
  Nondairy, liquid, *1 tablespoon*
  Nondairy, powdered, *2 teaspoons*
- Honey mustard, *1 tablespoon*
- Jam or jelly (light or no sugar added), *2 teaspoons*
- Ketchup, *1 tablespoon*
- Margarine spread:
  Fat-free, *1 tablespoon*
  Reduced-fat, *1 teaspoon*
- Mayonnaise:
  Fat-free, *1 tablespoon*
  Reduced-fat, *1 teaspoon*
- Parmesan cheese (freshly grated), *1 tablespoon*

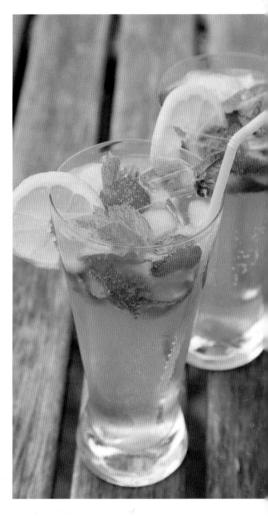

- Pickle relish, *1 tablespoon*
- Salad dressing:
  Fat-free or low-fat, *1 tablespoon*
  Fat-free Italian, *2 tablespoons*
- Salsa, *$\frac{1}{4}$ cup*
- Sour cream: Fat-free or reduced-fat, *1 tablespoon*
- Sweet and sour sauce, *2 teaspoons*
- Soy sauce, *1 tablespoon*
- Sweet chili sauce, *1 tablespoon*
- Syrup (sugar-free), *2 tablespoons*
- Taco sauce, *1 tablespoon*
- Whipped topping:
  Light or fat-free, *2 tablespoons*
  Regular, *1 tablespoon*

Six-Week Meal Plan

The following pages take the work out of calorie counting by offering a **complete six-week meal plan.** Each day suggests three meals and two snacks, totaling roughly 1,400 calories. **Feel free to substitute foods or mix and match the meals from various days.** Be sure, however, to pay attention to calories. To plan future weeks, **record what you're eating and track calories** using the blank Do-It-Yourself worksheets found on pages 470-471.

Comfort Food Diet Strategies:

- The great thing about the Comfort Food Diet is that you can serve incredible meals to your family members...and they won't even realize they're eating healthy! Look through the recipes in this book and immediately begin the meal plan by swapping in the dishes you know they'll enjoy most.

- The Comfort Food Diet tracks calories per day to make it easier to stay within the 1,400 calorie guidelines. If you should exceed that limit one day, however, simply plan on consuming fewer calories the following day. Keeping a food/calorie journal will help you track such instances.

- Consider making extras and freezing the leftovers for busy days or work lunches. When preparing large-batch recipes, stash a few items in the freezer for low-calorie snacks and desserts.

- Review the items on the Free Foods List (p. 41), and use them to satisfy hunger between meals. They're also tasty ways to round out a menu without adding too many calories.

- Try to get the most nutrients from calories. In other words, a couple tablespoons of chocolate-covered raisins have nearly the same amount of calories as four dates. The dates offer more health benefits than the chocolate treats, but feel free to enjoy the raisins if your sweet tooth is begging for a little attention.

day 1

BREAKFAST:

- Berry & Yogurt Phyllo Nest (p. 92)
  72 calories
- 1 large scrambled egg
  101 calories
- 1 slice whole wheat toast
  69 calories
- with 1 teaspoon reduced-fat margarine spread
  free food
- 1 cup fat-free milk
  86 calories
- Hot tea (with sugar substitute if desired)
  free food

  BREAKFAST TOTAL: 328 CALORIES

LUNCH:

- 1¾ cups Zesty Hamburger Soup (p. 177)
  251 calories
- 1 whole wheat dinner roll
  76 calories
- 1 medium banana
  100 calories
- Mineral water
  free food

  LUNCH TOTAL: 427 CALORIES

DINNER & DESSERT:

- 1 serving Tomato Walnut Tilapia (p. 223)
  205 calories
- 1 whole wheat dinner roll
  76 calories
- with 1 teaspoon reduced-fat margarine spread
  free food
- Shredded cabbage topped with 1 tablespoon reduced-fat salad dressing
  free food
- Ice water
  free food
- 1 piece Ice Cream Sandwich Dessert (p. 428)
  244 calories

  DINNER TOTAL: 525 CALORIES

SNACKS:

- 1 cup whole strawberries
  45 calories
- 1 piece string cheese
  80 calories

  WEEK 1, DAY 1 TOTAL: 1,405 CALORIES

day 2

BREAKFAST:

- 1 slice Crustless Spinach Quiche (p. 110)
  197 calories
- 1 slice whole wheat toast
  69 calories
- with 1 tablespoon no-sugar-added jam
  free food
- Hot tea (with sugar substitute if desired)
  free food
- ½ cup orange juice
  55 calories

  BREAKFAST TOTAL: 321 CALORIES

LUNCH:

- 1 cup Salmon Chowder (p. 145)
  198 calories
- 4 saltine crackers
  52 calories
- ⅔ cup red grapes
  86 calories
- 1 cup fat-free milk
  86 calories

  LUNCH TOTAL: 422 CALORIES

DINNER & DESSERT:

- 1 cup Zippy Spaghetti Sauce (p. 456)
  220 calories
- served over 1 cup cooked spaghetti
  100 calories
- 1 big green salad (see Free Foods List on p. 41) with 1 tablespoon reduced-fat salad dressing
  free food
- 1 cup fat-free milk
  86 calories
- 1 Chocolate Peanut Butter Parfait (p. 411)
  146 calories
- Coffee (with sugar substitute and 1 tablespoon liquid non-dairy creamer if desired)
  free food

  DINNER TOTAL: 552 CALORIES

SNACKS:

- 1 piece string cheese
  80 calories
- 1 medium peach or plum
  40 calories

  WEEK 1, DAY 2 TOTAL: 1,415 CALORIES

day 3

BREAKFAST:

- 2 servings Vegetable Scrambled Eggs (p. 87)
  180 calories
- 2 mini bagels (2½ inch diameter)
  144 calories
- with 1 tablespoon whipped cream cheese
  35 calories
- Coffee (with sugar substitute and 1 tablespoon liquid nondairy creamer if desired)
  free food

  BREAKFAST TOTAL: 359 CALORIES

LUNCH:

- 1 California Chicken Wrap (p. 167)
  300 calories
- 1 medium banana
  100 calories
- Diet soft drink
  free food

  LUNCH TOTAL: 400 CALORIES

DINNER & DESSERT:

- 1 serving Grilled Stuffed Pork Tenderloin (p. 281)
  296 calories
- Steamed fresh or frozen green beans topped with 1 teaspoon reduced-fat margarine spread
  free food
- 1 big green salad (see Free Foods List on p. 41) with 1 tablespoon reduced-fat salad dressing
  free food
- 1 cup fat-free milk
  86 calories
- 1 Mini Apple Strudel (p. 395)
  100 calories
- Hot tea (with sugar substitute if desired)
  free food

  DINNER TOTAL: 482 CALORIES

SNACKS:

- ½ cup sugar-free chocolate pudding (prepared with fat-free milk) topped with a crushed chocolate wafer
  99 calories
- ½ cup fresh blueberries
  41 calories

WEEK 1, DAY 3 TOTAL: 1,381 CALORIES

day 4

BREAKFAST:

- 2 Yogurt Pancakes (p. 139)
  242 calories
- with 1 teaspoon reduced-fat margarine spread
  free food
- drizzled with 1 tablespoon maple syrup
  52 calories
- ½ cup orange juice
  55 calories

  BREAKFAST TOTAL: 349 CALORIES

LUNCH:

- 1 cup Southwestern Chicken Soup (p. 445)
  143 calories
- 1 half-sandwich made with 1 piece whole wheat bread and 2 slices deli smoked turkey breast with 1 teaspoon fat-free mayonnaise
  89 calories
- 1 piece string cheese
  80 calories
- 1 medium banana
  100 calories
- Sugar-free flavored water
  free food

  LUNCH TOTAL: 412 CALORIES

DINNER & DESSERT:

- 1 Makeover Li'l Cheddar Meat Loaf (p. 213)
  187 Calories
- 1 medium baked russet potato
  161 calories
- Steamed fresh broccoli florets
  free food
- 1 cup fat-free milk
  86 calories
- 1 piece Chunky Fruit 'n' Nut Fudge (p. 401)
  92 calories
- Coffee (with sugar substitute and 1 tablespoon liquid nondairy creamer if desired)
  free food

  DINNER TOTAL: 526 CALORIES

SNACKS:

- 1 medium peach or plum
  40 calories
- ⅓ cup 1% cottage cheese with ¼ cup unsweetened pineapple tidbits
  81 calories

WEEK 1, DAY 4 TOTAL: 1,408 CALORIES

day 5

BREAKFAST:

- ½ cup Raisin Oatmeal Mix (p. 104)
  186 calories
- 1 Turkey Breakfast Sausage Patty (p. 93)
  85 calories
- ½ cup cubed fresh pineapple
  37 calories
- 1 cup fat-free milk
  86 calories

BREAKFAST TOTAL: 394 CALORIES

LUNCH:

- 1 Open-Faced Portobello Sandwich (p. 146)
  236 calories
- 1 piece string cheese
  80 calories
- 1 medium pear
  96 calories
- Celery sticks with 1 tablespoon fat-free ranch salad dressing
  free food
- Mineral water
  free food

LUNCH TOTAL: 412 CALORIES

DINNER & DESSERT:

- 1 serving Smothered Chicken Italiano (p. 279)
  252 calories
- 1 big green salad (see Free Foods List on p. 41) with 1 tablespoon reduced-fat salad dressing
  free food
- 2 sesame bread sticks (5g each)
  40 calories
- 1 serving Broccoli with Lemon Sauce (p. 350)
  76 calories
- Diet soft drink
  free food
- 1 piece Chunky Fruit 'n' Nut Fudge (p. 401)
  92 calories
- Hot tea (with sugar substitute if desired)
  free food

DINNER TOTAL: 460 CALORIES

SNACKS:

- ⅔ cup Cheerios with ¼ cup fat-free milk
  93 calories
- ½ cup sliced strawberries with 2 tablespoons reduced-fat frozen whipped topping
  47 calories

WEEK 1, DAY 5 TOTAL: 1,406 CALORIES

day 6

BREAKFAST:

- 1 cup Cappuccino Smoothie (p. 115)
  166 calories
- 1 Turkey Breakfast Sausage Patty (p. 93)
  85 calories
- 1 mini bagel (2½ inch diameter)
  72 calories
- with 1 tablespoon whipped cream cheese
  35 calories
- Hot tea (with sugar substitute if desired)
  free food

BREAKFAST TOTAL: 358 CALORIES

LUNCH:

- 1 Simon's Famous Tuna Salad (p. 161)
  271 calories
- ⅓ cup red grapes
  43 calories
- 1 cup fat-free milk
  86 calories

LUNCH TOTAL: 400 CALORIES

DINNER & DESSERT:

- 1 serving Grilled Pork Chops with Cilantro Salsa (p. 230)
  240 calories
- 1 small baked sweet potato
  128 calories
- with 1 teaspoon reduced-fat margarine spread
  free food
- 1 cup Grilled Broccoli & Cauliflower (p. 352)
  47 calories
- Ice water
  free food
- 1 Chocolate Pudding Sandwich (p. 407)
  73 calories
- Coffee (with sugar substitute and 1 tablespoon liquid nondairy creamer if desired)
  free food

DINNER TOTAL: 488 CALORIES

SNACKS:

- ½ small apple with 2 tablespoons fat-free caramel ice cream topping
  93 calories
- 1 medium plum
  40 calories

WEEK 1, DAY 6 TOTAL: 1,379 CALORIES

day 7

BREAKFAST:

- 2 Nutmeg Waffles (p. 99)
  196 Calories
- with 1 teaspoon reduced-fat margarine spread
  free food
- drizzled with 1 tablespoon maple syrup
  52 calories
- ½ cup cubed fresh pineapple
  37 calories
- ¾ cup orange juice
  83 calories

BREAKFAST TOTAL: 368 CALORIES

LUNCH:

- 1 California Pizza (p. 148)
  245 calories
- 1 big green salad (see Free Foods List on p. 41)
  with 1 tablespoon reduced-fat salad dressing
  free food
- ¾ cup fresh blueberries
  62 calories
- 1 cup Watermelon Cooler (p. 75)
  82 calories

LUNCH TOTAL: 389 CALORIES

DINNER & DESSERT:

- 1 serving Cornmeal Oven-Fried Chicken (p. 209)
  244 calories
- ¾ cup Potato Vegetable Medley (p. 345)
  59 calories
- 1 slice whole wheat bread
  69 calories
- with 1 teaspoon reduced-fat margarine spread
  free food
- 1 cup fat-free milk
  86 calories
- 1 Chocolate Pudding Sandwich (p. 407)
  73 calories

DINNER TOTAL: 531 CALORIES

SNACKS:

- 1 cup Strawberry Mango Smoothie (p. 83)
  100 calories
- Baby carrots
  free food
- 1 cup prepared sugar-free gelatin
  8 calories

WEEK 1, DAY 7 TOTAL: 1,396 CALORIES

day 1

BREAKFAST:

- 1 serving Baked Eggs with Cheddar & Bacon (p. 119)
  107 calories
- 1 mini bagel (2½ inch diameter)
  72 calories
- with 1 tablespoon fat-free cream cheese
  free food
- ⅔ cup red grapes
  86 calories
- ½ cup orange juice
  55 calories
- Hot tea (with sugar substitute if desired)
  free food

BREAKFAST TOTAL: 320 CALORIES

LUNCH:

- 1⅓ cups Lasagna Soup (p. 185)
  280 calories
- 1 whole wheat dinner roll
  69 calories
- with 1 teaspoon reduced-fat margarine spread
  free food
- 1 cup fat-free milk
  86 calories

LUNCH TOTAL: 435 CALORIES

DINNER & DESSERT:

- 1 Tex-Mex Beef Barbecue sandwich (p. 452)
  294 calories
- Steamed green beans
  free food
- Ice water
  free food
- 1 serving Blackberry Cobbler (p. 441)
  199 calories

DINNER TOTAL: 493 CALORIES

SNACKS:

- ¾ cup skinny latte (made with fat-free milk)
  60 calories
- 1 Apple Skewer (p. 65)
  80 calories

WEEK 2, DAY 1, TOTAL: 1,388 CALORIES

day 2

BREAKFAST:

- 1 Scrambled Egg Muffin (p. 110)
133 calories
- ½ cup Orange Fruit Cup (p. 94)
80 calories
- 1 cup fat-free milk
86 calories
- Hot tea (with sugar substitute if desired)
free food

BREAKFAST TOTAL: 299 CALORIES

LUNCH:

- ⅔ cup Brunch Risotto (p. 130)
279 calories
- ¾ cup fresh blueberries
62 calories
- 1 whole wheat dinner roll
69 calories
- with 1 teaspoon reduced-fat margarine spread
free food
- Sugar-free flavored water
free food

LUNCH TOTAL: 410 CALORIES

DINNER & DESSERT:

- 1 serving Oven-Fried Fish Nuggets (p. 210)
171 calories
- 1 medium baked russet potato
161 calories
- 1 big green salad (see Free Foods List on p. 41) with 1 tablespoon reduced-fat salad dressing
free food
- 1 cup fat-free milk
86 calories
- 1 Cherry Chocolate Parfait (p. 417)
146 calories
- Coffee (with sugar substitute and liquid nondairy creamer if desired)
free food

DINNER TOTAL: 564 CALORIES

SNACKS:

- 1 cup Parmesan Popcorn (p. 75)
49 calories
- 1 cup cubed watermelon
40 calories
- ½ piece string cheese
40 calories

WEEK 2, DAY 2, TOTAL: 1,402 CALORIES

day 3

BREAKFAST:

- ¾ cup prepared oatmeal (made with water)
109 calories
- with 2 tablespoons raisins
54 calories
- 1 medium banana
100 calories
- 1 cup fat-free milk
86 calories
- Coffee (with sugar substitute and liquid nondairy creamer if desired)
free food

BREAKFAST TOTAL: 349 CALORIES

LUNCH:

- 1 sandwich made with 2 pieces whole wheat bread and 4 slices deli smoked turkey breast spread with 2 teaspoons fat-free mayonnaise
178 calories
- Baby carrots
free food
- 1 cup red grapes
129 calories
- 1 cup fat-free milk
86 calories

LUNCH TOTAL: 393 CALORIES

DINNER & DESSERT:

- 1 serving Country Chicken with Gravy (p. 270)
274 calories
- ½ cup prepared brown rice
108 calories
- ½ cup Wilted Garlic Spinach (p. 357)
66 calories
- 2 chocolate kisses
49 calories
- Hot tea (with sugar substitute if desired)
free food

DINNER TOTAL: 497 CALORIES

SNACKS:

- 1 Granola-To-Go Bar (p. 101)
130 calories
- Red and green pepper strips with 1 tablespoon reduced-fat ranch salad dressing
free food
- ½ cup sliced fresh strawberries
27 calories
- 1 cup prepared sugar-free gelatin
8 calories

WEEK 2, DAY 3, TOTAL: 1,404 CALORIES

day 4

BREAKFAST:

- 1 Colorful Cheese Omelet (p. 99)
  167 calories
- 1 medium apple
  72 calories
- 1 cup fat-free milk
  86 calories

BREAKFAST TOTAL: 325 CALORIES

LUNCH:

- 1½ cups Fruity Crab Pasta Salad (p. 168)
  322 calories
- 1 whole wheat dinner roll
  69 calories
- with 1 teaspoon reduced-fat margarine spread
  free food
- ⅓ cup red grapes
  43 calories
- Sugar-free flavored water
  free food

LUNCH TOTAL: 434 CALORIES

DINNER & DESSERT:

- 1 serving Stuffed Steak Spirals (p. 220)
  214 calories
- ¾ cup Seasoned Yukon Gold Wedges (p. 372)
  121 calories
- Steamed green beans with 1 teaspoon reduced-fat margarine spread
  free food
- Iced tea (with sugar substitute if desired)
  free food
- 1 Pina Colada Pudding Cup (p. 435)
  171 calories
- Coffee (with sugar substitute and 1 tablespoon liquid nondairy creamer if desired)
  free food

DINNER TOTAL: 506 CALORIES

SNACKS:

- ½ cup chocolate soy milk
  67 calories
- 1 medium plum
  40 calories

WEEK 2, DAY 4, TOTAL: 1,372 CALORIES

day 5

BREAKFAST:

- ½ cup Apple-Cinnamon Oatmeal Mix (p. 115)
  176 calories
- with 1 tablespoon maple syrup
  52 calories
- ½ cup blueberries
  41 calories
- 1 cup fat-free milk
  86 calories

BREAKFAST TOTAL: 355 CALORIES

LUNCH:

- 1 slice Chicken Alfredo Veggie Pizza (p. 178)
  317 calories
- 1 medium peach
  40 calories
- Mineral water
  free food

LUNCH TOTAL: 357 CALORIES

DINNER & DESSERT:

- 1 serving Broccoli-Turkey Casserole (p. 259)
  303 calories
- ¾ cup Sauteed Corn with Tomatoes & Basil (p. 346)
  85 calories
- 1 big green salad (see Free Foods List on p. 41) with 1 tablespoon reduced-fat salad dressing
  free food
- 1 cup fat-free milk
  86 calories
- ¾ cup Vanilla Tapioca Pudding (p. 412)
  133 calories
- Coffee (with sugar substitute and liquid non-dairy creamer if desired)
  free food

DINNER TOTAL: 607 CALORIES

SNACKS:

- ¾ cup air-popped popcorn
  24 calories
- 1 cup fresh raspberries
  60 calories

WEEK 2, DAY 5, TOTAL: 1,403 CALORIES

day 6

BREAKFAST:

- 1 serving Caramel Cream Crepes (p. 128)
  206 calories
- ½ cup sliced fresh strawberries
  27 calories
- 1 medium plum
  40 calories
- 1 cup fat-free milk
  86 calories
- Coffee (with sugar substitute and liquid non-dairy creamer if desired)
  free food

  BREAKFAST TOTAL: 359 CALORIES

LUNCH:

- 1½ cups Italian Sausage Bean Soup (p. 185)
  339 calories
- 1 whole wheat dinner roll
  69 calories
- with 1 teaspoon reduced-fat margarine spread
  free food
- ⅓ cup red grapes
  43 calories
- Ice water
  free food

  LUNCH TOTAL: 451 CALORIES

DINNER & DESSERT:

- 4 ounces beef tenderloin steak, broiled
  200 calories
- 1 small baked sweet potato
  128 calories
- ½ cup Parmesan Roasted Carrots (p. 362)
  82 calories
- Ice water
  free food
- 1 cup fat-free milk
  86 calories
- Hot tea (with sugar substitute if desired)
  free food

  DINNER TOTAL: 496 CALORIES

SNACKS:

- 9 tiny twist fat-free pretzels with 1 tablespoon honey mustard for dipping
  50 calories
- 1 cup prepared sugar-free gelatin
  8 calories
- 1 small orange
  45 calories

WEEK 2, DAY 6, TOTAL: 1,409 CALORIES

day 7

BREAKFAST:

- 1½ cup Wheaties
  161 calories
- with 1 cup fat-free milk
  86 calories
- 1 medium grapefruit
  92 calories
- Coffee (with sugar substitute and liquid non-dairy creamer if desired)
  free food

  BREAKFAST TOTAL: 339 CALORIES

LUNCH:

- 1 Grecian Gold Medal Wrap (p. 173)
  279 calories
- ½ cup cubed fresh pineapple
  37 calories
- 1 cup fat-free milk
  86 calories

  LUNCH TOTAL: 402 CALORIES

DINNER & DESSERT:

- 1 serving Sirloin Roast with Gravy (p. 185)
  185 calories
- 1 serving Golden au Gratin Potatoes (p. 375)
  167 calories
- 1 big green salad (see Free Foods List on p. 41) with 1 tablespoon reduced-fat salad dressing
  free food
- Ice water
  free food
- 1 piece Raspberry Pie with Oat Crust (p. 434)
  167 calories
- Hot tea (with sugar substitute if desired)
  free food

  DINNER TOTAL: 519 CALORIES

SNACKS:

- ¾ cup air-popped popcorn
  24 calories
- 1 cup whole fresh strawberries
  54 calories
- 1 medium apple
  72 calories

WEEK 2, DAY 7, TOTAL: 1,410 CALORIES

day 1

BREAKFAST:

- 3 slices Sweet Berry Bruschetta (p. 89)
  276 calories
- ½ cup orange juice
  55 calories
- Coffee (with sugar substitute and 1 tablespoon liquid nondairy creamer if desired)
  free food

BREAKFAST TOTAL: 331 CALORIES

LUNCH:

- 1 serving Tuna Artichoke Melts (p. 183)
  335 calories
- ¾ cup red grapes
  108 calories
- Iced tea (with sugar substitute if desired)
  free food

LUNCH TOTAL: 443 CALORIES

DINNER & DESSERT:

- 1 serving Balsamic-Seasoned Steak (p. 224)
  188 calories
- ¾ cup Colorful Roasted Veggies (p. 345)
  88 calories
- ½ small baked russet potato
  69 calories
- with 1 teaspoon reduced-fat margarine spread
  free food
- 1 Double Chocolate Cupcake (p. 416)
  139 calories
- ½ cup fat-free milk
  48 calories

DINNER TOTAL: 532 CALORIES

SNACKS:

- Baby carrots
  free food
- 1½ cups air-popped popcorn
  47 calories
- 2 chocolate kisses
  49 calories

WEEK 3, DAY 1 TOTAL: 1,402 CALORIES

day 2

BREAKFAST:

- 2 Overnight Yeast Waffles (p. 136)
  220 Calories
- drizzled with 4 teaspoons of maple syrup
  69 calories
- 1 Sage Breakfast Patty (p. 95)
  78 calories
- Hot tea (with sugar substitute if desired)
  free food

BREAKFAST TOTAL: 367 CALORIES

LUNCH:

- 1½ cups Vegetable Beef Stew (p. 467)
  278 calories
- 1 big green salad (see Free Foods List on p. 41) with 1 tablespoon reduced-fat salad dressing
  free food
- 1 cup fat-free milk
  86 calories

LUNCH TOTAL: 364 CALORIES

DINNER & DESSERT:

- 1 serving Chicken Marsala (p. 222)
  247 calories
- 1 serving Savory Asparagus (p. 362)
  74 calories
- ½ cup cooked long-grain white rice
  103 calories
- 1 Marbled Chocolate Cheesecake Bar (p. 406)
  95 calories
- Coffee (with sugar substitute and 1 tablespoon liquid nondairy creamer if desired)
  free food

DINNER TOTAL: 519 CALORIES

SNACKS:

- ½ cup sliced fresh strawberries with 2 tablespoons reduced-fat whipped topping
  47 calories
- ½ cup 1% cottage cheese with ¼ cup unsweetened pineapple tidbits
  108 calories

WEEK 3, DAY 2 TOTAL: 1,405 CALORIES

day 3

BREAKFAST:

- 1 Lemon-Blueberry Oat Muffin (p. 116)
  166 calories
- 1 medium banana
  100 calories
- 1 cup fat-free milk
  86 calories

BREAKFAST TOTAL: 352 CALORIES

LUNCH:

- 1 Taco Salad Wrap (p. 175)
  345 calories
- 8 white corn tortilla chips
  93 calories
- with ¼ cup salsa
  free food
- Diet soft drink
  free food

LUNCH TOTAL: 438 CALORIES

DINNER & DESSERT:

- 1 serving Glazed Pork Medallions (p. 221)
  200 calories
- ¾ cup Stir-Fried Carrots (p. 384)
  106 calories
- 1 big green salad (see Free Foods List on p. 41) with 1 tablespoon reduced-fat salad dressing
  free food
- Ice water
  free food
- 1 piece Fudgy Chocolate Dessert (p. 442)
  200 calories

DINNER TOTAL: 506 CALORIES

SNACKS:

- 1 small orange
  45 calories
- ½ piece string cheese
  40 calories

WEEK 3, DAY 3 TOTAL: 1,381 CALORIES

day 4

BREAKFAST:

- 6 ounces nonfat fruit yogurt
  160 calories
- topped with ¼ cup Toasted Almond Granola (p. 141)
  106 calories
- 1 slice whole wheat toast
  69 calories
- with 1 teaspoon reduced-fat margarine spread
  free food
- Hot tea (with sugar substitute if desired)
  free food

BREAKFAST TOTAL: 335 CALORIES

LUNCH:

- 1½ cups Zippy Corn Chowder (p. 145)
  285 calories
- 4 saltine crackers
  52 calories
- 1 big green salad (see Free Foods List on p. 41) with 1 tablespoon reduced-fat salad dressing
  free food
- 1 medium pear
  96 calories
- Sugar-free flavored water
  free food

LUNCH TOTAL: 433 CALORIES

DINNER & DESSERT:

- 1 serving Easy Chicken Potpie (p. 284)
  335 calories
- Ice water
  free food
- 1 Tiramisu Parfait (p. 431)
  189 calories
- Coffee (with sugar substitute and 1 tablespoon liquid nondairy creamer if desired)
  free food

DINNER TOTAL: 524 CALORIES

SNACKS:

- 1 miniature bagel with 1 tablespoon reduced-fat chive and onion cream cheese
  63 calories
- 1 medium plum
  40 calories

WEEK 3, DAY 4 TOTAL: 1,395 CALORIES

day 5

BREAKFAST:

- 1 serving Mushroom Spinach Omelet (p. 112)
  110 calories
- 2 slices Canadian bacon
  44 calories
- 1 slice whole wheat toast
  69 calories
- with 1 tablespoon no-sugar-added jam
  free food
- 1 cup cubed fresh pineapple
  74 calories
- Hot tea (with sugar substitute if desired)
  free food

BREAKFAST TOTAL: 297 CALORIES

LUNCH:

- Teriyaki Chicken Salad with Poppy Seed Dressing
  361 calories
- 1 whole wheat dinner roll
  76 calories
- with 1 teaspoon reduced-fat margarine spread
  free food
- Ice water
  free food

LUNCH TOTAL: 437 CALORIES

DINNER & DESSERT:

- 1 serving Southwest Pasta Bake (p. 265)
  328 calories
- Steamed fresh broccoli florets topped with
  1 teaspoon reduced-fat margarine spread
  free food
- 1 cup fat-free milk
  86 calories
- 2 Banana Chocolate Chip Cookies (p. 399)
  132 calories

DINNER TOTAL: 546 CALORIES

SNACKS:

- ½ English muffin topped with 1 slice tomato
  and 2 tablespoons shredded part-skim
  mozzarella cheese, broiled
  105 calories
- 1 cup prepared sugar-free flavored gelatin
  8 calories
- Baby carrots
  free food

WEEK 3, DAY 5 TOTAL: 1,393 CALORIES

day 6

BREAKFAST:

- 1 serving Fruited Dutch Baby (p. 127)
  203 calories
- with 1 tablespoon whipped cream
  26 calories
- 1 serving Peach Smoothie (p. 66)
  68 calories

BREAKFAST TOTAL: 297 CALORIES

LUNCH:

- 1 slice Baked Deli Focaccia Sandwich (p. 143)
  240 calories
- 20 baked potato chips
  200 calories
- Mineral water
  free food

LUNCH TOTAL: 440 CALORIES

DINNER & DESSERT:

- 1 serving Chicken with Mustard Gravy (p. 261)
  262 calories
- ⅔ cup Caramelized Onion Mashed
  Potatoes (p. 383)
  200 calories
- 1 big green salad (see Free Foods List on p. 41)
  with 1 tablespoon reduced-fat salad dressing
  free food
- 1 Wonton Sundae (p. 402)
  83 calories
- Hot tea (with sugar substitute if desired)
  free food

DINNER TOTAL: 545 CALORIES

SNACKS:

- Celery sticks with 1 tablespoon
  fat-free ranch salad dressing
  free food
- 1 cup fresh blueberries
  104 calories

WEEK 3, DAY 6 TOTAL: 1,386 CALORIES

day 7

BREAKFAST:

- 1 serving Ham 'n' Cheese Squares (p. 101)
  141 calories
- 1 Custard Berry Parfait (p. 119)
  119 calories
- 1 slice whole wheat toast
  69 calories
- with 1 teaspoon reduced-fat margarine spread
  free food
- Coffee (with sugar substitute and 1 tablespoon liquid nondairy creamer if desired)
  free food

BREAKFAST TOTAL: 329 CALORIES

LUNCH:

- 1 Spicy Buffalo Chicken Wrap (p. 186)
  273 calories
- 1 big green salad (see Free Foods List on p. 41)
  free food
- with 3 tablespoons of reduced-fat blue cheese salad dressing
  42 calories
- Diet soft drink
  free food

LUNCH TOTAL: 315 CALORIES

DINNER & DESSERT:

- 1 serving Swiss Steak (p. 275)
  255 calories
- ½ cup cooked long-grain white rice
  103 calories
- Steamed fresh or frozen green beans
  free food
- Iced tea
  (with sugar substitute if desired)
  free food
- 1 slice Yummy Chocolate Cake (p. 437)
  197 calories

DINNER TOTAL: 555 CALORIES

SNACKS:

- 1 cup Cajun Popcorn (p. 71)
  77 calories
- ½ medium pear and ½ ounce reduced-fat cheddar cheese
  94 calories
- 1 chocolate kiss
  25 calories

WEEK 3, DAY 7 TOTAL: 1,395 CALORIES

day 1

BREAKFAST:

- 3 pancakes from Homemade Pancake Mix (p. 140)
  258 calories
- with 2 tablespoons sugar-free syrup
  free food
- ⅔ cup red grapes
  86 calories
- Coffee (with sugar substitute and liquid nondairy creamer if desired)
  free food

BREAKFAST TOTAL: 344 CALORIES

LUNCH:

- 1 Presto Chicken Taco (p. 147)
  215 calories
- with 1 tablespoon taco sauce and 1 tablespoon reduced-fat sour cream
  free food
- 1 medium pear
  96 calories
- Steamed broccoli florets
  free food
- 1 cup fat-free milk
  86 calories
- Coffee (with sugar substitute and liquid nondairy creamer if desired)
  free food

LUNCH TOTAL: 397 CALORIES

DINNER & DESSERT:

- 1 BBQ Beef Sandwich (p. 448)
  354 calories
- ⅔ cup Home-Style Coleslaw (p. 361)
  88 calories
- 1 cup fat-free milk
  86 calories
- Hot tea (with sugar substitute if desired)
  free food

DINNER TOTAL: 528 CALORIES

SNACKS:

- ¼ cup pretzel sticks with 1 tablespoon honey mustard
  77 calories
- 1 clementine
  35 calories
- Red and green pepper strips with 1 tablespoon reduced-fat ranch salad dressing
  free food

WEEK 4, DAY 1, TOTAL: 1,381 CALORIES

day 2

BREAKFAST:

- 1 piece Monterey Quiche (p. 138)
265 calories
- ⅔ cup red grapes
86 calories
- 1 cup fat-free milk
86 calories
- Hot tea (with sugar substitute if desired)
free food

BREAKFAST TOTAL: 437 CALORIES

LUNCH:

- 1 sandwich made with 2 pieces whole wheat bread and 4 slices deli smoked turkey breast spread with 2 teaspoons fat-free mayonnaise
178 calories
- 10 baked potato chips
100 calories
- 1 cup fat-free milk
86 calories
- Diet soft drink
free food

LUNCH TOTAL: 364 CALORIES

DINNER & DESSERT:

- 1 serving Tilapia with Grapefruit Salsa (p. 293)
264 calories
- 1 big green salad (see Free Foods List on p. 41) with 1 tablespoon reduced-fat salad dressing
free food
- ½ Grandma's Stuffed Yellow Squash (p. 378)
103 calories
- Ice water
free food
- 1 serving Broiled Fruit Dessert (p. 395)
80 calories
- Hot tea (with sugar substitute if desired)
free food

DINNER TOTAL: 447 CALORIES

SNACKS:

- ½ cup fat-free vanilla frozen yogurt
95 calories
- 1 cup sliced fresh strawberries
54 calories

WEEK 4, DAY 2, TOTAL: 1,397 CALORIES

day 3

BREAKFAST:

- 2 frozen waffles
196 calories
- with 1 tablespoon sugar-free syrup
free food
- 1 cup sliced fresh strawberries
54 calories
- 1 cup fat-free milk
86 calories
- Coffee (with sugar substitute and 1 tablespoon liquid nondairy creamer if desired)
free food

BREAKFAST TOTAL: 336 CALORIES

LUNCH:

- 1 serving Ratatouille with Polenta (p. 156)
195 calories
- 1 piece Tropical Meringue Tart (p. 427)
145 calories
- Ice water
free food

LUNCH TOTAL: 340 CALORIES

DINNER & DESSERT:

- 1 serving Pork Medallions with Dijon Sauce (p. 284)
323 calories
- ¾ cup Herbed Potato Salad (p. 368)
142 calories
- Shredded cabbage topped with 1 tablespoon reduced-fat salad dressing
free food
- 1 sliced medium apple with cinnamon
72 calories
- Hot tea (with sugar substitute if desired)
free food

DINNER TOTAL: 537 CALORIES

SNACKS:

- 1 ice cream cake cone filled with ⅓ cup fat-free strawberry yogurt and ¼ cup blueberries
81 calories
- 1 piece string cheese
80 calories
- 1 clementine
35 calories

WEEK 4, DAY 3, TOTAL: 1,409 CALORIES

day 4

BREAKFAST:

- 1 Hawaiian Breakfast Cup (p. 123)
  131 calories
- 1 cup orange juice
  110 calories
- 1 cup fresh raspberries
  60 calories
- Coffee (with sugar substitute and liquid nondairy creamer if desired)
  free food

BREAKFAST TOTAL: 301 CALORIES

LUNCH:

- 1 Garbanzo Bean Pita (1 filled pita half) (p. 105)
  241 calories
- 1 serving Basil Cherry Tomatoes (p. 347)
  42 calories
- 1 clementine
  35 calories
- 1 cup fat-free milk
  86 calories

LUNCH TOTAL: 404 CALORIES

DINNER & DESSERT:

- 1 serving Burgundy Beef Stew with 1 cup noodles (p. 326)
  388 calories
- Steamed broccoli florets with 1 teaspoon reduced-fat margarine spread
  free food
- 1 cup fat-free milk
  86 calories
- ½ cup Cappuccino Pudding (p. 422)
  105 calories
- Iced tea (with sugar substitute if desired)
  free food

DINNER TOTAL: 579 CALORIES

SNACKS:

- 1 medium kiwifruit
  46 calories
- 1 crisp ladyfinger cookie
  30 calories
- ½ cup cheese popcorn
  40 calories

WEEK 4, DAY 4, TOTAL: 1,400 CALORIES

day 5

BREAKFAST:

- 1 serving Baked Blueberry & Peach Oatmeal (p. 99)
  277 calories
- 1 cup fat-free milk
  86 calories
- Hot tea (with sugar substitute if desired)
  free food

BREAKFAST TOTAL: 363 CALORIES

LUNCH:

- 1 Grilled Fish Sandwich (p. 152)
  241 calories
- 1 medium peach
  40 calories
- 1 dill pickle spear
  free food
- ½ cup fat-free milk
  43 calories
- Club soda
  free food

LUNCH TOTAL: 324 CALORIES

DINNER & DESSERT:

- 4 ounce salmon fillet, broiled
  184 calories
- 1 whole wheat dinner roll
  69 calories
- with 1 teaspoon reduced-fat margarine spread
  free food
- ½ cup Peas a la Francaise (p. 379)
  112 calories
- 1 big green salad (see Free Foods List on p. 41) with 1 tablespoon reduced-fat salad dressing
  free food
- Ice water
  free food
- 1 serving Coconut Custard Pie (p. 443)
  214 calories
- Coffee (with sugar substitute and liquid nondairy creamer if desired)
  free food

DINNER TOTAL: 579 CALORIES

SNACKS:

- ½ medium apple with ½ ounce sharp cheddar cheese
  93 calories
- ½ cup fat-free milk
  43 calories

WEEK 4, DAY 5, TOTAL: 1,402 CALORIES

day 6

BREAKFAST:

- 1½ cups Cheerios
  167 calories
- with ½ cup fat-free milk
  43 calories
- ½ medium banana
  50 calories
- ½ cup orange juice
  55 calories
- Coffee (with sugar substitute and liquid nondairy creamer if desired)
  free food

BREAKFAST TOTAL: 315 CALORIES

LUNCH:

- 1⅓ cup Chicken Caesar Pasta Toss (p. 188)
  363 calories
- 1 whole wheat dinner roll
  76 calories
- with 1 teaspoon reduced-fat margarine spread
  free food
- ½ cup fat-free milk
  43 calories

LUNCH TOTAL: 482 CALORIES

DINNER & DESSERT:

- 1 serving Grilled Pork Tenderloin (p. 238)
  171 calories
- 1 serving Coconut-Pecan Sweet Potatoes (p. 463)
  211 calories
- Steamed green beans
  free food
- 1 cup cubed watermelon
  40 calories
- 1 piece Lemon Fluff Dessert (p. 413)
  135 Calories

DINNER TOTAL: 557 CALORIES

SNACKS:

- Baby carrots and celery sticks with 1 tablespoon reduced-fat ranch salad dressing
  free food
- 1 cup prepared sugar-free gelatin
  8 calories
- 9 tiny twist fat-free pretzels with 1 tablespoon honey mustard
  50 calories

WEEK 4, DAY 6, TOTAL: 1,412 CALORIES

day 7

BREAKFAST:

- 1½ cups Wheaties
  161 calories
- with 1 cup fat-free milk
  86 calories
- ½ cup blueberries
  41 calories
- ½ cup sliced fresh strawberries
  27 calories
- Coffee (with sugar substitute and liquid nondairy creamer if desired)
  free food

BREAKFAST TOTAL: 315 CALORIES

LUNCH:

- 1 Super Flatbread Wrap (p. 182)
  348 calories
- Red and green pepper strips with 1 tablespoon reduced-fat ranch sald dressing
  free food
- 1 cup fat-free milk
  86 calories

LUNCH TOTAL: 434 CALORIES

DINNER & DESSERT:

- 1 serving Crunchy Onion Barbecue Chicken (p. 277)
  286 calories
- 1 small baked russet potato
  138 calories
- 1 big green salad (see Free Foods List on p. 41) with 1 tablespoon reduced-fat salad dressing
  free food
- Ice water
  free food
- 1 serving Sangria Gelatin Dessert (p. 405)
  95 calories
- Hot tea (with sugar substitute if desired)
  free food

DINNER TOTAL: 519 CALORIES

SNACKS:

- ⅓ cup Strawberry-Raspberry Ice (p. 423)
  79 calories
- 7 miniature caramel-flavored rice cakes
  60 calories

WEEK 4, DAY 7, TOTAL: 1,407 CALORIES

day 1

BREAKFAST:

- 1 piece Crustless Spinach Quiche (p. 110)
197 calories
¾ cup tomato juice
31 calories
- ⅔ cup red grapes
86 calories
- Ice water
free food

BREAKFAST TOTAL: 314 CALORIES

LUNCH:

- 1 California Pizza (p. 148)
245 calories
- 1 serving Basil Cherry Tomatoes (p. 347)
42 calories
- ¾ cup minestrone soup
90 calories
- 1 cup fresh raspberries
60 calories
- 1 big green salad (see Free Food List on p. 41)
with 1 tablespoon reduced-fat salad dressing
free food
- Diet soft drink
free food

LUNCH TOTAL: 437 CALORIES

DINNER & DESSERT:

- 1 cup Jambalaya (p. 469)
228 calories
- 1 cup Garlic Oregano Zucchini (p. 362)
90 calories
- 1 big green salad (see Free Food List on p. 53)
with 1 tablespoon reduced-fat salad dressing
free food
- Carbonated water
free food
- ¾ cup Makeover Toffee Crunch Dessert (p. 435)
177 calories

DINNER TOTAL: 495 CALORIES

SNACKS:

- 1 Cordon Bleu Appetizer (p. 65)
86 calories
- ½ frozen waffle with 1 tablespoon sugar-free syrup
58 calories

WEEK 5, DAY 1, TOTAL: 1,390 CALORIES

day 2

BREAKFAST:

- 2 Blueberry Oat Pancakes (p. 125)
221 calories
- with 2 tablespoons sugar-free syrup
free food
- 1 medium banana
100 calories
- Coffee (with sugar substitute and 1 tablespoon liquid nondairy creamer if desired)
free food

BREAKFAST TOTAL: 321 CALORIES

LUNCH:

- 1 sandwich Simon's Famous Tuna Salad (p. 161)
271 calories
- 1 serving Grapefruit Orange Medley (p. 103)
140 calories
- Baby carrots
free food
- Iced tea (with sugar substitute if desired)
free food

LUNCH TOTAL: 411 CALORIES

DINNER & DESSERT:

- 1 Sizzling Beef Kabob (p. 218)
227 calories
- ¾ cup Steamed Kale (p. 360)
61 calories
- 1 whole wheat dinner roll
76 calories
- Mineral water
free food
- 1 Tortilla Dessert Cup (p. 426)
130 calories
- Hot tea (with sugar substitute if desired)
free food

DINNER TOTAL: 494 CALORIES

SNACKS:

- 7 miniature caramel-flavored rice cakes
60 calories
- ½ medium apple with ½ ounce sharp cheddar cheese
93 calories

WEEK 5, DAY 2, TOTAL: 1,379 CALORIES

day 3

BREAKFAST:

- 1 serving Too-Yummy-To-Share Scramble (p. 104)
  136 calories
- 1 Turkey Breakfast Sausage Patty (p. 93)
  85 calories
- 1 cup orange juice
  110 calories

BREAKFAST TOTAL: 331 CALORIES

LUNCH:

- 1 Roasted Red Pepper Sandwich (p.160)
  404 calories
- ½ cup sliced fresh strawberries
  27 calories
- Ice water
  free food

LUNCH TOTAL: 431 CALORIES

DINNER & DESSERT:

- 1 serving Tilapia & Lemon Sauce (p. 302)
  334 calories
- ¾ cup Savory Brussels Sprouts (p. 364)
  76 calories
- 1 big green salad (see Free Food List on p. 41) with 1 tablespoon reduced-fat salad dressing
  free food
- Diet soft drink
  free food
- 1 cup Strawberry Banana Delight (p. 405)
  78 calories
- Coffee (with sugar substitute and 1 tablespoon liquid nondairy creamer if desired)
  free food

DINNER TOTAL: 488 CALORIES

SNACKS:

- 2 Jalapenos with Olive-Cream Filling (p. 75)
  58 calories
- ½ small pear, sliced with 1 tablespoon caramel ice cream topping
  92 calories

WEEK 5, DAY 3, TOTAL: 1,400 CALORIES

day 4

BREAKFAST:

- 2 Nutmeg Waffles (p. 99)
  196 calories
- 1 large scrambled egg
  101 calories
- 1 small orange
  45 calories
- Coffee (with sugar substitute and 1 tablespoon liquid nondairy creamer if desired)
  free food

BREAKFAST TOTAL: 342 CALORIES

LUNCH:

- 1 California Chicken Wrap (p. 167)
  300 calories
- ½ cup sliced strawberries with 2 tablespoons reduced-fat frozen whipped topping
  47 calories
- ½ cup fat-free vanilla frozen yogurt
  95 calories
- 1 glass club soda
  free food

LUNCH TOTAL: 442 CALORIES

DINNER & DESSERT:

- 1 cup Skillet Tacos (p. 305)
  267 calories
- ¾ cup Corn and Broccoli in Cheese Sauce (p. 449)
  148 calories
- Iced tea (with sugar substitute if desired)
  free food
- 1 serving Lemon Pudding Cup (p. 406)
  84 calories
- Hot tea (with sugar substitute if desired)
  free food

DINNER TOTAL: 499 CALORIES

SNACKS:

- 1 piece Chunky Fruit and Nut Fudge (p. 407)
  92 calories
- 2 pineapple rings
  41 calories

WEEK 5, DAY 4, TOTAL: 1,416 CALORIES

day 5

BREAKFAST:

- ½ cup Raisin Oatmeal Mix (p. 104)
  186 calories
- 1 slice whole wheat toast
  69 calories
- with 1 teaspoon reduced-fat margarine spread
  free food
- ½ small banana with 2 teaspoons reduced-fat creamy peanut butter
  99 calories
- Ice water
  free food

  BREAKFAST TOTAL: **354 CALORIES**

LUNCH:

- 1 Slow-Cooked Pork Taco (p. 446)
  301 calories
- ½ cup cooked long-grain white rice
  103 calories
- 1 cup cubed watermelon
  40 calories
- Steamed fresh or frozen green beans topped with 1 teaspoon reduced-fat margarine spread
  free food
- Sugar-free flavored water
  free food

  LUNCH TOTAL: **444 CALORIES**

DINNER & DESSERT:

- 1 serving Chipotle-Rubbed Beef Tenderloin (p. 225)
  195 calories
- ¾ cup Corn 'n' Red Pepper Medley (p. 382)
  130 calories
- 1 whole wheat dinner roll
  76 calories
- Ice water
  free food
- 1 piece Chunky Fruit and Nut Fudge (p. 401)
  92 calories
- Hot tea (with sugar substitute if desired)
  free food

  DINNER TOTAL: **493 CALORIES**

SNACKS:

- 3 Caprese Tomato Bites (p. 72)
  63 calories
- 2 chocolate kisses
  49 calories

WEEK 5, DAY 5, TOTAL: 1,403 CALORIES

day 6

BREAKFAST:

- 1 piece Harvest Vegetable Tart (p. 131)
  256 calories
- ½ cup strawberry-flavored 1% milk
  75 calories
- Ice water
  free food

  BREAKFAST TOTAL: **331 CALORIES**

LUNCH:

- 1 serving Honey-Dijon Chicken Salad (p. 171)
  301 calories
- ⅔ cups Spiced Glazed Carrots (p. 350)
  83 calories
- ½ cup fat-free milk
  43 calories

  LUNCH TOTAL: **427 CALORIES**

DINNER & DESSERT:

- 1 serving Pot Roast with Vegetables (p. 315)
  417 calories
- Ice water
  free food
- 1 Trail Mix Cluster (p. 82)
  79 calories
- Hot tea (with sugar substitute if desired)
  free food

  DINNER TOTAL: **496 CALORIES**

SNACKS:

- 1 Icy Fruit Pop (p. 69)
  66 calories
- 1 clementine
  35 calories
- 2 tablespoons tuna with 3 wheat crackers
  50 calories

WEEK 5, DAY 6, TOTAL: 1,405 CALORIES

day 7

BREAKFAST:

- 1 Mini Ham 'n' Cheese Frittata (p. 113)
106 calories
- 1 cup Sunrise Slushy (p. 95)
73 calories
- 1 slice cinnamon-raisin toast with 1 teaspoon honey
91 calories
- 1 cup cubed fresh pineapple
74 calories
- Coffee (with sugar substitute and 1 tablespoon liquid nondairy creamer if desired)
free food

BREAKFAST TOTAL: 344 CALORIES

LUNCH:

- 2 Open-Faced Veggie Sandwiches (p. 144)
249 calories
- 10 baked potato chips
100 calories
- 1 medium banana
100 calories
- 1 dill pickle spear
free food
- Ice water
free food

LUNCH TOTAL: 449 CALORIES

DINNER & DESSERT:

- 1 serving Tender Chicken Nuggets (p. 224)
194 calories
- ¾ cup Broccoli with Lemon Sauce (p. 350)
76 calories
- 1 big green salad (see the Free Food List on p. 41) with 1 tablespoon reduced-fat salad dressing
free food
- 1 piece Hot Berries 'n' Brownie Ice Cream Cake (p. 433)
233 calories
- Coffee (with sugar substitute and 1 tablespoon liquid nondairy creamer if desired)
free food

DINNER TOTAL: 503 CALORIES

SNACKS:

- 1 ounce deli turkey breast with 3 slices snack rye bread
84 calories
- 1 cup cubed watermelon
40 calories

WEEK 5, DAY 7, TOTAL: 1,420 CALORIES

day 1

BREAKFAST:

- 2 Ham and Apricot Crepes (p. 137)
258 calories
- 1 small orange
45 calories
- ½ cup fat-free milk
43 calories
- Coffee (with sugar substitute and 1 tablespoon liquid nondairy creamer if desired)
free food

BREAKFAST TOTAL: 346 CALORIES

LUNCH:

- 1 serving Vegetable Soup with Dumplings (p.178)
258 calories
- 1 medium banana
100 calories
- 1 cup fat-free milk
86 calories

LUNCH TOTAL: 444 CALORIES

DINNER & DESSERT:

- 1 serving German-Style Short Ribs (p. 450)
302 calories
- served with ⅔ cup prepared egg noodles
147 calories
- 1 big green salad (see Free Foods List on p. 41) with 1 tablespoon reduced-fat salad dressing
free food
- 1 Banana-Chip Mini Cupcake (p. 400)
65 calories
- Iced tea (with sugar substitute if desired)
free food

DINNER TOTAL: 514 CALORIES

SNACKS:

- 9 tiny twist fat-free pretzels
50 calories
- with 1 tablespoon honey mustard for dipping
free food
- 1 medium peach or plum
40 calories

WEEK 6, DAY 1, TOTAL: 1,394 CALORIES

day 2

BREAKFAST:

- 1 cup prepared Spiced Oatmeal Mix (p. 139)
  210 calories
- ½ a small grapefruit with 1 teaspoon sugar
  48 calories
- 1 slice whole wheat toast
  69 calories
- with 1 tablespoon no-sugar-added jam
  free food
- Hot tea (with sugar substitute if desired)
  free food

BREAKFAST TOTAL: 327 CALORIES

LUNCH:

- 1 Ranch Chicken Salad Sandwich (p. 172)
  257 calories
- 1 serving Grape Tomato Mozzarella Salad
  (p. 358)
  85 calories
- ½ cup cubed fresh pineapple
  37 calories
- Sugar-free flavored water
  free food

LUNCH TOTAL: 379 CALORIES

DINNER & DESSERT:

- 1¼ cups Mushroom Pepper Steak (p. 240)
  241 calories
- ½ cup prepared long-grain white rice
  103 calories
- 1 big green salad (see Free Foods List on p. 41)
  with 1 tablespoon reduced-fat salad dressing
  free food
- 1 cup fat-free milk
  86 calories
- 1 Mother Lode Pretzel (p. 426)
  114 calories

DINNER TOTAL: 544 CALORIES

SNACKS:

- 1 slice Sangria Gelatin Ring (p. 409)
  80 calories
- 1 mini bagel with 1 tablespoon reduced-fat
  chive and onion cream cheese
  63 calories

WEEK 6, DAY 2, TOTAL: 1,393 CALORIES

day 3

BREAKFAST:

- 1 Sage Breakfast Patty (p. 95)
  78 calories
- 1 large scrambled egg
  101 calories
- 1 slice whole wheat toast
  69 calories
- with 1 teaspoon reduced-fat margarine spread
  free food
- 1 cup orange juice
  110 calories

BREAKFAST TOTAL: 358 CALORIES

LUNCH:

- 1½ cups Ham 'n' Chickpea Soup (p. 174)
  312 calories
- 1 piece string cheese
  80 calories
- ⅓ cup red grapes
  43 calories
- Ice water
  free food

LUNCH TOTAL: 435 CALORIES

DINNER & DESSERT:

- 1½ cups Chicken Rice Dish (p. 290)
  247 calories
- 1 big green salad (see Free Foods List on p. 41)
  with 1 tablespoon reduced-fat salad dressing
  free food
- 1 cup fat-free milk
  86 calories
- 2 Chocolate Gingersnaps (p. 409)
  138 calories
- Hot tea (with sugar substitute if desired)
  free food

DINNER TOTAL: 471 CALORIES

SNACKS:

- ½ cup cubed fresh pineapple
  37 calories
- 1 cup prepared sugar-free gelatin
  8 calories
- with 2 tablespoons fat-free frozen
  whipped topping
  free food
- 3 chocolate kisses
  75 calories

WEEK 6, DAY 3, TOTAL: 1,384 CALORIES

day 4

BREAKFAST:

- 1 serving Cheese Tomato Egg Bake (p. 102)
110 calories
- 1 mini bagel (2½ inch diameter)
72 calories
- with 1 tablespoons whipped cream cheese
35 calories
- 1 cup cubed fresh pineapple
74 calories
- 1 cup fat-free milk
86 calories

BREAKFAST TOTAL: 377 CALORIES

LUNCH:

- 1½ cups Shrimp Pasta Salad (p. 195)
391 calories
- Baby carrots
free food
- 1 medium plum
40 calories
- Sugar-free flavored water
free food

LUNCH TOTAL: 431 CALORIES

DINNER & DESSERT:

- 1 serving Rosemary Turkey Breast (p. 212)
148 calories
- Steamed fresh or frozen green beans topped with 1 teaspoon reduced-fat margarine spread
free food
- ⅔ cup Cranberry Cornmeal Dressing (p. 288)
205 calories
- Iced tea (with sugar substitute if desired)
free food
- 1 slice Sangria Gelatin Ring (p. 409)
80 calories
- Coffee (with sugar substitute and 1 tablespoon liquid nondairy creamer if desired)
free food

DINNER TOTAL: 433 CALORIES

SNACKS:

- 1 piece string cheese
80 calories
- ¾ cup fresh blueberries
63 calories

WEEK 6, DAY 4, TOTAL: 1,384 CALORIES

day 5

BREAKFAST:

- 2 cups Strawberry Tofu Smoothie (p. 111)
272 calories
- 1 slice whole wheat toast
69 calories
- with 1 teaspoon reduced-fat margarine spread
free food

BREAKFAST TOTAL: 341 CALORIES

LUNCH:

- 1 Veggie Cheese Sandwich (p. 147)
168 calories
- 1⅓ cups Broccoli Chowder (p. 154)
233 calories
- Diet soft drink
free food

LUNCH TOTAL: 401 CALORIES

DINNER & DESSERT:

- 1 cup Mushroom Turkey Tetrazzini (p. 338)
362 calories
- Steamed fresh or frozen pea pods topped with 1 teaspoon reduced-fat margarine spread
free food
- 1 big green salad (see Free Foods List on p. 41) with 1 tablespoon reduced-fat salad dressing
free food
- 1 cup fat-free milk
86 calories
- 1 Mother Lode Pretzel (p. 426)
114 calories

DINNER TOTAL: 562 CALORIES

SNACKS:

- 1 medium peach or plum
40 calories
- 9 tiny twist fat-free pretzels
50 calories

WEEK 6, DAY 5, TOTAL: 1,394 CALORIES

day 6

BREAKFAST:

- 1 wedge Fajita Frittata (p. 117)
  137 calories
- served with ¼ cup salsa
  free food
- 1 cup Mint Berry Blast (p. 95)
  65 calories
- 2 slices whole wheat toast
  138 calories
- with 1 tablespoon no-sugar-added jam
  free food
- Hot tea (with sugar substitute if desired)
  free food

BREAKFAST TOTAL: 340 CALORIES

LUNCH:

- 1 Tangy Tuna Bunwich (p.169)
  336 calories
- Baby carrots
  free food
- ¾ cup fresh blueberries
  63 calories
- 1 dill pickle spear
  free food
- Ice water
  free food

LUNCH TOTAL: 399 CALORIES

DINNER & DESSERT:

- 1 Corny Chicken Wrap (p. 340)
  363 calories
- 1 big green salad (see Free Foods List on p. 41)
  with 1 tablespoon reduced-fat salad dressing
  free food
- 2 sesame breadsticks (5g each)
  40 calories
- 1 cup fat-free milk
  86 calories
- 1 Chocolate Gingersnap (p. 409)
  69 calories
- Hot tea (with sugar substitute if desired)
  free food

DINNER TOTAL: 558 CALORIES

SNACKS

- 1 medium apple
  72 calories
- 1½ cups air-popped popcorn
  47 calories

WEEK 6, DAY 6, TOTAL: 1,416 CALORIES

day 7

BREAKFAST:

- ¼ cup Paradise Granola (p. 122)
  132 calories
- sprinkled onto 6 ounces nonfat fruit yogurt
  160 calories
- ½ cup orange juice
  55 calories
- Coffee (with sugar substitute and
  1 tablespoon liquid nondairy creamer
  if desired)
  free food

BREAKFAST TOTAL: 347 CALORIES

LUNCH:

- 1¾ cups Chicken Spaghetti Salad (p. 172)
  329 calories
- ⅓ cup red grapes
  43 calories
- Iced tea (with sugar substitute if desired)
  free food

LUNCH TOTAL: 372 CALORIES

DINNER & DESSERT:

- 1 Braised Pork Chop (p. 241)
  180 calories
- ⅔ cup Spanish Rice (p. 371)
  156 calories
- Steamed fresh or frozen green beans topped
  with 1 teaspoon reduced-fat margarine spread
  free food
- 1 big green salad (see Free Foods List on p. 41)
  with 1 tablespoon reduced-fat salad dressing
  free food
- 1 cup fat-free milk
  86 calories
- 1 Dark Chocolate Butterscotch Brownie (p. 425)
  110 calories

DINNER TOTAL: 532 CALORIES

SNACKS:

- 1 cup fresh raspberries
  60 calories
- 3 pieces snack rye bread topped with 1 tablespoon
  reduced-fat garden vegetable cream cheese and
  6 cucumber slices
  89 calories

WEEK 6, DAY 7, TOTAL: 1,400 CALORIES

Snacks

It's easy to **avoid cravings** when you indulge in a snack between meals. If you're a woman, enjoy **100 calories worth of snacks per day**. Men should eat snacks totaling **no more than 200 calories**.

CONTENTS

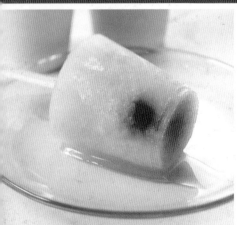

ICY FRUIT POPS
PAGE 69

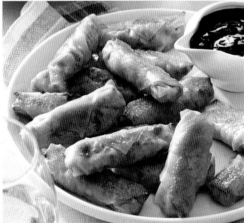

CRISPY BAKED WONTONS
PAGE 71

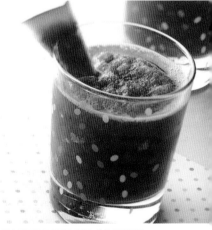

WATERMELON COOLER
PAGE 75

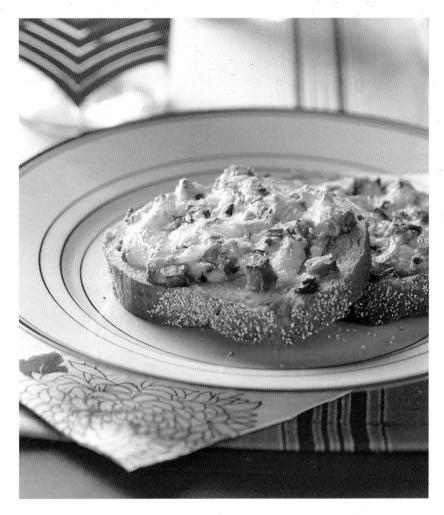

80 CALORIES Apple Skewers

We enjoy these flavorful grilled apples with a lightly spiced coating all year. Best of all, they're a cinch to grill, and cleanup is a breeze.
—**DORIS SOWERS** HUTCHINSON, KS

START TO FINISH: 30 MIN.
MAKES: 4 SERVINGS

- 4 **medium apples, peeled and quartered**
- 4 **teaspoons sugar**
- 1¼ **teaspoons ground cinnamon**

1. Thread apples on four metal or soaked wooden skewers. Lightly spray with cooking spray. Combine sugar and cinnamon; sprinkle over apples.

2. Moisten a paper towel with cooking oil; using long-handled tongs, lightly coat the grill rack. Grill, covered, over medium heat for 6-8 minutes or until golden. Turn; cook 8-10 minutes longer or until golden and tender. Serve warm.

PER SERVING *1 skewer equals 80 cal., trace fat (trace sat. fat), 0 chol., trace sodium, 21 g carb., 2 g fiber, trace pro.* **Diabetic Exchange:** *1 fruit.*

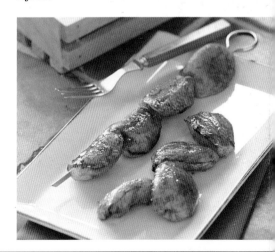

86 CALORIES
Cordon Bleu Appetizers

Looking for a cheesy snack with mass appeal? Adults and kids alike love these satisfying appetizers!
—**SUSAN MELLO** JACKSON HEIGHTS, NY

START TO FINISH: 30 MIN.
MAKES: 1½ DOZEN

- 4 **ounces cream cheese, softened**
- 1 **teaspoon Dijon mustard**
- 1 **cup (4 ounces) shredded Swiss cheese**
- ¾ **cup diced fully cooked ham**
- ½ **cup minced chives, divided**
- 18 **slices French bread (½ inch thick)**

1. In a small bowl, beat cream cheese and mustard until smooth. Stir in the Swiss cheese, ham and ¼ cup chives. Spread 1 tablespoon mixture over each bread slice; place on an ungreased baking sheet.

2. Bake at 350° for 12-15 minutes or until lightly browned. Sprinkle with remaining chives.

PER SERVING *1 appetizer equals 86 cal., 5 g fat (3 g sat. fat), 16 mg chol., 185 mg sodium, 7 g carb., trace fiber, 4 g pro.* **Diabetic Exchanges:** *1 fat, ½ starch.*

44 CALORIES

Tex-Mex Popcorn

Spicy Southwest seasoning makes my snackin' good popcorn ideal for any fiesta.
—**KATIE ROSE** PEWAUKEE, WI

START TO FINISH: 15 MIN.
MAKES: 4 QUARTS

- ½ **cup popcorn kernels**
- 3 **tablespoons canola oil**
- ½ **teaspoon cumin seeds**
  Refrigerated butter-flavored spray
- ¼ **cup minced fresh cilantro**
- 1 **teaspoon salt**
- 1 **teaspoon chili powder**
- ½ **teaspoon garlic powder**
- ⅛ **teaspoon smoked paprika**

1. In a Dutch oven over medium heat, cook the popcorn kernels, oil and cumin seeds until oil begins to sizzle. Cover and shake for 2-3 minutes or until popcorn stops popping.

2. Transfer to a large bowl; spritz with butter-flavored spray. Add remaining ingredients and toss to coat. Continue spritzing and tossing until popcorn is coated.

PER SERVING *1 cup equals 44 cal., 3 g fat (trace sat. fat), 0 chol., 150 mg sodium, 5 g carb., 1 g fiber, 1 g pro.*

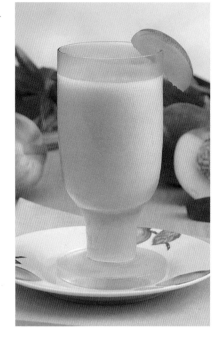

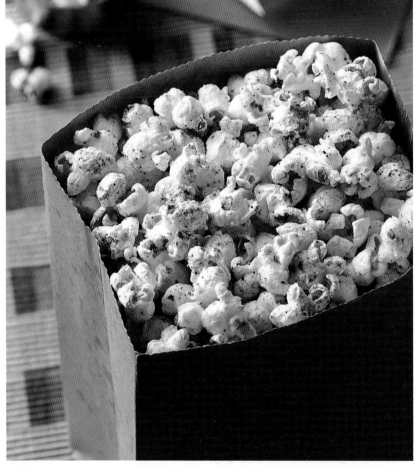

68 CALORIES

Peach Smoothie

Whip up this creamy treat as a refreshing and nutritious snack or a quick chilled breakfast. Because you can use frozen fruit, you don't have to wait until peaches are in season to enjoy the delicious drink.
—**MARTHA POLASEK** MARKHAM, TX

START TO FINISH: 5 MIN.
MAKES: 2 SERVINGS

- ½ **cup peach or apricot nectar**
- ½ **cup sliced fresh or frozen peaches**
- ¼ **cup fat-free vanilla yogurt**
- 2 **ice cubes**

In a blender, combine all the ingredients. Cover and process until blended. Pour into chilled glasses; serve immediately.

PER SERVING *¾ cup equals 68 cal., trace fat (trace sat. fat), 1 mg chol., 4 mg sodium, 16 g carb., 1 g fiber, 2 g pro.* **Diabetic Exchange:** *1 starch.*

Garlic Pumpkin Seeds

What to do with all those pumpkin seeds from your pumpkin-carving party? This microwave-easy recipe will have folks eating 'em up by crunchy handfuls! Save a few for yourself before they're gone.

—IOLA EGLE BELLA VISTA, AR

START TO FINISH: 25 MIN.
MAKES: 2 CUPS

- 1 **tablespoon canola oil**
- ½ **teaspoon celery salt**
- ½ **teaspoon garlic powder**
- ½ **teaspoon seasoned salt**
- 2 **cups fresh pumpkin seeds**

1. In a small bowl, combine the oil, celery salt, garlic powder and seasoned salt. Add pumpkin seeds; toss to coat. Spread a quarter of the seeds in a single layer on a microwave-safe plate.

2. Microwave, uncovered, on high for 1 minute; stir. Microwave for 2-3 minutes longer or until seeds are crunchy and lightly browned, stirring after each minute.

3. Repeat with remaining pumpkin seeds. Serve warm, or cool before storing in an airtight container.

NOTE *This recipe was tested in a 1,100-watt microwave.*

PER SERVING *¼ cup equals 87 cal., 5 g fat (1 g sat. fat), 0 chol., 191 mg sodium, 9 g carb., 1 g fiber, 3 g pro.* **Diabetic Exchanges:** *1 fat, ½ starch.*

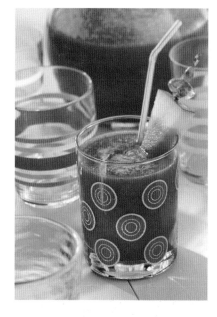

Strawberry
Watermelon Slush

We like to relax on the back porch after a long hot day with glasses of my slush. What could be more refreshing in the heat of summer?

—PATTY HOWSE GREAT FALLS, MT

START TO FINISH: 10 MIN.
MAKES: 5 CUPS

- 2 **cups cubed seedless watermelon**
- 1 **pint fresh strawberries, halved**
- ⅓ **cup sugar**
- ⅓ **cup lemon juice**
- 2 **cups ice cubes**

In a blender, combine the watermelon, strawberries, sugar and lemon juice; cover and process on high until smooth. While processing, gradually add the ice cubes and process until slushy. Pour into chilled glasses and serve immediately.

PER SERVING *1 cup equals 89 cal., trace fat (trace sat. fat), 0 chol., 3 mg sodium, 24 g carb., 2 g fiber, 1 g pro.*

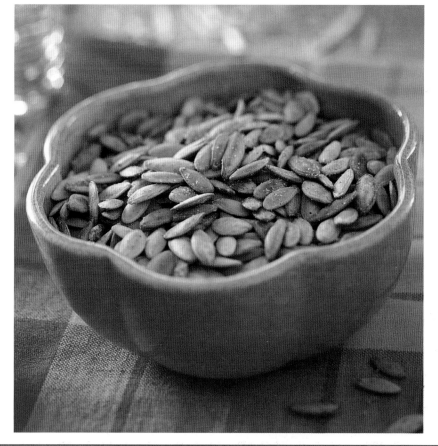

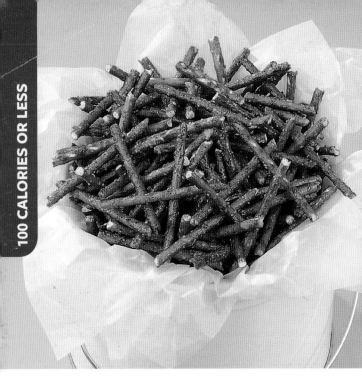

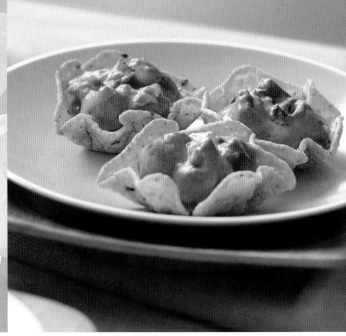

98 CALORIES

Spiced Honey Pretzels

If your tastes run to sweet and spicy, you'll love these zesty pretzels with a twist. The coating is so yummy, you won't need a fattening dip to enjoy them!

—MARY LOU MOON BEAVERTON, OR

START TO FINISH: 15 MIN.
MAKES: 8 SERVINGS

- 4 **cups thin pretzel sticks**
- 3 **tablespoons honey**
- 2 **teaspoons butter, melted**
- 1 **teaspoon onion powder**
- 1 **teaspoon chili powder**

1. Line a 15-in. x 10-in. x 1-in. baking pan with foil; coat the foil with cooking spray. Place pretzels in a large bowl.

2. In a small bowl, combine the honey, butter, onion powder and chili powder. Pour over pretzels; toss to coat evenly. Spread into prepared pan.

3. Bake at 350° for 8 minutes, stirring once. Cool on a wire rack, stirring gently several times to separate.

PER SERVING *½ cup equals 98 cal., 1 g fat (1 g sat. fat), 3 mg chol., 487 mg sodium, 20 g carb., 1 g fiber, 2 g pro.* **Diabetic Exchange:** *1½ starch.*

66 CALORIES

Chili con Queso Dip

Chilies and garlic kick up the flavor of my dip, making it a real crowd-pleaser. You'd never guess it's low in fat.

—SARAH MOHRMAN FORT WAYNE, IN

START TO FINISH: 25 MIN. • **MAKES:** 3 CUPS

- 1 **can (14½ ounces) no-salt-added diced tomatoes**
- 1 **can (10 ounces) diced tomatoes and green chilies**
- 1 **small onion, chopped**
- 1 **teaspoon olive oil**
- 2 **garlic cloves, minced**
- 1 **package (8 ounces) fat-free cream cheese, cubed**
- 6 **ounces reduced-fat process cheese (Velveeta), cubed**
- 1 **teaspoon chili powder**
- 2 **tablespoons minced fresh cilantro**
  Baked tortilla chip scoops

1. Pour both cans of tomatoes into a colander over a bowl; drain, reserving ⅓ cup liquid. Discard remaining liquid or save it for another use.

2. In a large skillet, saute onion in oil until tender. Add garlic; cook 1 minute longer. Stir in cream cheese until melted. Add tomatoes, process cheese, chili powder and reserved liquid. Cook and stir over low heat until cheese is melted. Stir in cilantro. Serve warm with chips.

PER SERVING *¼ cup (calculated without chips) equals 66 cal., 2 g fat (1 g sat. fat), 7 mg chol., 411 mg sodium, 6 g carb., 1 g fiber, 6 g pro.* **Diabetic Exchanges:** *½ starch, ½ fat.*

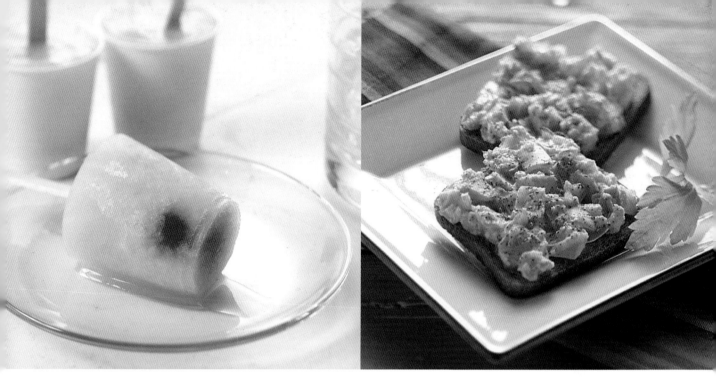

Icy Fruit Pops

My grandmother made these pineapple treats for my brother and me when we were little. Today, the pops remain a cool and refreshing snack that delights kids of all ages.

—LEANN KANE FORSYTH, IL

PREP: 20 MIN. + FREEZING
MAKES: 2 DOZEN

- 1 can (20 ounces) crushed pineapple, undrained
- 1 cup water
- ¾ cup thawed orange juice concentrate
- ¾ cup thawed lemonade concentrate
  Sugar substitute equivalent to ½ cup sugar
- 5 medium firm bananas, cut into ¼-inch slices and quartered
- 1 can (12 ounces) diet ginger ale
- 24 maraschino cherries or fresh strawberries
- 24 wooden pop sticks

1. In a large bowl, combine the pineapple, water, orange juice concentrate, lemonade concentrate and sugar substitute. Stir in the bananas and ginger ale.

2. Place a cherry in each of twenty-four 3-oz. paper cups; fill with pineapple mixture. Insert wooden pop sticks. Cover and freeze until firm.

NOTE *This recipe was tested with Splenda no-calorie sweetener.*

PER SERVING *1 pop equals 66 cal., trace fat (trace sat. fat), 0 chol., 5 mg sodium, 17 g carb., 1 g fiber, 1 g pro.* **Diabetic Exchange:** *1 fruit.*

Artichoke Rye Toasts

Quick, light and cheesy, these tasty artichoke bites make irresistible finger food for guests and partygoers.

—JO ANN GUZOLIK
WEST LEECHBURG, PA

PREP: 30 MIN. • **BAKE:** 10 MIN.
MAKES: 2 DOZEN

- 24 slices snack rye bread
  Refrigerated butter-flavored spray
- 1 can (14 ounces) water-packed artichoke hearts, rinsed, drained and chopped
- ½ cup grated Parmesan cheese
- ¼ cup shredded cheddar cheese
- ⅛ teaspoon cayenne pepper
- 4 egg whites
- ¼ teaspoon paprika

1. Place the bread on ungreased baking sheets; spritz with butter-flavored spray. In a small bowl, combine the artichokes, cheeses and cayenne. In another bowl, beat egg whites until stiff; fold into artichoke mixture.

2. Spread over bread; sprinkle with paprika. Bake at 400° for 10-12 minutes or until golden brown. Serve warm. Refrigerate leftovers.

PER SERVING *2 slices equals 78 cal., 2 g fat (1 g sat. fat), 5 mg chol., 270 mg sodium, 9 g carb., 1 g fiber, 5 g pro.*

❝I have the Comfort Food Diet Cookbook and use a lot of the recipes. I've started to lose weight even in the first few weeks. I'm doing it the healthy way so it will stay off. No rebounding for me!❞

—RUTH WOODMAN YORK

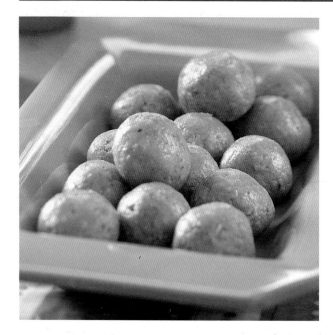

70 CALORIES

No-Bake Peanut Butter Treats

My quick and tasty dessert is perfect for a road trip. The treats won't stick to your hands. Keep them in the refrigerator for an easy snack anytime.

—**SONIA ROHDA** WAVERLY, NE

START TO FINISH: 10 MIN. • **MAKES:** 15 TREATS

- ⅓ **cup chunky peanut butter**
- ¼ **cup honey**
- ½ **teaspoon vanilla extract**
- ⅓ **cup nonfat dry milk powder**
- ⅓ **cup quick-cooking oats**
- 2 **tablespoons graham cracker crumbs**

In a small bowl, combine the peanut butter, honey and vanilla. Stir in the milk powder, oats and graham cracker crumbs. Shape into 1-in. balls. Cover and refrigerate until serving.

PER SERVING *1 treat equals 70 cal., 3 g fat (1 g sat. fat), 1 mg chol., 46 mg sodium, 9 g carb., 1 g fiber, 3 g pro. Diabetic Exchanges: ½ starch, ½ fat.*

55 CALORIES Spiced Coffee with Cream

This recipe was a wonderful discovery! I serve it to company or whip it up as a treat for my husband and me.

—**ALPHA WILSON** ROSWELL, NM

PREP: 10 MIN. + FREEZING • **MAKES:** 2 SERVINGS

- ¼ **cup evaporated milk**
- 2¼ **teaspoons confectioners' sugar**
- ¼ **teaspoon ground cinnamon**
- ⅛ **teaspoon vanilla extract**
- 1 **cup hot strong brewed coffee**
  Ground nutmeg
- 2 **cinnamon sticks**

1. Pour milk into a small bowl; place mixer beaters in the bowl. Cover and freeze for 30 minutes or until ice crystals begin to form.

2. Add the sugar, cinnamon and vanilla; beat until thick and fluffy. Divide mixture between two mugs; add coffee. Garnish with nutmeg and cinnamon sticks. Serve immediately.

PER SERVING *1 cup equals 55 cal., 2 g fat (2 g sat. fat), 10 mg chol., 32 mg sodium, 7 g carb., trace fiber, 2 g pro.*

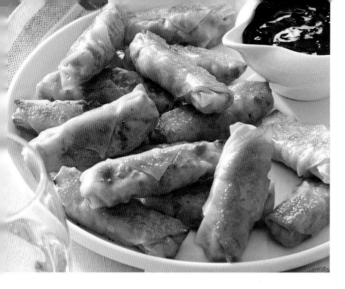

38 CALORIES Crispy Baked Wontons

Quick and versatile, these wontons are great as a snack or paired with a bowl of soothing soup on a cold day. I like to make a large batch, freeze half on a floured baking sheet, then store in an airtight container.
—**BRIANNA SHADE** BEAVERTON, OR

PREP: 30 MIN. • **BAKE:** 10 MIN. • **MAKES:** ABOUT 4 DOZEN

- ½ pound ground pork
- ½ pound extra-lean ground turkey
- 1 small onion, chopped
- 1 can (8 ounces) sliced water chestnuts, drained and chopped
- ⅓ cup reduced-sodium soy sauce
- ¼ cup egg substitute
- 1½ teaspoons ground ginger
- 1 package (12 ounces) wonton wrappers
  Cooking spray
  Sweet-and-sour sauce, optional

1. In a large skillet, cook the pork, turkey and onion over medium heat until meat is no longer pink; drain. Transfer to a large bowl. Stir in the water chestnuts, soy sauce, egg substitute and ginger.
2. Position a wonton wrapper with one point toward you. (Keep remaining wrappers covered with a damp paper towel until ready to use.) Place 2 heaping teaspoons of filling in the center of wrapper. Fold bottom corner over filling; fold sides toward center over filling. Roll toward the remaining point. Moisten top corner with water; press to seal. Repeat with remaining wrappers and filling.

3. Place on baking sheets coated with cooking spray; lightly coat wontons with additional cooking spray.
4. Bake at 400° for 10-12 minutes or until golden brown, turning once. Serve warm with sweet-and-sour sauce if desired.
PER SERVING *1 wonton (calculated without sweet-and-sour sauce) equals 38 cal., 1 g fat (trace sat. fat), 5 mg chol., 103 mg sodium, 5 g carb., trace fiber, 3 g pro.*

77 CALORIES Cajun Popcorn

Authentic Cajun popcorn is actually deep-fried crawfish tails seasoned with peppery spices. But we like this lighter, simpler version made with real popcorn. It's our favorite TV snack.
—**RUBY WILLIAMS** BOGALUSA, LA

START TO FINISH: 10 MIN. • **MAKES:** 3 QUARTS

- 1 teaspoon salt
- ½ teaspoon ground cumin
- ½ teaspoon garlic powder
- ½ teaspoon dried basil
- ½ teaspoon dried thyme
- ½ teaspoon paprika
- ¼ teaspoon pepper
- ⅛ teaspoon cayenne pepper
- 2 tablespoons canola oil
- 3 quarts popped popcorn

In a small bowl, combine the first eight ingredients; set aside. In a small saucepan, heat oil over medium heat for 1 minute; add seasonings. Cook and stir over low heat for 1 minute. Place the popcorn in a large bowl; add seasoning mixture and toss to coat.
PER SERVING *1 cup equals 77 cal., 5 g fat (1 g sat. fat), 0 chol., 294 mg sodium, 7 g carb., 1 g fiber, 1 g pro.*

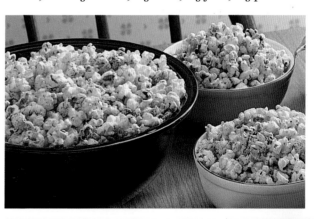

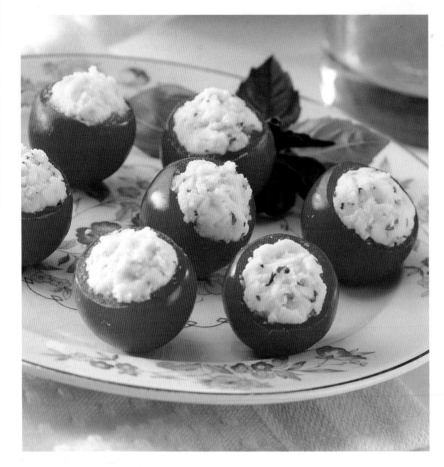

63 CALORIES

White Chocolate Pretzel Snack

I make these sweet crunchy treats often during holidays. They're nice to have on hand to serve or to take as a hostess gift. This recipe is extremely easy to make, and my children love to help.

—ESTELLE CUMMINGS CAMBRIDGE, MD

START TO FINISH: 20 MIN.
MAKES: 1 DOZEN

- ½ **cup pretzel sticks**
- ½ **cup salted peanuts**
- ½ **cup crisp rice cereal**
- 4 **ounces white baking chocolate, chopped**
- 1 **teaspoon shortening**

1. In a large bowl, combine the pretzels, peanuts and cereal. In a microwave, melt chocolate and shortening, stir until smooth.
2. Pour over pretzel mixture; toss to coat evenly. Drop by heaping tablespoonfuls onto waxed paper; allow to cool.

PER SERVING *1 piece equals 63 cal., 4 g fat (1 g sat. fat), 1 mg chol., 67 mg sodium, 5 g carb., 1 g fiber, 2 g pro.*

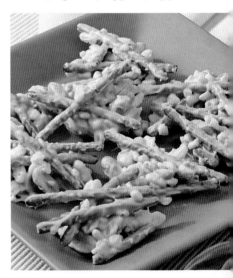

63 CALORIES

Caprese Tomato Bites

I love the classic combination of tomatoes, mozzarella and basil in these bite-size appetizers. They give you a genuine taste of summertime.

—CRYSTAL WILLIAMS BROOKLYN, NY

START TO FINISH: 30 MIN.
MAKES: ABOUT 3½ DOZEN

- 1 **pint cherry tomatoes, halved**
- 3 **tablespoons heavy whipping cream**
- ½ **pound fresh mozzarella cheese, sliced**
- 6 **fresh basil leaves**
- 1 **garlic clove, minced**
- 1 **tablespoon balsamic vinegar**

1. Scoop out and discard pulp of cherry tomatoes. Invert tomatoes onto paper towels to drain.
2. In a food processor, combine the cream, mozzarella cheese, basil and garlic; cover and process mixture until blended.
3. Cut a small hole in the corner of a pastry or heavy-duty resealable plastic bag; fill with cheese mixture.
4. Turn tomato halves over and drizzle with vinegar. Pipe cheese mixture into tomatoes. Refrigerate until serving.

PER SERVING *3 appetizers equals 63 cal., 5 g fat (3 g sat. fat), 17 mg chol., 27 mg sodium, 2 g carb., trace fiber, 3 g pro.*

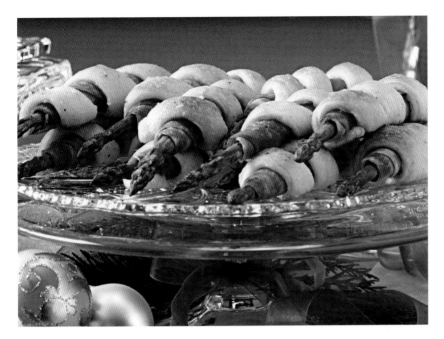

Ham Asparagus Spirals

Just three ingredients are all you need to prepare these impressive-looking hors d'oeuvres. They are a welcome addition to the table.
—**ROSIE HUFFER** WESTMINSTER, CA

PREP: 20 MIN. • **BAKE:** 15 MIN.
MAKES: 20 APPETIZERS

- 20 **fresh asparagus spears, trimmed**
- 20 **thin slices deli ham**
- 1 **package (10.6 ounces) refrigerated Italian breadsticks and garlic spread**

1. In a large skillet, bring ½ in. of water to a boil; add asparagus. Reduce heat; cover and simmer for 2 minutes. Drain and immediately place asparagus in ice water; drain and pat dry.
2. Wrap a slice of ham around each asparagus spear. Unroll breadstick dough; spread with garlic spread. Cut each breadstick in half lengthwise. Wrap one piece of dough, garlic spread side in, around each ham-wrapped asparagus spear.
3. Place on an ungreased baking sheet. Bake at 375° for 13-15 minutes or until golden brown. Serve immediately.
PER SERVING *1 spiral equals 49 cal., 2 g fat (trace sat. fat), trace chol., 154 mg sodium, 7 g carb., trace fiber, 2 g pro.*

Cheesy Pita Crisps

I first made these golden wedges when my college roommates and I wanted garlic bread but only had pitas on hand. My husband likes this skinny version even better than the original!
—**CHRISTINE MATTIKO**
DALLASTOWN, PA

START TO FINISH: 25 MIN.
MAKES: 8 SERVINGS

- 4 **whole wheat pita pocket halves**
- ¼ **cup reduced-fat margarine, melted**
- ½ **teaspoon garlic powder**
- ½ **teaspoon onion powder**
- ¼ **teaspoon salt**
- ¼ **teaspoon pepper**
- 3 **tablespoons grated Parmesan cheese**
- ½ **cup shredded part-skim mozzarella cheese**

1. Split each pita pocket in half. Cut each into two triangles; place split side up on a baking sheet coated with cooking spray.
2. In bowl, combine the margarine, garlic powder, onion powder, salt and pepper; stir in the Parmesan cheese. Spread over triangles. Sprinkle with mozzarella cheese.
3. Bake at 400° for 12-15 minutes or until golden brown.
PER SERVING *2 triangles equals 95 cal., 5 g fat (2 g sat. fat), 6 mg chol., 264 mg sodium, 9 g carb., 1 g fiber, 4 g pro.* **Diabetic Exchanges:** *1 fat, ½ starch.*

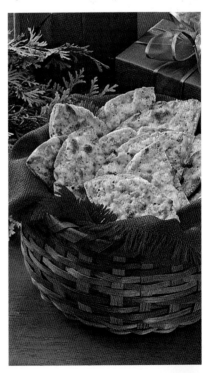

" Once a week, I had a 'splurge' meal where I could eat whatever sounded good to me. Because of my healthier habits, I found that when these meals came around, I was eating less and getting more enjoyment from my food. "

—ASHLEY LATIMER

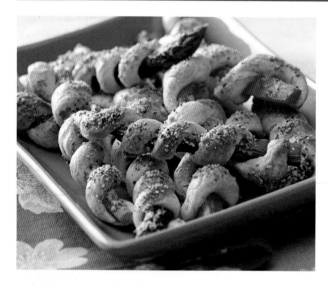

97 CALORIES Vegetable Spiral Sticks

I love to serve these savory wrapped vegetable sticks for parties or special occasions. They're a simple but impressive appetizer.

—TERI ALBRECHT MOUNT AIRY, MD

START TO FINISH: 30 MIN. • **MAKES:** 2 DOZEN

- 3 **medium carrots**
- 12 **fresh asparagus spears, trimmed**
- 1 **tube (11 ounces) refrigerated breadsticks**
- 1 **egg white, lightly beaten**
- ¼ **cup grated Parmesan cheese**
- ½ **teaspoon dried oregano**

1. Cut carrots lengthwise into quarters. In a large skillet, bring 2 in. of water to a boil. Add carrots; cook for 3 minutes. Add asparagus; cook 2-3 minutes longer. Drain and rinse with cold water; pat dry.

2. Cut each piece of breadstick dough in half. Roll each piece into a 7-in. rope. Wrap one rope in a spiral around each vegetable. Place on a baking sheet coated with cooking spray; tuck ends of dough under vegetables to secure.

3. Brush with egg white. Combine cheese and oregano; sprinkle over sticks. Bake at 375° for 12-14 minutes or until golden brown. Serve warm.

PER SERVING *2 sticks equals 97 cal., 2 g fat (trace sat. fat), 2 mg chol., 247 mg sodium, 15 g carb., 1 g fiber, 4 g pro.* **Diabetic Exchanges:** *1 starch, 1 vegetable.*

0 CALORIES Spicy Mint Tea

In the old days, mint tea was said to dispel headaches and indigestion. I don't know about that, but I do know that this tea refreshes me every time.

—IONE BANKS JEFFERSON, OR

START TO FINISH: 15 MIN. • **MAKES:** 6 SERVINGS

- 6 **cups water**
- 2 **cinnamon sticks**
- 4 **whole cloves**
- 4 **whole allspice**
- 2 **cups fresh mint leaves**
  Honey, optional

Bring the water, cinnamon, cloves and allspice to a boil. Boil for 1 minute. Stir in mint leaves. Remove from heat and steep for 5 minutes. Strain into cups. Sweeten with honey if desired.

PER SERVING *1 cup (calculated without honey) equals 0 cal., trace fat (trace sat. fat), 0 chol., 0 mg sodium, 0 g carb., 0 g fiber, 0 g pro.* **Diabetic Exchange:** *Free food.*

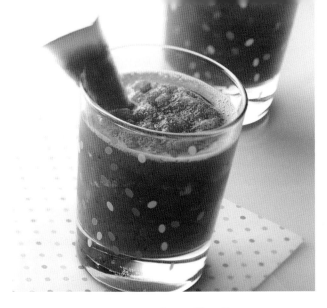

Place popcorn in a large bowl. Drizzle with butter. Combine the remaining ingredients; sprinkle over popcorn and toss to coat.

PER SERVING *1 cup equals 49 cal., 2 g fat (1 g sat. fat), 5 mg chol., 146 mg sodium, 7 g carb., 1 g fiber, 2 g pro.* **Diabetic Exchange:** *½ starch.*

58 CALORIES

Jalapenos with Olive-Cream Filling

Whenever I need something for a get-together or potluck, I take these yummy jalapenos. I get many requests for them.
—KRISTAL PETERSON WALKER, LA

START TO FINISH: 25 MIN. • **MAKES:** 32 APPETIZERS

- 1 package (8 ounces) cream cheese, softened
- ¼ cup chopped pimiento-stuffed olives
- 2 tablespoons olive juice
- 16 large jalapeno peppers, halved lengthwise and seeded

In a small bowl, combine the cream cheese, olives and olive juice. Spoon about 2 teaspoons into each jalapeno half. Serve immediately or refrigerate.

NOTE *Wear disposable gloves when cutting hot peppers; the oils can burn skin. Avoid touching your face.*
PER SERVING *2 appetizers equals 58 cal., 5 g fat (3 g sat. fat), 16 mg chol., 103 mg sodium, 1 g carb., trace fiber, 1 g pro.*

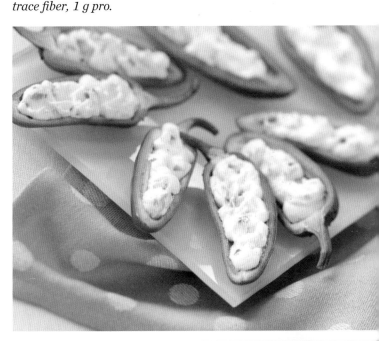

82 CALORIES # Watermelon Cooler

Cool down on a sweltering day with this special blend that features summer's favorite fruit. It's lovely and refreshing.
—TASTE OF HOME TEST KITCHEN

START TO FINISH: 10 MIN. • **MAKES:** 2 SERVINGS

- 1 cup ginger ale, chilled
- 2 fresh mint leaves
- 2 cups cubed seedless watermelon, frozen

In a blender, cover and process ginger ale and mint for 15 seconds or until finely chopped. Add watermelon; cover and process until slushy. Pour into chilled glasses; serve immediately.

PER SERVING *1 cup equals 82 cal., 0 fat (0 sat. fat), 0 chol., 14 mg sodium, 24 g carb., 1 g fiber, 1 g pro.* **Diabetic Exchanges:** *1 fruit, ½ starch.*

49 CALORIES # Parmesan Popcorn

Give popcorn a new twist with my fun and tasty recipe. It's great for watching movies or as an on-the-go snack. Kids seem to gobble it up with as much enjoyment as adults.
—BETSY KING DULUTH, MN

START TO FINISH: 10 MIN. • **MAKES:** 2 QUARTS

- 8 cups air-popped popcorn
- 2 tablespoons reduced-fat butter, melted
- 2 tablespoons grated Parmesan cheese
- ¼ teaspoon salt
- ¼ teaspoon dried oregano
- ⅛ teaspoon garlic salt

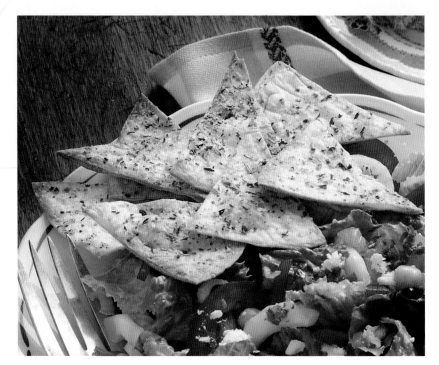

2 cups fresh pumpkin seeds
5 teaspoons butter, melted
1 teaspoon Worcestershire sauce
1 teaspoon sugar
½ teaspoon salt
¼ teaspoon garlic powder
⅛ to ¼ teaspoon cayenne pepper

1. In a bowl, toss pumpkin seeds with butter and Worcestershire sauce. Combine the sugar, salt, garlic powder and cayenne; sprinkle over seeds and toss to coat.

2. Line a 15-in. x 10-in. x 1-in. baking pan with foil; coat foil with cooking spray. Spread seeds in pan. Bake at 250° for 45-60 minutes or until seeds are dry and lightly browned, stirring every 15 minutes. Cool completely. Store in an airtight container.

PER SERVING *¼ cup equals 95 cal., 5 g fat (2 g sat. fat), 6 mg chol., 181 mg sodium, 9 g carb., 1 g fiber, 3 g pro.* **Diabetic Exchanges:** *1 fat, ½ starch.*

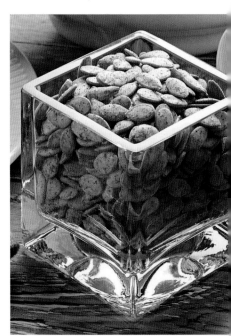

94 CALORIES
Herbed Tortilla Chips

I dreamed these up when I found several packages of tortilla shells while cleaning out my freezer. They make an inexpensive, low-calorie treat for my husband and me.

—ANGELA CASE MONTICELLO, AR

START TO FINISH: 20 MIN.
MAKES: 3 SERVINGS

2 teaspoons grated Parmesan cheese
½ teaspoon dried oregano
½ teaspoon dried parsley flakes
½ teaspoon dried rosemary, crushed
¼ teaspoon garlic powder
⅛ teaspoon kosher salt
Dash pepper
2 flour tortillas (6 inches)
2 teaspoons olive oil

1. In a small bowl, combine the first seven ingredients. Brush tortillas with oil; cut each tortilla into six wedges. Arrange in a single layer on a baking sheet coated with cooking spray.

2. Sprinkle wedges with seasoning mixture. Bake at 425° for 5-7 minutes or until golden brown. Cool for 5 minutes.

PER SERVING *4 chips equals 94 cal., 5 g fat (1 g sat. fat), 1 mg chol., 245 mg sodium, 9 g carb., trace fiber, 3 g pro.* **Diabetic Exchanges:** *1 fat, ½ starch.*

95 CALORIES
Light Roasted Pumpkin Seeds

Try this zippy twist on a Halloween tradition the next time you have an abundance of pumpkin seeds. It's got just enough heat to take the chill off autumn afternoons and snackers!

—TASTE OF HOME TEST KITCHEN

PREP: 10 MIN. • **BAKE:** 45 MIN. + COOLING
MAKES: 2 CUPS

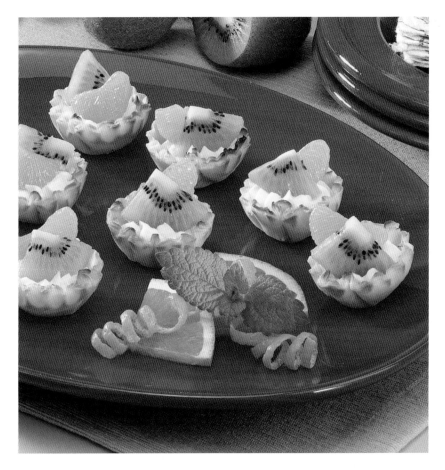

Mini Polenta Pizzas

With just four ingredients, you can be the talk of the party! These tasty bites are special enough for a fancy gathering and no one will know they're healthful.
—**LILY JULOW** GAINESVILLE, FL

START TO FINISH: 30 MIN.
MAKES: 2 DOZEN

- 2 tubes (1 pound each) polenta
- ½ cup grated Parmesan cheese
- 12 oil-packed sun-dried tomatoes, halved
- ¼ cup prepared pesto

1. Cut polenta into 24 slices; place on ungreased baking sheets. Sprinkle with half of the cheese. Top each with a tomato half and ½ teaspoon pesto; sprinkle with remaining cheese.
2. Bake at 450° for 7-10 minutes or until cheese is melted.
PER SERVING *1 mini pizza equals 57 cal., 2 g fat (1 g sat. fat), 2 mg chol., 182 mg sodium, 8 g carb., 1 g fiber, 2 g pro.* **Diabetic Exchanges:** *½ starch, ½ fat.*

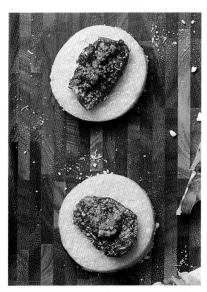

Cheesecake Phyllo Cups

I've been making these colorful and fruity cheesecake bites for years. Topped with kiwifruit and mandarin oranges, they are just delicious.
—**LORRAINE CHEVALIER** MERRIMAC, MA

START TO FINISH: 25 MIN.
MAKES: 2½ DOZEN

- 4 ounces reduced-fat cream cheese
- ½ cup reduced-fat sour cream
  Sugar substitute equivalent to 2 tablespoons sugar
- 1 teaspoon vanilla extract
- 2 packages (2.1 ounces each) frozen miniature phyllo tart shells, thawed
- 1 can (11 ounces) mandarin oranges slices, drained
- 1 kiwifruit, peeled, sliced and cut into quarters

1. In a small bowl, beat the cream cheese, sour cream, sugar substitute and vanilla until smooth.
2. Pipe or spoon filling into phyllo shells. Top each with an orange segment and kiwi piece. Refrigerate until serving.
NOTE *This recipe was tested with Splenda sugar blend.*
PER SERVING *1 phyllo cup equals 46 cal., 2 g fat (1 g sat. fat), 4 mg chol., 29 mg sodium, 5 g carb., trace fiber, 1 g pro.*

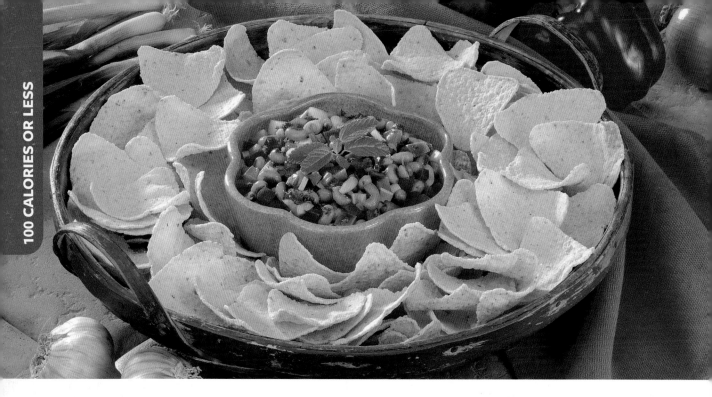

77 CALORIES Texas Caviar

My neighbor gave me a container of this zippy salsa one Christmas, and I had to have the recipe! Now I fix it regularly for get-togethers and never have leftovers.
—**KATHY FARIS** LYTLE, TX

PREP: 15 MIN. + CHILLING • **MAKES:** 4 CUPS

- 1 can (15½ ounces) black-eyed peas, rinsed and drained
- ¾ cup chopped sweet red pepper
- ¾ cup chopped green pepper
- 1 medium onion, chopped
- 3 green onions, chopped
- ¼ cup minced fresh parsley
- 1 jar (2 ounces) diced pimientos, drained
- 1 garlic clove, minced
- 1 bottle (8 ounces) fat-free Italian salad dressing
  Tortilla chips

In a large bowl, combine the peas, peppers, onions, parsley, pimientos and garlic. Pour salad dressing over pea mixture; stir gently to coat. Cover and refrigerate for 24 hours. Serve with tortilla chips.

PER SERVING *½ cup (calculated without chips) equals 77 cal., trace fat (trace sat. fat), 1 mg chol., 482 mg sodium, 15 g carb., 3 g fiber, 4 g pro.* **Diabetic Exchange:** *1 starch.*

94 CALORIES Veggie Tortilla Pinwheels

These bite-size snacks are delicious any time of the day. Simply combine cream cheese, dried beef, chopped vegetables and salad dressing mix, then roll into tortillas, chill, slice and serve.
—**DORIS ANN YODER** ARTHUR, IL

PREP: 15 MIN. + CHILLING
MAKES: ABOUT 5 DOZEN

- 1 package (8 ounces) cream cheese, softened
- 4 teaspoons ranch salad dressing mix
- 1 package (2¼ ounces) dried beef, chopped
- ½ cup chopped fresh broccoli
- ½ cup chopped fresh cauliflower
- ¼ cup chopped green onions
- ¼ cup sliced pimiento-stuffed olives
- 5 flour tortillas (8 inches), room temperature
  Salsa, optional

1. In a large bowl, beat the cream cheese and salad dressing mix until blended. Stir in the beef, broccoli, cauliflower, onions and olives.
2. Spread over tortillas; roll up tightly and wrap in plastic wrap. Refrigerate for at least 2 hours.
3. Unwrap and cut into ½-in. slices. Serve with salsa if desired.
PER SERVING *3 pieces equals 94 cal., 5 g fat (3 g sat. fat), 14 mg chol., 527 mg sodium, 9 g carb., trace fiber, 3 g pro.*

66 CALORIES Six-Vegetable Juice

You might say our family and friends enjoy my vegetable garden by the glassful. My husband likes spicy foods, and after one sip, he proclaimed this juice perfect! For more delicate palates, you can leave out the hot peppers.

—DEBORAH MOYER LIBERTY, PA

PREP: 35 MIN. • **COOK:** 30 MIN. + CHILLING • **MAKES:** 2 QUARTS

- 5 pounds ripe tomatoes, peeled and chopped
- ½ cup water
- ¼ cup chopped green pepper
- ¼ cup chopped carrot
- ¼ cup chopped celery
- ¼ cup lemon juice
- 2 tablespoons chopped onion
- 1 tablespoon salt
- 1 to 1½ small serrano peppers

1. In a Dutch oven, combine the first eight ingredients. Remove stems and seeds if desired from the serrano peppers; add to tomato mixture. Bring to a boil. Reduce heat; cover and simmer for 30 minutes or until vegetables are tender. Cool.

2. Press mixture through a food mill or fine sieve. Refrigerate until chilled or freeze. Shake or stir juice well before serving.

NOTE *Wear disposable gloves when cutting hot peppers; the oils can burn skin. Avoid touching your face.*

PER SERVING *1 cup equals 66 cal., 1 g fat (trace sat. fat), 0 chol., 915 mg sodium, 15 g carb., 3 g fiber, 3 g pro.*

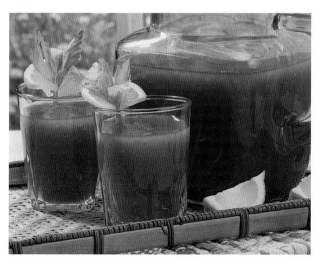

Looking for a post-workout **snack**?

Check out these favorites from our readers! For other satisfying ideas, see our list of low-calorie snacks on pages 84 and 85, and the free foods listed on page 41.

"100-calorie microwave popcorn. The whole *bag* is only 100 calories!"**—MELISSA DRIVER-ALGREN**

"An apple or a banana...usually an apple, because it takes longer to eat!"**—KATHY SCHAEFER**

"Half a serving of zero-fat Greek yogurt on fresh or frozen fruit."**—MARY OBERG ARNESON**

"Tomato with fresh mozzarella, basil, olive oil, a little garlic and a sprinkle of balsamic vinegar."
—LINDA BOLGER

"A 100-calorie ice cream sandwich."
—DELANE HANSEN KEMPF

"Celery with low-fat peanut butter."**—JOHN CELESTRE**

"Fresh cucumbers and tomatoes from the garden."
—BARBARA BUSH

"Two light string cheese sticks."**—AMY LEFAVOUR**

"Cottage cheese with pineapple."**—CINDY JOHOSKY**

"A chewy granola bar. It tastes good and takes the edge off my hunger."**—CINDY DUPIN**

"A package of sweet and salty 100-calorie snack mix."**—BRITTANY NIKOLAS**

"Sour cream and onion cracker chips."
—SUZANNE HOLIFIELD

"Orange creme yogurt."**—MICHELE LENZ**

"Roasted red pepper hummus with veggies."
—CECILIA DENNY

80 CALORIES Frappe Mocha

Coffee ice cubes add punched-up flavor and body to this refreshing drink. What a treat on a warm day!

—BEVERLY COYDE GASPORT, NY

PREP: 5 MIN. + FREEZING
MAKES: 2 SERVINGS

- 1 **teaspoon instant coffee granules**
- ¼ **cup boiling water**
- 1 **cup fat-free milk**
- 4½ **teaspoons chocolate syrup**
- ½ **cup crushed ice**
  Whipped topping and additional chocolate syrup, optional

1. In a small bowl, dissolve coffee granules in water. Pour into an ice cube tray; freeze.

2. In a blender, combine the milk, chocolate syrup and coffee ice cubes. Cover and process until smooth. Add crushed ice; blend. Pour into chilled glasses; serve immediately. Garnish with whipped topping and additional chocolate syrup if desired.

PER SERVING *1 cup (calculated without garnishes) equals 80 cal., trace fat (trace sat. fat), 2 mg chol., 61 mg sodium, 15 g carb., 0 fiber, 5 g pro.*

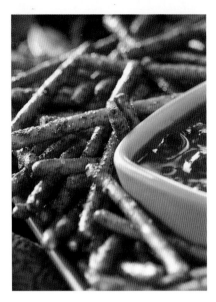

98 CALORIES Pretzel Bones

Just grab a bag of pretzel sticks, season them and you'll have a tasty snack in no time at all! These sweet and savory treats are perfect for anytime munching.

—TASTE OF HOME TEST KITCHEN

START TO FINISH: 15 MIN.
MAKES: 12 CUPS

- ¼ **cup honey**
- 2½ **tablespoons butter**
- 2 **tablespoons chili powder**
- 1 **tablespoon onion powder**
- 1 **package (15 ounces) pretzel sticks**

1. In a Dutch oven, melt honey and butter; stir in chili powder and onion powder. Add pretzels; toss to coat. Spread in a single layer in 15-in. x 10-in. x 1-in. baking pans coated with cooking spray.

2. Bake at 300° for 5 minutes, stirring once. Cool in pans on wire racks. Store in an airtight container.

PER SERVING *½ cup equals 98 cal., 2 g fat (1 g sat. fat), 3 mg chol., 305 mg sodium, 19 g carb., 1 g fiber, 2 g pro.* **Diabetic Exchange:** *1 starch.*

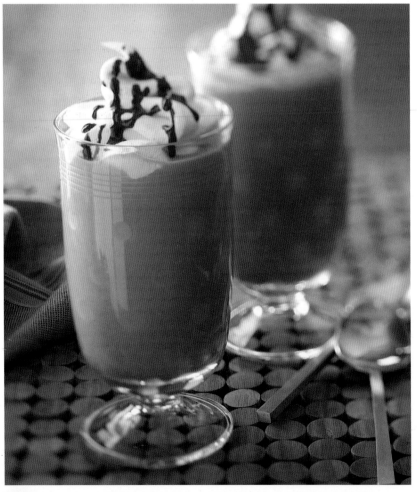

Chocolate Fruit Dip

My grandma helped me experiment with different chocolate sauce and yogurt combinations to create this fruit dip for a tea party we had. Our guests said it was a sweet way to start the meal.

—ABIGAIL SIMS TERRELL, TX

PREP: 10 MIN. + CHILLING
COOK: 5 MIN. + COOLING • **MAKES:** 1 CUP

- 1½ **cups plain yogurt**
- 2 **tablespoons fat-free milk**
- 10 **miniature marshmallows**
- 2 **tablespoons semisweet chocolate chips**
- **Assorted fresh fruit**

1. Line a strainer with four layers of cheesecloth or one coffee filter and place over a bowl. Place yogurt in prepared strainer; cover yogurt with edges of cheesecloth. Refrigerate for 8 hours or overnight.
2. In a small heavy saucepan, combine the milk, marshmallows and chocolate chips. Cook and stir until chips are melted and mixture is smooth. Transfer to a small bowl; cool to room temperature.
3. Remove yogurt from cheesecloth and discard liquid from bowl. Gradually stir yogurt into milk mixture. Refrigerate until serving. Serve with fruit.

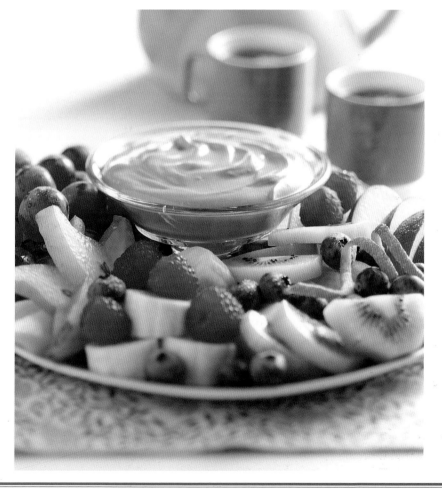

PER SERVING ¼ cup (calculated without fruit) equals 88 cal., 5 g fat (3 g sat. fat), 12 mg chol., 47 mg sodium, 9 g carb., trace fiber, 4 g pro. *Diabetic Exchanges:* 1 fat, ½ starch.

Sunflower Popcorn Bars

Kansas is called the Sunflower State because of the wild sunflowers that grow abundantly here. Cultivated varieties of sunflowers are now becoming an important crop for many Kansas farmers.

—KAREN ANN BLAND GOVE, KS

START TO FINISH: 25 MIN.
MAKES: 4 DOZEN

- 1 **cup sugar**
- ½ **cup light corn syrup**
- ½ **cup honey**
- ½ **cup peanut butter**
- ¼ **cup butter, softened**
- 1 **teaspoon vanilla extract**
- 1 **cup salted sunflower kernels**
- 4 **quarts popped popcorn**

1. In a large saucepan over medium heat, bring the sugar, corn syrup and honey to a boil, stirring often. Boil for 2 minutes. Remove from the heat; stir in the peanut butter, butter and vanilla until smooth. Add sunflower kernels.
2. Place the popcorn in a large bowl. Add syrup and stir to coat. Press into two greased 13-in. x 9-in. pans. Cut into bars. Store in an airtight container.
NOTE *Reduced-fat peanut butter is not recommended for this recipe.*
PER SERVING 1 bar equals 96 cal., 5 g fat (1 g sat. fat), 3 mg chol., 76 mg sodium, 13 g carb., 1 g fiber, 2 g pro.

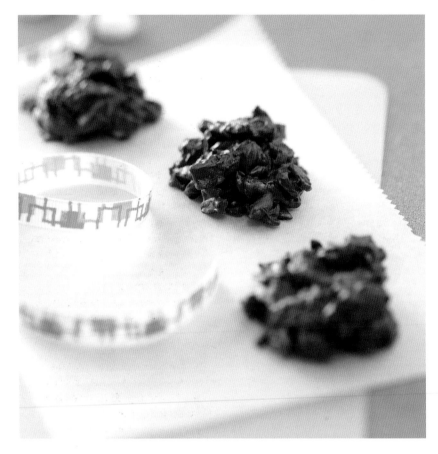

81 CALORIES

Mini Rice Cake Snacks

We had a ball dressing up sweet bite-size rice cakes with a simple spread and a variety of colorful fruits. Try these!

—TASTE OF HOME TEST KITCHEN

START TO FINISH: 10 MIN.
MAKES: 2 DOZEN

- 3 **ounces reduced-fat cream cheese**
- ¼ **cup orange marmalade**
- 24 **miniature honey-nut or cinnamon-apple rice cakes**
- 2 **medium fresh strawberries, sliced**
- 3 **tablespoons fresh blueberries**
- 3 **tablespoons mandarin orange segments**
- 3 **tablespoons pineapple tidbits**

In a small bowl, combine the cream cheese and marmalade until blended. Spread over rice cakes; top with fruit.

PER SERVING *3 rice cakes equals 81 cal., 2 g fat (1 g sat. fat), 6 mg chol., 57 mg sodium, 15 g carb., 1 g fiber, 2 g pro.* **Diabetic Exchanges:** *1½ starch, ½ fruit.*

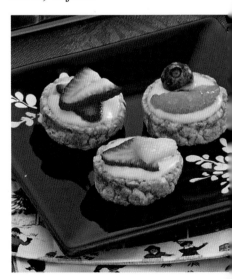

79 CALORIES

Trail Mix Clusters

These delicious snacks make great gifts because they look and taste like they came from an expensive chocolate shop. Packed with heart-healthy dried fruits, seeds and nuts, they're full of fiber and couldn't be more guilt-free. Bet you can't eat just one!

—ALINA NIEMI HONOLULU, HI

PREP: 25 MIN. + CHILLING
MAKES: 4 DOZEN

- 2 **cups (12 ounces) semisweet chocolate chips**
- ½ **cup unsalted sunflower kernels**
- ½ **cup salted pumpkin seeds or pepitas**
- ½ **cup coarsely chopped cashews**
- ½ **cup coarsely chopped pecans**
- ¼ **cup flaked coconut**
- ¼ **cup finely chopped dried apricots**
- ¼ **cup dried cranberries**
- ¼ **cup dried cherries or blueberries**

1. In a large microwave-safe bowl, melt chocolate chips; stir until smooth. Stir in the remaining ingredients.

2. Drop by tablespoonfuls onto waxed paper-lined baking sheets. Refrigerate until firm. Store in the refrigerator.

PER SERVING *1 piece equals 79 cal., 6 g fat (2 g sat. fat), 0 chol., 26 mg sodium, 8 g carb., 1 g fiber, 2 g pro.* **Diabetic Exchanges:** *1 fat, ½ starch.*

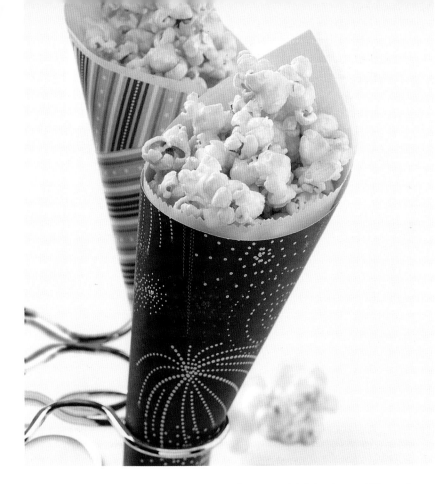

100 CALORIES Strawberry Mango Smoothies

Sometimes artificial sweeteners make food taste exactly that, artificial. But that's not the case with these smoothies. They're delicious and creamy with lots of strawberry and mango flavor.
—TASTE OF HOME TEST KITCHEN

START TO FINISH: 10 MIN.
MAKES: 4 SERVINGS

- 1 cup fat-free milk
- ½ cup vanilla yogurt
- 1½ cups halved fresh strawberries
- 1 medium mango, peeled and chopped
- 4 to 6 ice cubes
  Sugar substitute equivalent to 1 tablespoon sugar

In a blender, combine all the ingredients; cover and process for 30-45 seconds or until smooth. Stir if necessary. Pour into chilled glasses; serve immediately.
NOTE *This recipe was tested with Splenda no-calorie sweetener.*
PER SERVING *1 cup equals 100 cal., 1 g fat (trace sat. fat), 3 mg chol., 47 mg sodium, 21 g carb., 2 g fiber, 4 g pro.* **Diabetic Exchanges:** *1 fruit, ½ fat-free milk.*

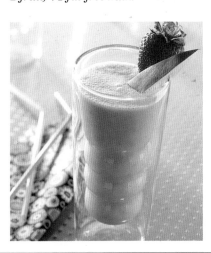

91 CALORIES
Sweet 'n' Salty Popcorn

This popcorn recipe is a family favorite on weekend movie nights, thanks to the classic salty-sweet flavor.
—HILARY KERR HAWKS, MI

PREP: 10 MIN. • **BAKE:** 25 MIN. + COOLING
MAKES: 10 CUPS

- 10 cups air-popped popcorn
- 1 tablespoon butter
- 5 tablespoons instant vanilla pudding mix
- ⅓ cup light corn syrup
- 1 teaspoon vanilla extract
  Dash salt

1. Place popcorn in a large bowl. In a small microwave-safe bowl, melt butter; whisk in the pudding mix, corn syrup, vanilla and salt until smooth.
2. Microwave, uncovered, for 45 seconds or until bubbly. Pour over popcorn; toss to coat. Spread in two 15-in. x 10-in. x 1-in. baking pans coated with cooking spray.
3. Bake at 250° for 25-30 minutes or until crisp, stirring once. Remove popcorn from pan to waxed paper to cool. Break into clusters. Store in airtight containers.
NOTE *This recipe was tested in a 1,100-watt microwave.*
PER SERVING *1 cup equals 91 cal., 2 g fat (1 g sat. fat), 3 mg chol., 83 mg sodium, 19 g carb., 1 g fiber, 1 g pro.* **Diabetic Exchange:** *1 starch.*

When hunger comes calling, **treat yourself to a simple bite** that's fast and easy but won't pack on the pounds. Each item is an ideal way to satisfy a **serious snack attack**!

50 calories or less

- ¾ cup tomato juice, **31 CALORIES**

- ½ cup blackberries, **31 CALORIES**

- 1 cup air-popped popcorn sprinkled with Italian seasoning, **31 CALORIES**

- 2 apricots, **34 CALORIES**

- 1 clementine, **35 CALORIES**

- ½ cinnamon graham cracker, **35 CALORIES**

- ⅓ cup unsweetened applesauce sprinkled with cinnamon, **35 CALORIES**

- ½ cup cubed pineapple, **37 CALORIES**

- 1 medium peach, **40 CALORIES**

- 1 medium plum, **40 CALORIES**

- 1 cup cubed watermelon, **40 CALORIES**

- ½ cup cheese popcorn, **40 CALORIES**

- 8 sweet cherries, **41 CALORIES**

- 2 pineapple rings, **41 CALORIES**

- ½ miniature bagel with 2 teaspoons fat-free cream cheese, **42 CALORIES**

- 1 mini box (.5 ounces) raisins, **42 CALORIES**

- ⅓ cup grapes with 1 tablespoon fat-free whipped topping, **45 CALORIES**

- 1 cup whole strawberries, **45 CALORIES**

- 1 medium kiwifruit, **46 CALORIES**

- ½ cup baby carrots with 1 tablespoon hummus, **48 CALORIES**

- Mixed salad greens with 1 tablespoon crumbled feta cheese and 1 tablespoon fat-free creamy Caesar salad dressing, **49 CALORIES**

- 1 small cucumber, sliced, with 2 tablespoons reduced-fat French onion dip, **49 CALORIES**

- 2 chocolate kisses, **49 CALORIES**

- 2 tablespoons tuna with 3 wheat crackers, **50 CALORIES**

- ½ medium banana, **50 CALORIES**

- 1 cup reduced-sodium V8 juice, **50 CALORIES**

- 10 large olives, **50 CALORIES**

51-100 calories

- ¼ cup dried apples, **52 CALORIES**

- ½ cup broccoli florets with 2 tablespoons fat-free ranch salad dressing, **58 CALORIES**

- ½ frozen waffle with 1 tablespoon sugar-free syrup, **58 CALORIES**

- ½ cup canned peaches (drained), **58 CALORIES**

- 2 crisp lady finger cookies, **60 CALORIES**

- 7 miniature caramel-flavored rice cakes, **60 CALORIES**

- ¾ cup skinny latte (made with fat-free milk), **60 CALORIES**

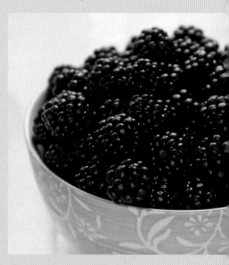

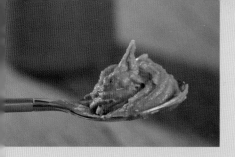

- 1 cup raspberries, **60 CALORIES**

- 1 medium orange, **62 CALORIES**

- ½ cup red or green grapes, **65 CALORIES**

- 1 fun-size Snickers candy bar, **71 CALORIES**

- 1 medium apple, **72 CALORIES**

- ½ cup Honey Nut Cheerios, **74 CALORIES**

- ½ cup strawberry-flavored 1% milk, **75 CALORIES**

- ½ cup fruit cocktail (drained), **75 CALORIES**

- 2 California roll slices, **75 CALORIES**

- 30 whole grain cheddar Goldfish Crackers, **76 CALORIES**

- 5 medium cooked shrimp with 2 tablespoons cocktail sauce, **77 CALORIES**

- ¼ cup pretzel sticks with 1 tablespoon honey mustard, **77 CALORIES**

- 10 medium cashews, **78 CALORIES**

- 1 piece of string cheese, **80 CALORIES**

- 1 Hunt's Fat-Free Snack Pack tapioca pudding, **80 CALORIES**

- 4 ounces diced peaches in 100% fruit juice, **80 CALORIES**

- ½ cup raspberries with 1 tablespoon chocolate syrup, **80 CALORIES**

- 1 ice cream cake cone filled with ⅓ cup fat-free strawberry yogurt and ¼ cup blueberries, **81 CALORIES**

- ½ cup 1% cottage cheese sprinkled with chives or dill weed, **81 CALORIES**

- 1 ounce deli turkey breast with 3 slices snack rye bread, **84 CALORIES**

- 24 pistachios, **85 CALORIES**

- ½ cup 1% chocolate milk, **85 CALORIES**

- ½ ounce Swiss cheese and 2 Ritz crackers, **87 CALORIES**

- 8 animal crackers, **88 CALORIES**

- 3 pieces snack rye bread topped with 1 tablespoon reduced-fat garden vegetable cream cheese and 6 cucumber slices, **89 CALORIES**

- ⅓ cup baked beans, **89 CALORIES**

- ¼ cup miniature marshmallows with 1 tablespoon semisweet chocolate chips, **90 CALORIES**

- 1 crisp rice cereal bar (22 g package), **90 CALORIES**

- ½ small pear with 1 tablespoon caramel ice cream topping, **92 CALORIES**

- ¾ cup sugar-free hot cocoa prepared with fat-free milk, **92 CALORIES**

- 1 cup mandarin orange segments, **92 CALORIES**

- 7 walnut halves, **93 CALORIES**

- 2 tablespoons chocolate-covered raisins, **93 CALORIES**

- ½ medium apple with ½ ounce sharp cheddar cheese, **93 CALORIES**

- ½ small apple with 2 tablespoons caramel ice cream topping, **93 CALORIES**

- 3 cups air-popped popcorn, **94 CALORIES**

- 4 dates, **94 CALORIES**

- 13 almonds, **95 CALORIES**

- ½ cup fat-free vanilla frozen yogurt, **95 CALORIES**

- 1 tablespoon peanut butter, **96 CALORIES**

- 6 Ritz Crackers, **97 CALORIES**

- ½ cup plain fat-free yogurt with ¼ cup blueberries, **98 CALORIES**

- ½ small banana with 2 teaspoons reduced-fat creamy peanut butter, **99 CALORIES**

- ½ cup sugar-free chocolate pudding (prepared with fat-free milk) topped with 1 crushed chocolate wafer, **99 CALORIES**

- 1 container Weight Watchers Berries 'n Cream Yogurt (6 ounces), **100 CALORIES**

Breakfasts

Mom told us all along —and she was right! **Breakfast is the most important meal of the day.** It gets your body going for the morning ahead and whatever it may bring. Try to consume roughly **350 calories at breakfast,** and you'll have fewer cravings the rest of the day.

CONTENTS

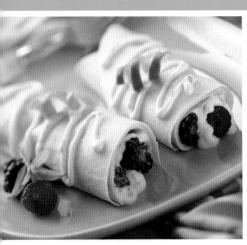

BREAKFAST CREPES WITH BERRIES
PAGE 102

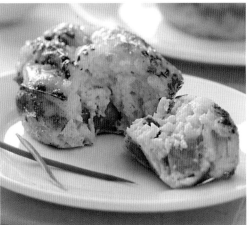
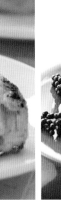

MINI HAM & CHEESE FRITTATAS
PAGE 113

BLUEBERRY OAT PANCAKES
PAGE 125

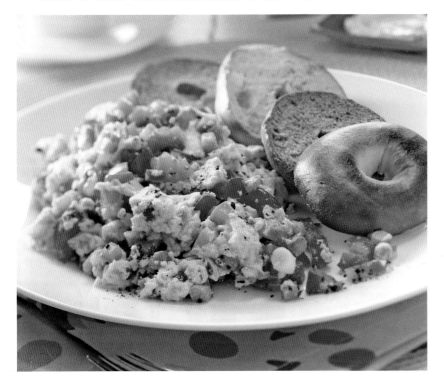

These easy, healthy sausages taste great, and they make an elegant brunch dish. The recipe is also very versatile. It's easily doubled or tripled for a crowd, and the sausage freezes well either cooked or raw.

—ANGELA BUCHANAN LONGMONT, CO

START TO FINISH: 25 MIN.
MAKES: 8 PATTIES

- 1 **large tart apple, peeled and diced**
- 2 **teaspoons poultry seasoning**
- 1 **teaspoon salt**
- ¼ **teaspoon pepper**
- 1 **pound ground chicken**

1. In a large bowl, combine the apple, poultry seasoning, salt and pepper. Crumble chicken over mixture and mix well. Shape into eight 3-in. patties.
2. In a large skillet coated with cooking spray, cook patties over medium heat for 5-6 minutes on each side or until no longer pink.
PER SERVING *1 sausage patty equals 92 cal., 5 g fat (1 g sat. fat), 38 mg chol., 328 mg sodium, 4 g carb., 1 g fiber, 9 g pro.* **Diabetic Exchange:** *1 medium-fat meat.*

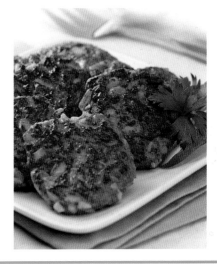

90 CALORIES Vegetable Scrambled Eggs

Try these scrambled eggs packed with a variety of veggies. They'll give you an instant healthy start to your day.

—MARILYN IPSON ROGERS, AR

START TO FINISH: 10 MIN.
MAKES: 2 SERVINGS

- 1 **cup egg substitute**
- ½ **cup chopped green pepper**
- ¼ **cup sliced green onions**
- ¼ **cup fat-free milk**
- ¼ **teaspoon salt**
- ⅛ **teaspoon pepper**
- 1 **small tomato, chopped and seeded**

1. In a small bowl, combine the egg substitute, green pepper, onions, milk, salt and pepper.
2. Pour into a nonstick skillet coated with cooking spray. Cook and stir over medium heat until eggs are nearly set. Add tomato; cook and stir until completely set.
PER SERVING *1 serving equals 90 cal., trace fat (trace sat. fat), 1 mg chol., 563 mg sodium, 8 g carb., 2 g fiber, 14 g pro.* **Diabetic Exchanges:** *2 lean meat, 1 vegetable.*

69 CALORIES Asparagus Ham Roll-Ups

Havarti cheese, asparagus and red peppers make these tasty roll-ups ideal for a spring celebration. Fresh chive ties give them a fussed-over look, but they're a cinch to make!

—**RHONDA STRUTHERS** OTTAWA, ON

START TO FINISH: 25 MIN.
MAKES: 16 SERVINGS

- 16 **fresh asparagus spears, trimmed**
- 1 **medium sweet red pepper, cut into 16 strips**
- 8 **ounces Havarti cheese, cut into 16 strips**
- 8 **thin slices deli ham or prosciutto, cut in half lengthwise**
- 16 **whole chives**

1. In a large skillet, bring 1 in. of water to a boil. Add asparagus; cover and cook for 3 minutes. Drain and immediately place asparagus in ice water. Drain and pat dry.

2. Place an asparagus spear, red pepper strip and cheese strip on each piece of ham. Roll up tightly; tie with a chive. Refrigerate until serving.

PER SERVING *1 roll-up equals 69 cal., 5 g fat (3 g sat. fat), 18 mg chol., 180 mg sodium, 2 g carb., trace fiber, 6 g pro.* **Diabetic Exchanges:** *1 fat, ½ vegetable.*

82 CALORIES Cinnamon-Raisin Bites

These sconelike snacks are wonderful right out of the oven, but they're also good at room temperature when you're on the way to work or school.

—**HANNAH BARRINGER** LOUDON, TN

START TO FINISH: 25 MIN.
MAKES: 2 DOZEN

- 2 **cups all-purpose flour**
- 3 **teaspoons baking powder**
- ½ **teaspoon salt**
- ½ **teaspoon ground cinnamon**

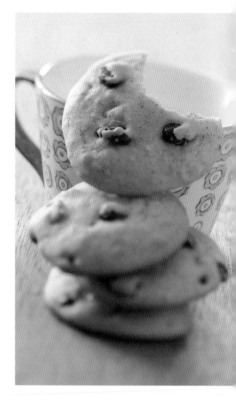

- ¼ **teaspoon ground nutmeg**
- 1 **cup fat-free milk**
- ¼ **cup canola oil**
- ¼ **cup honey**
- ½ **cup raisins**

1. In a large bowl, combine the flour, baking powder, salt, cinnamon and nutmeg.

2. In a small bowl, combine the milk, oil and honey; add to the dry ingredients and stir just until moistened. Stir in raisins.

3. Drop by tablespoonfuls onto baking sheets coated with cooking spray. Bake at 425° for 8-10 minutes or until lightly browned. Remove to wire racks.

PER SERVING *1 piece equals 82 cal., 2 g fat (trace sat. fat), trace chol., 104 mg sodium, 14 g carb., trace fiber, 2 g pro.* **Diabetic Exchanges:** *1 starch, ½ fat.*

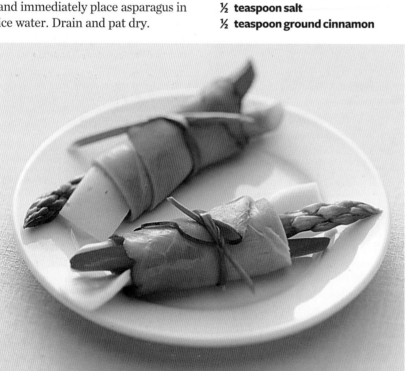

92 CALORIES Sweet Berry Bruschetta

I've made this recipe by toasting the bread on a grill at cookouts, but any way I serve it, I never have any leftovers. The bruschetta is sweet instead of savory, and guests enjoy the change.
—PATRICIA NIEH PORTOLA VALLEY, CA

START TO FINISH: 20 MIN.
MAKES: 10 PIECES

- **10 slices French bread (½ inch thick)**
  Cooking spray
- **5 teaspoons sugar, divided**
- **6 ounces fat-free cream cheese**
- **½ teaspoon almond extract**
- **¾ cup fresh blackberries**
- **¾ cup fresh raspberries**
- **¼ cup slivered almonds, toasted**
- **2 teaspoons confectioners' sugar**

1. Place bread on an ungreased baking sheet; lightly coat with cooking spray. Sprinkle with 2 teaspoons sugar.
2. Broil 3-4 in. from the heat for 1-2 minutes or until the bread is lightly browned.
3. In a small bowl, combine the cream cheese, extract and remaining sugar. Spread over toasted bread. Top with berries and almonds; dust with confectioners' sugar. Serve immediately.
PER SERVING *1 piece equals 92 cal., 2 g fat (trace sat. fat), 1 mg chol., 179 mg sodium, 14 g carb., 2 g fiber, 4 g pro.* **Diabetic Exchanges:** *1 starch, ½ fat.*

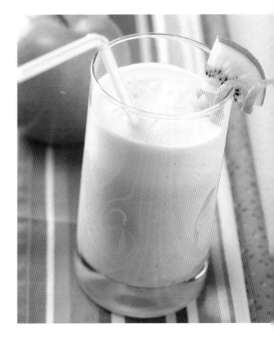

70 CALORIES Orange Soy Milk Frappes

Light, frothy and filled with natural goodness, this creamy orange smoothie takes just a few ingredients...but makes a wholesome morning eye-opener.
—TASTE OF HOME TEST KITCHEN

START TO FINISH: 10 MIN.
MAKES: 2 SERVINGS

- **½ cup vanilla soy milk**
- **½ cup orange juice**
- **5 ice cubes**
- **2 teaspoons sugar**
- **¼ teaspoon vanilla extract**
  Dash salt

In a blender, combine all the ingredients; cover and process for 30-45 seconds or until smooth. Pour into chilled glasses; serve immediately.
PER SERVING *1 cup equals 70 cal., 1 g fat (0 sat. fat), 0 chol., 98 mg sodium, 13 g carb., 0 fiber, 2 g pro.* **Diabetic Exchanges:** *½ starch, ½ fruit.*

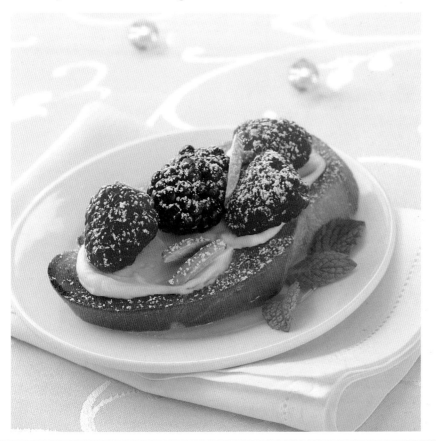

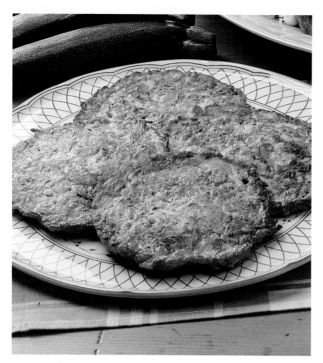

88 CALORIES Zucchini Pancakes

A tasty change of pace from ordinary potato pancakes, these can be paired with any main dish. They also make a budget-friendly way to round out a brunch.

—CHARLOTTE GOLDBERG HONEY GROVE, PA

START TO FINISH: 20 MIN. • **MAKES:** 4 SERVINGS

- 1½ **cups shredded zucchini**
- 2 **tablespoons biscuit/baking mix**
- 3 **tablespoons grated Parmesan cheese**
  Dash pepper
- 1 **egg, lightly beaten**
- 1 **tablespoon canola oil**

1. In a sieve or colander, drain the zucchini, squeezing to remove excess liquid. Pat dry; set aside. In a small bowl, combine the baking mix, cheese and pepper. Stir in egg until blended. Add the zucchini; toss to coat.

2. In a large skillet, heat oil over medium heat; drop ¼ cupfuls of batter into skillet and press lightly to flatten. Fry for 2 minutes on each side or until golden brown. Drain on paper towels.

PER SERVING *1 pancake equals 88 cal., 6 g fat (2 g sat. fat), 56 mg chol., 134 mg sodium, 4 g carb., 1 g fiber, 4 g pro.*

63 CALORIES

Cinnamon-Honey Grapefruit

Although grapefruit is naturally delicious, it gains even more great flavor with this recipe. I like to prepare this as a light breakfast, but it also makes an appealing addition to eggs or granola.

—CARSON SADLER SOURIS, MB

START TO FINISH: 10 MIN. • **MAKES:** 2 SERVINGS

- 1 **medium grapefruit**
- 2 **teaspoons honey**
  Dash ground cinnamon

1. Cut each grapefruit in half. With a sharp knife, cut around each section to loosen fruit. Place cut side up in a baking pan.

2. Drizzle each half with 1 teaspoon honey; sprinkle with cinnamon. Broil 4 in. from heat for 2-3 minutes or until bubbly. Serve warm.

PER SERVING *½ grapefruit equals 63 cal., trace fat (trace sat. fat), 0 chol., trace sodium, 16 g carb., 1 g fiber, 1 g pro.* **Diabetic Exchanges:** *½ starch, ½ fruit.*

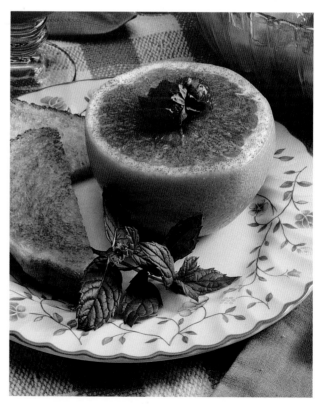

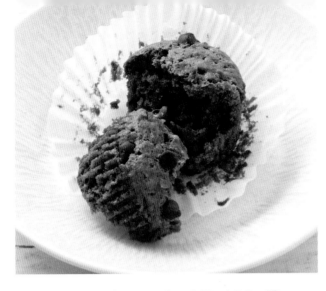

81 CALORIES Cafe Mocha Mini Muffins

These sweet little bites are a good choice for many different occasions—including a quiet morning with a cup of coffee and the newspaper. They freeze well so it's always easy to keep some on hand. And they're just the right size for snacking!

—TINA SAWCHUK ARDMORE, AB

PREP: 20 MIN. • **BAKE:** 15 MIN. • **MAKES:** 1½ DOZEN

- 2 teaspoons instant coffee granules
- ⅓ cup boiling water
- ¼ cup quick-cooking oats
- 3 tablespoons butter, softened
- ¼ cup sugar
- 3 tablespoons brown sugar
- 1 egg yolk
- ½ teaspoon vanilla extract
- ½ cup all-purpose flour
- 1 tablespoon baking cocoa
- ½ teaspoon baking powder
- ⅛ teaspoon baking soda
- ⅛ teaspoon salt
- ½ cup miniature semisweet chocolate chips, divided

1. In a small bowl, dissolve coffee granules in water. Stir in the oats; set aside. In another bowl, cream butter and sugars. Beat in egg yolk, vanilla and oat mixture. Combine the flour, cocoa, baking powder, baking soda and salt; add to oat mixture just until moistened. Stir in ⅓ cup chocolate chips.

2. Fill foil- or paper-lined miniature muffin cups three-fourths full. Sprinkle with remaining chips. Bake at 350° for 12-15 minutes or until a toothpick inserted near the center comes out clean. Cool for 5 minutes before removing from pans to wire racks.

NOTE *Muffins may be frozen for up to 2 months.*
PER SERVING *1 muffin equals 81 cal., 4 g fat (2 g sat. fat), 17 mg chol., 53 mg sodium, 12 g carb., 1 g fiber, 1 g pro.* **Diabetic Exchanges:** *1 starch, ½ fat.*

100 CALORIES Sun-Kissed Smoothies

Grapefruit, banana, pineapple and peaches flavor this refreshing, satisfying smoothie. It makes a healthy treat any time of day.

—TASTE OF HOME TEST KITCHEN

START TO FINISH: 10 MIN. • **MAKES:** 3 SERVINGS

- ¾ cup ruby red grapefruit juice
- 1 medium ripe banana, cut into chunks and frozen
- ½ cup cubed fresh pineapple
- ½ cup frozen unsweetened peach slices
- 4 ice cubes
- 1 tablespoon sugar

In a blender, combine all ingredients; cover and process for 30-45 seconds or until smooth. Pour into chilled glasses; serve immediately.

PER SERVING *¾ cup equals 100 cal., trace fat (trace sat. fat), 0 chol., 2 mg sodium, 25 g carb., 2 g fiber, 1 g pro.* **Diabetic Exchanges:** *1 fruit, ½ starch.*

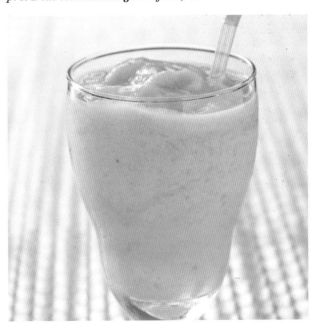

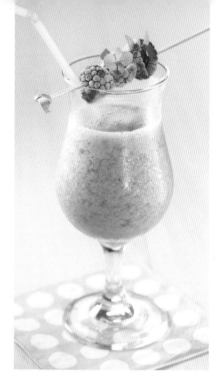

Berry & Yogurt Phyllo Nests

72 CALORIES

This elegant treat lends a special touch to any meal. Add variety by using your own favorite combination of flavored yogurt and fresh fruit.

—TASTE OF HOME TEST KITCHEN

PREP: 25 MIN. + COOLING
MAKES: 6 SERVINGS

- 6 **sheets phyllo dough (14 inches x 9 inches)**
  Butter-flavored cooking spray
- 2½ **teaspoons sugar, divided**
- ⅓ **cup vanilla yogurt**
- 1 **teaspoon grated orange peel**
- 1 **teaspoon orange juice**
- ½ **cup halved fresh strawberries**
- ½ **cup fresh raspberries**
- ½ **cup fresh blueberries**
  Fresh mint leaves, optional

1. Place one sheet of phyllo dough on a work surface; spritz with butter-flavored spray. Top with a another sheet of phyllo; spritz with spray. Cut into six squares. (Keep remaining phyllo covered with plastic wrap to avoid drying out.) Repeat with remaining phyllo.

2. Stack three squares of layered phyllo in each of six muffin cups coated with cooking spray, rotating squares so corners do not overlap. Sprinkle ¼ teaspoon sugar into each cup. Spritz with cooking spray. Bake at 375° for 6-8 minutes or until golden brown. Cool on a wire rack.

3. Meanwhile, in a small bowl, whisk the yogurt, orange peel and juice, and remaining sugar. Spoon yogurt mixture into cups; top with berries. Garnish with mint if desired.

PER SERVING *1 serving equals 72 cal., 1 g fat (trace sat. fat), 1 mg chol., 54 mg sodium, 14 g carb., 2 g fiber, 2 g pro.* **Diabetic Exchange:** *1 starch.*

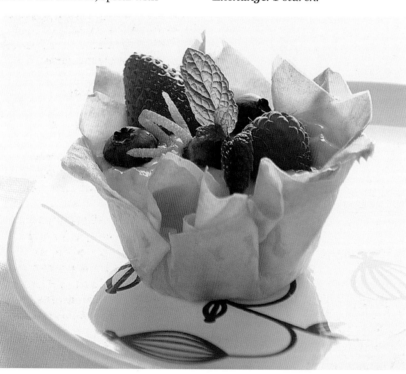

Fruit Smoothies

97 CALORIES

With its combination of fruits, this delicious, quick-to-fix smoothie is a powerhouse of nutrition.

—BRYCE SICKICH
NEW PORT RICHEY, FL

START TO FINISH: 5 MIN.
MAKES: 3 SERVINGS

- ¾ **cup fat-free milk**
- ½ **cup orange juice**
- ½ **cup unsweetened applesauce**
- 1 **small ripe banana, halved**
- ½ **cup frozen unsweetened raspberries**
- 7 **to 10 ice cubes**

In a blender, combine all ingredients; cover and process until smooth. Pour into chilled glasses; serve immediately.

PER SERVING *1 cup equals 97 cal., trace fat (trace sat. fat), 1 mg chol., 33 mg sodium, 22 g carb., 2 g fiber, 3 g pro.* **Diabetic Exchange:** *1½ fruit.*

63 CALORIES Fruit Cup with Citrus Sauce

Here's a medley of fresh fruits so elegant that I serve it in my prettiest crystal bowls. With its dressed-up flavor, it's perfect for a special event.
—**EDNA LEE** GREELEY, CO

PREP: 10 MIN. + CHILLING
MAKES: 6 SERVINGS

- ¾ cup orange juice
- ¼ cup white wine or white grape juice
- 2 tablespoons lemon juice
- 1 tablespoon sugar
- 1½ cups fresh or frozen cantaloupe balls
- 1 cup halved green grapes
- 1 cup halved fresh strawberries
  Fresh mint, optional

1. In a small bowl, combine the orange juice, wine, lemon juice and sugar. In a large bowl, combine the fruit; add the juice mixture and toss to coat.
2. Cover and refrigerate for 2-3 hours, stirring occasionally. Garnish with mint if desired.
PER SERVING ¾ cup equals 63 cal., trace fat (trace sat. fat), 0 chol., 5 mg sodium, 14 g carb., 1 g fiber, 1 g pro. **Diabetic Exchange:** 1 fruit.

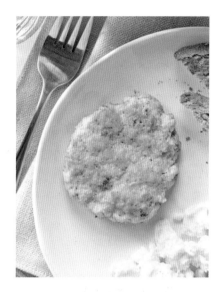

85 CALORIES Turkey Breakfast Sausage

These hearty sausage patties are loaded with flavor but contain a fraction of the sodium and fat found in commercial pork sausage.
—**JUDY CULBERTSON** DANSVILLE, NY

START TO FINISH: 20 MIN.
MAKES: 8 SERVINGS

- 1 pound lean ground turkey
- ¾ teaspoon salt
- ½ teaspoon rubbed sage
- ½ teaspoon pepper
- ¼ teaspoon ground ginger

1. Crumble turkey into a large bowl. Add the salt, sage, pepper and ginger. Shape into eight 2-in. patties.
2. In a nonstick skillet coated with cooking spray, cook patties over medium heat for 4-6 minutes on each side or until a thermometer reads 165° and juices run clear.
PER SERVING 1 patty equals 85 cal., 5 g fat (1 g sat. fat), 45 mg chol., 275 mg sodium, trace carb., trace fiber, 10 g pro. **Diabetic Exchanges:** 1 lean meat, ½ fat.

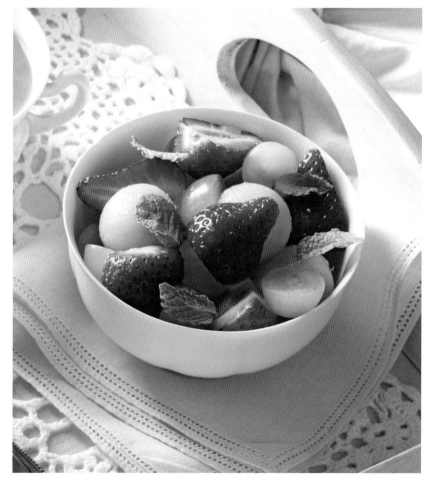

91 CALORIES

Applesauce Oatmeal Pancakes

My recipe makes light, fluffy pancakes that will have the entire family asking for seconds. They're wonderful for those on restricted diets. Try them topped with a little applesauce for a tasty breakfast that's low in calories.
—MARTHA CAGE WHEELING, WV

START TO FINISH: 30 MIN.
MAKES: 5 SERVINGS (2 PANCAKES EACH)

- 1 cup quick-cooking oats
- ¼ cup whole wheat flour
- ¼ cup all-purpose flour
- 1 tablespoon baking powder
- 1 cup fat-free milk
- 2 tablespoons unsweetened applesauce
- 4 egg whites

1. In a bowl, combine the oats, flours and baking powder. In another bowl, combine milk, applesauce and egg whites; add to dry ingredients and mix well.
2. Pour batter by ¼ cupfuls onto a heated griddle coated with cooking spray. Cook until bubbles appear on the top; turn and cook until lightly browned.
PER SERVING *2 pancakes equals 91 cal., 1 g fat (0 sat. fat), 1 mg chol., 323 mg sodium, 15 g carb., 0 fiber, 5 g pro.* **Diabetic Exchange:** *1 starch.*

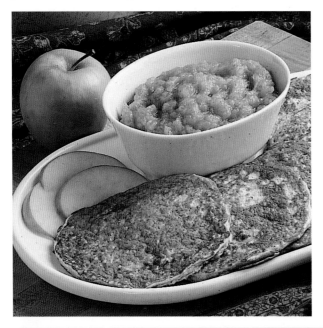

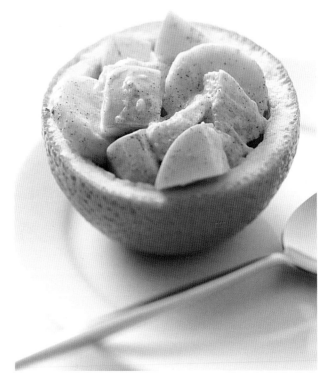

80 CALORIES Orange Fruit Cups

This recipe is always a favorite with children who come to visit. It's a wonderful treat that's healthy, fast and easy to make.
—SUSAN WIENER SPRING HILL, FL

START TO FINISH: 20 MIN. • **MAKES:** 4 SERVINGS

- 2 medium navel oranges, halved
- 1 small apple, chopped
- 1 small banana, sliced
- ¼ cup plain yogurt
- ¼ teaspoon ground cinnamon
  Additional ground cinnamon, optional

1. Using a paring or grapefruit knife and a spoon, scoop out pulp from oranges, leaving a shell. Separate orange sections and chop; transfer to a small bowl.
2. Add the apple, banana, yogurt and cinnamon. Fill orange shells with fruit mixture. Sprinkle with additional cinnamon if desired. Serve immediately.
PER SERVING *½ cup fruit equals 80 cal., 1 g fat (trace sat. fat), 2 mg chol., 8 mg sodium, 19 g carb., 3 g fiber, 2 g pro.* **Diabetic Exchange:** *1 fruit.*

❝ I eat egg whites with veggies or oatmeal with fruit and nuts for breakfast. I also have coffee or green tea every day, since it seems to help increase my metabolism. ❞
—MARY LAJOIE

65 CALORIES Mint Berry Blast

What's better than a bowl of fresh-picked berries? A bowl of berries enhanced with mint, lemon juice and a dollop of whipped topping! It's quick, easy and so refreshing.
—**DIANE HARRISON** MECHANICSBURG, PA

START TO FINISH: 10 MIN. • **MAKES:** 4 SERVINGS

- 1 **cup each fresh raspberries, blackberries, blueberries and halved strawberries**
- 1 **tablespoon minced fresh mint**
- 1 **tablespoon lemon juice**
  Whipped topping, optional

In a large bowl, combine the berries, mint and lemon juice; gently toss to coat. Cover and refrigerate until serving. Garnish with whipped topping if desired.
PER SERVING *1 cup (calculated without whipped topping) equals 65 cal., 1 g fat (trace sat. fat), 0 chol., 1 mg sodium, 16 g carb., 6 g fiber, 1 g pro.* **Diabetic Exchange:** *1 fruit.*

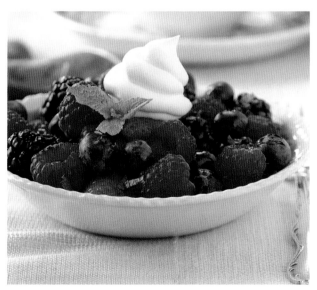

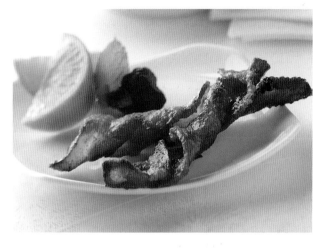

75 CALORIES Spiced Bacon Twists

A sweet and savory rub makes this tasty bacon delicious and worth the bit of extra work. Extend the cooking time just a little if you like your bacon crispy.
—**GLENDA EVANS WITTNER** JOPLIN, MO

PREP: 10 MIN. • **BAKE:** 25 MIN. • **MAKES:** 5 SERVINGS

- ¼ **cup packed brown sugar**
- 1½ **teaspoons ground mustard**
- ⅛ **teaspoon ground cinnamon**
- ⅛ **teaspoon ground nutmeg**
  Dash cayenne pepper
- 10 **center-cut bacon strips**

1. Combine the first five ingredients; rub over bacon on both sides. Twist bacon; place on a rack in a 15-in. x 10-in. x 1-in. baking pan.
2. Bake at 350° for 25-30 minutes or until firm; bake longer if desired.
PER SERVING *2 bacon twists equals 75 cal., 4 g fat (1 g sat. fat), 15 mg chol., 212 mg sodium, 6 g carb., trace fiber, 5 g pro.* **Diabetic Exchanges:** *1 high-fat meat, ½ starch.*

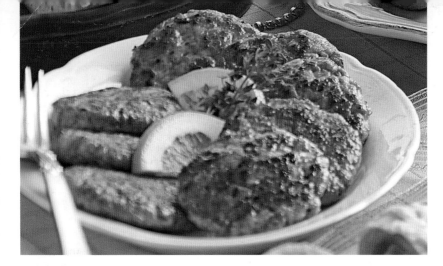

73 CALORIES
Sunrise Slushies

My teenage daughters are perpetual dieters, and I sometimes worry about their nutrition. So I came up with this yummy breakfast beverage full of fruity goodness, and they love it!

—**LINDA EVANCOE-COBLE** LEOLA, PA

START TO FINISH: 10 MIN.
MAKES: 8 SERVINGS

- 2 **cups orange juice**
- 1 **cup reduced-calorie reduced-sugar cranberry juice**
- 1 **medium tart apple, chopped**
- ½ **cup cubed peeled mango**
- 2 **kiwifruit, peeled, sliced and quartered**
- 2 **cups halved fresh strawberries**
- 8 **to 10 ice cubes**

In a blender, place half of each ingredient; cover and process until smooth. Pour into chilled glasses. Repeat with remaining ingredients. Serve immediately.

PER SERVING *1 cup equals 73 cal., trace fat (trace sat. fat), 0 chol., 2 mg sodium, 18 g carb., 2 g fiber, 1 g pro.* **Diabetic Exchange:** *1 fruit.*

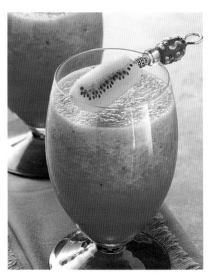

78 CALORIES
Sage Breakfast Patties

You'll want to skip store-bought breakfast patties once you try my simple recipe. It combines ground turkey and pork with plenty of sage and other seasonings for down-home flavor.

—**LAURA MCDOWELL** LAKE VILLA, IL

START TO FINISH: 30 MIN.
MAKES: 1½ DOZEN

- 2 **teaspoons rubbed sage**
- 2 **teaspoons minced chives**
- ¾ **teaspoon salt**
- ¾ **teaspoon white pepper**
- ¼ **teaspoon onion powder**
- ¼ **teaspoon chili powder**
- ⅛ **teaspoon dried thyme**
- 1 **pound ground turkey**
- ½ **pound ground pork**

1. In a large bowl, combine the first seven ingredients. Crumble turkey and pork over mixture and mix well.

2. Shape into eighteen 2-in. patties. In a large skillet, cook patties over medium heat for 3-4 minutes on each side or until a thermometer reads 165°. Drain on paper towels.

PER SERVING *1 patty equals 78 cal., 6 g fat (2 g sat. fat), 26 mg chol., 131 mg sodium, trace carb., trace fiber, 6 g pro.* **Diabetic Exchange:** *1 medium-fat meat.*

100 CALORIES Homemade Egg Substitute

Egg substitute can be used to replace whole eggs in many recipes with good results, especially in frittatas, omelets and quiches. This egg substitute is easy to whip up.

—**TASTE OF HOME TEST KITCHEN**

START TO FINISH: 5 MIN.
MAKES: ¼ CUP EGG SUBSTITUTE EQUIVALENT TO 1 LARGE EGG, 1 SERVING

- 2 **large egg whites, lightly beaten**
- 1 **tablespoon nonfat dry milk powder**
- 1 **teaspoon canola oil**
- 4 **drops yellow food coloring, optional**

In a small bowl, whisk the egg whites, milk powder and oil until well blended. Add food coloring if desired.

NOTE *The cholesterol in 1 large whole fresh egg is 213 mg.*
PER SERVING *¼ cup equals 100 cal., 5 g fat (1 g sat. fat), 1 mg chol., 150 mg sodium, 5 g carb.,0 fiber, 10 g pro.* **Diabetic Exchanges:** *1 lean meat, 1 fat.*

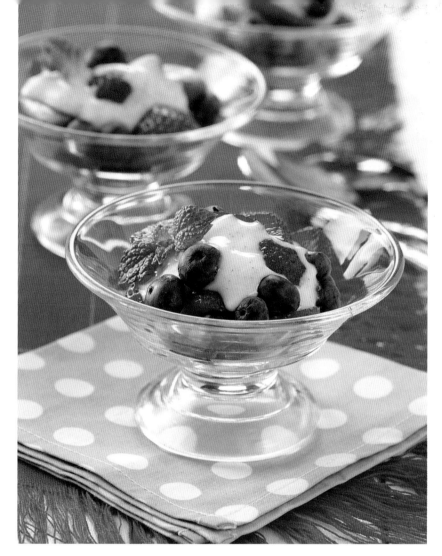

75 CALORIES

Hard-Cooked Eggs

Here's a nice, easy way to make hard-cooked eggs. They're good for snacking or can be used in various recipes.

—TASTE OF HOME TEST KITCHEN

PREP: 20 MIN. + COOLING
MAKES: 12 SERVINGS

12 eggs
Cold water

1. Place eggs in a single layer in a large saucepan; add enough cold water to cover by 1 in. Cover and quickly bring to a boil. Remove from the heat. Let stand 15 minutes for large eggs (18 minutes for extra-large eggs and 12 minutes for medium eggs).
2. Rinse eggs in cold water and place in ice water until completely cooled. Drain and refrigerate.

PER SERVING *1 egg equals 75 cal., 5 g fat (2 g sat. fat), 213 mg chol., 63 mg sodium, 1 g carb., 0 fiber, 6 g pro.*

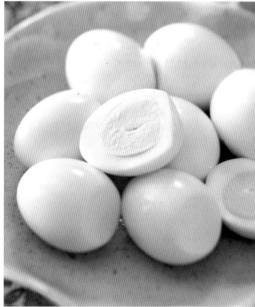

98 CALORIES

Berry Yogurt Cups

Blueberries and strawberries jazz up plain yogurt in this perfect-for-summer easy dessert. Use this combination, or any of your favorite fruits!

—SHANNON MINK COLUMBUS, OH

START TO FINISH: 10 MIN.
MAKES: 4 SERVINGS

- 1½ **cups sliced fresh strawberries**
- 1½ **cups fresh blueberries**
- ¾ **cup (6 ounces) vanilla yogurt**
- 1 **teaspoon sugar**
- ⅛ **to ¼ teaspoon ground cinnamon**

Divide strawberries and blueberries among four individual serving dishes. In a small bowl, combine the yogurt, sugar and cinnamon; spoon over fruit.

PER SERVING *¾ cup fruit with 3 tablespoons yogurt equals 98 cal., 2 g fat (1 g sat. fat), 4 mg chol., 29 mg sodium, 20 g carb., 3 g fiber, 3 g pro.* **Diabetic Exchanges:** *1 fruit, ½ milk.*

101-200 CALORIES

Orange Whole Wheat Pancakes

Friends and family will flip over these light whole wheat pancakes. I adapted them from a traditional pancake recipe, and they feature a sunny twist of citrus. Mix raisins or dried cranberries into the batter to add a bit of chewy sweetness.
—**EARL BRUNNER** LAS VEGAS, NV

START TO FINISH: 25 MIN. • **MAKES:** 16 PANCAKES

- 3 **egg whites**
- 1 **cup orange juice**
- ⅓ **cup unsweetened applesauce**
- ¼ **teaspoon orange extract**
- 1¼ **cups whole wheat flour**
- 2 **tablespoons sugar**
- 2 **teaspoons baking powder**
- ½ **teaspoon salt**
- ½ **cup orange marmalade**

1. In a blender, combine the first four ingredients. Cover and process until smooth. In a large bowl, combine the flour, sugar, baking powder and salt; make a well. Add orange juice mixture; stir just until moistened.

2. Pour batter by 2 tablespoonfuls onto a hot griddle coated with cooking spray. Turn when bubbles form on top of pancake; cook until second side is golden brown. Serve with marmalade.

PER SERVING *2 pancakes with 1 tablespoon marmalade equals 150 cal., trace fat (trace sat. fat), 0 chol., 238 mg sodium, 35 g carb., 3 g fiber, 4 g pro.* **Diabetic Exchange:** *2 starch.*

Chewy Granola Bars

For a satisfying snack that's both soft and crispy, try my recipe. These bars make a tempting, nutritious treat.
—**VIRGINIA KRITES** CRIDERSVILLE, OH

PREP: 10 MIN. • **BAKE:** 25 MIN. • **MAKES:** 2 DOZEN

- ½ **cup butter, softened**
- 1 **cup packed brown sugar**
- ¼ **cup sugar**
- 2 **tablespoons honey**
- ½ **teaspoon vanilla extract**
- 1 **egg**
- 1 **cup all-purpose flour**
- 1 **teaspoon ground cinnamon**
- ½ **teaspoon baking powder**
- ¼ **teaspoon salt**
- 1½ **cups quick-cooking oats**
- 1¼ **cups crisp rice cereal**
- 1 **cup chopped nuts**
- 1 **cup raisins or semisweet chocolate chips, optional**

1. In a large bowl, cream butter and sugars until light and fluffy. Add the honey, vanilla and egg; mix well. Combine the flour, cinnamon, baking powder and salt; gradually add to creamed mixture. Stir in oats, cereal, nuts and raisins or chocolate chips if desired.

2. Press into a greased 13-in. x 9-in. baking pan. Bake at 350° for 25-30 minutes or until the top is lightly browned. Cool on a wire rack. Cut into bars.

PER SERVING *1 bar equals 160 cal., 7 g fat (3 g sat. fat), 19 mg chol., 91 mg sodium, 22 g carb., 1 g fiber, 3 g pro.* **Diabetic Exchanges:** *1½ starch, 1½ fat.*

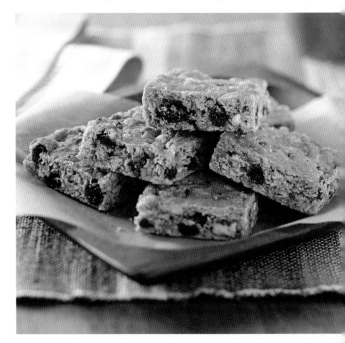

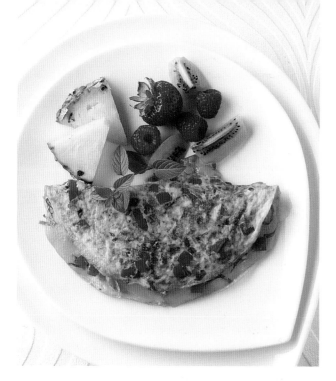

167 CALORIES Colorful Cheese Omelet

When I start my day with this omelet, I'm able to go nonstop all morning and know I'm getting the valuable nutrients I need.
—**LYNDA O'DELL LYNCH** PORT HURON, MI

START TO FINISH: 20 MIN. • **MAKES:** 1 SERVING

- 1 egg
- 2 egg whites
- 2 tablespoons chopped fresh baby spinach
- 1/8 teaspoon hot pepper sauce
- 2 tablespoons chopped sweet red pepper
- 1 green onion, chopped
- 2 tablespoons shredded cheddar cheese

1. In a small bowl, whisk the egg, egg whites, spinach and pepper sauce; set aside. In a small nonstick skillet coated with cooking spray, saute red pepper and onion until tender. Reduce heat to medium.
2. Add egg mixture to skillet (mixture should set immediately at edges). As eggs set, push cooked edges toward the center, letting uncooked portion flow underneath. When the eggs are set, sprinkle with cheese; fold other side over filling. Slide omelet onto a plate.
PER SERVING 1 omelet equals 167 cal., 9 g fat (5 g sat. fat), 227 mg chol., 276 mg sodium, 4 g carb., 1 g fiber, 17 g pro. *Diabetic Exchange:* 2 medium-fat meat.

196 CALORIES Nutmeg Waffles

Bake an extra batch of these tender, golden waffles on the weekend. Freeze them in packages of two to pop in the toaster and reheat on hurried mornings.
—**JAMES CHRISTENSEN** ST. ANTHONY, ID

START TO FINISH: 15 MIN. • **MAKES:** 8 WAFFLES

- 1¼ cups all-purpose flour
- 1 teaspoon baking powder
- 1 teaspoon ground cinnamon
- ½ teaspoon salt
- ½ teaspoon ground nutmeg
- ¼ teaspoon baking soda
- 1 egg, lightly beaten
- 1 cup fat-free milk
- 1 teaspoon canola oil
- 1 teaspoon vanilla extract
  Butter and maple syrup, optional

1. In a small bowl, combine the flour, baking powder, cinnamon, salt, nutmeg and baking soda. In another bowl, combine the egg, milk, oil and vanilla; stir into dry ingredients until smooth.
2. Bake in a preheated waffle iron according to manufacturer's directions until golden brown. Serve with butter and syrup if desired.
PER SERVING 2 waffles (calculated without butter and syrup) equals 196 cal., 3 g fat (1 g sat. fat), 54 mg chol., 518 mg sodium, 34 g carb., 1 g fiber, 8 g pro. *Diabetic Exchanges:* 2 starch, ½ fat.

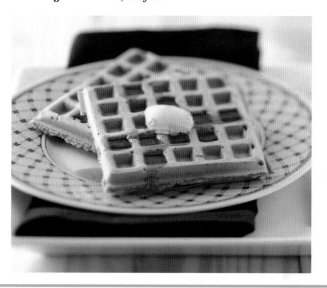

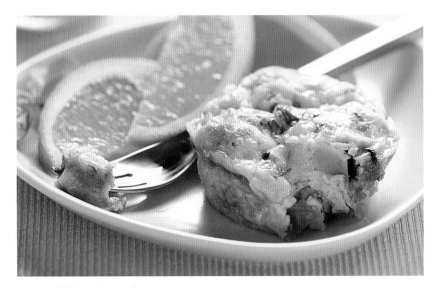

158 CALORIES

Apple Yogurt Parfaits

Get the morning started right with this super-simple, four-ingredient parfait. Try using chunky applesauce for an easy variation.

—REBEKAH RADEWAHN
WAUWATOSA, WI

START TO FINISH: 10 MIN.
MAKES: 4 SERVINGS

- 1 cup sweetened applesauce
  Dash ground nutmeg
- ½ cup granola with raisins
- 1⅓ cups vanilla yogurt

In a small bowl, combine applesauce and nutmeg. Spoon 1 tablespoon granola into each of four parfait glasses. Layer each with ⅓ cup yogurt and ¼ cup applesauce; sprinkle with remaining granola. Serve immediately.

PER SERVING *1 parfait equals 158 cal., 2 g fat (1 g sat. fat), 4 mg chol., 70 mg sodium, 30 g carb., 1 g fiber, 5 g pro.*

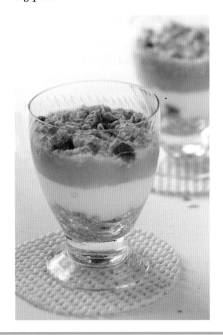

172 CALORIES

Italian Mini Frittatas

While these individual frittatas contain prosciutto, cheese and butter, the amounts are small so each portion stays slimming. They're easy to prepare, easy to serve and will certainly become a brunch favorite.

—MICHELLE ANDERSON EAGLE, ID

PREP: 25 MIN. • **BAKE:** 25 MIN.
MAKES: 1 DOZEN

- 2 tablespoons chopped sun-dried tomatoes (not packed in oil)
- ½ cup boiling water
- 2 thin slices prosciutto, finely chopped
- ¼ cup chopped shallots
- 1 teaspoon butter
- 2 garlic cloves, minced
- ¼ cup all-purpose flour
- 1½ cups fat-free milk
- 4 egg whites
- 2 eggs
- 1 cup (4 ounces) shredded part-skim mozzarella cheese
- ¼ cup shredded Asiago cheese
- ½ cup canned water-packed artichoke hearts, rinsed, drained and chopped
- 2 tablespoons minced fresh basil or 2 teaspoons dried basil
- ¾ teaspoon salt
- ½ teaspoon white pepper

1. Place tomatoes in a bowl; add boiling water. Cover and let stand for 5 minutes. Drain and set aside.
2. In a small nonstick skillet, saute prosciutto and shallots in butter until shallots are tender. Add garlic; cook 1 minute longer. Remove from the heat; set aside.
3. In a large bowl, whisk flour and milk until smooth; whisk in the egg whites and eggs until blended. Stir in the cheeses, artichokes, basil, salt, pepper, and reserved tomatoes and prosciutto mixture.
4. Coat 12 muffin cups with cooking spray; fill with egg mixture. Bake at 350° for 25-30 minutes or until a knife inserted near the center comes out clean. Carefully run a knife around edges to loosen; remove from pan. Serve warm.

PER SERVING *2 frittatas equals 172 cal., 7 g fat (4 g sat. fat), 93 mg chol., 642 mg sodium, 11 g carb., trace fiber, 15 g pro.*

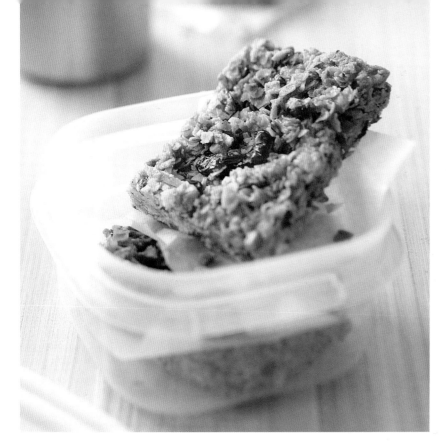

Ham 'n' Cheese Squares

So easy to prepare, this appetizing egg dish is loaded with ham, Swiss cheese and caraway flavor. It cuts nicely into squares, making it an ideal addition to a brunch buffet.

—SUE ROSS CASA GRANDE, AZ

PREP: 15 MIN. • **BAKE:** 20 MIN.
MAKES: 9 SERVINGS

- 1½ cups cubed fully cooked ham
- 1 carton (6 ounces) plain yogurt
- ¼ cup crushed saltines (about 6)
- ¼ cup shredded Swiss cheese
- 2 tablespoons butter, melted
- 2 teaspoons caraway seeds
- 6 eggs

1. In a large bowl, combine the first six ingredients. In a small bowl, beat eggs until thickened and lemon-colored; fold into ham mixture. Transfer to a greased 8-in. square baking dish.
2. Bake at 375° for 20-25 minutes or until a knife inserted near the center comes out clean. Let stand for 5 minutes before cutting.

PER SERVING *1 serving equals 141 cal., 9 g fat (4 g sat. fat), 166 mg chol., 404 mg sodium, 3 g carb., trace fiber, 10 g pro.*

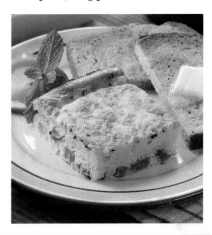

130 CALORIES

Granola-To-Go Bars

These grab-and-go bars make a handy portable breakfast or hearty snack for a long day out. They're chewy, fruity, sweet and really satisfy!

—SALLY HAEN MENOMONEE FALLS, WI

PREP: 30 MIN. • **BAKE:** 15 MIN. + COOLING
MAKES: 3 DOZEN

- 3½ cups quick-cooking oats
- 1 cup chopped almonds
- 1 egg, lightly beaten
- ⅔ cup butter, melted
- ½ cup honey
- 1 teaspoon vanilla extract
- ½ cup sunflower kernels
- ½ cup flaked coconut
- ½ cup chopped dried apples
- ½ cup dried cranberries
- ½ cup packed brown sugar
- ½ teaspoon ground cinnamon

1. Preheat oven to 350°. Combine oats and almonds in a 15x10x1-in. baking pan coated with cooking spray. Bake 15 minutes or until toasted, stirring occasionally.
2. In a large bowl, combine egg, butter, honey and vanilla. Stir in sunflower kernels, coconut, apples, cranberries, brown sugar and cinnamon. Stir in oat mixture.
3. Firmly press into a 15-in. x 10-in. x 1-in. baking pan coated with cooking spray. Bake at 350° for 3-18 minutes or until set and edges are lightly browned. Cool on a wire rack. Cut into bars. Store in an airtight container.

PER SERVING *1 bar equals 130 cal., 7 g fat (3 g sat. fat), 15 mg chol., 40 mg sodium, 16 g carb., 2 g fiber, 2 g pro.*

182 CALORIES

Breakfast Crepes with Berries

After a long day of blackberry picking, I whipped up a sauce to dress up some crepes I had on hand. The crepes make an elegant addition to brunch, but the sauce is also delectable over waffles.

—JENNIFER WEISBRODT OCONOMOWOC, WI

START TO FINISH: 20 MIN. • **MAKES:** 8 SERVINGS

- 1½ cups fresh raspberries
- 1½ cups fresh blackberries
- 1 cup (8 ounces) sour cream
- ½ cup confectioners' sugar
- 1 carton (6 ounces) orange creme yogurt
- 1 tablespoon lime juice
- 1½ teaspoons grated lime peel
- ½ teaspoon vanilla extract
- ⅛ teaspoon salt
- 8 prepared crepes (9 inches)

1. In a large bowl, combine raspberries and blackberries; set aside. In a small bowl, combine sour cream and confectioners' sugar until smooth. Stir in the yogurt, lime juice, lime peel, vanilla and salt.

2. Spread 2 tablespoons sour cream mixture over each crepe; top with about ⅓ cup berries. Roll up; drizzle with remaining sour cream mixture. Serve immediately.

PER SERVING *1 crepe equals 182 cal., 7 g fat (4 g sat. fat), 27 mg chol., 144 mg sodium, 27 g carb., 3 g fiber, 3 g pro.* **Diabetic Exchanges:** *1½ starch, 1½ fat.*

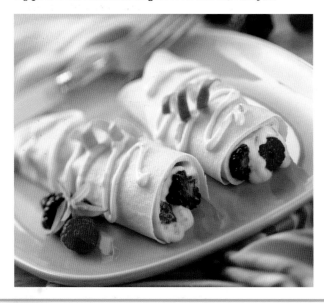

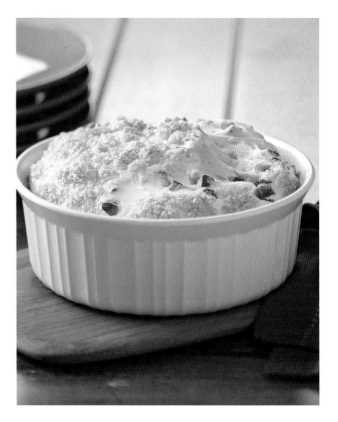

110 CALORIES Cheese Tomato Egg Bake

While making eggs one day, I wanted something different, so I created this special egg bake. We loved it! I hope you will, too.

—JONATHAN MILLER NAUGATUCK, CT

PREP: 10 MIN. • **BAKE:** 25 MIN. • **MAKES:** 2 SERVINGS

- ¾ cup egg substitute
- 2 tablespoons reduced-fat ranch salad dressing
- ⅛ teaspoon garlic powder
- 1 plum tomato, seeded and diced
- 1 slice process American cheese

1. In a large bowl, whisk the egg substitute, salad dressing and garlic powder. Spray the bottom of a 3-cup round baking dish with cooking spray. Pour half of the egg mixture into dish; top with tomato and cheese. Pour the remaining egg mixture on top.

2. Bake at 350° for 22-26 minutes or until completely set and a knife comes out clean.

PER SERVING *1 serving equals 110 cal., 4 g fat (1 g sat. fat), 7 mg chol., 442 mg sodium, 6 g carb., trace fiber, 12 g pro.*

Spinach Omelet Brunch Roll

This recipe uses the combination of veggies from one of my favorite recipes and the rolling technique of another. The result is this stunning presentation that tastes as good as it looks.

—LAINE BEAL TOPEKA, KS

PREP: 20 MIN. • **BAKE:** 15 MIN.
MAKES: 8 SERVINGS

- 2 cups egg substitute
- 4 eggs
- ½ teaspoon salt
- ⅛ teaspoon hot pepper sauce
- 1 package (10 ounces) frozen chopped spinach, thawed and squeezed dry
- ¼ cup chopped red onion
- 1 teaspoon Italian seasoning
- 5 turkey bacon strips, diced and cooked, divided
- 1 pound sliced fresh mushrooms
- 2 teaspoons canola oil
- 1 cup (4 ounces) shredded part-skim mozzarella cheese, divided

1. Line a 15-in. x 10-in. x 1-in. baking pan with parchment paper; coat paper with cooking spray and set aside. In a large bowl, whisk the egg substitute, eggs, salt and pepper sauce. Stir in the spinach, onion, Italian seasoning and ¼ cup bacon.

2. Pour into prepared pan. Bake at 375° for 15-20 minutes or until set. Meanwhile, in a large nonstick skillet, saute mushrooms in oil for 6-8 minutes or until tender. Drain on paper towels; blot to remove excess moisture. Keep warm.

3. Turn omelet onto a work surface; peel off parchment paper. Sprinkle omelet with mushrooms and ¾ cup cheese; roll up jelly-roll style, starting with a short side. Place on a serving platter. Sprinkle with remaining cheese and bacon.

PER SERVING *1 slice equals 160 cal., 8 g fat (3 g sat. fat), 122 mg chol., 505 mg sodium, 6 g carb., 2 g fiber, 17 g pro.* ***Diabetic Exchanges:** 2 lean meat, 1 vegetable, ½ fat.*

Grapefruit Orange Medley

Let the fruits' natural flavors shine through with a refreshing recipe that will brighten up any morning!

—TASTE OF HOME TEST KITCHEN

PREP: 10 MIN. • **COOK:** 20 MIN. + CHILLING
MAKES: 5 SERVINGS

- 2 tablespoons sugar
- 1 tablespoon cornstarch
- ½ cup lemon-lime soda
- 2 cans (11 ounces each) mandarin oranges, drained
- 2 medium grapefruit, peeled and sectioned
- 1½ cups green grapes

1. In a saucepan, combine sugar and cornstarch. Whisk in soda until smooth. Bring to a boil; cook and stir for 1 minute or until thickened. Cover and refrigerate until cool.

2. In a large bowl, combine the oranges, grapefruit and grapes. Add sauce; stir to coat.

PER SERVING *½ cup equals 140 cal., trace fat (trace sat. fat), 0 chol., 8 mg sodium, 36 g carb., 2 g fiber, 1 g pro.*

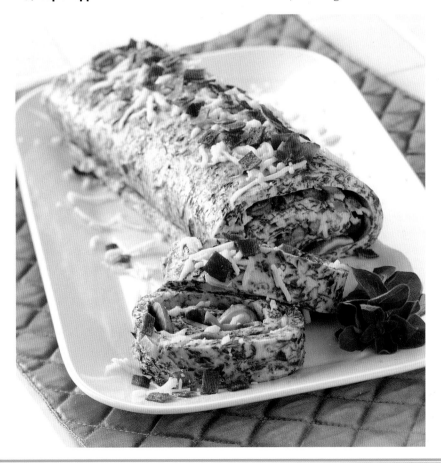

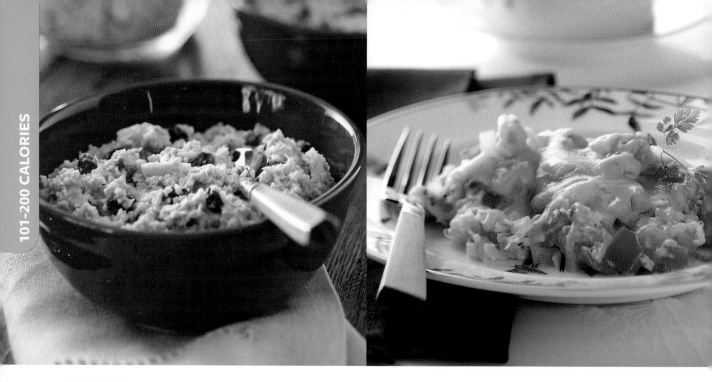

Raisin Oatmeal Mix

We like the sweet cinnamony flavor of oatmeal. The mix makes it convenient to warm a bowl in the microwave for a speedy breakfast.

—**ROBERT CAUMMISAR** GRAYSON, KY

START TO FINISH: 10 MIN.
MAKES: 14 SERVINGS (7 CUPS MIX)

- 6 **cups quick-cooking oats**
- ½ **cup raisins**
- ½ **cup chopped dried apples or dried banana chips**
- ¼ **cup sugar**
- ¼ **cup packed brown sugar**
- 3 **teaspoons ground cinnamon**
- 1 **teaspoon salt**

**ADDITIONAL INGREDIENT
(FOR EACH SERVING)**

- **3/4 cup water**

In a large bowl, combine the first seven ingredients. Store in an airtight container in a cool dry place for up to 1 month.

TO PREPARE OATMEAL *In a deep microwave-safe bowl, combine ½ cup oatmeal mix and ¾ cup water. Microwave, uncovered, on high for 45 seconds; stir. Cook 30-45 seconds longer or until bubbly. Let stand 1-2 minutes.*
NOTE *This recipe was tested in a 1,100-watt microwave.*
PER SERVING *1 serving equals 186 cal., 2 g fat (trace sat. fat), 0 chol., 175 mg sodium, 36 g carb., 4 g fiber, 6 g pro.* **Diabetic Exchange:** *2½ starch.*

Too-Yummy-To-Share Scramble

Pamper yourself some sunny morning with this scrumptious single-serving egg dish...you're worth it! I've gotten many compliments on this recipe; basil gives it an extra-fresh flavor.

—**VICKEY ABATE** GREEN ISLAND, NY

START TO FINISH: 15 MIN.
MAKES: 1 SERVING

- ¼ **cup chopped sweet onion**
- ¼ **cup chopped tomato**
- ⅛ **teaspoon dried basil**
  Dash salt and pepper
- 1 **egg**
- 1 **tablespoon water**
- 2 **tablespoons shredded reduced-fat cheddar cheese**

1. In a small nonstick skillet coated with cooking spray, cook and stir onion over medium heat until tender. Add the tomato, basil, salt and pepper; cook 1 minute longer.
2. In a small bowl, whisk egg and water. Add egg mixture to the pan; cook and stir until the egg is completely set.
3. Remove from the heat. Sprinkle with cheese; cover and let stand until cheese is melted.
PER SERVING *1 serving equals 136 cal., 8 g fat (4 g sat. fat), 222 mg chol., 310 mg sodium, 7 g carb., 1 g fiber, 11 g pro.*

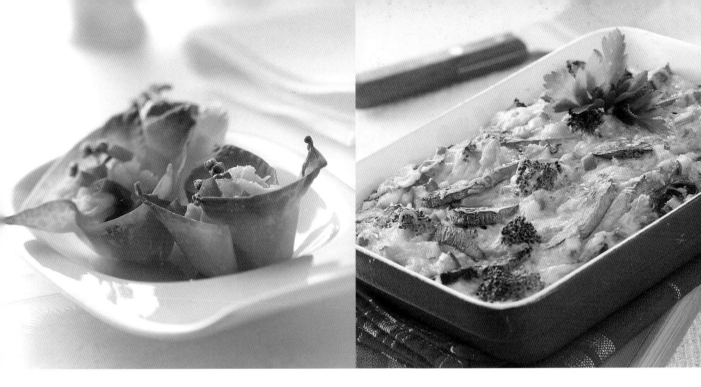

Wake-Up Wonton Cups

Dainty, delectable and delightfully different, these yummy breakfast bites add a fun touch to a healthy morning meal. Pepper sauce lends just a bit of heat and can be adjusted to your liking.
—**GINA BERRY** CHANHASSEN, MN

START TO FINISH: 20 MIN.
MAKES: 10 WONTON CUPS

- 10 **wonton wrappers**
  Cooking spray
- 4 **eggs**
- ½ **teaspoon garlic powder**
- ¼ **teaspoon salt**
- 1 **medium tomato, seeded and chopped**
- 10 **drops hot pepper sauce**

1. Press wonton wrappers into miniature muffin cups coated with cooking spray. Spritz wrappers with cooking spray. Bake at 350° for 10-12 minutes or until lightly browned.

2. Meanwhile, in a small bowl, whisk the eggs, garlic powder and salt. Heat a small nonstick skillet coated with cooking spray until hot. Add egg mixture; cook and stir over medium heat until eggs are completely set.

3. Spoon eggs into cups. Top each with chopped tomato and a drop of pepper sauce.
PER SERVING *2 wonton cups equals 110 cal., 4 g fat (1 g sat. fat), 171 mg chol., 269 mg sodium, 11 g carb., 1 g fiber, 7 g pro.* **Diabetic Exchanges:** *1 starch, 1 medium-fat meat.*

Vegetable Frittata

Looking for a way to incorporate fresh veggies into your breakfast? I think this dish is the perfect solution.
—**PAULINE HOWARD** LAGO VISTA, TX

PREP: 15 MIN. • **BAKE:** 20 MIN.
MAKES: 2 SERVINGS

- 1 **cup egg substitute**
- 1 **cup sliced fresh mushrooms**
- ½ **cup chopped fresh broccoli**
- ¼ **cup shredded reduced-fat cheddar cheese**
- 2 **tablespoons finely chopped onion**
- 2 **tablespoons finely chopped green pepper**
- 2 **tablespoons grated Parmesan cheese**
- ⅛ **teaspoon salt**
  Dash pepper

1. In a large bowl, combine all ingredients. Pour into a shallow 2-cup baking dish coated with cooking spray.

2. Bake, uncovered, at 350° for 20-25 minutes or until a knife inserted near the center comes out clean. Serve immediately.
PER SERVING *½ frittata equals 141 cal., 5 g fat (3 g sat. fat), 14 mg chol., 571 mg sodium, 6 g carb., 1 g fiber, 19 g pro.* **Diabetic Exchange:** *3 lean meat.*

❝Exercise first thing in the morning. Get it over with! If you wait until later in the day, there will always be something that gets in the way, or you will just blow it off because you are beat.❞
—MELISSA LUCZAK KAFKA

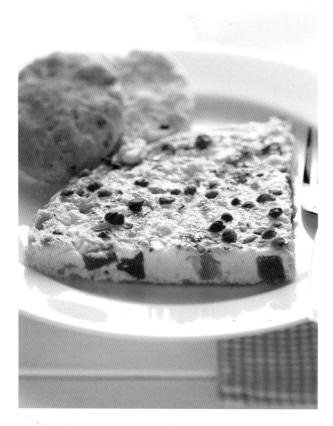

138 CALORIES Anytime Frittata

We enjoy frittatas often at our house. They're a great way to use up leftover vegetables, cheese and meat. You can even serve the hearty recipe with fruit and biscuits for a light supper.
—**LYNNE VAN WAGENEN** SALT LAKE CITY, UTAH

START TO FINISH: 30 MIN. • **MAKES:** 4 SERVINGS

1¼ cups egg substitute
2 eggs
½ teaspoon dried oregano
⅛ teaspoon pepper
1 small onion, chopped
1 garlic clove, minced
1 teaspoon butter
3 plum tomatoes, chopped
½ cup crumbled feta cheese
2 tablespoons capers, drained

1. In a small bowl, whisk the egg substitute, eggs, oregano and pepper; set aside. In a 10-in. oven-proof skillet, saute onion and garlic in butter for 2 minutes. Stir in tomatoes; heat through.
2. Pour reserved egg mixture into skillet. Reduce heat; cover and cook for 4-6 minutes or until nearly set.
3. Sprinkle with cheese and capers. Broil 3-4 in. from the heat for 2-3 minutes or until eggs are completely set. Let stand for 5 minutes. Cut into wedges.
PER SERVING *1 wedge equals 138 cal., 6 g fat (3 g sat. fat), 116 mg chol., 465 mg sodium, 6 g carb., 2 g fiber, 14 g pro.* **Diabetic Exchanges:** *2 lean meat, 1 vegetable, ½ fat.*

200 CALORIES Baked Blueberry Pancake

While fixing supper, I sometimes prepare this huge pancake for breakfast the next day. I cut it into squares before storing it in the refrigerator, then simply top the squares with butter and syrup before placing them in the microwave in the morning. This takes most of the fuss out of making breakfast!
—**NORNA DETIG** LINDENWOOD, IL

START TO FINISH: 20 MIN. • **MAKES:** 6 SERVINGS

2 cups pancake mix
1½ cups fat-free milk
1 egg
1 tablespoon canola oil
1 teaspoon ground cinnamon
1 cup fresh or frozen blueberries
Butter and maple syrup

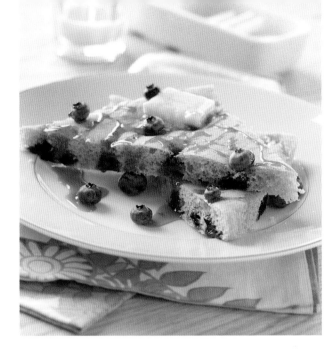

1. In a large bowl, combine the pancake mix, milk, egg, oil and cinnamon just until blended (batter will be lumpy). Fold in blueberries.

2. Spread into a greased 15-in. x 10-in. x 1-in. baking pan. Bake at 400° for 10-12 minutes or until golden brown. Serve with butter and syrup.

NOTE *If using frozen blueberries, use without thawing to avoid discoloring the batter.*

PER SERVING *1 serving equals 200 cal., 4 g fat (1 g sat. fat), 36 mg chol., 527 mg sodium, 34 g carb., 3 g fiber, 7 g pro.* **Diabetic Exchanges:** *2 starch, 1 fat.*

181 CALORIES Raspberry Streusel Muffins

Whether people like raspberries or not, these muffins always receive rave reviews. Pecans, brown sugar and a sweet yummy glaze make them seem anything but light.
—KRISTIN STANK INDIANAPOLIS, IN

PREP: 25 MIN. • **BAKE:** 20 MIN. • **MAKES:** 1 DOZEN

- 1½ cups all-purpose flour
- ¼ cup sugar
- ¼ cup packed brown sugar
- 2 teaspoons baking powder
- 1 teaspoon ground cinnamon
- ¼ teaspoon salt
- 1 egg, lightly beaten
- ½ cup plus 2 tablespoons fat-free milk
- 2 tablespoons butter, melted
- 1¼ cups fresh or frozen raspberries
- 1 teaspoon grated lemon peel

TOPPING
- ¼ cup chopped pecans
- ¼ cup packed brown sugar
- 2 tablespoons all-purpose flour
- 1 teaspoon ground cinnamon
- 1 teaspoon grated lemon peel
- 1 tablespoon butter, melted

GLAZE
- ¼ cup confectioners' sugar
- 1½ teaspoons lemon juice

1. In a large bowl, combine the first six ingredients. Combine egg, milk and butter; stir into dry ingredients until just moistened. Fold in raspberries and lemon peel. Coat muffin cups with cooking spray or use paper liners; fill three-fourths full with batter.

2. Combine topping ingredients; sprinkle about 1 tablespoon over each muffin. Bake at 350° for 18-22 minutes or until a toothpick comes out clean. Cool for 5 minutes before removing from pan to a wire rack. Combine glaze ingredients; drizzle over muffins.

NOTE *If using frozen raspberries, use without thawing to avoid discoloring the batter.*

PER SERVING *1 muffin equals 181 cal., 5 g fat (2 g sat. fat), 26 mg chol., 133 mg sodium, 31 g carb., 2 g fiber, 3 g pro.* **Diabetic Exchanges:** *2 starch, 1 fat.*

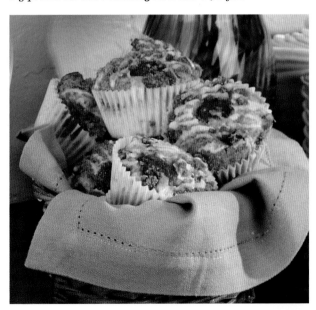

195 CALORIES Banana Blueberry Pancakes

This recipe is a favorite in our home. My kids don't even realize how healthy it is!

—KELLY REINICKE
WISCONSIN RAPIDS, WI

PREP: 15 MIN. • **COOK:** 5 MIN./BATCH
MAKES: 14 PANCAKES

- 1 cup whole wheat flour
- ½ cup all-purpose flour
- 2 tablespoons sugar
- 2 teaspoons baking powder
- ½ teaspoon salt
- 1 egg, lightly beaten
- 1¼ cups fat-free milk
- 3 medium ripe bananas, mashed
- 1 teaspoon vanilla extract
- 1½ cups fresh or frozen blueberries
  Maple syrup, optional

1. In a bowl, combine the flours, sugar, baking powder and salt. In separate bowl, combine egg, milk, bananas and vanilla; stir into dry ingredients just until moistened.

2. Pour batter by ¼ cupfuls onto a hot griddle coated with cooking spray; sprinkle with blueberries. Turn when bubbles form on top; cook until second side is golden brown. Serve with syrup if desired.

NOTE *If using frozen blueberries, use without thawing to avoid discoloring the batter.*

PER SERVING *2 pancakes (calculated without syrup) equals 195 cal., 2 g fat (trace sat. fat), 31 mg chol., 317 mg sodium, 41 g carb., 4 g fiber, 6 g pro.* **Diabetic Exchanges:** *1½ starch, 1 fruit.*

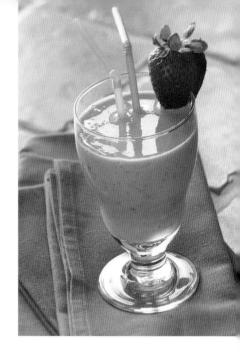

120 CALORIES Orange Strawberry Smoothies

My family and friends were so surprised when I told them that this refreshing, healthy drink has a secret ingredient... tofu! Believe it or not, my dad even requests it for dessert!

—JAN GILREATH WINNEBAGO, MN

START TO FINISH: 5 MIN.
MAKES: 6 SERVINGS

- 2¼ cups orange juice
- 1 package (12.3 ounces) silken reduced-fat firm tofu
- 3 cups halved frozen unsweetened strawberries
- 1½ cups sliced ripe bananas

In a food processor, combine the orange juice, tofu, strawberries and bananas; cover and pulse until blended. Pour into chilled glasses; serve immediately.

PER SERVING *1 cup equals 120 cal., 1 g fat (trace sat. fat), 0 chol., 51 mg sodium, 25 g carb., 3 g fiber, 5 g pro.* **Diabetic Exchanges:** *1½ fruit, 1 lean meat.*

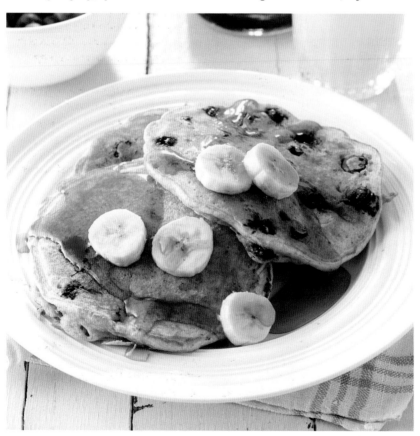

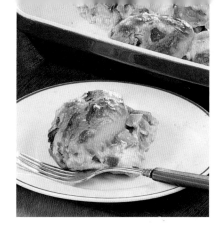

179 CALORIES Egg 'n' Bacon Sandwiches

Here's a healthy, homemade take on a fast-food favorite. My son-in-law created this recipe so my grandchildren could have a quick yet nutritious breakfast before school.

—SHARON PICKETT AURORA, IN

START TO FINISH: 5 MIN.
MAKES: 2 SERVINGS

- 2 eggs
- 1 teaspoon fat-free milk
- ¼ teaspoon salt
- ⅛ teaspoon pepper
- 2 slices Canadian bacon (½ ounce each)
- 1 English muffin, split and toasted
- 2 tablespoons shredded reduced-fat cheddar cheese

1. In a small bowl, whisk the eggs, milk, salt and pepper. Divide between two 10-oz. microwave-safe custard cups coated with cooking spray. Microwave, uncovered, on high for 20 seconds. Stir; microwave 20-25 seconds longer or until center of egg is almost set.

2. Place a slice of bacon on each muffin half; top with egg and sprinkle with cheese. Microwave, uncovered, for 10-13 seconds or until cheese is melted. Let stand for 20-30 seconds before serving.

NOTE *This recipe was tested in a 1,100-watt microwave.*

PER SERVING *1 sandwich equals 179 cal., 8 g fat (3 g sat. fat), 223 mg chol., 673 mg sodium, 14 g carb., 1 g fiber, 12 g pro.* **Diabetic Exchanges:** *1 starch, 1 lean meat.*

160 CALORIES Special Brunch Bake

This eye-opener features buttermilk biscuits. If you don't have Canadian bacon, try it with turkey bacon or ham.

—NICKI WOODS SPRINGFIELD, MO

PREP: 10 MIN. • **BAKE:** 30 MIN.
MAKES: 12 SERVINGS

- 2 tubes (4 ounces each) refrigerated buttermilk biscuits
- 3 cartons (8 ounces each) egg substitute
- 7 ounces Canadian bacon, chopped
- 1 cup (4 ounces) shredded reduced-fat cheddar cheese
- 1 cup (4 ounces) shredded part-skim mozzarella cheese
- ½ cup chopped fresh mushrooms
- ½ cup finely chopped onion
- ¼ teaspoon pepper

1. Arrange biscuits in a 13-in. x 9-in. baking dish coated with cooking spray. In a large bowl, combine the remaining ingredients; pour over biscuits.

2. Bake, uncovered, at 350° for 30-35 minutes or until a knife inserted near the center comes out clean.

PER SERVING *1 serving equals 160 cal., 5 g fat (3 g sat. fat), 20 mg chol., 616 mg sodium, 13 g carb., 1 g fiber, 15 g pro.*

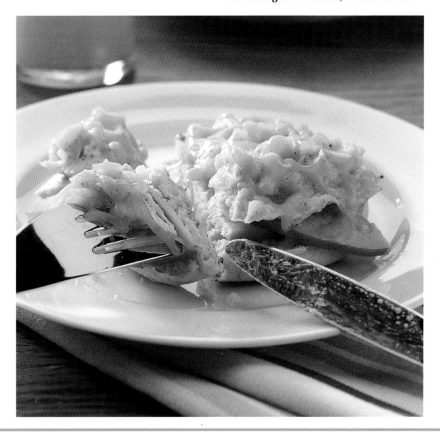

197 CALORIES Crustless Spinach Quiche

My daughter is a vegetarian, so I eliminated the ham called for in the original recipe. Wedges of this wholesome quiche make a flavorful brunch, lunch or even light supper.

—VICKI SCHRUPP ST. CLOUD, MN

PREP: 15 MIN. • **BAKE:** 45 MIN. • **MAKES:** 8 SERVINGS

- 3 ounces reduced-fat cream cheese, softened
- 1 cup fat-free milk
- 1 cup egg substitute
- ¼ teaspoon pepper
- 3 cups (12 ounces) shredded reduced-fat cheddar cheese
- 3 cups frozen chopped spinach, thawed and squeezed dry
- 1 cup frozen chopped broccoli, thawed and well drained
- 1 small onion, finely chopped
- 5 fresh mushrooms, sliced

1. In a small bowl, beat cream cheese. Add the milk, egg substitute and pepper; beat until smooth. Stir in remaining ingredients.

2. Transfer to a 10-in. quiche pan coated with cooking spray. Bake at 350° for 45-50 minutes or until a knife inserted near the center comes out clean.

PER SERVING *1 piece equals 197 cal., 12 g fat (8 g sat. fat), 38 mg chol., 439 mg sodium, 8 g carb., 3 g fiber, 18 g pro.* **Diabetic Exchanges:** *2 medium-fat meat, 1 vegetable.*

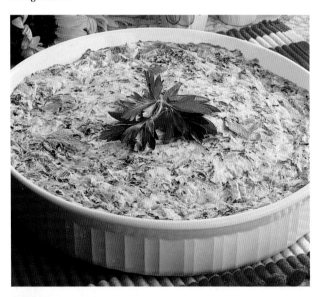

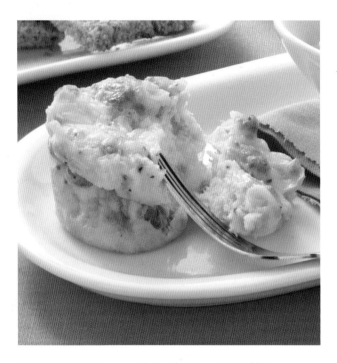

133 CALORIES Scrambled Egg Muffins

After enjoying scrambled egg muffins at a local restaurant, I came up with this savory version that my husband likes even better. Freeze the extras to reheat on busy mornings.

—CATHY LARKINS MARSHFIELD, MO

START TO FINISH: 30 MIN. • **MAKES:** 1 DOZEN

- ½ pound bulk pork sausage
- 12 eggs
- ½ cup chopped onion
- ¼ cup chopped green pepper
- ½ teaspoon salt
- ¼ teaspoon garlic powder
- ¼ teaspoon pepper
- ½ cup shredded cheddar cheese

1. Preheat oven to 350°. In a large skillet, cook sausage over medium heat until no longer pink; drain.

2. In a large bowl, beat eggs. Add onion, green pepper, salt, garlic powder and pepper. Stir in sausage and cheese.

3. Spoon by ⅓ cupfuls into muffin cups coated with cooking spray. Bake 20-25 minutes or until a knife inserted near the center comes out clean.

PER SERVING *1 muffin equals 133 cal., 10 g fat (4 g sat. fat), 224 mg chol., 268 mg sodium, 2 g carb., trace fiber, 9 g pro.*

136 CALORIES Strawberry Tofu Smoothies

Here's a sweet way to get more soy in your diet. It's light, tasty and portable— I take one with me every morning in an insulated mug for an energizing breakfast-on-the-go.
—**DEBBIE STEPP** OCALA, FL

START TO FINISH: 10 MIN.
MAKES: 2 SERVINGS

- **1 cup unsweetened apple juice**
- **1½ cups frozen unsweetened strawberries**
- **4 ounces silken firm tofu, cubed**
- **1 teaspoon sugar**

In a blender, combine all the ingredients; cover and process for 45-60 seconds or until smooth. Pour into chilled glasses; serve immediately.
PER SERVING *1 cup equals 136 cal., 2 g fat (trace sat. fat), 0 chol., 25 mg sodium, 26 g carb., 3 g fiber, 5 g pro. **Diabetic Exchanges:** 1½ fruit, 1 lean meat.*

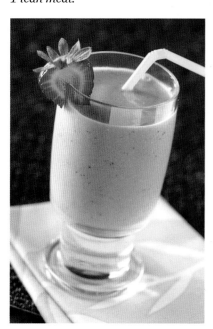

Here are some typical **breakfast foods** and the numbers of calories they contain. Use this list as a reference when combining morning mainstays to keep within your goal of a **350-calorie breakfast**.

- ½ cup fat-free vanilla yogurt topped with 2 tablespoons Wheaties, **86 CALORIES**

- ½ cup fat-free plain yogurt topped with 1½ teaspoons honey, **109 CALORIES**

- ½ cup fat-free plain yogurt topped with 4 strawberries or ¼ cup blueberries, **109 CALORIES**

- 6 ounces fat-free fruit-flavored yogurt, **160 CALORIES**

- 1 slice whole wheat toast, **69 CALORIES**

- 1 scrambled egg, **101 CALORIES**

- 1 plain mini bagel, **72 CALORIES**

- 1 tablespoon whipped cream cheese, **35 CALORIES**

- ½ toasted whole wheat English muffin with 1 tablespoon peanut butter, **157 CALORIES**

- 1 frozen waffle, **98 CALORIES**

- 1 pancake (6" diameter prepared from dry pancake mix), **149 CALORIES**

- 1 cup Cheerios, **111 CALORIES**

- 1 cup Wheaties, **107 CALORIES**

- ¾ cup plain oatmeal (made with water), **109 CALORIES**

- ⅓ cup frosted bite-size Shredded Wheat with ⅓ cup fat-free milk, **89 CALORIES**

- 1 cup orange juice, **110 CALORIES**

- 1 cup fat-free milk, **86 CALORIES**

- 1 cup skinny latte (made with fat-free milk), **80 CALORIES**

- ½ small grapefruit with 1 teaspoon sugar, **48 CALORIES**

- 1 medium banana, **100 CALORIES**

- ½ cup cooked grits, **76 CALORIES**

- 1 medium apple with 1 tablespoon peanut butter, **161 CALORIES**

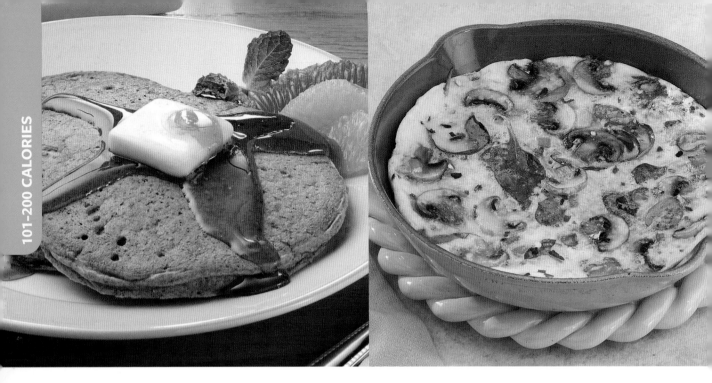

195 CALORIES Buttermilk Buckwheat Pancakes

We created this recipe using buckwheat flour. It produces light, tender pancakes.

—TASTE OF HOME TEST KITCHEN

START TO FINISH: 25 MIN.
MAKES: 4 SERVINGS

- 1 **cup buckwheat flour**
- 2 **tablespoons brown sugar**
- 1 **teaspoon baking powder**
- ½ **teaspoon baking soda**
- ½ **teaspoon salt**
- ⅛ **teaspoon each ground cinnamon, nutmeg and cloves**
- 1 **egg**
- 1 **cup buttermilk**
- 1 **tablespoon butter, melted**

1. In a large bowl, combine the flour, brown sugar, baking powder, baking soda, salt, cinnamon, nutmeg and cloves. Whisk the egg, buttermilk and butter; stir into dry ingredients just until moistened.
2. Pour batter by ¼ cupfuls onto a hot nonstick griddle coated with cooking spray. Turn when bubbles form on top of pancakes; cook until second side is golden brown.

PER SERVING *2 pancakes equals 195 cal., 6 g fat (3 g sat. fat), 63 mg chol., 667 mg sodium, 31 g carb., 3 g fiber, 7 g pro.*

110 CALORIES Mushroom Spinach Omelet

For a change of pace, I like to add some diced celery and a bit of fresh parsley.

—ARLENE HAMMONDS GRAY, TN

START TO FINISH: 20 MIN.
MAKES: 2 SERVINGS

- 1 **egg**
- 3 **egg whites**
- 1 **tablespoon grated Parmesan cheese**
- 1 **tablespoon shredded cheddar cheese**
- ¼ **teaspoon salt**
- ⅛ **teaspoon crushed red pepper flakes**
- ⅛ **teaspoon garlic powder**
- ⅛ **teaspoon pepper**
- ½ **cup sliced fresh mushrooms**
- 2 **tablespoons finely chopped green pepper**
- 1 **tablespoon finely chopped onion**
- ½ **teaspoon olive oil**
- 1 **cup torn fresh spinach**

1. In a small bowl, beat the egg and egg whites. Add cheeses, salt, pepper flakes, garlic powder and pepper; mix well. Set aside.
2. In an 8-in. nonstick skillet, saute the mushrooms, green pepper and onion in oil for 4-5 minutes or until tender. Add spinach; cook and stir until spinach is wilted. Add egg mixture. As eggs set, lift edges, letting uncooked portion flow underneath. Cut into wedges. Serve immediately.

PER SERVING *1 serving equals 110 cal., 6 g fat (2 g sat. fat), 112 mg chol., 489 mg sodium, 4 g carb., 1 g fiber, 11 g pro.*

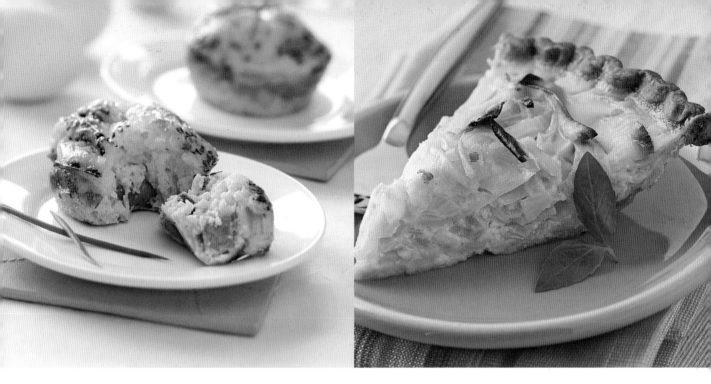

106 CALORIES Mini Ham & Cheese Frittatas

Control serving sizes easily with these nutritious mini frittatas that make breakfast fun again!

—SUSAN WATT BASKING RIDGE, NJ

PREP: 15 MIN. • **BAKE:** 25 MIN.
MAKES: 8 FRITTATAS

- ¼ **pound cubed fully cooked ham**
- 1 **cup (4 ounces) shredded fat-free cheddar cheese**
- 6 **eggs**
- 4 **egg whites**
- 3 **tablespoons minced chives**
- 2 **tablespoons fat-free milk**
- ¼ **teaspoon salt**
- ¼ **teaspoon pepper**

1. Divide ham among eight muffin cups coated with cooking spray; top with cheese. In a large bowl, beat eggs and whites. Beat in chives, milk, salt and pepper. Pour over cheese, filling each muffin cup three-fourths full.

2. Bake at 375° for 22-25 minutes or until a knife inserted near the center comes out clean. Carefully run a knife around edges to loosen; remove from pan. Serve warm.

PER SERVING *1 frittata equals 106 cal., 4 g fat (1 g sat. fat), 167 mg chol., 428 mg sodium, 2 g carb., trace fiber, 14 g pro.* **Diabetic Exchange:** *2 medium-fat meat.*

187 CALORIES Sweet Onion Pie

Chock-full of onions, this creamy, quichelike pie makes a scrumptious addition to a brunch buffet. By using less butter to cook the onions and taking advantage of light ingredients, I cut calories and fat in this tasty dish.

—BARBARA REESE CATAWISSA, PA

PREP: 35 MIN. • **BAKE:** 20 MIN.
MAKES: 8 SERVINGS

- 2 **sweet onions, halved and sliced**
- 1 **tablespoon butter**
- 1 **unbaked pastry shell (9 inches)**
- 1 **cup egg substitute**
- 1 **cup fat-free evaporated milk**
- 1 **teaspoon salt**
- ¼ **teaspoon pepper**

1. In a large nonstick skillet, cook onions in butter over medium-low heat for 30 minutes or until very tender. Meanwhile, line unpricked pastry shell with a double thickness of heavy-duty foil.

2. Bake at 450° for 6 minutes. Remove foil; cool on a wire rack. Reduce heat to 425°.

3. Spoon onions into pastry shell. In a small bowl, whisk the egg substitute, milk, salt and pepper; pour over onions. Bake for 20-25 minutes or until knife inserted near center comes out clean. Let stand for 5-10 minutes before cutting.

PER SERVING *1 piece equals 187 cal., 9 g fat (4 g sat. fat), 10 mg chol., 510 mg sodium, 20 g carb., 1 g fiber, 7 g pro.* **Diabetic Exchanges:** *1 starch, 1 lean meat, 1 fat.*

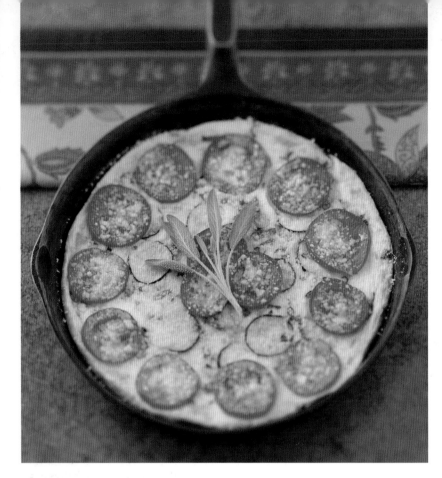

Raspberry Pancakes

Sometimes we have these pancakes for dinner because they are so rich. They're the best on a cool summer night!

—**KAREN EDLAND** MCHENRY, ND

START TO FINISH: 25 MIN.
MAKES: 4 SERVINGS

- ⅔ **cup all-purpose flour**
- 1 **tablespoon sugar**
- 1 **teaspoon baking powder**
- ¾ **teaspoon baking soda**
- ⅓ **cup plain yogurt**
- 1 **large egg, beaten lightly**
- 1 **tablespoon butter, melted and cooled**
- ½ **cup milk**
- 1 **cup fresh raspberries**
  Raspberry jam
  Confectioners' sugar

1. Whisk together flour, sugar, baking powder and soda. (Add a pinch of salt if desired.) Set aside.
2. In large bowl, whisk together yogurt, egg, butter and milk. Add to flour mixture; stir just until combined. Fold in raspberries.
3. Heat a griddle over moderately high heat; brush with additional melted butter. Drop scant ¼ cupfuls of batter onto griddle; cook for 1 minute or until bubbles form on top. Turn and cook 1 minute more. Serve with raspberry jam and sugar.
PER SERVING *2 pancakes (calculated without jam and confectioners' sugar) equals 178 cal., 6 g fat (3 g sat. fat), 68 mg chol., 405 mg sodium, 25 g carb., 3 g fiber, 6 g pro.* **Diabetic Exchanges:** *1½ starch, 1 fat.*

Italian Garden Frittata

I like to serve this pretty frittata with melon wedges for a colorful breakfast or brunch.

—**SALLY MALONEY** DALLAS, GA

START TO FINISH: 30 MIN.
MAKES: 4 SERVINGS

- 6 **egg whites**
- 4 **eggs**
- ½ **cup grated Romano cheese, divided**
- 1 **tablespoon minced fresh sage**
- ½ **teaspoon salt**
- ¼ **teaspoon pepper**
- 1 **small zucchini, sliced**
- 2 **green onions, sliced**
- 1 **teaspoon olive oil**
- 2 **plum tomatoes, thinly sliced**

1. In a large bowl, whisk the egg whites, eggs, ¼ cup Romano cheese, sage, salt and pepper; set aside.
2. In a 10-in. ovenproof skillet coated with cooking spray, saute zucchini and onions in oil for 2 minutes. Add egg mixture; cover and cook for 4-6 minutes or until eggs are nearly set.
3. Uncover; top with tomato slices and remaining cheese. Broil 3-4 in. from the heat for 2-3 minutes or until the eggs are completely set. Let stand for 5 minutes. Cut into wedges.
PER SERVING *1 wedge equals 183 cal., 11 g fat (5 g sat. fat), 228 mg chol., 655 mg sodium, 4 g carb., 1 g fiber, 18 g pro.*

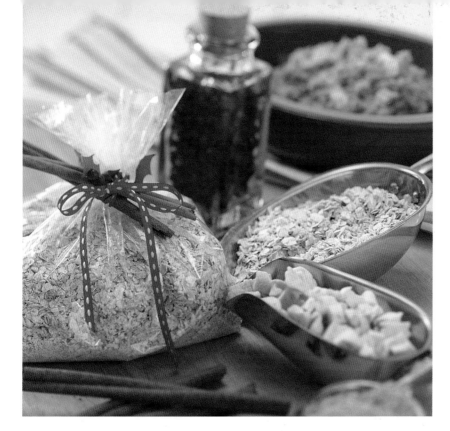

Cappuccino Smoothies

This icy cappuccino is a sweet change of pace from fruit smoothies. My mom and I created it looking to fix an easy snack.
—**MICHELLE CLUNEY** LAKE MARY, FL

START TO FINISH: 5 MIN.
MAKES: 3 SERVINGS

- 1 **cup (8 ounces) cappuccino or coffee yogurt**
- ⅓ **cup milk**
- 3 **tablespoons confectioners' sugar, optional**
- 1 **tablespoon chocolate syrup**
- 1½ **cups ice cubes**
- ½ **cup miniature marshmallows, divided**

In a blender, combine the yogurt, milk, sugar if desired and chocolate syrup. Add ice cubes and ¼ cup marshmallows; cover and process until blended. Pour into chilled glasses; top with the remaining marshmallows. Serve immediately.
PER SERVING *1 cup equals 166 cal., 3 g fat (2 g sat. fat), 11 mg chol., 69 mg sodium, 30 g carb., trace fiber, 5 g pro.*

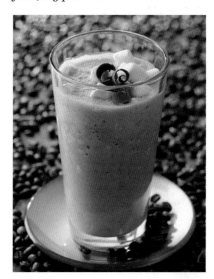

Apple-Cinnamon Oatmeal Mix

Oatmeal is a breakfast staple at our house. It's a warm, nutritious start to the day that keeps us going all morning. We used to buy oatmeal mixes, but now think our homemade version is better! You can substitute raisins or other dried fruit for the apples.
—**LYNNE VAN WAGENEN**
SALT LAKE CITY, UTAH

START TO FINISH: 5 MIN.
MAKES: 16 SERVINGS (8 CUPS MIX)

- 6 **cups quick-cooking oats**
- 1⅓ **cups nonfat dry milk powder**
- 1 **cup dried apples, diced**
- ¼ **cup sugar**
- ¼ **cup packed brown sugar**
- 1 **tablespoon ground cinnamon**
- 1 **teaspoon salt**
- ¼ **teaspoon ground cloves**

ADDITIONAL INGREDIENT
(FOR EACH SERVING)

- ½ **cup water**

In a large bowl, combine the first eight ingredients. Store in an airtight container in a cool dry place for up to 6 months.
TO PREPARE OATMEAL *Shake mix well. In a small saucepan, bring water to a boil; slowly stir in ½ cup mix for each serving. Cook and stir over medium heat for 1 minute. Remove from the heat. Cover and let stand for 1 minute or until oatmeal reaches desired consistency.*
PER SERVING *1 serving equals 176 cal., 2 g fat (trace sat. fat), 1 mg chol., 185 mg sodium, 33 g carb., 4 g fiber, 7 g pro.* **Diabetic Exchange:** *2 starch.*

163 CALORIES Festive French Pancakes

Not quite as thin as true crepes, these light-as-a-feather pancakes are topped with preserves and a dusting of confectioners' sugar. They're elegant and so easy to make!

—**DIANE AUNE** NINE MILE FALLS, WA

START TO FINISH: 15 MIN. • **MAKES:** 8 PANCAKES

- ⅔ cup milk
- 2 eggs
- ⅓ cup water
- ½ teaspoon vanilla extract
- ¾ cup all-purpose flour
- 2 tablespoons confectioners' sugar
- 1 teaspoon baking powder
- ½ teaspoon salt
  Preserves of your choice, optional
  Additional confectioners' sugar, optional

1. In a blender, combine the milk, eggs, water and vanilla; cover and process until well blended. Combine the flour, confectioners' sugar, baking powder and salt; add to egg mixture. Cover and process until smooth.

2. Heat a lightly greased 8-in. nonstick skillet over medium heat; pour 2 tablespoons batter into the center of skillet. Lift and tilt pan to coat bottom evenly. Cook until top appears dry; turn and cook 15-20 seconds longer. Remove to a wire rack.

3. Repeat with remaining batter, greasing skillet as

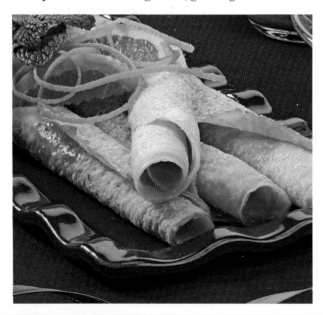

needed. Spread preserves over pancakes if desired; roll up. Sprinkle with confectioners' sugar if desired.

PER SERVING *2 pancakes (calculated without preserves and confectioners' sugar) equals 163 cal., 4 g fat (2 g sat. fat), 112 mg chol., 447 mg sodium, 24 g carb., 1 g fiber, 7 g pro.* **Diabetic Exchanges:** *1½ starch, ½ fat.*

166 CALORIES
Lemon-Blueberry Oat Muffins

My yummy oatmeal muffins showcase juicy blueberries and a zesty lemon flavor. They're the perfect mid-morning snack.

—**JAMIE BROWN** WALDEN, CO

PREP: 15 MIN. • **BAKE:** 20 MIN. • **MAKES:** 1 DOZEN

- 1 cup quick-cooking oats
- 1 cup all-purpose flour
- ½ cup sugar
- 3 teaspoons baking powder
- ¼ teaspoon salt
- 1 egg
- 1 egg white
- 1 cup fat-free milk
- 2 tablespoons butter, melted
- 1 teaspoon grated lemon peel
- 1 teaspoon vanilla extract
- 1 cup fresh or frozen blueberries

TOPPING
- ½ cup quick-cooking oats
- 2 tablespoons brown sugar
- 1 tablespoon butter, softened

1. In a large bowl, combine the first five ingredients. In another bowl, combine the egg, egg white, milk, butter, lemon peel and vanilla. Add to dry ingredients just until moistened. Fold in berries.

2. Coat muffin cups with cooking spray or use paper liners; fill two-thirds full. Combine topping ingredients; sprinkle over batter.

3. Bake at 400° for 20-22 minutes or until a toothpick inserted in the muffin comes out clean. Cool 5 minutes before removing from pan to a wire rack to cool completely.

NOTE *If using frozen blueberries, use without thawing to avoid discoloring the batter.*

PER SERVING *1 muffin equals 166 cal., 4 g fat (2 g sat. fat), 26 mg chol., 158 mg sodium, 28 g carb., 2 g fiber, 4 g pro.* **Diabetic Exchanges:** *1½ starch, 1 fat.*

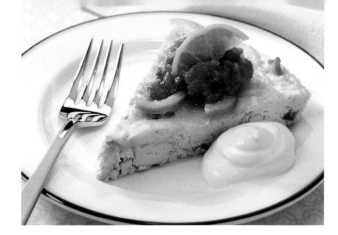

137 CALORIES Fajita Frittata

Here is a super-flavorful and quick entree. It takes me just a few minutes to prepare. Though you could serve it for brunch, whenever I ask my family what they want for dinner, this is their most popular request.
—MARY ANN IRVINE LOMBARD, IL

START TO FINISH: 25 MIN. • **MAKES:** 8 SERVINGS
- ½ **pound boneless skinless chicken breast, cut into strips**
- 1 **small onion, cut into thin strips**
- ½ **medium green pepper, cut into thin strips**
- 1 **teaspoon lime juice**
- ½ **teaspoon salt**
- ½ **teaspoon ground cumin**
- ½ **teaspoon chili powder**
- 2 **tablespoons canola oil**
- 2 **cups egg substitute**
- 1 **cup (4 ounces) shredded reduced-fat Colby-Monterey Jack cheese**
    Salsa and sour cream, optional

1. In a large ovenproof skillet, saute the chicken, onion, green pepper, lime juice, salt, cumin and chili powder in oil until chicken is no longer pink.
2. Pour egg substitute over chicken mixture. Cover and cook over medium-low heat for 8-10 minutes or until nearly set. Uncover; broil 6 in. from the heat for 2-3 minutes or until eggs are set.
3. Sprinkle with cheese. Cover and let stand for 1 minute or until cheese is melted. Serve with salsa and sour cream if desired.
PER SERVING *1 serving (calculated without salsa and sour cream) equals 137 cal., 7 g fat (2 g sat. fat), 23 mg chol., 393 mg sodium, 3 g carb., trace fiber, 15 g pro.*
***Diabetic Exchanges:** 2 lean meat, 1 fat.*

170 CALORIES Bacon-Broccoli Quiche Cups

Packed with veggies and melted cheese, this comforting and colorful egg bake has become a holiday brunch classic in our home.
—IRENE STEINMEYER DENVER, CO

PREP: 10 MIN. • **BAKE:** 25 MIN. • **MAKES:** 2 SERVINGS
- 4 **bacon strips, diced**
- ¼ **cup fresh broccoli florets**
- ¼ **cup chopped onion**
- 1 **garlic clove, minced**
- ¾ **cup egg substitute**
- 1 **tablespoon dried parsley flakes**
- ⅛ **teaspoon seasoned salt, optional**
    Dash pepper
- ¼ **cup shredded reduced-fat cheddar cheese**
- 2 **tablespoons chopped tomato**

1. In a large skillet, cook bacon over medium heat until crisp. Using a slotted spoon, remove to paper towels; drain, reserving 1 teaspoon drippings. In the drippings, cook broccoli and onion over medium heat for 2-3 minutes or until vegetables are tender. Add garlic; cook 1 minute longer.
2. In a small bowl, beat the egg substitute, parsley, seasoned salt if desired and pepper. Stir in bacon and broccoli mixture; add cheese and tomato.
3. Pour into two 10-oz. ramekins or custard cups coated with cooking spray. Bake at 400° for 22-25 minutes or until a knife inserted near the center comes out clean.
PER SERVING *1 quiche equals 170 cal., 8 g fat (4 g sat. fat), 24 mg chol., 576 mg sodium, 6 g carb., 1 g fiber, 18 g pro.*

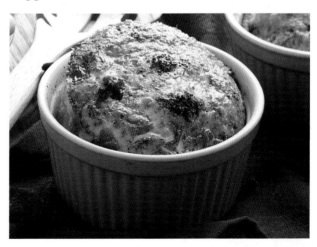

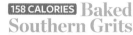 **Chocolate Chip Banana Muffins**

These yummy treats have lots of banana flavor. The chocolate chips disguise the whole wheat taste in the tender muffins. They're ideal for breakfast or an anytime snack with coffee.
—**LAUREN D. HEYN** OAK CREEK, WI

PREP: 15 MIN. • **BAKE:** 20 MIN.
MAKES: 1 DOZEN

- ¾ cup all-purpose flour
- ¾ cup whole wheat flour
- ½ cup wheat bran
- ½ cup packed brown sugar
- 1 teaspoon baking powder
- ¾ teaspoon baking soda
- ½ teaspoon salt
- 2 eggs, lightly beaten
- ¼ cup fat-free milk
- 1⅓ cups mashed ripe bananas (2 to 3 medium)
- ⅓ cup unsweetened applesauce
- 1 teaspoon vanilla extract
- ½ cup miniature chocolate chips
- ⅓ cup chopped pecans

1. In a large bowl, combine the first seven ingredients. In another bowl, combine the eggs, milk, bananas, applesauce and vanilla. Stir into dry ingredients just until moistened. Fold in chocolate chips.
2. Coat muffin cups with cooking spray; fill three-fourths full with batter. Sprinkle with pecans.
3. Bake at 375° for 18-22 minutes or until a toothpick inserted near the center comes out clean. Cool for 5 minutes before removing from pan to a wire rack. Serve warm.
PER SERVING *1 muffin equals 191 cal., 6 g fat (2 g sat. fat), 36 mg chol., 236 mg sodium, 33 g carb., 4 g fiber, 4 g pro.* **Diabetic Exchanges:** *2 starch, ½ fat.*

158 CALORIES **Baked Southern Grits**

I turn a Southern favorite into a tasty low-fat dish with this recipe. Jalapeno peppers add a welcome kick, while reduced-fat cheese creates a rich texture.
—**KAREN MAU** JACKSBORO, TN

PREP: 20 MIN. • **BAKE:** 30 MIN.
MAKES: 8 SERVINGS

- 4 cups water
- 1 cup quick-cooking grits
- 4 egg whites
- 2 eggs
- 1½ cups (6 ounces) shredded reduced-fat cheddar cheese
- ½ cup fat-free milk
- 1 to 2 jalapeno peppers, seeded and chopped
- ½ teaspoon garlic salt
- ¼ teaspoon white pepper
- 4 green onions, chopped, divided

1. In a large saucepan, bring water to a boil. Add grits; cook and stir over medium heat for 5 minutes or until thickened. Remove from the heat.
2. In a small bowl, whisk egg whites and eggs. Stir a small amount of hot grits into eggs; return all to the pan, stirring constantly. Stir in the cheese, milk, jalapenos, garlic salt, pepper and half of the onions.
3. Transfer to a 2-qt. baking dish coated with cooking spray. Bake, uncovered, at 350° for 30-35 minutes or until golden brown. Sprinkle with remaining onions.
NOTE *Wear disposable gloves when cutting hot peppers; the oils can burn skin. Avoid touching your face.*
PER SERVING *¾ cup equals 158 cal., 6 g fat (3 g sat. fat), 68 mg chol., 300 mg sodium, 17 g carb., 1 g fiber, 11 g pro.* **Diabetic Exchanges:** *1 starch, 1 lean meat, ½ fat.*

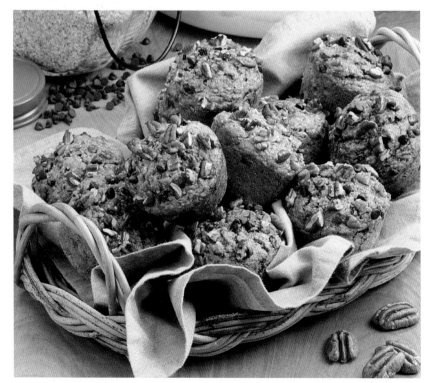

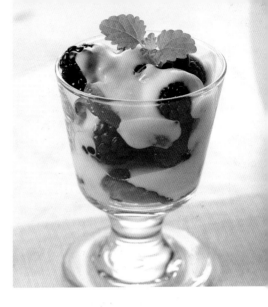

Baked Eggs with Cheddar and Bacon

Perfect for two, these little cups are super-easy to make and just the thing for a special breakfast. They're also very nice for a casual dinner. The smoky cheese and bacon elevate eggs to another level!

—CATHERINE WILKINSON DEWEY, AZ

START TO FINISH: 25 MIN.
MAKES: 2 SERVINGS

- 2 **eggs**
- 2 **tablespoons fat-free milk, divided**
- 1 **tablespoon shredded smoked cheddar cheese**
- 1 **teaspoon minced fresh parsley**
- ⅛ **teaspoon salt**
  Dash pepper
- 1 **bacon strip**

1. Coat two 4-oz. ramekins with cooking spray; break an egg into each dish. Spoon 1 tablespoon milk over each egg. Combine the cheese, parsley, salt and pepper; sprinkle over tops.

2. Bake, uncovered, at 325° for 12-15 minutes or until whites are completely set and yolks begin to thicken but are not firm.

3. Meanwhile, in a small skillet, cook bacon over medium heat until crisp. Remove to paper towels to drain. Crumble bacon and sprinkle over eggs.

PER SERVING *1 serving equals 107 cal., 7 g fat (3 g sat. fat), 219 mg chol., 319 mg sodium, 1 g carb., trace fiber, 9 g pro.*

Custard Berry Parfaits

Here's a low-fat dessert that captures the flavors of fresh-berry season. The homemade custard comes together in minutes, but seems like you fussed.

—TRISHA KRUSE EAGLE, ID

PREP: 25 MIN. + CHILLING
MAKES: 6 SERVINGS

- ¼ **cup sugar**
- 4 **teaspoons cornstarch**
- ¼ **teaspoon salt**
- 1⅔ **cups 1% milk**
- 2 **egg yolks, lightly beaten**
- ¾ **teaspoon vanilla extract**
- 3 **cups mixed fresh berries**

1. In a small saucepan, combine the sugar, cornstarch and salt. Stir in milk until smooth. Cook and stir over medium-high heat until thickened and bubbly. Reduce heat; cook and stir 2 minutes longer. Remove from the heat.

2. Stir a small amount of hot filling into egg yolks; return all to the pan, stirring constantly. Bring to a gentle boil; cook and stir 2 minutes longer. Remove from the heat.

3. Gently stir in vanilla. Cool to room temperature without stirring. Transfer to a bowl; press plastic wrap onto surface of custard. Refrigerate for at least 1 hour.

4. Just before serving, spoon ¼ cup of berries into each parfait glass; top with 2 tablespoons of custard. Repeat layers.

PER SERVING *½ cup berries with ¼ cup custard equals 119 cal., 3 g fat (1 g sat. fat), 74 mg chol., 137 mg sodium, 21 g carb., 3 g fiber, 4 g pro.* **Diabetic Exchanges:** *1 fruit, ½ starch, ½ fat.*

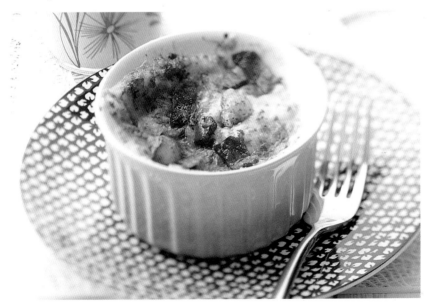

> ❝ I pack my gym bag the night before so I can just grab it in the morning and go to the gym right after work. ❞
> —NEO SENKGE

147 CALORIES Cherry Yogurt

Serve wholesome granola over our thick, rich yogurt for a quick breakfast. Or layer it in a parfait glass with granola and fruit. It will keep in the refrigerator for the week. Look for 100% cherry juice at the store, since the cocktail blends have added sugar.
—TASTE OF HOME TEST KITCHEN

PREP: 10 MIN. + CHILLING • **MAKES:** 3 CUPS

- 4 cups (32 ounces) reduced-fat plain yogurt
- 1 cup frozen pitted dark sweet cherries, thawed and quartered
- ½ cup cherry juice
- 3 tablespoons confectioners' sugar
- 1½ teaspoons vanilla extract

1. Line a strainer with four layers of cheesecloth or one coffee filter and place over a bowl. Place yogurt in prepared strainer; cover yogurt with edges of cheesecloth. Refrigerate for 8 hours or overnight.

2. Remove yogurt from cheesecloth and discard liquid from bowl. Place yogurt in a small bowl; stir in the remaining ingredients. Cover and refrigerate until serving.
PER SERVING *½ cup equals 147 cal., 3 g fat (2 g sat. fat), 10 mg chol., 115 mg sodium, 22 g carb., 1 g fiber, 9 g pro.* **Diabetic Exchanges:** *1 reduced-fat milk, ½ fruit.*

176 CALORIES Frittata Florentine

This recipe has huge flavor and is good for you! Thanks to the eggs, cheese and spinach, you get a dose of phosphorus and calcium, too, which contribute to healthier bones.
—JENNY FLAKE NEWPORT BEACH, CA

START TO FINISH: 30 MIN. • **MAKES:** 4 SERVINGS

- 6 egg whites
- 3 eggs
- ½ teaspoon dried oregano
- ¼ teaspoon garlic powder
- ¼ teaspoon salt
- ¼ teaspoon pepper
- 1 small onion, finely chopped
- ¼ cup finely chopped sweet red pepper
- 2 turkey bacon strips, chopped
- 1 tablespoon olive oil
- 1 cup fresh baby spinach
- 3 tablespoons thinly sliced fresh basil leaves
- ½ cup shredded part-skim mozzarella cheese

1. In a small bowl, whisk the first six ingredients; set aside. In an 8-in. ovenproof skillet, saute onion, red pepper and bacon in oil until tender. Reduce heat; top with spinach.

2. Pour reserved egg mixture over spinach. As eggs set, push cooked edges toward the center, letting uncooked portion flow underneath until eggs are nearly set. Sprinkle with basil and cheese.

3. Broil 3-4 in. from the heat for 2-3 minutes or until eggs are completely set. Let stand for 5 minutes. Cut into wedges.
PER SERVING *1 wedge equals 176 cal., 11 g fat (4 g sat. fat), 174 mg chol., 451 mg sodium, 4 g carb., 1 g fiber, 15 g pro.*

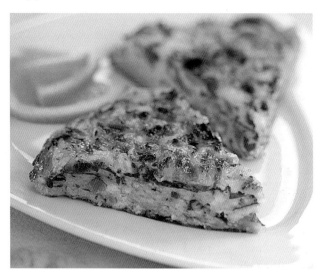

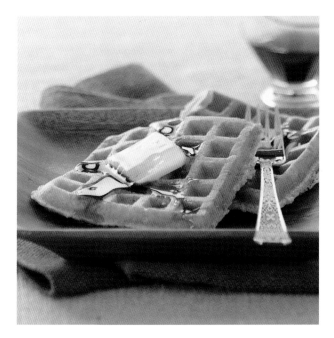

2. Bake in a preheated waffle iron according to manufacturer's directions until golden brown. Serve with butter and syrup if desired.

PER SERVING *2 waffles (calculated without butter and syrup) equals 187 cal., 7 g fat (2 g sat. fat), 52 mg chol., 336 mg sodium, 25 g carb., 2 g fiber, 7 g pro.* **Diabetic Exchanges:** *1½ starch, 1 fat.*

186 CALORIES Garlic Cheese Grits

Looking for the perfect brunch side dish? These grits are smooth, creamy, and full of flavor from the cheese and garlic.
—**ROSE TUTTLE** OVIEDO, FL

START TO FINISH: 20 MIN. • **MAKES:** 2 SERVINGS

- 1 cup water
- ¼ cup quick-cooking grits
- ½ cup reduced-fat process cheese (Velveeta)
- ¼ teaspoon garlic powder
- ¼ cup cornflakes, coarsely crushed
- 1 teaspoon butter, melted

1. In a saucepan, bring water to a boil. Slowly stir in grits. Reduce heat; cook and stir for 4-5 minutes or until thickened. Add cheese and garlic powder; stir until cheese is melted. Pour into greased 2-cup baking dish.
2. In a small bowl, combine cornflakes and butter; sprinkle over grits. Bake, uncovered, at 350° for 10-15 minutes or until firm and top is lightly toasted.

PER SERVING *¾ cup equals 186 cal., 7 g fat (4 g sat. fat), 20 mg chol., 662 mg sodium, 24 g carb., 1 g fiber, 9 g pro.* **Diabetic Exchanges:** *1½ starch, 1 medium-fat meat, ½ fat.*

187 CALORIES
Makeover Multigrain Waffles
These multigrain waffles are crispy, airy and lower in fat, calories and cholesterol than traditional butter-laden waffles. They don't, however, lack any of the great taste of the originals.
—**BETTY BLAIR** BARTLETT, TN

PREP: 15 MIN. • **COOK:** 5 MIN./BATCH • **MAKES:** 28 WAFFLES

- 1 cup all-purpose flour
- 1 cup whole wheat flour
- 1 cup cornmeal
- 1 tablespoon sugar
- 1 tablespoon baking powder
- ¾ teaspoon baking soda
- ½ teaspoon salt
- 3 eggs
- 4 egg whites
- 3 cups buttermilk
- ½ cup unsweetened applesauce
- 3 tablespoons canola oil
- 2 tablespoons butter, melted
  Butter and maple syrup, optional

1. In a large bowl, combine the first seven ingredients. In another bowl, whisk the eggs, egg whites, buttermilk, applesauce, oil and butter; whisk into dry ingredients just until blended.

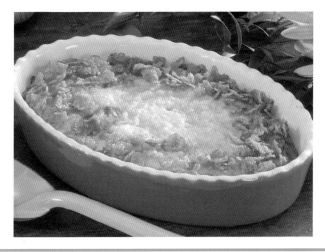

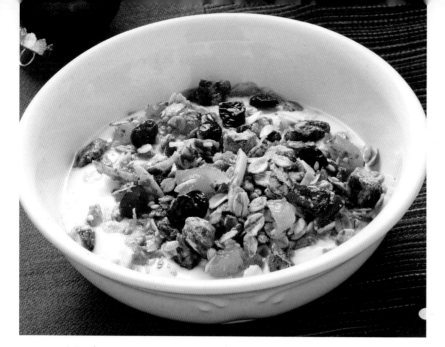

1 tube (12 ounces) refrigerated buttermilk biscuits
1 cup cubed fully cooked ham
1 cup leftover mashed potatoes
1 cup (4 ounces) shredded cheddar cheese, divided
½ teaspoon dried parsley flakes
¼ teaspoon garlic powder

1. Press each biscuit onto the bottom and up the sides of a greased muffin cup. In a large bowl, combine the ham, potatoes, ½ cup cheese, parsley and garlic powder.
2. Spoon ¼ cup into each prepared cup. Sprinkle with the remaining cheese. Bake at 350° for 20-25 minutes or until lightly browned. Serve warm. Refrigerate leftovers.
PER SERVING *1 potato puff equals 165 cal., 5 g fat (3 g sat. fat), 20 mg chol., 592 mg sodium, 21 g carb., trace fiber, 8 g pro.* **Diabetic Exchanges:** *1½ starch, 1 fat.*

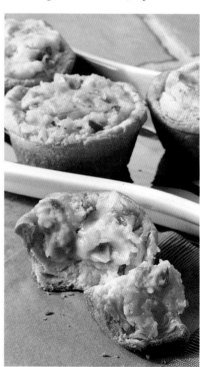

132 CALORIES
Paradise Granola

Even our 4-year-old, who isn't fond of dried fruit, enjoys this granola. It's low in fat, full of fiber and just plain delicious!
—**ROBYN LARABEE** LUCKNOW, ON

PREP: 20 MIN. • **BAKE:** 20 MIN. + COOLING
MAKES: 7 CUPS

2 cups old-fashioned oats
½ cup flaked coconut
½ cup toasted wheat germ
¼ cup oat bran
¼ cup sunflower kernels
¼ cup slivered almonds
¼ cup chopped pecans
2 tablespoons sesame seeds
¼ cup honey
2 tablespoons canola oil
2 tablespoons grated orange peel
1 teaspoon vanilla extract
½ teaspoon salt
1 cup dried cranberries
¾ cup chopped dates
½ cup chopped dried figs
½ cup chopped dried apricots
3 tablespoons raisins

1. In a large bowl, combine first eight ingredients. In a small bowl, whisk the honey, oil, orange peel, vanilla and salt; pour over oat mixture and mix well. Spread evenly into an ungreased 15-in. x 10-in. x 1-in. baking pan.
2. Bake at 350° for 20-25 minutes or until golden brown, stirring once. Cool completely on a wire rack. Stir in dried fruits. Store in an airtight container.
PER SERVING *¼ cup equals 132 cal., 5 g fat (1 g sat. fat), 0 chol., 57 mg sodium, 23 g carb., 3 g fiber, 3 g pro.* **Diabetic Exchanges:** *1 starch, ½ fruit, ½ fat.*

165 CALORIES
Ham Potato Puffs

Here's a different way to use up leftover mashed potatoes. It was an instant hit with our teenagers. They're also great for lunch with steamed green beans.
—**BRAD EICHELBERGER** YORK, PA

PREP: 20 MIN. • **BAKE:** 20 MIN.
MAKES: 10 PUFFS

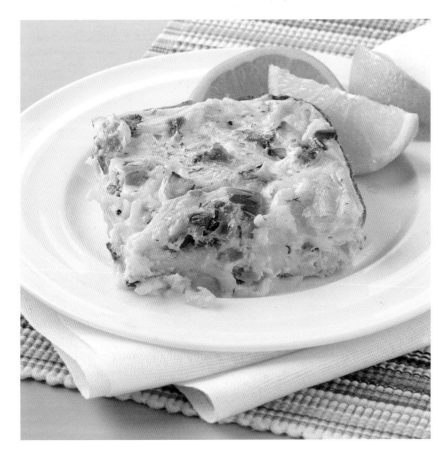

3. Transfer to a 13-in. x 9-in. baking dish coated with cooking spray. Bake, uncovered, at 350° for 30-35 minutes or until a knife inserted near the center comes out clean.

PER SERVING *1 piece equals 181 cal., 8 g fat (3 g sat. fat), 122 mg chol., 591 mg sodium, 11 g carb., 1 g fiber, 16 g pro.* **Diabetic Exchanges:** *2 lean meat, 1 starch.*

131 CALORIES Hawaiian Breakfast Cups

In Hawaii, this dish is called Hua Moa Pua'a lpu, meaning flower, cup and egg. The sweet and savory ham cup has a nice surprise inside with just a touch of mild salsa and sharp cheddar cheese.

—JUDY REAGAN HANNIBAL, MO

PREP: 15 MIN. • **BAKE:** 20 MIN.
MAKES: 6 SERVINGS

- 6 **thin slices deli ham**
- ¼ **cup shredded cheddar cheese**
- 2 **tablespoons mild salsa**
- 6 **canned pineapple slices**
- 6 **eggs**
- ½ **teaspoon salt-free seasoning blend**

1. Line six greased 8-oz. ramekins with ham. Layer each with cheese, salsa and pineapple. Crack an egg into the center of each cup; sprinkle with seasoning blend.

2. Place the ramekins on a baking sheet. Bake at 350° for 20-25 minutes or until the egg whites are completely set and the yolks still soft.

PER SERVING *1 breakfast cup equals 131 cal., 7 g fat (3 g sat. fat), 226 mg chol., 320 mg sodium, 6 g carb., trace fiber, 11 g pro.* **Diabetic Exchanges:** *2 medium-fat meat, ½ starch.*

181 CALORIES

Makeover Sunday Brunch Casserole

The *Taste of Home* Test Kitchen dramatically improved the nutritional value of my recipe for this hearty brunch item. It's wonderful because the staff managed to keep the casserole's core flavors and ingredients intact!
—ALICE HOFMANN SUSSEX, WI

PREP: 20 MIN. • **BAKE:** 30 MIN.
MAKES: 8 SERVINGS

- 6 **bacon strips**
- 1 **small onion, chopped**
- 1 **small green pepper, chopped**
- 1 **teaspoon canola oil**
- 2 **cartons (8 ounces each) egg substitute**
- 4 **eggs**
- 1 **cup fat-free milk**
- 4 **cups frozen shredded hash brown potatoes, thawed**
- 1 **cup (4 ounces) shredded reduced-fat cheddar cheese**
- ¾ **teaspoon salt**
- ½ **teaspoon pepper**
- ¼ **teaspoon dill weed**

1. In a large skillet, cook bacon over medium heat until crisp. Remove to paper towels; drain. Crumble bacon and set aside. In the same skillet, saute onion and green pepper in oil until tender; remove with a slotted spoon.

2. In a large bowl, whisk the egg substitute, eggs and milk. Stir in the hash browns, cheese, salt, pepper, dill, onion mixture and reserved bacon.

201-300 CALORIES

202 CALORIES Makeover Toasted Granola

My family likes this granola in so many ways. We sprinkle it over yogurt and ice cream, we eat it with milk like cereal, and we love to just eat it right from the container!

—SUSAN LAJEUNESSE COLCHESTER, VT

PREP: 20 MIN. • **BAKE:** 1¼ HOURS + COOLING • **MAKES:** 10½ CUPS

- 1 cup packed brown sugar
- ⅓ cup water
- 4 cups old-fashioned oats
- 2 cups bran flakes
- 1 jar (12 ounces) toasted wheat germ
- 2 tablespoons all-purpose flour
- ¾ teaspoon salt
- ⅓ cup canola oil
- 2 teaspoons vanilla extract

1. In a large saucepan, bring brown sugar and water to a boil. Cook and stir until sugar is dissolved. Remove from heat; set aside. In a large bowl, combine oats, bran flakes, wheat germ, flour and salt. Stir oil and vanilla into sugar mixture; pour over oat mixture and toss to coat.

2. Transfer to two 15-in. x 10-in. x 1-in. baking pans coated with cooking spray. Bake at 250° for 1¼ to 1½ hours or until dry and lightly browned, stirring every 15 minutes. Cool completely on wire racks. Store in an airtight container.

PER SERVING *½ cup equals 202 cal., 6 g fat (1 g sat. fat), 0 chol., 118 mg sodium, 32 g carb., 4 g fiber, 8 g pro.* **Diabetic Exchanges:** *2 starch, 1 fat.*

277 CALORIES

Baked Blueberry & Peach Oatmeal

Baked oatmeal is a staple in our home. It's very easy to prepare the night before—just keep the dry and wet ingredients separate until ready to bake. I've tried a variety of fruits, but blueberry and peach is our favorite combination.

—ROSEMARIE WELESKI NATRONA HEIGHTS, PA

PREP: 20 MIN. • **BAKE:** 35 MIN. • **MAKES:** 9 SERVINGS

- 3 cups old-fashioned oats
- ½ cup packed brown sugar
- 2 teaspoons baking powder
- ½ teaspoon salt
- 2 egg whites
- 1 egg
- 1¼ cups fat-free milk
- ¼ cup canola oil
- 1 teaspoon vanilla extract
- 1 can (15 ounces) sliced peaches in juice, drained and chopped
- 1 cup fresh or frozen blueberries
- ⅓ cup chopped walnuts
  Additional fat-free milk, optional

1. In a large bowl, combine the oats, brown sugar, baking powder and salt. Whisk the egg whites, egg, milk, oil and vanilla; add to dry ingredients and stir until blended. Let stand for 5 minutes. Stir in peaches and blueberries.

2. Transfer to an 11-in. x 7-in. baking dish coated with cooking spray. Sprinkle with walnuts. Bake, uncovered, at 350° for 35-40 minutes or until top is lightly browned and a thermometer reads 160°. Serve with additional milk if desired.

PER SERVING *1 serving (calculated without additional milk) equals 277 cal., 11 g fat (1 g sat. fat), 24 mg chol., 263 mg sodium, 38 g carb., 3 g fiber, 8 g pro.* **Diabetic Exchanges:** *2 starch, 2 fat, ½ fruit.*

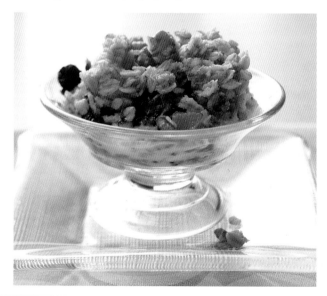

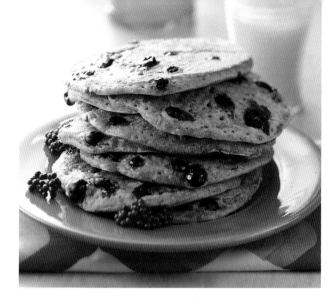

221 CALORIES Blueberry Oat Pancakes

I grind my own oats for this recipe, which makes the pancakes light and fluffy. And, you get plenty of bursting-with-flavor blueberries in every bite!
—**CANDY SUMMERHILL** ALEXANDER, AR

PREP: 20 MIN. • **COOK:** 5 MIN./BATCH • **MAKES:** 10 PANCAKES

- ¾ **cup quick-cooking oats, divided**
- 3 **tablespoons orange juice**
- 1 **egg, lightly beaten**
- ⅔ **cup fat-free evaporated milk**
- ¼ **cup reduced-fat sour cream**
- 2 **tablespoons unsweetened applesauce**
- ½ **teaspoon vanilla extract**
- ½ **cup whole wheat flour**
- ¼ **cup all-purpose flour**
- 3 **tablespoons brown sugar**
- 1 **teaspoon baking powder**
- ½ **teaspoon ground cinnamon**
- ¼ **teaspoon salt**
- ¼ **teaspoon baking soda**
- 1 **cup fresh or frozen unsweetened blueberries**

1. In a small bowl, combine ¼ cup oats and orange juice; let stand for 5 minutes. Stir in the egg, milk, sour cream, applesauce and vanilla; set aside.
2. Place remaining oats in a small food processor; cover and process until ground. Place in a large bowl; add flours, brown sugar, baking powder, cinnamon, salt and baking soda. Stir in wet ingredients just until moistened.
3. Pour batter by ¼ cupfuls onto a hot griddle coated with cooking spray; sprinkle with blueberries. Turn when bubbles form on top; cook until second side is golden brown.
PER SERVING *2 pancakes equals 221 cal., 3 g fat (1 g sat. fat), 48 mg chol., 327 mg sodium, 41 g carb., 4 g fiber, 9 g pro.* **Diabetic Exchanges:** *2 starch, ½ fruit, ½ fat.*

237 CALORIES Mango Smoothies

Treat yourself to this yummy blend of mango, pineapple, banana and honey. The yogurt makes it rich and creamy, but it only has 2 grams of fat!
—**TASTE OF HOME TEST KITCHEN**

START TO FINISH: 10 MIN. • **MAKES:** 2 SERVINGS

- ½ **cup unsweetened pineapple juice**
- 2 **cups frozen chopped peeled mangoes**
- ½ **medium ripe banana**
- ½ **cup reduced-fat plain yogurt**
- 1 **tablespoon honey**

In a blender, combine all ingredients; cover and process until smooth. Pour into chilled glasses; serve immediately.
PER SERVING *1 cup equals 237 cal., 2 g fat (1 g sat. fat), 4 mg chol., 48 mg sodium, 56 g carb., 4 g fiber, 5 g pro.*

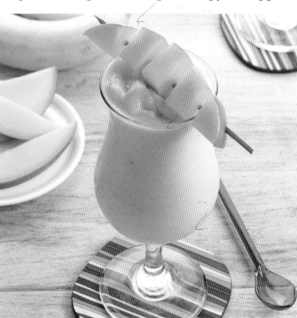

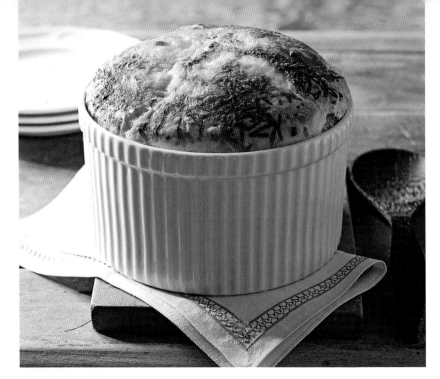

223 CALORIES Florence-Inspired Souffle

This souffle is not only absolutely delicious, but also light and beautiful. Your guests will be impressed every time it is served. So grab your fork and dig in to this little taste of Florence!

—JENNY FLAKE NEWPORT BEACH, CA

PREP: 35 MIN. • **BAKE:** 35 MIN.
MAKES: 4 SERVINGS

- 6 egg whites
- ¾ cup onion and garlic salad croutons
- 1 small onion, finely chopped
- ¼ cup finely chopped sweet red pepper
- 2 ounces thinly sliced prosciutto, chopped
- 2 teaspoons olive oil
- 2 cups fresh baby spinach
- 1 garlic clove, minced
- ⅓ cup all-purpose flour
- ½ teaspoon salt
- ¼ teaspoon pepper
- 1¼ cups fat-free milk
- 1 egg yolk, lightly beaten
- ¼ teaspoon cream of tartar
- ¼ cup shredded Italian cheese blend

1. Place egg whites in a large bowl; let stand at room temperature for 30 minutes.
2. In a food processor, process croutons until ground. Sprinkle evenly onto the bottom and 1 in. up the sides of a greased 2-qt. souffle dish; set aside.
3. In a large saucepan, saute the onion, red pepper and prosciutto in oil until vegetables are crisp-tender. Add the spinach and garlic; cook just until spinach is wilted. Stir in the flour, salt and pepper until blended. Gradually add milk. Bring to a boil; cook and stir for 2 minutes or until thickened.
4. Transfer to a large bowl. Stir a small amount of hot mixture into egg yolk; return all to the bowl, stirring constantly. Cool slightly.
5. Add cream of tartar to egg whites; beat until stiff peaks form. Fold into vegetable mixture. Transfer to prepared dish; sprinkle with cheese.
6. Bake at 350° for 35-40 minutes or until top is puffed and center appears set. Serve immediately.

PER SERVING 1 serving equals 223 cal., 9 g fat (3 g sat. fat), 73 mg chol., 843 mg sodium, 20 g carb., 2 g fiber, 16 g pro. **Diabetic Exchanges:** 2 lean meat, 1½ starch.

228 CALORIES Dried Fruit Muesli

Give your day a healthful start by enjoying this old-fashioned chilled cereal. Filled with wholesome ingredients, it sits in the fridge overnight for the perfect morning pick-me-up. Switch up the nuts or fruit to your liking.

—TASTE OF HOME TEST KITCHEN

PREP: 10 MIN. + CHILLING
MAKES: 4 SERVINGS

- 1 cup quick-cooking oats
- 1 cup fat-free milk
- ¼ cup orange juice
- ¼ cup chopped dried apricots
- ¼ cup dried cranberries
- ¼ cup chopped dried apples
- 2 tablespoons chopped almonds
- 2 tablespoons honey
- ⅛ teaspoon salt
- ⅛ teaspoon ground cinnamon

In a large bowl, combine all ingredients. Cover and refrigerate for at least 8 hours or overnight.

PER SERVING ½ cup equals 228 cal., 4 g fat (trace sat. fat), 1 mg chol., 112 mg sodium, 43 g carb., 4 g fiber, 7 g pro. **Diabetic Exchanges:** 1½ starch, 1 fruit, ½ fat-free milk, ½ fat.

Fruited Dutch Baby

Here's a sensational way to showcase fruit for a holiday breakfast or brunch. If you prefer, sprinkle the oven-baked pancake with powdered sugar or serve it with canned pie filling or other fruit.
—**SHIRLEY ROBERTSON** VERSAILLES, MO

START TO FINISH: 30 MIN.
MAKES: 6 SERVINGS

- 1 **tablespoon butter**
- ¾ **cup all-purpose flour**
- 1 **tablespoon sugar**
- ¼ **teaspoon salt**
- 3 **eggs, lightly beaten**
- ¾ **cup 2% milk**
- 1½ **cups sliced fresh strawberries**
- 2 **medium firm bananas, sliced**
  Whipped cream, optional
- ¼ **cup flaked coconut, toasted**

1. Place butter in a 9-in. pie plate. Place in a 400° oven for 5 minutes or until melted. Meanwhile, in a large bowl, combine the flour, sugar and salt. Stir in eggs and milk until smooth. Pour into prepared pie plate. Bake for 15-20 minutes or until golden brown.

2. In a large bowl, combine strawberries and bananas. Using a slotted spoon, place fruit in center of pancake. Top with whipped cream if desired. Sprinkle with coconut. Serve immediately.

PER SERVING *1 piece (calculated without whipped cream) equals 203 cal., 7 g fat (4 g sat. fat), 114 mg chol., 170 mg sodium, 30 g carb., 2 g fiber, 7 g pro.* **Diabetic Exchanges:** *1½ starch, 1 fat, ½ fruit.*

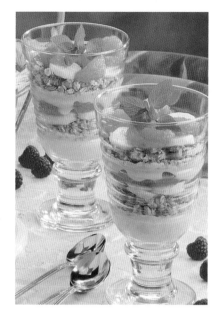

Breakfast Sundaes

Kids of all ages will love the layers of creamy yogurt, crunchy granola, banana slices and mandarin oranges in this dish. It sweetens the morning meal but is just as refreshing as a healthful dessert or after-school snack.
—**LINDA FRANCESCHI** ELDRED, NY

START TO FINISH: 10 MIN.
MAKES: 4 SERVINGS

- 2 **cups (16 ounces) fat-free raspberry yogurt or flavored yogurt of your choice**
- 1 **cup reduced-fat granola cereal**
- 2 **medium firm bananas, sliced**
- 1 **can (15 ounces) mandarin oranges, drained**

In four parfait glasses or bowls, layer half of the yogurt, granola, bananas and oranges. Repeat layers. Serve immediately.

PER SERVING *1 serving equals 266 cal., 2 g fat (trace sat. fat), 3 mg chol., 130 mg sodium, 57 g carb., 6 g fiber, 9 g pro.*

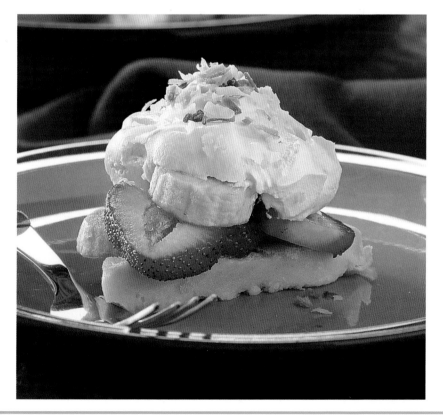

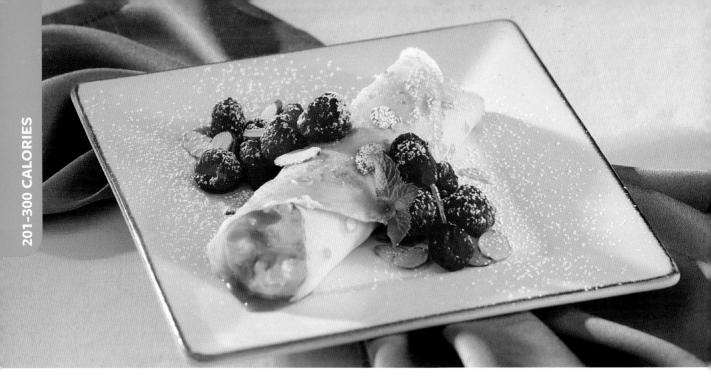

206 CALORIES

Caramel Cream Crepes

These lovely homemade crepes with a creamy caramel filling are a cinch to whip up. And they boast a flavor that guests are sure to rave about.

—TASTE OF HOME TEST KITCHEN

PREP: 20 MIN. + CHILLING
COOK: 15 MIN. • **MAKES:** 6 SERVINGS

- 6 tablespoons fat-free milk
- 6 tablespoons egg substitute
- 1½ teaspoons butter, melted
- ½ teaspoon vanilla extract
- 6 tablespoons all-purpose flour
- 6 ounces fat-free cream cheese
- 3 tablespoons plus 6 teaspoons fat-free caramel ice cream topping, divided
- 2¼ cups reduced-fat whipped topping
- 1½ cups fresh raspberries
- ⅓ cup white wine or unsweetened apple juice
- 3 tablespoons sliced almonds, toasted

1. In a blender, combine the milk, egg substitute, butter and vanilla; cover and process until blended. Add the flour; cover and process until blended. Cover and refrigerate for 1 hour.

2. Lightly coat a 6-in. nonstick skillet with cooking spray; heat over medium heat. Pour about 2 tablespoons of batter into center of skillet; lift and tilt pan to evenly coat bottom. Cook until top appears dry and bottom is golden; turn and cook 15-20 seconds longer. Remove to a wire rack. Repeat with remaining batter. Stack cooled crepes with waxed paper or paper towels in between.

3. In a small bowl, beat cream cheese and 3 tablespoons caramel topping until smooth. Fold in whipped topping. Spoon down the center of each crepe. Drizzle with remaining caramel topping; roll up.

4. In a small microwave-safe bowl, combine raspberries and wine.

Microwave on high 30-60 seconds or until warm. Using a slotted spoon, place berries over crepes. Sprinkle with almonds.

PER SERVING *1 serving equals 206 cal., 6 g fat (4 g sat. fat), 5 mg chol., 227 mg sodium, 25 g carb., 3 g fiber, 8 g pro.* **Diabetic Exchanges:** *1½ starch, 1 lean meat, 1 fat.*

267 CALORIES # Peach-Stuffed French Toast

With make-ahead convenience and scrumptious flavor, my recipe is ideal for holiday brunches. It's great for busy hostesses with a crowd to feed!

—JULIE ROBINSON LITTLE CHUTE, WI

PREP: 25 MIN. + CHILLING
BAKE: 25 MIN. • **MAKES:** 10 SERVINGS

- 1 loaf (1 pound) French bread, cut into 20 slices
- 1 can (15 ounces) sliced peaches in extra-light syrup, drained and chopped
- ¼ cup chopped pecans

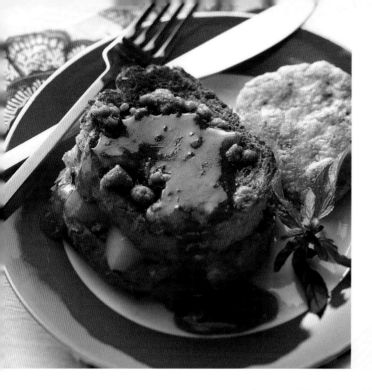
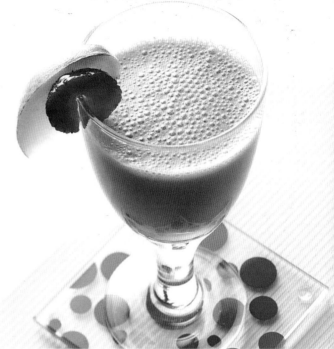

4 eggs
4 egg whites
1½ cups fat-free milk
3 tablespoons sugar
1¼ teaspoons ground cinnamon, divided
1 teaspoon vanilla extract
¼ cup all-purpose flour
2 tablespoons brown sugar
2 tablespoons cold butter
Reduced-calorie pancake syrup, optional

1. Arrange half of the bread in a 13-in. x 9-in. baking dish coated with cooking spray. Top with peaches, pecans and remaining bread.
2. In a small bowl, whisk the eggs, egg whites, milk, sugar, 1 teaspoon cinnamon and vanilla; pour over bread. Cover and refrigerate for 8 hours or overnight.
3. Remove from the refrigerator 30 minutes before baking. Bake, uncovered, at 400° for 20 minutes.

4. In a small bowl, combine the flour, brown sugar and remaining cinnamon; cut in butter until crumbly. Sprinkle over French toast. Bake 5-10 minutes longer or until a knife inserted near the center comes out clean. Serve with syrup if desired.

PER SERVING *1 piece (calculated without syrup) equals 267 cal., 8 g fat (3 g sat. fat), 92 mg chol., 368 mg sodium, 39 g carb., 2 g fiber, 10 g pro.* **Diabetic Exchanges:** *2½ starch, 1½ fat.*

`225 CALORIES`
Yogurt Fruit Smoothies

There's nothing more refreshing for a quick morning meal than a cold fruit smoothie. This is one recipe you will keep in the front of your cookbook because you'll want to use it for all different occasions! I'm thrilled to share it with fellow cooks who love to wow their brunch guests.
—**JENNY FLAKE** NEWPORT BEACH, CA

START TO FINISH: 10 MIN.
MAKES: 6 SERVINGS

1 can (11½ ounces) frozen strawberry breeze juice concentrate, thawed
1 cup (8 ounces) vanilla yogurt
½ cup milk
1 tablespoon honey
1 teaspoon vanilla extract
1 pint fresh strawberries, hulled
1 large banana, cut into chunks
1 cup chopped peeled fresh or frozen peaches
1 cup crushed ice

Place half of all ingredients in a blender; cover and process for 15 seconds or until smooth. Pour into chilled glasses. Repeat with the remaining ingredients. Serve smoothies immediately.

PER SERVING *¾ cup equals 225 cal., 1 g fat (1 g sat. fat), 4 mg chol., 38 mg sodium, 51 g carb., 2 g fiber, 4 g pro.*

258 CALORIES Brunch Enchiladas

Here's a fun change-of-pace way to start the day! Hostesses with overnight guests will love its make-ahead convenience.

—**GAIL SYKORA** MENOMONEE FALLS, WI

PREP: 15 MIN. + CHILLING • **BAKE:** 40 MIN. + STANDING
MAKES: 10 SERVINGS

- 2 **cups cubed fully cooked ham**
- ½ **cup chopped green onions**
- 10 **fat-free flour tortillas (8 inches)**
- 2 **cups (8 ounces) shredded reduced-fat cheddar cheese**
- 1 **tablespoon all-purpose flour**
- 2 **cups fat-free milk**
- 1½ **cups egg substitute**

1. Combine ham and onions; place about ⅓ cup down the center of each tortilla. Top with 2 tablespoons of cheese. Roll up and place seam side down in a greased 13-in. x 9-in. baking dish.

2. In a large bowl, whisk the flour, milk and eggs until smooth. Pour over tortillas. Cover and refrigerate for 8 hours or overnight.

3. Remove from the refrigerator 30 minutes before baking. Cover and bake at 350° for 25 minutes. Uncover; bake 10 minutes longer. Sprinkle with remaining cheese; bake for 3 minutes or until cheese is melted. Let stand for 10 minutes before serving.

PER SERVING *1 enchilada equals 258 cal., 7 g fat (4 g sat. fat), 32 mg chol., 838 mg sodium, 29 g carb., 1 g fiber, 19 g pro.*

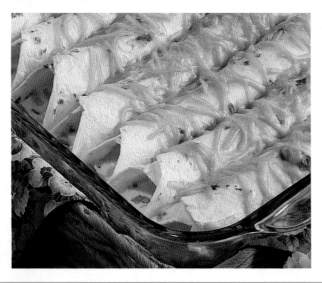

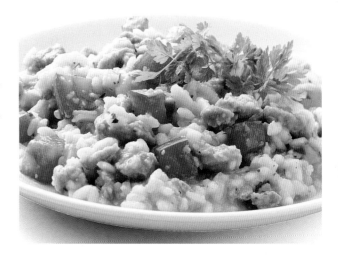

279 CALORIES Brunch Risotto

This light, flavorful and inexpensive risotto makes a surprising addition to a traditional brunch menu. It's gotten lots of compliments from my friends.

—**JENNIFER DINES** BRIGHTON, MA

PREP: 10 MIN. • **COOK:** 30 MIN. • **MAKES:** 8 SERVINGS

- 5¼ to 5¾ **cups reduced-sodium chicken broth**
- ¾ **pound Italian turkey sausage links, casings removed**
- 2 **cups uncooked arborio rice**
- 1 **garlic clove, minced**
- ¼ **teaspoon pepper**
- 1 **tablespoon olive oil**
- 1 **medium tomato, chopped**

1. In a large saucepan, heat broth and keep warm. In a large nonstick skillet, cook sausage until no longer pink; drain and set aside.

2. In the same skillet, saute the rice, garlic and pepper in oil for 2-3 minutes. Return sausage to skillet. Carefully stir in 1 cup heated broth. Cook and stir until all of the liquid is absorbed.

3. Add remaining broth, ½ cup at a time, stirring constantly. Allow liquid to absorb between additions. Cook just until risotto is creamy and rice is almost tender. Total cooking time is about 20 minutes. Add tomato and heat through. Serve immediately.

PER SERVING *⅔ cup equals 279 cal., 6 g fat (2 g sat. fat), 23 mg chol., 653 mg sodium, 42 g carb., 1 g fiber, 12 g pro.* **Diabetic Exchanges:** *2½ starch, 1 lean meat, ½ fat.*

256 CALORIES Harvest Vegetable Tart

When guests lay eyes on this lightened-up veggie tart, they immediately approve. I've been serving it for over 30 years. The robust taste and attractive appearance always get a warm reception.

—RUTH LEE TROY, ON

PREP: 45 MIN. + CHILLING • **BAKE:** 30 MIN. • **MAKES:** 6 SERVINGS

- ½ cup all-purpose flour
- ¼ cup whole wheat flour
- ¼ cup cornmeal
- 2 tablespoons grated Parmesan cheese
- ½ teaspoon salt
- ⅛ teaspoon cayenne pepper
- ¼ cup cold butter, cubed
- 3 to 4 tablespoons cold water

FILLING
- ½ cup thinly sliced green onions
- 2 garlic cloves, minced
- 1 tablespoon olive oil
- 5 slices peeled eggplant (3½ inches x ¼ inch)
- 2 tablespoons grated Parmesan cheese, divided
- 1 small tomato, cut into ¼-inch slices
- 3 green pepper rings
- 3 sweet red pepper rings
- ½ cup frozen corn
- 2 eggs, lightly beaten
- ⅔ cup fat-free evaporated milk
- ¾ teaspoon salt
- ¼ teaspoon pepper

1. In a bowl, combine the first six ingredients. Cut in butter until crumbly. Gradually add water, tossing with a fork until dough forms a ball. Cover and refrigerate for at least 30 minutes.

2. Roll out pastry to fit a 9-in. tart pan with removable bottom. Transfer pastry to pan; trim even with edge of pan. Line unpricked pastry shell with a double thickness of heavy-duty foil. Bake at 450° for 8 minutes. Remove foil; bake 5 minutes longer.

3. In a large nonstick skillet coated with cooking spray, cook onions and garlic in oil for 2 minutes. Add eggplant; cook for 4-5 minutes or until softened. Cool for 5 minutes. Spoon into crust. Sprinkle with 1 tablespoon Parmesan cheese. Top with tomato slices and pepper rings. Sprinkle with corn.

4. In a small bowl, whisk the eggs, milk, salt and pepper; pour over vegetables. Sprinkle with remaining Parmesan cheese. Bake at 350° for 30-35 minutes or until a knife inserted near the center comes out clean.

PER SERVING *1 piece equals 256 cal., 13 g fat (6 g sat. fat), 95 mg chol., 691 mg sodium, 27 g carb., 3 g fiber, 9 g pro.* **Diabetic Exchanges:** *2 fat, 1½ starch, 1 vegetable.*

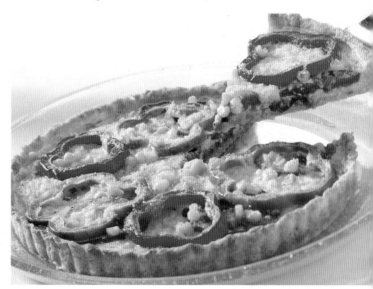

216 CALORIES Eggs Benedict

My mock hollandaise sauce is smooth and creamy—and so much healthier than the regular version.

—REBECCA BAIRD SALT LAKE CITY, UT

PREP: 25 MIN. • **COOK:** 15 MIN.
MAKES: 8 SERVINGS

- 8 slices Canadian bacon
- 8 eggs

HOLLANDAISE SAUCE
- 2 tablespoons all-purpose flour
- ¼ teaspoon salt
- ¼ teaspoon ground mustard
- ⅛ teaspoon cayenne pepper
- ½ cup fat-free milk
- ½ cup fat-free evaporated milk
- 1 egg yolk, lightly beaten
- 1 tablespoon butter-flavored sprinkles
- 1 tablespoon lemon juice
- 4 whole wheat English muffins, split and toasted

1. In a large nonstick skillet coated with cooking spray, brown bacon on both sides; remove and keep warm.
2. Place 2-3 in. of water in a large skillet with high sides. Bring to a boil; reduce heat and simmer gently. Break cold eggs, one at a time, into a custard cup or saucer; holding the cup close to the surface of the water, slip each egg into water. Cook, uncovered, until whites are completely set and yolks begin to thicken but are not hard, about 4 minutes.
3. Meanwhile, in a small saucepan, combine the flour, salt, mustard and cayenne. Gradually stir in milk and evaporated milk until smooth. Bring to a boil; cook and stir for 1-2 minutes or until thickened. Remove from the heat.
4. Stir a small amount of sauce into egg yolk; return all to the pan, stirring constantly. Bring to a gentle boil; cook and stir for 2 minutes. Remove from the heat; stir in butter-flavored sprinkles and lemon juice.
5. With a slotted spoon, lift each egg out of the water. Top each muffin half with a slice of bacon, an egg and 2 tablespoons sauce. Serve immediately.

NOTE *This recipe was tested with Molly McButter. Look for it in the spice aisle.*

PER SERVING *1 serving equals 216 cal., 8 g fat (3 g sat. fat), 252 mg chol., 752 mg sodium, 19 g carb., 2 g fiber, 17 g pro.* **Diabetic Exchanges:** *2 medium-fat meat, 1 starch.*

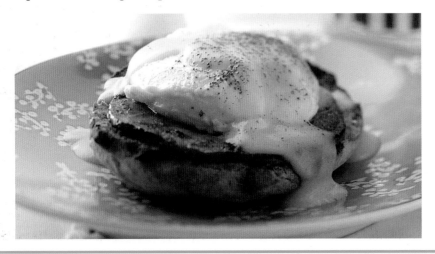

249 CALORIES Puffy Apple Omelet

This is one omelet you won't forget because of its unique and delicious flavors. Yum!

—MELISSA DAVENPORT CAMPBELL, MN

PREP: 15 MIN. • **BAKE:** 20 MIN.
MAKES: 2 SERVINGS

- 3 tablespoons all-purpose flour
- ¼ teaspoon baking powder
- 2 eggs, separated
- 3 tablespoons fat-free milk
- 1 tablespoon lemon juice
- 3 tablespoons sugar

TOPPING
- 1 large tart apple, peeled and thinly sliced
- 1 teaspoon sugar
- ¼ teaspoon ground cinnamon

1. In a small bowl, combine flour and baking powder. In another bowl, whisk egg yolks, milk and lemon juice; add to dry ingredients and mix well. Set aside.
2. In a small bowl, beat egg whites on medium speed until soft peaks form. Gradually beat in the sugar, 1 tablespoon as a time, on high until stiff peaks form. Fold into yolk mixture.
3. Pour into a shallow 1½-qt. baking dish coated with cooking spray. Arrange apple slices on top. Combine sugar and cinnamon; sprinkle over apples.
4. Bake, uncovered, at 375° for 18-20 minutes or until a knife inserted near center comes out clean. Cut in half.

PER SERVING *1 serving equals 249 cal., 5 g fat (2 g sat. fat), 212 mg chol., 130 mg sodium, 44 g carb., 2 g fiber, 9 g pro.* **Diabetic Exchanges:** *2 starch, 1 lean meat, 1 fruit.*

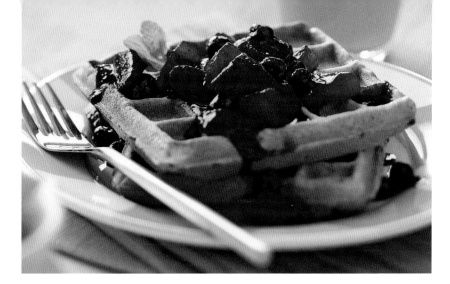

251 CALORIES Waffles with Peach-Berry Compote

I created my compote recipe one summer Sunday when I was looking for a more healthful alternative to butter and maple syrup to top my waffles. I was amazed at the results!

—**BRANDI WATERS** FAYETTEVILLE, AR

PREP: 25 MIN. • **COOK:** 5 MIN./BATCH
MAKES: 12 WAFFLES (1½ CUPS COMPOTE)

- 1 **cup chopped peeled fresh or frozen peaches**
- ½ **cup orange juice**
- 2 **tablespoons brown sugar**
- ¼ **teaspoon ground cinnamon**
- 1 **cup fresh or frozen blueberries**
- ½ **cup sliced fresh or frozen strawberries**

BATTER

- 1¼ **cups all-purpose flour**
- ½ **cup whole wheat flour**
- 2 **tablespoons flaxseed**
- 1 **teaspoon baking powder**
- 1 **teaspoon baking soda**
- ½ **teaspoon ground cinnamon**
- 1 **cup buttermilk**
- ¾ **cup orange juice**
- 1 **tablespoon canola oil**
- 1 **teaspoon vanilla extract**

1. In a small saucepan, combine the peaches, orange juice, brown sugar and cinnamon; bring to a boil over medium heat. Add berries; cook and stir for 8-10 minutes or until compote is thickened.

2. In a large bowl, combine the flours, flaxseed, baking powder, baking soda and cinnamon. Combine the buttermilk, orange juice, oil and vanilla; stir into dry ingredients just until moistened.

3. Bake in a preheated waffle iron according to manufacturer's directions until golden brown. Serve with compote.

PER SERVING *2 waffles with ¼ cup compote equals 251 cal., 4 g fat (1 g sat. fat), 2 mg chol., 324 mg sodium, 47 g carb., 4 g fiber, 7 g pro.* **Diabetic Exchanges:** *2½ starch, ½ fruit, ½ fat.*

285 CALORIES Blueberry French Toast

The original recipe called for heavy cream and whole eggs, but my lightened-up version still has plenty of delicious taste.

—**NANCY ARGO** UNIONTOWN, OH

PREP: 20 MIN. • **BAKE:** 20 MIN.
MAKES: 6 SERVINGS

- ½ **cup sugar**
- 2½ **teaspoons cornstarch**
- 1 **teaspoon ground cinnamon**
- ¼ **teaspoon ground allspice**
- ¾ **cup water**
- 4 **cups fresh or frozen blueberries**
- 1 **cup egg substitute**
- 1 **cup fat-free milk**
- 1 **teaspoon vanilla extract**
- ½ **teaspoon salt**
- 12 **slices French bread (1 inch thick)**

1. In a large bowl, combine the sugar, cornstarch, cinnamon and allspice; stir in water until smooth. Add blueberries; mix well. Transfer to a 13-in. x 9-in. baking dish coated with cooking spray.

2. In a large bowl, beat the egg substitute, milk, vanilla and salt. Dip each slice of bread into egg mixture; arrange slices over berries.

3. Bake at 400° for 20-25 minutes or until toast is golden brown and blueberries are bubbly.

PER SERVING *2 slices with about ½ cup blueberries equals 285 cal., 2 g fat (trace sat. fat), 1 mg chol., 575 mg sodium, 58 g carb., 4 g fiber, 10 g pro.*

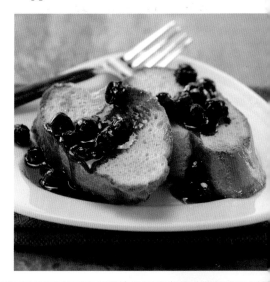

211 CALORIES — Silver Dollar Oat Pancakes

I combined two of my grandson Joshua's favorite foods—applesauce and oatmeal—into these wholesome little pancakes. He likes their fun size.
—MARGARET WILSON SUN CITY, CA

START TO FINISH: 25 MIN. • **MAKES:** 4 SERVINGS

- ½ cup all-purpose flour
- ½ cup quick-cooking oats
- 1½ teaspoons sugar
- 1 teaspoon baking powder
- ½ teaspoon baking soda
- ½ teaspoon salt
- 1 egg
- ¾ cup buttermilk
- ½ cup cinnamon applesauce
- 2 tablespoons butter, melted
  Maple syrup or topping of your choice

1. In a large bowl, combine the dry ingredients. In a small bowl, beat the egg, buttermilk, applesauce and butter; stir into dry ingredients just until moistened.

2. Pour batter by 2 tablespoonfuls onto a hot griddle coated with cooking spray; turn when bubbles form on top. Cook until second side is golden brown. Serve with maple syrup.

PER SERVING *5 pancakes (calculated without syrup) equals 211 cal., 8 g fat (4 g sat. fat), 70 mg chol., 660 mg sodium, 29 g carb., 2 g fiber, 6 g pro.* **Diabetic Exchanges:** *2 starch, 1½ fat.*

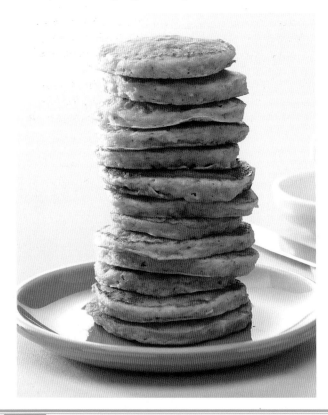

207 CALORIES — Confetti Scrambled Egg Pockets

This sunny specialty is a definite crowd-pleaser. My eight grandchildren often enjoy these egg-packed pitas for Saturday morning brunch...or with a light salad for supper. They love the combination of fresh veggies and scrambled eggs tucked inside fun-to-eat sandwiches.
—DIXIE TERRY GOREVILLE, IL

START TO FINISH: 20 MIN. • **MAKES:** 6 SERVINGS

- 1 cup fresh or frozen corn
- ¼ cup chopped green pepper
- 2 tablespoons chopped onion
- 1 jar (2 ounces) diced pimientos, drained
- 1 tablespoon butter
- 1¼ cups egg substitute
- 3 eggs
- ¼ cup fat-free evaporated milk
- ½ teaspoon seasoned salt
- 1 medium tomato, seeded and chopped
- 1 green onion, sliced
- 6 whole wheat pita pocket halves

1. In a large nonstick skillet, saute the corn, green pepper, onion and pimientos in butter for 5-7 minutes or until tender.

2. In a large bowl, combine the egg substitute, eggs, milk and salt; pour into skillet. Cook and stir over medium heat until eggs are completely set. Stir in the tomato and green onion.

3. Spoon about ⅔ cup into each pita half. Serve sandwiches warm.

PER SERVING *1 filled pita half equals 207 cal., 6 g fat (2 g sat. fat), 112 mg chol., 538 mg sodium, 28 g carb., 4 g fiber, 13 g pro.* **Diabetic Exchanges:** *1½ starch, 1 lean meat, 1 vegetable, ½ fat.*

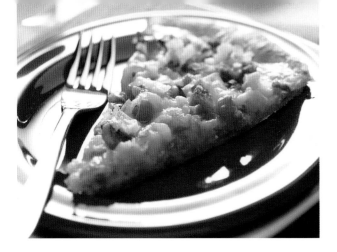

241 CALORIES Sausage and Egg Pizza

Using turkey sausage, fat-free cheddar cheese, egg substitute and reduced-fat crescent rolls really helped cut the calories and fat in this tasty recipe.
—**VICKI MEYERS** CASTALIA, OH

START TO FINISH: 30 MIN. • **MAKES:** 6 SLICES

- 1 tube (8 ounces) refrigerated reduced-fat crescent rolls
- ½ pound Italian turkey sausage links, casings removed
- 1¾ cups sliced fresh mushrooms
- 1¼ cups frozen shredded hash brown potatoes
- ¼ teaspoon garlic salt
- ¼ teaspoon pepper
- 2 green onions, chopped
- 2 tablespoons finely chopped sweet red pepper
- ½ cup shredded fat-free cheddar cheese
- ¾ cup egg substitute

1. Separate crescent dough into eight triangles; place on an ungreased 12-in. pizza pan with points toward the center. Press onto pan to form a crust, sealing perforations. Build up edges slightly. Bake at 375° for 8 minutes.
2. Meanwhile, crumble sausage into a large nonstick skillet coated with cooking spray. Add mushrooms; cook and stir over medium heat until meat is no longer pink. Drain and set aside. In the same skillet, cook potatoes, garlic salt and pepper over medium heat until browned.
3. Sprinkle sausage mixture over crust. Layer with potatoes, onions, red pepper and cheese; pour egg substitute over the top. Bake for 10-12 minutes or until egg is set and cheese is melted.
PER SERVING *1 slice equals 241 cal., 10 g fat (2 g sat. fat), 24 mg chol., 744 mg sodium, 22 g carb., 1 g fiber, 16 g pro.* **Diabetic Exchanges:** *2 lean meat, 1½ starch, ½ fat.*

219 CALORIES Breakfast Bake

I wanted to have scrambled eggs and hash browns one morning, and this is the dish I created. My wife loved it...and guess who's making breakfast more often ever since?
—**HOWARD ROGERS** EL PASO, TX

PREP: 15 MIN. • **BAKE:** 50 MIN. • **MAKES:** 6 SERVINGS

- 1½ cups egg substitute
- ½ cup fat-free milk
- 3½ cups frozen O'Brien potatoes, thawed
- 1⅓ cups shredded reduced-fat cheddar cheese, divided
- ½ cup chopped sweet onion
- 4 tablespoons crumbled cooked bacon, divided
- ½ teaspoon salt
- ½ teaspoon salt-free seasoning blend
- ¼ teaspoon chili powder
- 4 green onions, chopped

1. In a large bowl, whisk egg substitute and milk. Stir in the potatoes, 1 cup cheese, onion, 2 tablespoons bacon, salt, seasoning blend and chili powder. Pour into an 8-in. square baking dish coated with cooking spray.
2. Bake at 350° for 45-50 minutes or until a knife inserted near the center comes out clean. Sprinkle with remaining cheese and bacon. Bake 3-5 minutes longer or until cheese is melted. Sprinkle with green onions. Let stand for 5 minutes before cutting.
PER SERVING *1 piece equals 219 cal., 6 g fat (4 g sat. fat), 22 mg chol., 682 mg sodium, 25 g carb., 3 g fiber, 17 g pro.* **Diabetic Exchanges:** *2 lean meat, 1½ starch.*

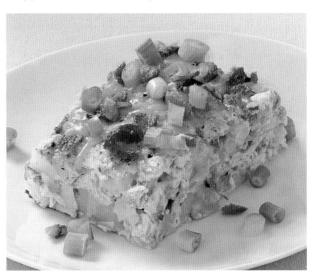

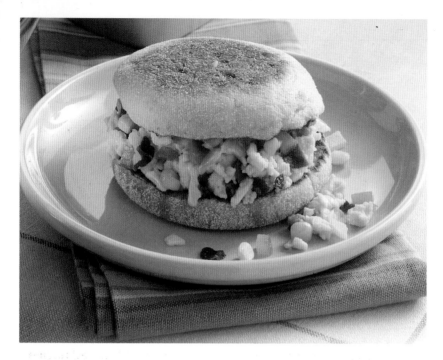

PREP: 15 MIN. + CHILLING
COOK: 5 MIN./BATCH
MAKES: 10 SERVINGS

- 1 **package (¼ ounce) active dry yeast**
- ½ **cup warm water (110° to 115°)**
- 1 **teaspoon sugar**
- 2 **cups warm milk (110° to 115°)**
- ½ **cup butter, melted**
- 2 **eggs, lightly beaten**
- 2 **cups all-purpose flour**
- 1 **teaspoon salt**

1. In a large bowl, dissolve yeast in warm water. Add sugar; let stand for 5 minutes. Add the milk, butter and eggs; mix well. Combine flour and salt; stir into milk mixture. Cover and refrigerate overnight.
2. Stir batter. Bake waffles in a preheated waffle iron according to manufacturer's directions until golden brown.
PER SERVING *2 waffles equals 220 cal., 12 g fat (7 g sat. fat), 74 mg chol., 366 mg sodium, 22 g carb., 1 g fiber, 6 g pro.*

248 CALORIES
Spicy Scrambled Egg Sandwiches

You'll love these energy-building sandwiches! When my daughters were young, I'd pile the tasty eggs onto English muffins, pour each girl a glass of juice, and let them eat together on the patio. They always chatted excitedly about the fun day ahead.
—HELEN VAIL GLENSIDE, PA

START TO FINISH: 30 MIN.
MAKES: 4 SERVINGS

- ⅓ **cup chopped green pepper**
- ¼ **cup chopped onion**
- 3 **eggs**
- 4 **egg whites**
- 1 **tablespoon water**
- ¼ **teaspoon salt**
- ¼ **teaspoon ground mustard**
- ⅛ **teaspoon pepper**
- ⅛ **teaspoon hot pepper sauce**
- ⅓ **cup fresh or frozen corn, thawed**
- ¼ **cup real bacon bits**
- 4 **English muffins, split and toasted**

1. In a 10-in. skillet coated with cooking spray, cook green pepper and onion over medium heat until tender, about 8 minutes.
2. In a large bowl, whisk the eggs, egg whites, water, salt, mustard, pepper and pepper sauce. Pour into skillet. Add corn and bacon; cook and stir until eggs are completely set. Spoon onto English muffin bottoms; replace tops. Serve sandwiches immediately.
PER SERVING *1 sandwich equals 248 cal., 6 g fat (2 g sat. fat), 164 mg chol., 739 mg sodium, 31 g carb., 2 g fiber, 16 g pro.* **Diabetic Exchanges:** *2 starch, 2 lean meat.*

220 CALORIES
Overnight Yeast Waffles

Starting the day with a hearty breakfast is a smart move when you're trying to follow a healthy eating plan. These waffles are so good that I freeze some ahead for breakfast on busy days.
—MARY BALCOMB FLORENCE, OR

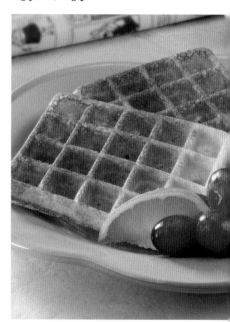

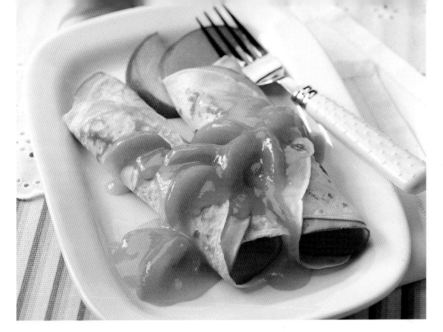

222 CALORIES
Orange Oatmeal

I like to make this for breakfast because it's quick, yet out of the ordinary. The orange flavor adds a little something extra to a weekday breakfast.
—**BERNICE HAACK** MILWAUKEE, WI

START TO FINISH: 10 MIN.
MAKES: 2 SERVINGS

- 1 cup water
- ¾ cup orange juice
- ⅛ teaspoon salt
- 1 cup quick-cooking oats
- ¼ teaspoon grated orange peel
- 1 to 2 tablespoons brown sugar

In a small saucepan, bring the water, orange juice and salt to a boil. Stir in oats and cook for 1 minute or until oatmeal reaches desired consistency. Stir in orange peel. Serve with brown sugar.
PER SERVING *1 serving (prepared with 1 tablespoon brown sugar) equals 222 cal., 3 g fat (trace sat. fat), 0 chol., 151 mg sodium, 43 g carb., 4 g fiber, 7 g pro.* **Diabetic Exchanges:** *2 starch, 1 fruit.*

258 CALORIES ## Ham and Apricot Crepes

A sweet apricot sauce complements these savory ham crepes.
—**CANDY EVAVOLD** SAMAMMISH, WA

PREP: 35 MIN. + CHILLING • **BAKE:** 20 MIN.
MAKES: 10 SERVINGS

- 1½ cups milk
- 2 eggs, lightly beaten
- 1 tablespoon butter, melted
- 1 cup all-purpose flour
- 20 thin slices deli ham

SAUCE
- 1 can (15¼ ounces) apricot halves
- ⅔ cup sugar
- 2 tablespoons cornstarch
- ⅛ teaspoon salt
- 2 cans (5½ ounces each) apricot nectar
- 2 tablespoons butter
- 2 teaspoons lemon juice

1. In a large bowl, beat the milk, eggs and butter. Add flour and beat until well combined. Cover and refrigerate for 1 hour.
2. Heat a lightly greased 8-in. nonstick skillet; pour 2 tablespoons batter into the center of skillet. Lift and tilt pan to evenly coat bottom. Cook until top appears dry; turn and cook 15-20 seconds longer. Remove to a wire rack. Repeat with remaining batter, greasing skillet as needed. When cool, stack crepes with waxed paper or paper towels in between.
3. Place a slice of ham on each crepe; roll up. Place in two greased 13-in. x 9-in. baking dishes. Bake, uncovered, at 350° for 20 minutes.
4. Meanwhile, drain apricots, reserving syrup. Cut apricots into ¼-in. slices; set aside. In a large saucepan, combine the sugar, cornstarch and salt. Add apricot nectar and reserved syrup; stir until smooth. Bring to a boil; cook and stir for 1-2 minutes or until thickened. Remove from the heat; stir in the butter, lemon juice and apricot slices. Serve with crepes.
PER SERVING *2 crepes with ¼ cup sauce equals 258 cal., 7 g fat (3 g sat. fat), 76 mg chol., 493 mg sodium, 39 g carb., 1 g fiber, 12 g pro.*

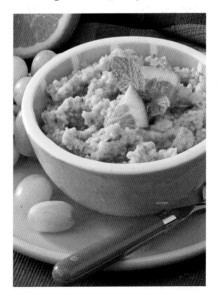

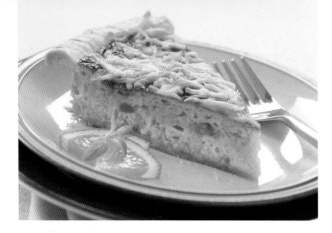

PER SERVING *1 piece equals 265 cal., 14 g fat (5 g sat. fat), 88 mg chol., 610 mg sodium, 21 g carb., 1 g fiber, 16 g pro.*

222 CALORIES Raspberry Key Lime Crepes

Key lime juice turns cream cheese into a refreshing filling for berry-topped crepes. Sometimes, I even pipe the sweet filling into phyllo-dough cones that I bake separately.
—**WOLFGANG HANAU** WEST PALM BEACH, FL

PREP: 20 MIN. + CHILLING • **MAKES:** 6 SERVINGS

- 3 **tablespoons Key lime juice**
- 1 **package (12.3 ounces) silken firm tofu, crumbled**
- 6 **ounces reduced-fat cream cheese, cubed**
- ⅔ **cup confectioners' sugar, divided**
- 2½ **teaspoons grated lime peel**
    Dash salt
    Dash ground nutmeg
- 6 **prepared crepes (9 inches)**
- 1½ **cups fresh raspberries**

1. In a blender, combine the lime juice, tofu and cream cheese; cover and process until smooth. Set aside 1 teaspoon confectioners' sugar. Add the lime peel, salt, nutmeg and remaining confectioners' sugar to tofu mixture; cover and process until blended. Refrigerate for at least 1 hour.

2. Spread cream cheese mixture over crepes. Sprinkle with raspberries; roll up. Dust with reserved confectioners' sugar.

PER SERVING *1 filled crepe equals 222 cal., 9 g fat (5 g sat. fat), 26 mg chol., 247 mg sodium, 28 g carb., 3 g fiber, 8 g pro.* **Diabetic Exchanges:** *1½ starch, 1 lean meat, 1 fat, ½ fruit.*

265 CALORIES Monterey Quiche

With its creamy goodness and Southwestern flair, this quiche is always a hit with my family. It's perfect for special brunches or for lunch with fresh fruit on the side.
—**PAM PRESSLY** BEACHWOOD, OH

PREP: 25 MIN. • **BAKE:** 45 MIN. + STANDING
MAKES: 2 QUICHES (6 SERVINGS EACH)

- ½ **cup chopped onion**
- 1 **tablespoon butter**
- 2 **garlic cloves, minced**
- 8 **egg whites, divided**
- 4 **eggs**
- 2 **cups (16 ounces) 1% small-curd cottage cheese**
- 2 **cups (8 ounces) shredded reduced-fat Mexican cheese blend, divided**
- 2 **cans (4 ounces each) chopped green chilies**
- ⅓ **cup all-purpose flour**
- ¾ **teaspoon baking powder**
- ¼ **teaspoon salt**
- 2 **unbaked deep-dish pastry shells (9 inches)**

1. In a small nonstick skillet, cook onion in butter over medium-low heat until tender, stirring occasionally. Add garlic; cook 1 minute longer.

2. In a large bowl, combine 6 egg whites, eggs, cottage cheese, 1½ cups shredded cheese, chilies, flour, baking powder, salt and onion mixture. In a large bowl, beat remaining egg whites until stiff peaks form. Fold into cheese mixture. Pour into pastry shells.

3. Bake at 400° for 10 minutes. Reduce heat to 350°; bake for 30 minutes. Sprinkle with remaining cheese; bake 5 minutes longer or until a knife inserted near the center comes out clean and cheese is melted. Let stand for 10 minutes before cutting.

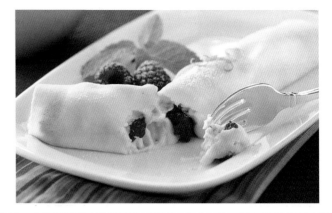

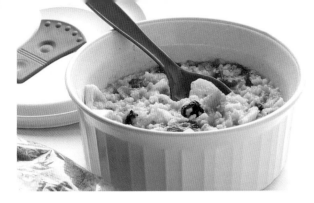

2 cups all-purpose flour
2 tablespoons sugar
2 teaspoons baking powder
1 teaspoon baking soda
2 eggs, lightly beaten
2 cups (16 ounces) plain yogurt
¼ cup water
  Semisweet chocolate chips, dried cranberries, sliced
    ripe bananas and coarsely chopped pecans, optional

210 CALORIES Spiced Oatmeal Mix

Oatmeal isn't just for breakfast anymore, thanks to this warm and cozy treat. Try it as a quick pick-me-up any time of day. Microwaving the mix makes it a snap to whip up.
—**LORETTA KLEINJAN** VOLGA, SD

START TO FINISH: 15 MIN. • **MAKES:** 18 SERVINGS

  8 **cups quick-cooking oats**
1½ **cups chopped mixed dried fruit**
  ½ **cup sugar**
  ½ **cup packed brown sugar**
2½ **teaspoons ground cinnamon**
  1 **teaspoon salt**
  ½ **teaspoon ground nutmeg**

In a large bowl, combine all of the ingredients. Store in an airtight container for up to 1 month.
TO PREPARE OATMEAL *Contents of mix may settle during storage. When preparing recipe, spoon mix into measuring cup. In a deep microwave-safe bowl, combine ½ cup oatmeal mix and 1 cup water. Microwave, uncovered, on high for 1-2 minutes or until bubbly, stirring every 30 seconds. Let stand for 1-2 minutes before serving.*
NOTE *This recipe was tested in a 1,100-watt microwave.*
PER SERVING *1 cup prepared oatmeal equals 210 cal., 3 g fat (trace sat. fat), 0 chol., 137 mg sodium, 42 g carb., 4 g fiber, 6 g pro.* **Diabetic Exchanges:** *2 starch, ½ fruit.*

242 CALORIES Yogurt Pancakes

Get your day off to a great start with delicious yogurt pancakes. Simply whip up a quick batch on the weekend—varying the fillings—and pop them in your freezer. Then savor the fluffy flapjacks one mouthwatering morning at a time. You might not even need syrup!
—**CHERYLL BABER** HOMEDALE, ID

PREP: 15 MIN. • **COOK:** 5 MIN./BATCH • **MAKES:** 12 PANCAKES

1. In a small bowl, combine the flour, sugar, baking powder and baking soda. In another bowl, whisk the eggs, yogurt and water. Stir into dry ingredients just until moistened.
2. Pour batter by ¼ cupfuls onto a hot griddle coated with cooking spray. Sprinkle with optional ingredients if desired. Turn when bubbles form on top; cook until the second side is golden brown.
3. To freeze, arrange cooled pancakes in a single layer on baking sheets. Freeze overnight or until frozen. Transfer to a resealable plastic freezer bag. May be frozen for up to 2 months.
TO USE FROZEN PANCAKES *Place pancakes on a microwave-safe plate; microwave on high for 40-50 seconds or until heated through.*
PER SERVING *2 pancakes (calculated without optional ingredients) equals 242 cal., 5 g fat (2 g sat. fat), 81 mg chol., 403 mg sodium, 40 g carb., 1 g fiber, 9 g pro.* **Diabetic Exchange:** *3 starch.*

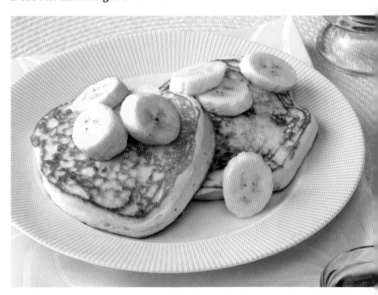

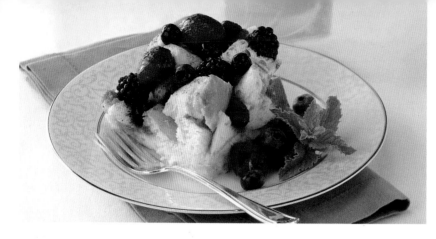

297 CALORIES · Mixed Berry French Toast Bake

Perfect for fuss-free holiday breakfasts or company, this recipe is scrumptious and so easy to put together the night before. I love it!

—AMY BERRY POLAND, ME

PREP: 20 MIN. + CHILLING • **BAKE:** 45 MIN.
MAKES: 8 SERVINGS

- 1 loaf (1 pound) French bread, cubed
- 6 egg whites
- 3 eggs
- 1¾ cups fat-free milk
- 1 teaspoon sugar
- 1 teaspoon ground cinnamon
- 1 teaspoon vanilla extract
- ¼ teaspoon salt
- 1 package (12 ounces) frozen unsweetened mixed berries
- 2 tablespoons cold butter
- ⅓ cup packed brown sugar

1. Place bread cubes in a 13-in. x 9-in. baking dish coated with cooking spray. In a large bowl, combine the egg whites, eggs, milk, sugar, cinnamon, vanilla and salt; pour over bread. Cover and refrigerate for 8 hours or overnight.
2. Thirty minutes before baking, remove the berries from the freezer and set aside, and remove the baking dish from the refrigerator.

Bake the French toast, covered, at 350° for 30 minutes.
3. In a small bowl, cut butter into brown sugar until crumbly. Sprinkle berries and brown sugar mixture over French toast. Bake, uncovered, for 15-20 minutes or until a knife inserted near center comes out clean.
PER SERVING 1 serving equals 297 cal., 7 g fat (3 g sat. fat), 88 mg chol., 545 mg sodium, 46 g carb., 3 g fiber, 12 g pro.

258 CALORIES · Homemade Pancake Mix

I use whole wheat flour to bring extra flavor to the flapjacks on my breakfast table. My family particularly likes the blueberry-banana variation.

—WENDY MINK HUNTINGTON, IN

START TO FINISH: 25 MIN.
MAKES: ABOUT 6¾ CUPS MIX

- 4 cups all-purpose flour
- 2 cups whole wheat flour
- ⅔ cup sugar
- 2 tablespoons baking powder
- 1 tablespoon baking soda

ADDITIONAL INGREDIENTS FOR PANCAKES
- 1 egg
- ¾ cup 2% milk

ADDITIONAL INGREDIENTS FOR BLUEBERRY BANANA PANCAKES
- 1 egg
- ¾ cup 2% milk
- 1 medium ripe banana, mashed
- ¾ cup blueberries

In large bowl, combine the first five ingredients. Store in an airtight container in cool dry place for up to 6 months. Makes: 6-7 batches of pancakes (about 6 pancakes per batch).

TO PREPARE PANCAKES *Contents of mix may settle during storage. When preparing recipe, spoon mix into a measuring cup. In a small bowl, whisk egg and milk. Whisk in 1 cup pancake mix. Pour batter by ¼ cupfuls onto a lightly greased hot griddle; turn when bubbles form on top of pancakes. Cook until second side is golden brown.*

TO PREPARE BLUEBERRY BANANA PANCAKES *Contents of mix may settle during storage. When preparing recipe, spoon mix into measuring cup. In a large bowl, combine the egg, milk and banana. Whisk in 1 cup pancake mix. Fold in blueberries. Cook as directed above.*

PER SERVING *3 plain pancakes equals 258 cal., 4 g fat (1 g sat. fat), 84 mg chol., 448 mg sodium, 47 g carb., 3 g fiber, 10 g pro.*

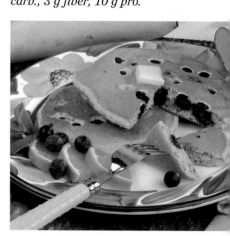

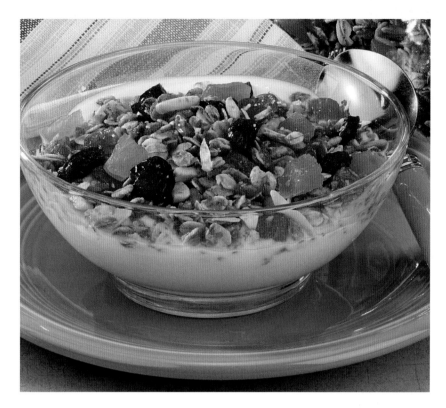

airtight container. Serve with yogurt if desired.

PER SERVING *½ cup equals 212 cal., 4 g fat (trace sat. fat), 0 chol., 88 mg sodium, 41 g carb., 3 g fiber, 6 g pro.*

267 CALORIES

Mediterranean Breakfast Pitas

These low-fat veggie pitas are great for any time of day, not just breakfast. They're loaded with spinach, bell pepper and other healthy ingredients.

—JOSIE-LYNN BELMONT
WOODBINE, GA

START TO FINISH: 25 MIN.
MAKES: 2 SERVINGS

- ¼ **cup chopped sweet red pepper**
- ¼ **cup chopped onion**
- 1 **cup egg substitute**
- ⅛ **teaspoon salt**
- ⅛ **teaspoon pepper**
- 1 **small tomato, chopped**
- ½ **cup torn fresh baby spinach**
- 1½ **teaspoons minced fresh basil**
- 2 **whole pita breads**
- 2 **tablespoons crumbled feta cheese**

1. In a small nonstick skillet coated with cooking spray, cook and stir red pepper and onion over medium heat for 3 minutes. Add the egg substitute, salt and pepper; cook and stir until set.

2. Combine the tomato, spinach and basil; spoon onto pitas. Top with egg mixture and sprinkle with feta cheese. Serve immediately.

PER SERVING *1 pita equals 267 cal., 2 g fat (1 g sat. fat), 4 mg chol., 798 mg sodium, 41 g carb., 3 g fiber, 20 g pro.* **Diabetic Exchanges:** *2 starch, 2 lean meat, 1 vegetable.*

212 CALORIES ## Toasted Almond Granola

I combined several granola recipes to come up with this crunchy cranberry-apricot treat. For fun, you can vary the kinds of fruits and nuts. The possibilities are endless.

—TRACY WEAKLY ALOHA, OR

PREP: 20 MIN. • **BAKE:** 20 MIN. + COOLING
MAKES: 8 CUPS

- 3 **cups old-fashioned oats**
- 2 **cups crisp rice cereal**
- ½ **cup toasted wheat germ**
- ½ **cup nonfat dry milk powder**
- ⅓ **cup slivered almonds**
- ¼ **cup packed brown sugar**
- 2 **tablespoons sunflower kernels**
- ¼ **teaspoon salt**
- ½ **cup orange juice**
- ¼ **cup honey**
- 2 **teaspoons canola oil**
- 2 **teaspoons vanilla extract**
- ½ **teaspoon almond extract**
- 1 **cup golden raisins**
- 1 **cup chopped dried apricots**
- ½ **cup dried cranberries**
  Fat-free plain yogurt, optional

1. In a large bowl, combine the oats, cereal, wheat germ, milk powder, almonds, brown sugar, sunflower kernels and salt. In a saucepan, combine the orange juice, honey and oil. Heat for 3-4 minutes over medium heat until honey is dissolved. Remove from the heat; stir in the extracts. Pour over the oat mixture; stir to coat.

2. Transfer to a 15-in. x 10-in. x 1-in. baking pan coated with cooking spray. Bake at 350° for 20-25 minutes or until crisp, stirring every 10 minutes. Remove and cool completely on a wire rack. Stir in dried fruits. Store in an

Lunches

A good midday meal is essential for keeping up your metabolism and avoiding excessive snacking. Try to stick to **450 calories when planning your lunch.**

CONTENTS

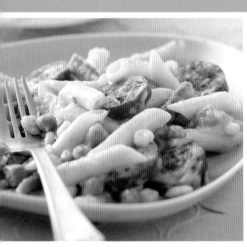

SPICY SAUSAGE AND PENNE
PAGE 144

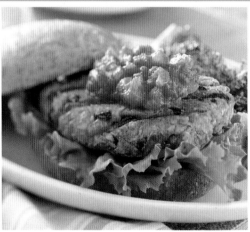

GRILLED BEAN BURGERS *PAGE 160*

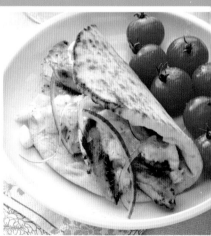

CHICKEN GYROS *PAGE 188*

250 CALORIES OR LESS

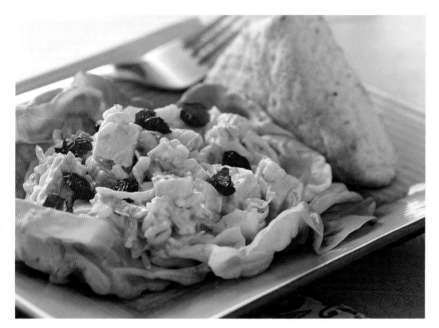

195 CALORIES Turkey Luncheon Salad

I received this recipe as a newlywed and made it healthier by using brown rice and fat-free mayo and sour cream. Think ladies' luncheon, with a light and refreshing Asian twist!

—JOAN CANNON NOBLESVILLE, IN

START TO FINISH: 25 MIN.
MAKES: 7 SERVINGS

- 2 cups cubed cooked turkey breast
- 2 cups cooked brown rice
- 1 can (14 ounces) bean sprouts, drained
- 1 can (8 ounces) sliced water chestnuts, drained
- 1 celery rib, chopped
- 1 small carrot, shredded
- ¼ cup finely chopped onion
- ½ cup fat-free mayonnaise
- ½ cup fat-free sour cream
- 1 tablespoon reduced-sodium soy sauce
- ¾ teaspoon salt
- 7 lettuce leaves
- ¼ cup dried cranberries

In a large bowl, combine the first seven ingredients. In a small bowl, combine the mayonnaise, sour cream, soy sauce and salt; pour over salad and gently stir to coat. Serve over lettuce leaves. Sprinkle each serving with cranberries.
PER SERVING *1 cup equals 195 cal., 2 g fat (trace sat. fat), 39 mg chol., 545 mg sodium, 29 g carb., 4 g fiber, 16 g pro.* **Diabetic Exchanges:** *1½ starch, 1 lean meat, 1 vegetable.*

240 CALORIES Baked Deli Focaccia Sandwich

Pesto and focaccia make this pretty sandwich deliciously different from most deli offerings. It's great to serve at football parties and other gatherings.

—MARY HUMENIUK-SMITH
PERRY HALL, MD

PREP: 10 MIN. • **BAKE:** 20 MIN. + STANDING
MAKES: 8 SERVINGS

- 1 loaf (12 ounces) focaccia bread
- ¼ cup prepared pesto
- ¼ pound sliced deli ham
- ¼ pound sliced deli smoked turkey
- ¼ pound sliced deli pastrami
- 5 slices process American cheese
- ⅓ cup thinly sliced onion
- 1 small tomato, sliced
- ¼ teaspoon Italian seasoning

1. Cut focaccia horizontally in half; spread pesto over cut sides. On bread bottom, layer the ham, turkey, pastrami, cheese, onion and tomato. Sprinkle with Italian seasoning. Replace bread top; wrap sandwich in foil. Place on a baking sheet.
2. Bake at 350° for 20-25 minutes or until heated through. Let stand for 10 minutes. Cut into wedges.
PER SERVING *1 serving equals 240 cal., 9 g fat (3 g sat. fat), 30 mg chol., 817 mg sodium, 26 g carb., 1 g fiber, 15 g pro.*

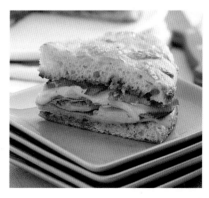

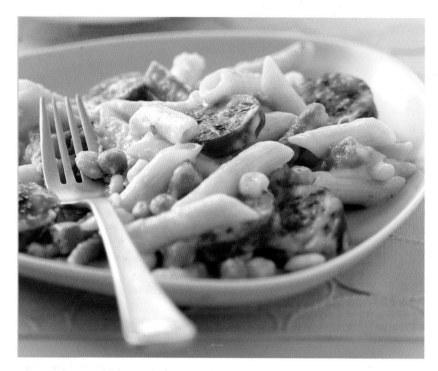

249 CALORIES Open-Faced Veggie Sandwiches

I'm a vegetarian and a big fan of these broiled sandwiches, but even non-vegetarians like their fresh taste. The topped English muffin halves make a great lunch or quick dinner.
—KAREN MELLO FAIRHAVEN, MA

START TO FINISH: 15 MIN.
MAKES: 4 SERVINGS

- 4 **teaspoons spicy brown or horseradish mustard**
- 4 **English muffins, split**
- ½ **cup each chopped fresh broccoli, cauliflower and sweet red pepper**
- 1 **cup (4 ounces) shredded cheddar cheese**

Spread mustard on cut sides of muffins. Top each with vegetables and cheese. Broil 4-6 in. from the heat for 3 minutes or until the cheese is melted.

PER SERVING *2 English muffin halves equals 249 cal., 9 g fat (6 g sat. fat), 30 mg chol., 506 mg sodium, 30 g carb., 2 g fiber, 11 g pro.* **Diabetic Exchanges:** *2 starch, 1 lean meat.*

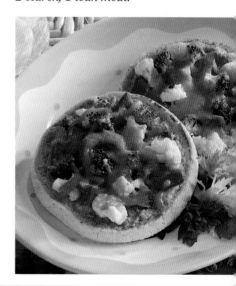

228 CALORIES Spicy Sausage and Penne

I got the inspiration for my original recipe from a dish at a local restaurant. It's a quick and easy lunch that I prepare often. You can substitute whatever pasta or veggies you have on hand for the versatile skillet meal.
—BRIAN ALBRIGHT SEWARD, NE

PREP: 10 MIN. • **COOK:** 25 MIN.
MAKES: 4 SERVINGS

- 1 **cup uncooked penne pasta**
- 1 **cup frozen mixed vegetables**
- ½ **pound smoked turkey sausage, cut into ¼-inch slices**
- 2 **tablespoons all-purpose flour**
- ¼ **teaspoon garlic powder**
- ¼ **teaspoon ground mustard**
- ¼ **teaspoon crushed red pepper flakes**
- 1¼ **cups fat-free milk**
- ⅓ **cup shredded part-skim mozzarella cheese**

1. Cook pasta in a large saucepan according to package directions, adding the vegetables during the last 6 minutes of cooking.
2. Meanwhile, in a large nonstick skillet coated with cooking spray, brown sausage; remove from skillet and keep warm.
3. In a small bowl, combine the flour, garlic powder, mustard and pepper flakes; gradually whisk in milk until smooth. Add milk mixture to the skillet, stirring to loosen browned bits from pan. Bring to a boil; cook and stir for 1-2 minutes or until thickened.
4. Drain pasta and vegetables; stir into the pan. Add cheese and reserved sausage; cook and stir until cheese is melted.

PER SERVING *1 cup equals 228 cal., 5 g fat (2 g sat. fat), 42 mg chol., 650 mg sodium, 27 g carb., 3 g fiber, 18 g pro.* **Diabetic Exchanges:** *2 lean meat, 1½ starch.*

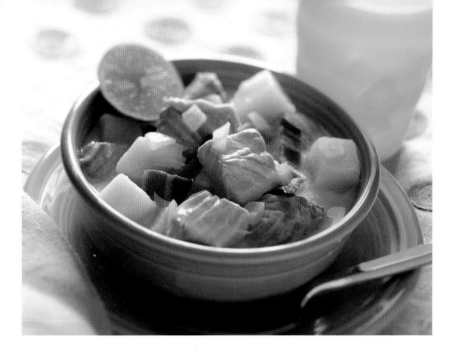

Salmon Chowder

The salmon in this recipe is a change from traditional chowder, but it certainly is delicious!

—**CINDY ST. MARTIN** PORTLAND, OR

PREP: 10 MIN. • **COOK:** 30 MIN.
MAKES: 14 SERVINGS

- 2 **pounds red potatoes, peeled and cubed**
- 1 **large onion, chopped**
- 6 **cups reduced-sodium chicken broth**
- 1 **pound salmon fillets, cut into 1-inch pieces**
- ½ **pound sliced bacon, cooked and crumbled**
- 2 **cups milk**
- 1 **cup half-and-half cream**
- 1 **tablespoon butter**
- ½ **teaspoon salt**
  Pepper to taste

1. In a Dutch oven, combine the potatoes, onion and broth. Bring to a boil. Reduce heat; cover and cook for 10-15 minutes or until potatoes are tender. Add salmon and bacon; cook over medium heat until fish flakes easily with a fork.

2. Reduce heat; stir in the milk, cream, butter, salt and pepper; heat through (do not boil). Thicken chowder if desired.

PER SERVING *1 cup equals 198 cal., 10 g fat (4 g sat. fat), 38 mg chol., 466 mg sodium, 14 g carb., 1 g fiber, 12 g pro.* **Diabetic Exchanges:** *1 starch, 1 lean meat, 1 fat.*

Zippy Corn Chowder

My zesty chowder was so well received the first time I made it that some of us had to go without seconds!

—**KERA BREDIN** VANCOUVER, BC

PREP: 15 MIN. • **COOK:** 30 MIN.
MAKES: 8 SERVINGS (2 QUARTS)

- 1 **medium onion, chopped**
- 1 **medium green pepper, chopped**
- 2 **tablespoons butter**
- 1 **can (14½ ounces) vegetable broth**
- 2 **large red potatoes, cubed**
- 1 **jalapeno pepper, chopped**
- 2 **teaspoons Dijon mustard**
- 1 **teaspoon salt**
- ½ **teaspoon paprika**
- ¼ **to ½ teaspoon crushed red pepper flakes**
- 3 **cups frozen corn**
- 4 **green onions, chopped**
- 3 **cups milk, divided**
- ¼ **cup all-purpose flour**

1. In a large saucepan, saute onion and green pepper in butter until tender. Add broth and potatoes. Bring to a boil. Reduce heat; cover and simmer for 15 minutes or until potatoes are almost tender. Stir in jalapeno, mustard and seasonings. Add corn, onions and 2½ cups milk. Bring to a boil.

2. Combine flour and remaining milk until smooth; gradually add to soup. Bring to a boil. Cook and stir 2 minutes or until thickened.

NOTE *Wear disposable gloves when cutting hot peppers; the oils can burn skin. Avoid touching your face.*

PER SERVING *1 cup equals 190 cal., 7 g fat (4 g sat. fat), 20 mg chol., 617 mg sodium, 28 g carb., 3 g fiber, 7 g pro.*

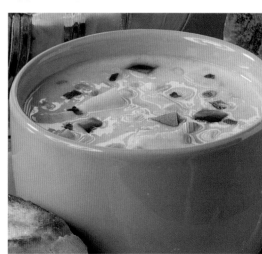

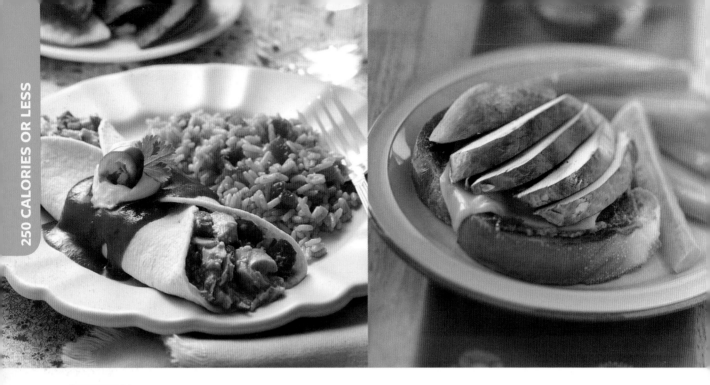

211 CALORIES
Soft Taco Wraps

The flavorful filling in these wraps has a definite kick, but you can adjust the jalapeno pepper to suit your taste.
—**MELISSA GREEN** LOUISVILLE, KY

START TO FINISH: 30 MIN.
MAKES: 6 SERVINGS

- 1 **can (10 ounces) diced tomatoes and green chilies, drained**
- 1 **can (9¾ ounces) chunk white chicken, drained**
- 1 **cup (4 ounces) shredded cheddar-Monterey Jack cheese**
- 2 **tablespoons diced jalapeno pepper**
- 2 **teaspoons taco seasoning**
- 6 **flour tortillas (6 inches), warmed**
  Taco sauce and sour cream, optional

1. In a bowl, combine the tomatoes, chicken, cheese, jalapeno and taco seasoning. Place about ⅓ cupful down the center of each tortilla.

Roll up and place seam side down in a greased 11-in. x 7-in. baking dish.
2. Bake, uncovered, at 350° for 10-15 minutes or until heated through. Serve with taco sauce and sour cream if desired.
NOTE *Wear disposable gloves when cutting hot peppers; the oils can burn skin. Avoid touching your face.*
PER SERVING *1 wrap (calculated without taco sauce and sour cream) equals 211 cal., 9 g fat (4 g sat. fat), 38 mg chol., 818 mg sodium, 17 g carb., 1 g fiber, 16 g pro.*

236 CALORIES
Open-Faced Portobello Sandwiches

These chewy, cheesy sandwiches skip the meat, yet are truly satisfying.
—**ROSEMARIE SMITH** BOUNTIFUL, UT

START TO FINISH: 15 MIN.
MAKES: 2 SERVINGS

- 4 **teaspoons prepared pesto**
- 2 **slices Italian bread (¾ inch thick), toasted**
- 3 **oil-packed sun-dried tomatoes, cut into strips**
- 2 **slices part-skim mozzarella cheese (¾ ounce each)**
- 2 **large portobello mushrooms, stems removed**

1. Spread pesto on toast; top with tomatoes and cheese. Place the mushrooms on a microwave-safe plate; cover with a paper towel. Microwave on high for 1 minute or until tender.
2. Cut mushrooms into ½-in. slices; place on cheese. Cook sandwiches on high for 15-20 seconds or until cheese is melted.
NOTE *This recipe was tested in a 1,100-watt microwave.*
PER SERVING *1 sandwich equals 236 cal., 11 g fat (4 g sat. fat), 15 mg chol., 382 mg sodium, 22 g carb., 3 g fiber, 12 g pro.* **Diabetic Exchanges:** *1 starch, 1 medium-fat meat, 1 vegetable, 1 fat.*

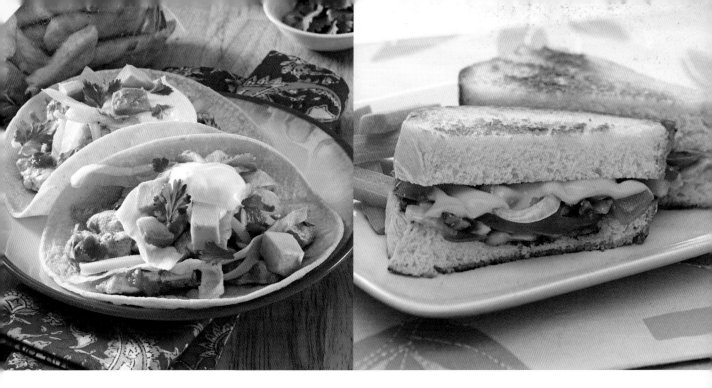

Presto Chicken Tacos

Slowly cooking the chicken with the seasonings is the key to perfection with this dish. The chicken mixture also makes a great salad topping.
—**NANETTE HILTON** LAS VEGAS, NV

PREP: 20 MIN. • **COOK:** 25 MIN.
MAKES: 12 SERVINGS

- 3 **pounds boneless skinless chicken breasts, cut into strips**
- 2 **tablespoons canola oil**
- 1 **garlic clove, minced**
- 2 **cans (14½ ounces each) diced tomatoes, undrained**
- 1 **teaspoon ground cumin**
- 1 **teaspoon chili powder**
- 12 **corn tortillas (6 inches), warmed**
  Optional toppings: shredded lettuce, shredded cheddar cheese, diced tomatoes, fresh cilantro leaves, sour cream and cubed avocado

1. In a Dutch oven, brown chicken in oil in batches. Add garlic; cook 1 minute longer. Add tomatoes, cumin and chili powder. Bring to a boil. Reduce heat; cover and simmer for 15-20 minutes or until chicken is no longer pink, stirring occasionally.

2. Fill each tortilla with about ½ cup chicken mixture. Serve with toppings of your choice.

PER SERVING *1 taco (calculated without toppings) equals 215 cal., 6 g fat (1 g sat. fat), 63 mg chol., 186 mg sodium, 16 g carb., 3 g fiber, 25 g pro.* **Diabetic Exchanges:** *3 lean meat, 1 starch.*

Veggie Cheese Sandwiches

Use whatever vegetables you have on hand the next time you need to clean out the vegetable drawer of your fridge.
—**BEVERLY LITTLE** MARIETTA, GA

START TO FINISH: 30 MIN.
MAKES: 4 SERVINGS

- ½ **cup sliced onion**
- ½ **cup julienned green pepper**
- ⅔ **cup chopped tomato**
- ½ **cup sliced fresh mushrooms**
- 8 **slices Italian bread (½ inch thick)**
- 4 **slices reduced-fat process American cheese product**
- 4 **teaspoons butter, softened**

1. In a small nonstick skillet coated with cooking spray, cook onion and green pepper for 2 minutes. Add tomato and mushrooms; cook and stir until tender; drain.

2. Divide the vegetable mixture over four slices of bread; top with cheese and remaining bread. Butter the top and bottom of each sandwich. In a skillet, toast sandwiches until lightly browned on both sides.

PER SERVING *1 sandwich equals 168 cal., 6 g fat (3 g sat. fat), 15 mg chol., 415 mg sodium, 20 g carb., 2 g fiber, 8 g pro.* **Diabetic Exchanges:** *1 starch, 1 lean meat, 1 vegetable, 1 fat.*

> "I make frequent trips up and down the stairs. And instead of asking my kids to bring me things, I get them myself. Remember to keep moving. Each step is burning more calories."

—PAM RICHARDSON

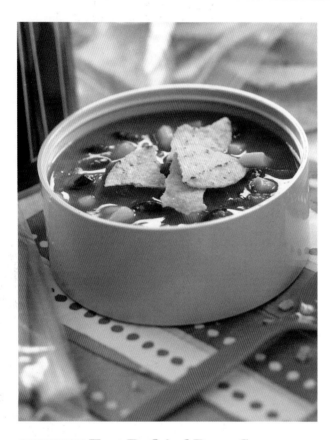

1 can (15 ounces) black beans, rinsed and drained
1 can (14½ ounces) chicken broth
1 can (14½ ounces) stewed tomatoes, cut up
½ cup water
1 can (4 ounces) chopped green chilies
¼ cup salsa
  Tortilla chips

In a large saucepan, combine the first eight ingredients. Bring to a boil. Reduce heat; simmer, uncovered, for 8-10 minutes or until heated through. Serve with tortilla chips.

PER SERVING *1 cup (calculated without chips) equals 117 cal., 1 g fat (trace sat. fat), 1 mg chol., 720 mg sodium, 21 g carb., 4 g fiber, 5 g pro.*

245 CALORIES California Pizzas

Here's a delicious lunch or light dinner for two. Tortillas make the convenient crust for little pizzas loaded with fresh veggies and cheese.

—**SHEILA MARTIN** LA QUINTA, CA

START TO FINISH: 20 MIN. • **MAKES:** 2 SERVINGS

½ cup chopped onion
½ cup chopped green pepper
2 teaspoons canola oil
2 flour tortillas (6 inches)
¼ teaspoon dried oregano
⅛ teaspoon garlic powder
1 medium tomato, sliced
½ cup shredded part-skim mozzarella cheese

1. In a small skillet, saute onion and green pepper in oil until tender. Place tortillas on an ungreased baking sheet. Top with onion mixture, oregano, garlic powder, tomato and cheese.

117 CALORIES Fast Refried Bean Soup

You'll love the way my recipe combines the ease of canned ingredients with the heartiness of chili. It's a perfect filler-upper on cold afternoons and a great last-minute lunch. If you like it spicier, use medium or hot green chilies instead of mild.

—**DARLENE BRENDEN** SALEM, OR

START TO FINISH: 25 MIN. • **MAKES:** 8 SERVINGS (2 QUARTS)

1 can (16 ounces) spicy fat-free refried beans
1 can (15¼ ounces) whole kernel corn, drained

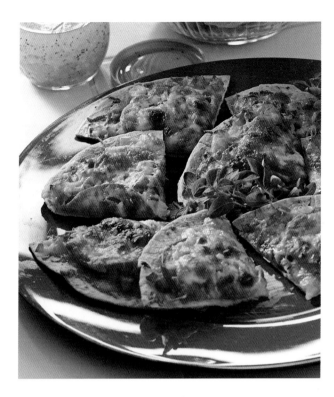

2. Bake at 400° for 8-10 minutes or until cheese is melted. Cut each pizza into four wedges.

PER SERVING *1 pizza equals 245 cal., 13 g fat (3 g sat. fat), 16 mg chol., 364 mg sodium, 23 g carb., 2 g fiber, 11 g pro.* **Diabetic Exchanges:** *1 starch, 1 medium-fat meat, 1 vegetable.*

218 CALORIES Bean and Pasta Soup

We're always on the lookout for good low-fat recipes, and this soup is a perennial favorite. Loaded with veggies and pasta, it's filling and delicious. Once school starts, I make it every week.
—**MARIA GOODING** ST. THOMAS, ON

PREP: 20 MIN. • **COOK:** 30 MIN. • **MAKES:** 5 SERVINGS

- 1 cup uncooked small pasta
- 2 celery ribs, thinly sliced
- 2 medium carrots, thinly sliced
- 1 medium onion, chopped
- 1 tablespoon olive oil
- 1 garlic clove, minced
- 2 cups water
- 1 can (14½ ounces) diced tomatoes, undrained
- 1¼ cups reduced-sodium chicken broth or vegetable broth
- 1 teaspoon dried basil
- ½ teaspoon dried rosemary, crushed
- ¼ teaspoon salt
- ⅛ teaspoon pepper
- 1 can (15 ounces) white kidney or cannellini beans, rinsed and drained
- 2 cups shredded fresh spinach
- ¼ cup shredded Parmesan cheese, optional

1. Cook pasta according to package directions. Meanwhile, in a large nonstick saucepan, saute the celery, carrots and onion in oil for 5 minutes. Add the garlic; cook 1 minute longer. Stir in water, tomatoes, broth, basil, rosemary, salt and pepper. Bring to a boil. Reduce heat; cover and simmer for 10 minutes or until carrots are tender.

2. Drain pasta; stir into vegetable mixture. Add the beans; heat through. Stir in spinach; cook until spinach is wilted, about 2 minutes. Sprinkle with Parmesan cheese if desired.

PER SERVING *1½ cups (calculated without cheese) equals 218 cal., 5 g fat (1 g sat. fat), 3 mg chol., 588 mg sodium, 35 g carb., 7 g fiber, 9 g pro.* **Diabetic Exchanges:** *2 vegetable, 1½ starch, 1 lean meat.*

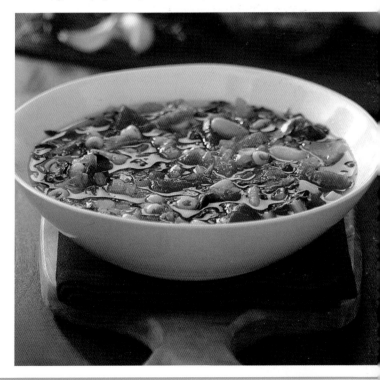

133 CALORIES ## Spiced Butternut Squash Soup

I like making this recipe all year long, but it's best in the fall and winter months when butternut squash is in season. I love it because it's not only hearty and filling, but very healthy and easy to make.
—**JULIE HESSION** LAS VEGAS, NV

PREP: 50 MIN. • **COOK:** 25 MIN.
MAKES: 12 SERVINGS (3 QUARTS)

- 2 **medium butternut squash (about 3 pounds each)**
- 2 **large onions, sliced**
- 1 **tablespoon olive oil**
- 1 **tablespoon butter**
- 2 **cinnamon sticks (3 inches)**
- 2 **tablespoons brown sugar**
- 1 **tablespoon minced fresh gingerroot**
- 2 **garlic cloves, minced**
- 3 **cans (14½ ounces each) reduced-sodium chicken broth**
- 2¼ **cups water**
- 1¼ **teaspoons salt**
- 1 **tablespoon minced fresh parsley**

1. Cut squash in half; discard seeds. Place squash cut side down in a 15-in. x 10-in. x 1-in. baking pan coated with cooking spray. Bake at 400° for 40-50 minutes or until tender. Cool slightly; scoop out pulp and set aside.

2. In a Dutch oven over medium heat, cook and stir onions in oil and butter for 2 minutes. Add the cinnamon, brown sugar, ginger and garlic; cook 2 minutes longer or until onions are tender. Stir in the broth, water, salt and reserved squash. Bring to a boil. Reduce heat; cover and simmer for 10 minutes.

3. Cool soup slightly. Discard cinnamon. In a blender, process soup in batches until smooth. Return all to the pan and heat through. Sprinkle each serving with parsley.
PER SERVING *1 cup equals 133 cal., 2 g fat (1 g sat. fat), 3 mg chol., 596 mg sodium, 28 g carb., 7 g fiber, 4 g pro.* **Diabetic Exchanges:** *2 starch, ½ fat.*

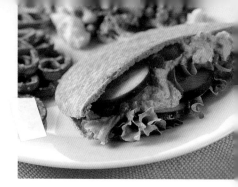

241 CALORIES ## Garbanzo Bean Pitas

Here's a wonderful meatless recipe for informal dinners and quick lunches alike. I add a little horseradish to my pitas for extra flavor.
—**SUSAN LE BRUN** SULPHUR, LA

START TO FINISH: 20 MIN.
MAKES: 4 SERVINGS

- 1 **can (15 ounces) garbanzo beans or chickpeas, rinsed and drained**
- ½ **cup fat-free mayonnaise**
- 1 **tablespoon water**
- 2 **tablespoons minced fresh parsley**
- 2 **tablespoons chopped walnuts**
- 1 **tablespoon chopped onion**
- 1 **garlic clove, minced**
- ⅛ **teaspoon pepper**
- 4 **whole wheat pita pocket halves**
- 4 **lettuce leaves**
- ½ **small cucumber, thinly sliced**
- 1 **small tomato, seeded and chopped**
- ¼ **cup fat-free ranch salad dressing, optional**

In a blender, combine the first eight ingredients; cover and process until blended. Spoon ⅓ cup of the bean mixture into each pita half. Top with lettuce, cucumber and tomato. Serve with ranch dressing if desired.
PER SERVING *1 filled pita half (calculated without dressing) equals 241 cal., 6 g fat (trace sat. fat), 3 mg chol., 552 mg sodium, 41 g carb., 8 g fiber, 9 g pro.* **Diabetic Exchanges:** *3 starch, 1 lean meat, 1 fat.*

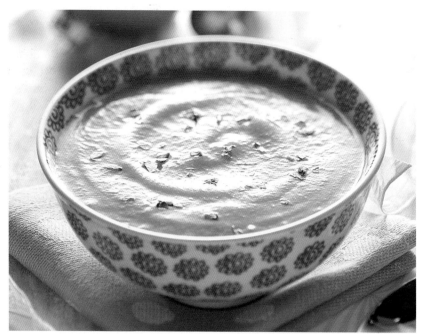

Italian Vegetable Soup

Laced with a splash of wine, my hearty soup is packed with garden-fresh nutrition and veggies! Substitute spinach or kale for the escarole if you wish.

—**LEA REITER** THOUSAND OAKS, CA

PREP: 15 MIN. • **COOK:** 25 MIN.
MAKES: 7 SERVINGS

- 2 **celery ribs, sliced**
- 1 **medium onion, chopped**
- 1 **medium carrot, halved and sliced**
- 1 **tablespoon olive oil**
- 2 **cups water**
- 1 **can (15 ounces) white kidney or cannellini beans, rinsed and drained**
- 1 **can (14½ ounces) diced tomatoes, undrained**
- 1 **can (14½ ounces) reduced-sodium chicken broth**
- ½ **cup Marsala wine or additional reduced-sodium chicken broth**
- 1 **teaspoon each dried basil, marjoram, oregano and thyme**
- ¼ **teaspoon salt**
- ¼ **teaspoon pepper**
- 1 **cup uncooked bow tie pasta**
- 6 **cups torn escarole**

1. In a Dutch oven, saute the celery, onion and carrot in oil until tender. Stir in the water, beans, tomatoes, broth, wine and seasonings. Bring to a boil. Stir in pasta.

2. Reduce heat; simmer, uncovered, for 13-15 minutes or until pasta is tender, adding escarole during the last 3 minutes of cooking.

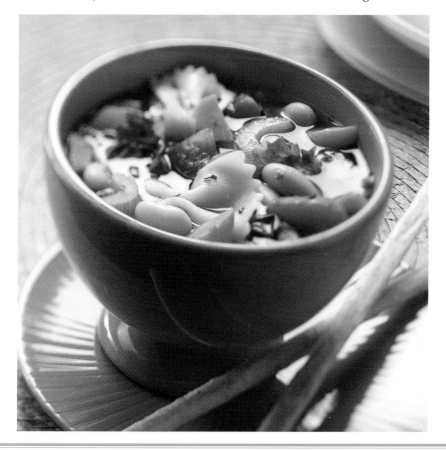

PER SERVING *1 cup equals 164 cal., 3 g fat (trace sat. fat), 0 chol., 426 mg sodium, 26 g carb., 5 g fiber, 6 g pro. **Diabetic Exchanges:** 1½ starch, 1 vegetable, ½ fat.*

Chicken Caesar Salad

Topping a delicious Caesar salad with tender grilled chicken breast ensures a healthy, filling lunch that satisfies.

—**KAY ANDERSEN** BEAR, DE

START TO FINISH: 25 MIN.
MAKES: 2 SERVINGS

- 2 **boneless skinless chicken breast halves (4 ounces each)**
- 2 **teaspoons olive oil**
- ¼ **teaspoon garlic salt**
- ¼ **teaspoon paprika**
- ¼ **teaspoon pepper**
- ⅛ **teaspoon dried basil**
- ⅛ **teaspoon dried oregano**
- 4 **cups torn romaine**
- 1 **small tomato, thinly sliced**
- ¼ **cup fat-free creamy Caesar salad dressing**
  Caesar salad croutons, optional

1. Brush chicken with oil. Combine the garlic salt, paprika, pepper, basil and oregano; sprinkle over chicken. Grill, covered, over medium heat or broil 4 in. from the heat for 4-7 minutes on each side or until a thermometer reads 170°.

2. Arrange romaine and tomato on plates. Cut chicken into strips; place over salads. Drizzle with dressing. Sprinkle with croutons if desired.

PER SERVING *1 serving (calculated without croutons) equals 236 cal., 8 g fat (1 g sat. fat), 63 mg chol., 653 mg sodium, 17 g carb., 4 g fiber, 26 g pro. **Diabetic Exchanges:** 3 lean meat, 2 vegetable, 1 starch, 1 fat.*

155 CALORIES

Makeover Mom's Clam Chowder

When we lived in Michigan, this was a perfect comforting soup when blustery winds blew into town. The steaming bowls of soup warmed us right down to the toes! The *Taste of Home* Test Kitchen created a lighter version for me.

—CHRISTINE SCHENHER SAN CLEMENTE, CA

PREP: 30 MIN. • **COOK:** 45 MIN.
MAKES: 12 SERVINGS (3 QUARTS)

- ¾ cup each chopped onion, celery and carrots
- ½ cup chopped green pepper
- ¼ cup butter, cubed
- 1 carton (32 ounces) reduced-sodium chicken broth
- 1 bottle (8 ounces) clam juice
- 2 teaspoons reduced-sodium chicken bouillon granules
- 1 bay leaf
- ½ teaspoon dried parsley flakes
- ½ teaspoon salt
- ¼ teaspoon curry powder
- ¼ teaspoon pepper
- 1 medium potato, peeled and cubed
- ⅔ cup all-purpose flour
- 2 cups 2% milk, divided
- 4 cans (6½ ounces each) minced clams, undrained
- 1 cup half-and-half cream

1. In a Dutch oven over medium heat, cook the onion, celery, carrots and green pepper in butter until tender. Stir in the broth, clam juice, bouillon and seasonings. Add potato. Bring to a boil. Reduce heat; simmer, uncovered, for 15-20 minutes or until potato is tender.

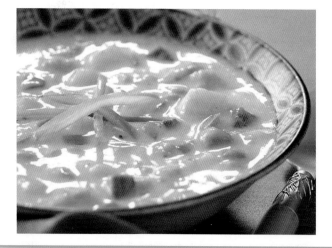

2. In a small bowl, combine flour and 1 cup milk until smooth. Gradually stir into soup. Bring to a boil; cook and stir for 1-2 minutes or until thickened.

3. Stir in the clams, cream and remaining milk; heat through (do not boil). Discard bay leaf before serving.
PER SERVING *1 cup equals 155 cal., 7 g fat (4 g sat. fat), 34 mg chol., 726 mg sodium, 15 g carb., 1 g fiber, 8 g pro.* **Diabetic Exchanges:** *1 starch, 1 lean meat, 1 fat.*

241 CALORIES Grilled Fish Sandwiches

These fish fillets are seasoned with lime juice and lemon-pepper before they're charbroiled on the grill. A simple honey-mustard mayo puts the sandwiches ahead of the rest.

—VIOLET BEARD MARSHALL, IL

START TO FINISH: 30 MIN. • **MAKES:** 4 SERVINGS

- 4 cod fillets (4 ounces each)
- 1 tablespoon lime juice
- ½ teaspoon lemon-pepper seasoning
- ¼ cup fat-free mayonnaise
- 2 teaspoons Dijon mustard
- 1 teaspoon honey
- 4 hamburger buns, split
- 4 lettuce leaves
- 4 tomato slices

1. Brush both sides of fillets with lime juice; sprinkle with lemon-pepper. Moisten a paper towel with cooking oil; using long-handled tongs, lightly coat the grill rack. Grill fillets, covered, over medium heat or broil 4 in. from the heat for 4-5 minutes on each side or until fish flakes easily with a fork.

2. In a small bowl, combine the mayonnaise, mustard and honey. Spread over the bottom of each bun. Top with a fillet, lettuce and tomato; replace bun tops.
PER SERVING *1 sandwich equals 241 cal., 3 g fat (1 g sat. fat), 49 mg chol., 528 mg sodium, 28 g carb., 2 g fiber, 24 g pro.* **Diabetic Exchanges:** *3 lean meat, 2 starch.*

230 CALORIES Mango Shrimp Pitas

Mango, ginger and curry combine with a splash of lime juice to coat this juicy grilled shrimp. Stuffed in pitas, the shrimp combo makes for a fabulous entree!

—BEVERLY OFERRALL LINKWOOD, MD

PREP: 15 MIN. + MARINATING • **GRILL:** 10 MIN. • **MAKES:** 4 SERVINGS

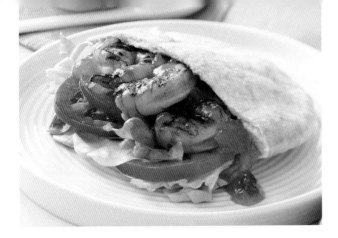

½ cup mango chutney
3 tablespoons lime juice
1 teaspoon grated fresh gingerroot
½ teaspoon curry powder
1 pound uncooked large shrimp, peeled and deveined
2 pita breads (6 inches), halved
8 Bibb or Boston lettuce leaves
1 large tomato, thinly sliced

1. In a small bowl, combine the chutney, lime juice, ginger and curry. Pour ½ cup marinade into a large resealable plastic bag; add the shrimp. Seal bag and turn to coat; refrigerate for at least 15 minutes. Cover and refrigerate remaining marinade.

2. Drain shrimp and discard marinade. Thread shrimp onto four metal or soaked wooden skewers. Moisten a paper towel with cooking oil; using long-handled tongs, lightly coat the grill rack.

3. Grill shrimp, covered, over medium heat or broil 4 in. from the heat for 6-8 minutes or until shrimp turn pink, turning frequently.

4. Fill pita halves with lettuce, tomato and shrimp; spoon reserved chutney mixture over filling.

PER SERVING *1 filled pita half equals 230 cal., 2 g fat (trace sat. fat), 138 mg chol., 410 mg sodium, 29 g carb., 1 g fiber, 22 g pro.* **Diabetic Exchanges:** *3 lean meat, 2 starch.*

238 CALORIES Black Bean-Pumpkin Soup

This is such a healthy recipe, packed with protein from the beans and vitamins from the pumpkin. The dollop of light sour cream adds a satisfying touch that feels indulgent.
—**JENNIFER FISHER** AUSTIN, TX

PREP: 30 MIN. • **COOK:** 30 MIN. • **MAKES:** 8 SERVINGS (2 QUARTS)

2 cans (15 ounces each) black beans, rinsed and drained
1 can (14½ ounces) diced tomatoes, drained
2 medium onions, finely chopped
1 teaspoon olive oil
3 garlic cloves, minced
1 teaspoon ground cumin
3 cups vegetable broth
1 can (15 ounces) solid-pack pumpkin
2 tablespoons cider vinegar
½ teaspoon pepper
2 tablespoons bourbon, optional
½ cup reduced-fat sour cream
½ cup thinly sliced green onions
½ cup roasted salted pumpkin seeds

1. Place beans and tomatoes in a food processor; cover and process until blended. Set aside.

2. In a Dutch oven, saute onions in oil until tender. Add garlic and cumin; saute 1 minute longer. Stir in the broth, pumpkin, vinegar, pepper and bean mixture. Bring to a boil. Reduce heat; cover and simmer for 20 minutes.

3. Stir in bourbon if desired. Garnish each serving with sour cream, green onions and pumpkin seeds.

PER SERVING *1 cup equals 238 cal., 8 g fat (2 g sat. fat), 5 mg chol., 716 mg sodium, 30 g carb., 9 g fiber, 13 g pro.* **Diabetic Exchanges:** *1½ starch, 1½ fat, 1 lean meat, 1 vegetable.*

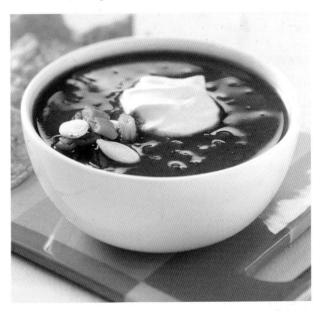

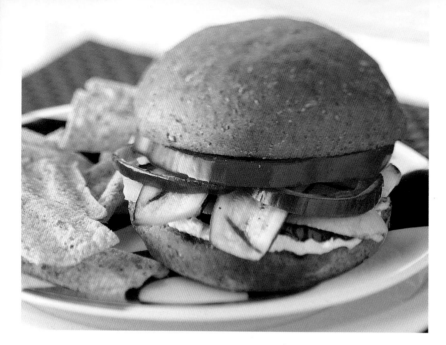

231 CALORIES Grilled
Veggie Sandwiches

Here's a fun recipe for using up those abundant summer garden veggies. Meat eaters won't even miss the meat with these hearty and fresh-tasting grilled sandwiches.

—**MELISSA WILBANKS** MEMPHIS, TN

START TO FINISH: 25 MIN.
MAKES: 4 SERVINGS

- 1 **small zucchini**
- 1 **small yellow summer squash**
- 1 **small eggplant**
  Cooking spray
- 1 **medium onion, sliced**
- 1 **large sweet red pepper, cut into rings**
- 4 **whole wheat hamburger buns, split**
- 3 **ounces fat-free cream cheese**
- ¼ **cup crumbled goat cheese**
- 1 **garlic clove, minced**
- ⅛ **teaspoon salt**
- ⅛ **teaspoon pepper**

1. Cut the zucchini, squash and eggplant into ¼-in.-thick strips;
spritz with cooking spray. Spritz the onion and the red pepper with cooking spray.

2. Grill vegetables, covered, over medium heat for 4-5 minutes on each side or until crisp-tender. Remove and keep warm. Grill buns, cut side down, over medium heat for 30-60 seconds or until toasted.

3. In a small bowl, combine the cheeses, garlic, salt and pepper; spread over bun bottoms. Top with vegetables. Replace bun tops.

PER SERVING *1 sandwich equals 231 cal., 6 g fat (2 g sat. fat), 10 mg chol., 438 mg sodium, 39 g carb., 10 g fiber, 11 g pro.* **Diabetic Exchanges:** *2½ starch, 1 fat.*

233 CALORIES
Broccoli Chowder

My family loves this original recipe for satisfying broccoli soup. The cheese makes it wonderfully creamy.

—**ESTHER SHANK** HARRISONBURG, VA

PREP: 20 MIN. • **COOK:** 15 MIN.
MAKES: 6 SERVINGS

- 4 **cups fresh small broccoli florets**
- 2 **medium potatoes, diced**
- 1½ **cups water**
- 2 **medium carrots, thinly sliced**
- 1 **large onion, chopped**
- 1 **celery rib, finely chopped**
- 4 **cups fat-free milk, divided**
- 2 **teaspoons reduced-sodium chicken bouillon granules**
- 1 **teaspoon Worcestershire sauce**
- ¾ **teaspoon salt**
- ½ **teaspoon pepper**
- ⅓ **cup all-purpose flour**
- 1 **cup cubed reduced-fat process cheese (Velveeta)**

1. In a large saucepan, combine the first six ingredients. Bring to a boil. Reduce heat; cover and simmer for 8-10 minutes or until vegetables are tender. Add 3 cups milk, bouillon, Worcestershire sauce, salt and pepper.

2. In a small bowl, combine flour and remaining milk until smooth; gradually stir into soup. Bring to a boil; cook and stir for 2 minutes or until thickened. Remove from heat; stir in cheese just until melted.

PER SERVING *1½ cups equals 233 cal., 3 g fat (2 g sat. fat), 11 mg chol., 838 mg sodium, 39 g carb., 6 g fiber, 15 g pro.*

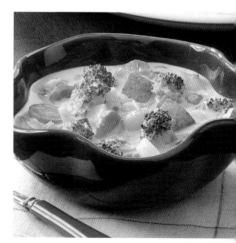

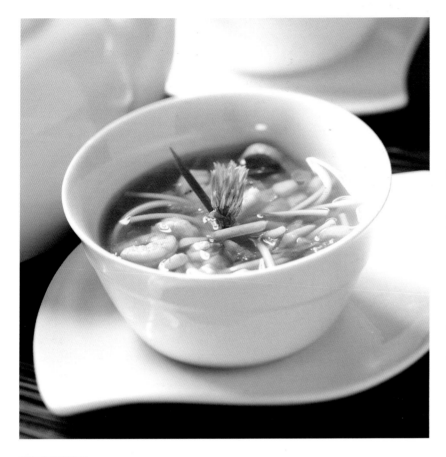

heat. Drain spaghetti. Add the spaghetti, lettuce, shrimp and green onion to the soup; heat through.

PER SERVING *1 cup equals 111 cal., 1 g fat (0.55 g sat. fat), 74 mg chol., 725 mg sodium, 13 g carb., 1 g fiber, 12 g pro.* **Diabetic Exchanges:** *1 starch, 1 lean meat.*

165 CALORIES Tuna Melts

I created this recipe when I got married years ago and have served it countless times since then. Sometimes I add a little chili powder to the tuna mixture, heap it over tortilla chips instead of English muffins, and microwave it for a plateful of hearty nachos.

—MARILYN SMELSER ALBANY, OR

START TO FINISH: 20 MIN.
MAKES: 8 SERVINGS

- 2 **cans (6 ounces each) light water-packed tuna, drained and flaked**
- ¾ **cup chopped sweet red pepper**
- ½ **cup chopped fresh mushrooms**
- ½ **cup shredded reduced-fat cheddar cheese**
- ¼ **cup sliced pimiento-stuffed olives**
- 4½ **teaspoons reduced-fat mayonnaise**
- 4 **English muffins, split and toasted**
- 8 **thin slices tomato**

1. In a large bowl, combine the tuna, red pepper, mushrooms, cheese and olives. Fold in mayonnaise. Spread over English muffin halves. Top each with a tomato slice.

2. Broil 6 in. from the heat for 7-9 minutes or until lightly browned. Serve immediately.

PER SERVING *1 serving equals 165 cal., 5 g fat (2 g sat. fat), 24 mg chol., 413 mg sodium, 16 g carb., 2 g fiber, 14 g pro.* **Diabetic Exchanges:** *2 lean meat, 1 starch.*

111 CALORIES

Asian Shrimp Soup

I make this soup so much, I've nicknamed it The House Specialty! It will appeal to anyone with a taste for Asian fare. If you don't have shrimp on hand, you can substitute chicken or pork.

—MICHELLE SMITH SYKESVILLE, MD

START TO FINISH: 20 MIN.
MAKES: 4 SERVINGS

- 1 **ounce uncooked thin spaghetti, broken into 1-inch pieces**
- 3 **cups plus 1 tablespoon water, divided**
- 3 **teaspoons reduced-sodium chicken bouillon granules**
- ½ **teaspoon salt**
- ½ **cup sliced fresh mushrooms**
- ½ **cup fresh or frozen corn**
- 1 **teaspoon cornstarch**
- 1½ **teaspoons reduced-sodium teriyaki sauce**
- 1 **cup thinly sliced romaine lettuce**
- 1 **can (6 ounces) small shrimp, rinsed and drained**
- 2 **tablespoons sliced green onion**

1. Cook spaghetti according to package directions.

2. In a large saucepan, combine 3 cups water, bouillon and salt; bring to a boil. Stir in mushrooms and corn. Reduce heat; cook, uncovered, until vegetables are tender.

3. Combine the cornstarch, teriyaki sauce and remaining water until smooth; stir into soup. Bring to a boil; cook and stir for 1-2 minutes or until slightly thickened. Reduce

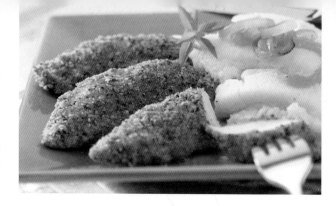

195 CALORIES Ratatouille with Polenta

Here's a hearty vegetarian meal inspired by the Provence region of France. Eggplant and other veggies are sauteed in olive oil and served over polenta.

—TASTE OF HOME TEST KITCHEN

PREP: 20 MIN. • **COOK:** 15 MIN. • **MAKES:** 4 SERVINGS

- ½ pound small fresh mushrooms, halved
- 1 medium sweet red pepper, chopped
- 1 small onion, chopped
- 4 teaspoons olive oil, divided
- 4 cups cubed peeled eggplant
- 1 small zucchini, chopped
- 1 cup cherry tomatoes
- 2 garlic cloves, minced
- 1½ teaspoons Italian seasoning
- ½ teaspoon salt
- 1 tube (1 pound) polenta, cut into ½-inch slices
  Grated Parmesan cheese, optional

1. In a large skillet, saute mushrooms, pepper and onion in 2 teaspoons oil until almost tender. Add the eggplant, zucchini, tomatoes, garlic, Italian seasoning and salt; cook 8-10 minutes longer or until tender.

2. In another skillet, cook polenta slices in remaining oil over medium-high heat for 3-4 minutes on each side or until lightly browned. Serve with ratatouille; sprinkle with cheese if desired.

PER SERVING *1½ cups ratatouille with 3 pieces of polenta equals 195 cal., 5 g fat (1 g sat. fat), 0 chol., 689 mg sodium, 34 g carb., 6 g fiber, 6 g pro.* **Diabetic Exchanges:** *2 starch, 1 fat.*

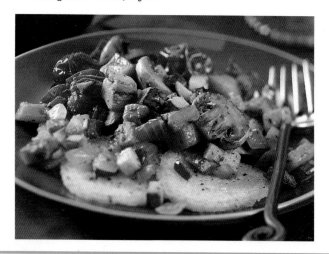

188 CALORIES Seasoned Chicken Strips

These strips are designed for kids, but tasty enough for company. The tender strips are moist and juicy and would also be great on a salad.

—BECKY OLIVER FAIRPLAY, CO

PREP/TOTAL TIME: 25 MIN. • **MAKES:** 4 SERVINGS

- ⅓ cup egg substitute
- 1 tablespoon prepared mustard
- 1 garlic clove, minced
- ¾ cup dry bread crumbs
- 2 teaspoons dried basil
- 1 teaspoon paprika
- ½ teaspoon salt
- ¼ teaspoon pepper
- 1 pound chicken tenderloins

1. In a shallow bowl, combine the egg substitute, mustard and garlic. In another shallow bowl, combine the bread crumbs, basil, paprika, salt and pepper. Dip chicken in egg mixture, then roll in crumbs.

2. Place on a baking sheet coated with cooking spray. Bake at 400° for 10-15 minutes or until golden brown and juices run clear.

PER SERVING *3 ounces cooked chicken equals 188 cal., 2 g fat (trace sat. fat), 67 mg chol., 525 mg sodium, 14 g carb., 1 g fiber, 30 g pro.* **Diabetic Exchanges:** *3 lean meat, 1 starch.*

225 CALORIES
Mediterranean Salad Sandwiches

These satisfying, fresh-flavored sandwiches taste like a summer salad on a bun. Add iced tea, sorbet for dessert, and call it an easy meal.

—CANDICE GARCIA WINTER HAVEN, FL

START TO FINISH: 30 MIN. • **MAKES:** 4 SERVINGS

2 tablespoons olive oil, divided
1 garlic clove, minced
¼ teaspoon salt
4 large portobello mushrooms, stems removed
2 cups spring mix salad greens
1 medium tomato, chopped
½ cup chopped roasted sweet red peppers
¼ cup crumbled reduced-fat feta cheese
2 tablespoons chopped pitted Greek olives
1 tablespoon red wine vinegar
½ teaspoon dried oregano
4 slices sourdough bread, toasted and halved

1. In a small bowl, combine 1 tablespoon oil, garlic and salt; brush over mushrooms.

2. Moisten a paper towel with cooking oil; using long-handled tongs, lightly coat the grill rack. Grill mushrooms, covered, over medium heat for 6-8 minutes on each side or until tender.

3. In a large bowl, combine the salad greens, tomato, peppers, cheese and olives. In a small bowl, whisk the vinegar, oregano and remaining oil. Pour over salad mixture; toss to coat.

4. Layer each of four half-slices of toast with a mushroom and ¾ cup salad mixture; top with remaining toast.

PER SERVING *1 serving equals 225 cal., 9 g fat (2 g sat. fat), 3 mg chol., 495 mg sodium, 26 g carb., 3 g fiber, 8 g pro.* **Diabetic Exchanges:** *2 vegetable, 2 fat, 1 starch.*

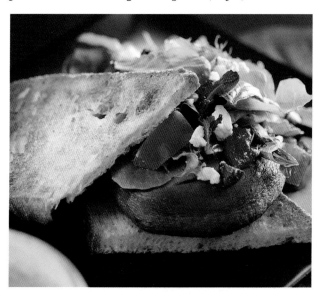

Below are some items you might use when **preparing a lunch**. When packing a lunch or adding to your afternoon menu, use this list to make sure you stick to your goal of **450 total calories**.

- 1 slice whole wheat bread, **69 CALORIES**
- 1 slice reduced-calorie bread, **48 CALORIES**
- 1 flour tortilla (6-in. diameter), **90 CALORIES**
- 1 corn tortilla (6-in. diameter), **58 CALORIES**
- 1 whole wheat dinner roll, **76 CALORIES**
- 1 hamburger bun, **79 CALORIES**
- 1 hard roll, **83 CALORIES**
- 1 slice American cheese (1 ounce), **93 CALORIES**
- 1 slice Swiss cheese (1 ounce), **106 CALORIES**
- 1 slice cheddar cheese (1 ounce), **113 CALORIES**
- ¼ cup diced cheddar cheese, **113 CALORIES**
- ½ cup 1% cottage cheese, **81 CALORIES**
- 1 tablespoon shredded Parmesan cheese, **21 CALORIES**
- 1 cup red or green grapes, **129 CALORIES**
- 1 medium orange, **62 CALORIES**
- 1 medium apple, **72 CALORIES**
- 1 cup mandarin orange segments, **92 CALORIES**
- 1 cup cubed watermelon, **40 CALORIES**
- ½ cup cubed pineapple, **37 CALORIES**
- 2 tablespoons peanut butter, **192 CALORIES**
- 1 ounce deli ham or turkey, **22 CALORIES**
- 20 baked potato chips, **200 CALORIES**
- ¾ cup miniature pretzel twists, **112 CALORIES**

For the calorie counts of other typical lunch side dishes, see the Snacks Calorie List on pages 84-85. Also check out the Free Foods List on page 41.

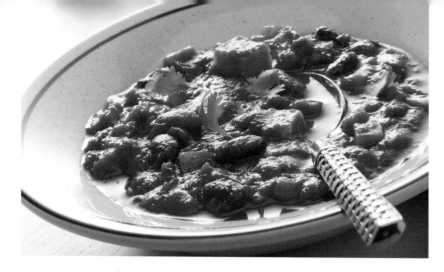

241 CALORIES

Anytime Turkey Chili

I created this unusual dish to grab the voters' attention at a chili contest we held in our backyard. With pumpkin, brown sugar and cooked turkey, it's like an entire Thanksgiving dinner in one bowl. It's the perfect food for a fall day.
—BRAD BAILEY CARY, NC

PREP: 20 MIN. • **COOK:** 1¼ HOURS
MAKES: 8 SERVINGS (2 QUARTS)

- ⅔ cup chopped sweet onion
- ½ cup chopped green pepper
- 1½ teaspoons dried oregano
- 1 teaspoon ground cumin
- 1 teaspoon olive oil
- 2 garlic cloves, minced
- 1 can (16 ounces) kidney beans, rinsed and drained
- 1 can (15½ ounces) great northern beans, rinsed and drained
- 1 can (15 ounces) solid-pack pumpkin
- 1 can (15 ounces) crushed tomatoes
- 1 can (14½ ounces) reduced-sodium chicken broth
- ½ cup water
- 2 tablespoons brown sugar
- 2 tablespoons chili powder
- ½ teaspoon pepper
- 3 cups cubed cooked turkey breast

1. In a large saucepan, saute onion, green pepper, oregano and cumin in oil until vegetables are tender. Add garlic; cook 1 minute longer.
2. Stir in the beans, pumpkin, tomatoes, broth, water, brown sugar, chili powder and pepper; bring to a boil. Reduce heat; cover and simmer for 1 hour. Add turkey; heat through.
PER SERVING *1 cup equals 241 cal., 2 g fat (trace sat. fat), 45 mg chol., 478 mg sodium, 32 g carb., 10 g fiber, 25 g pro.* **Diabetic Exchanges:** *3 lean meat, 1½ starch, 1 vegetable.*

141 CALORIES

Asian Linguine Salad

With loads of vegetables and a delicious dressing, this chilled pasta toss offers guilt-free enjoyment.
—PAT HILMER OSHKOSH, WI

PREP: 30 MIN. + CHILLING
MAKES: 8 SERVINGS

- 8 ounces uncooked linguine
- ⅓ cup reduced-sodium soy sauce
- ¼ cup water
- 2 tablespoons lemon juice
- 1½ teaspoons sesame oil
- 2 medium carrots, julienned
- ½ medium sweet red pepper, julienned
- 1½ teaspoons olive oil, divided
- ½ cup fresh snow peas
- 1 garlic clove, minced
- 1 small zucchini, julienned
- ½ cup canned bean sprouts
- 1 green onion, julienned

1. Cook linguine according to package directions; drain and place in a large bowl. Whisk the soy sauce, water, lemon juice and sesame oil. Refrigerate ¼ cup for dressing. Pour remaining mixture over hot linguine; toss to coat.
2. In a large nonstick skillet or wok coated with cooking spray, stir-fry carrots and red pepper in ¾ teaspoon olive oil for 2 minutes. Add snow peas and garlic; stir-fry 2 minutes longer. Add to linguine.
3. Stir-fry the zucchini, bean sprouts and onion in remaining olive oil for 2 minutes; add to linguine mixture. Cover and refrigerate for at least 2 hours. Just before serving, add dressing and toss to coat.
PER SERVING *1 serving equals 141 cal., 2 g fat (trace sat. fat), 0 chol., 415 mg sodium, 25 g carb., 2 g fiber, 5 g pro.* **Diabetic Exchanges:** *1½ starch, ½ fat.*

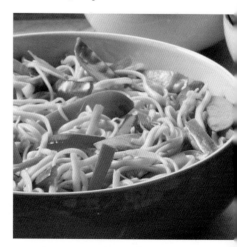

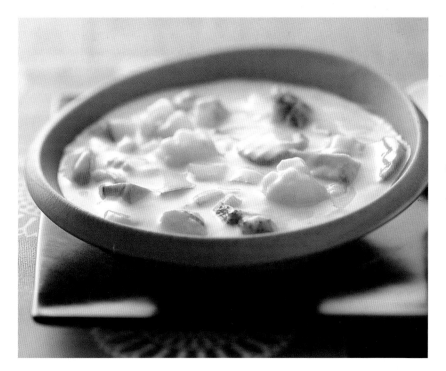

115 CALORIES
Veggie Cheese Soup

My niece makes this in a slow cooker by putting in all the ingredients but the cheese. When the veggies are tender, she adds the cubed cheese and has a nutritious meal ready 5 minutes later.
—JEAN HALL RAPID CITY, SD

PREP: 15 MIN. • **COOK:** 25 MIN.
MAKES: 9 SERVINGS

- 1 **medium onion, chopped**
- 1 **celery rib, chopped**
- 2 **small red potatoes, cut into ½-inch cubes**
- 2¾ **cups water**
- 2 **teaspoons reduced-sodium chicken bouillon granules**
- 1 **tablespoon cornstarch**
- ¼ **cup cold water**
- 1 **can (10¾ ounces) reduced-fat reduced-sodium condensed cream of chicken soup, undiluted**
- 3 **cups frozen California-blend vegetables, thawed**
- ½ **cup chopped fully cooked lean ham**
- 8 **ounces reduced-fat process cheese (Velveeta), cubed**

1. In a large nonstick saucepan coated with a cooking spray, cook onion and celery over medium heat until onion is tender. Stir in the potatoes, water and bouillon. Bring to a boil. Reduce heat; cover and simmer for 10 minutes.
2. Combine cornstarch and cold water until smooth; gradually stir into soup. Return to a boil; cook and stir for 1-2 minutes or until slightly thickened. Stir in the condensed soup until blended.
3. Reduce heat; add vegetables and ham. Cook and stir until vegetables are tender. Stir in cheese until melted.
PER SERVING *¾ cup equals 115 cal., 4 g fat (2 g sat. fat), 15 mg chol., 682 mg sodium, 13 g carb., 1 g fiber, 8 g pro.*

218 CALORIES Hot Swiss Chicken Sandwiches

I've been making these open-faced sandwiches for years, and people always ask for the recipe. I sometimes serve the filling on slices of sourdough or tucked into pitas.
—EDITH TABOR VANCOUVER, WA

START TO FINISH: 20 MIN.
MAKES: 6 SERVINGS

- ¼ **cup reduced-fat mayonnaise**
- ¼ **teaspoon salt**
- ¼ **teaspoon lemon juice**
- 1½ **cups diced cooked chicken breast**
- ⅔ **cup chopped celery**
- ½ **cup shredded reduced-fat Swiss cheese**
- 4 **teaspoons butter, softened**
- 6 **slices Italian bread (about ¾ inch thick)**
- 6 **slices tomato**
- ¾ **cup shredded lettuce**

1. In a large bowl, combine the mayonnaise, salt and lemon juice. Stir in the chicken, celery and cheese. Spread butter on each slice of bread; top each with ⅓ cup chicken mixture.
2. Place in a 15-in. x 10-in. x 1-in. baking pan. Broil 4-6 in. from the heat for 3-4 minutes or until heated through. Top sandwiches with tomato and lettuce.
PER SERVING *1 sandwich equals 218 cal., 9 g fat (3 g sat. fat), 44 mg chol., 438 mg sodium, 17 g carb., 1 g fiber, 17 g pro.*
Diabetic Exchanges: *2 lean meat, 1 starch, ½ fat.*

251-350 CALORIES

259 CALORIES Special Egg Salad

This recipe proves you don't have to sacrifice flavor to eat lighter. These yummy, satisfying egg salad sandwiches are sure to be well-received whenever you serve them.
—**JUDY NISSEN** SIOUX FALLS, SD

PREP: 15 MIN. + CHILLING • **MAKES:** 6 SERVINGS

- 3 ounces reduced-fat cream cheese
- ¼ cup fat-free mayonnaise
- ½ teaspoon sugar
- ¼ teaspoon onion powder
- ¼ teaspoon garlic powder
- ⅛ teaspoon salt
- ⅛ teaspoon pepper
- 6 hard-cooked eggs, chopped
- 12 slices whole wheat bread, toasted
- 6 lettuce leaves

In a small bowl, beat the cream cheese until smooth. Beat in the mayonnaise, sugar, onion powder, garlic powder, salt and pepper; fold in the eggs. Cover and refrigerate for 1 hour. Serve on toast with lettuce.
PER SERVING *1 serving equals 259 cal., 10 g fat (4 g sat. fat), 225 mg chol., 528 mg sodium, 30 g carb., 4 g fiber, 13 g pro.* **Diabetic Exchanges:** *2 starch, 1½ fat, 1 lean meat.*

307 CALORIES Grilled Bean Burgers

For a surefire meatless mainstay, I swear by these moist and delicious salsa-topped burgers. I first sampled them at an Eating Right session at our local library. And they can hold their own against any veggie burger you'd buy at the supermarket!
—**MARGUERITE SHAEFFER** SEWELL, NJ

PREP: 25 MIN. • **GRILL:** 10 MIN. • **MAKES:** 8 SERVINGS

- 1 large onion, finely chopped
- 1 tablespoon olive oil
- 4 garlic cloves, minced
- 1 medium carrot, shredded
- 1 to 2 teaspoons chili powder
- 1 teaspoon ground cumin
- 1 can (15 ounces) pinto beans, rinsed and drained
- 1 can (15 ounces) black beans, rinsed and drained
- 1½ cups quick-cooking oats
- 2 tablespoons Dijon mustard
- 2 tablespoons reduced-sodium soy sauce
- 1 tablespoon ketchup
- ¼ teaspoon pepper
- 8 whole wheat hamburger buns, split
- 8 lettuce leaves
- 8 tablespoons salsa

1. In a large nonstick skillet coated with cooking spray, saute onion in oil for 2 minutes. Add garlic; cook for 1 minute. Stir in the carrot, chili powder and cumin; cook 2 minutes longer or until carrot is tender. Remove from the heat; set aside.

2. In a large bowl, mash the pinto beans and black beans. Stir in oats. Add the mustard, soy sauce, ketchup, pepper and carrot mixture; mix well. Shape into eight 3½-in. patties.

3. Moisten a paper towel with cooking oil; using long-handled tongs, lightly coat the grill rack. Grill patties, covered, over medium heat or broil 4 in. from the heat for 4-5 minutes on each side or until heated through. Serve on buns with lettuce and salsa.
PER SERVING *1 burger equals 307 cal., 5 g fat (1 g sat. fat), 0 chol., 723 mg sodium, 53 g carb., 10 g fiber, 12 g pro.* **Diabetic Exchanges:** *3½ starch, 1 lean meat.*

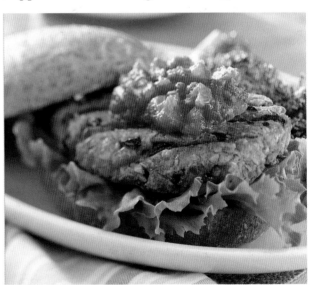

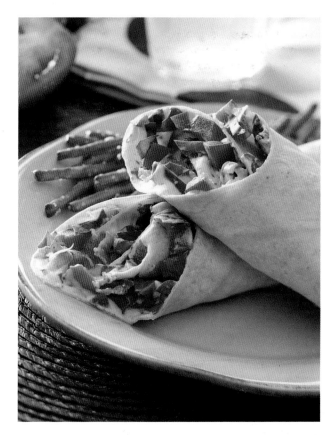

289 CALORIES Simon's Famous Tuna Salad

Crunchy carrots give this nicely seasoned tuna salad a unique and tasty twist you'll love. A simple and delicious lunch.

—SIMON SEITZ HIGHLAND, NY

START TO FINISH: 15 MIN. • **MAKES:** 5 SERVINGS

- 3 cans (5 ounces each) light water-packed tuna, drained and flaked
- ¾ cup fat-free mayonnaise
- ¼ cup chopped celery
- ¼ cup chopped carrot
- ½ teaspoon onion powder
- ½ teaspoon garlic powder
- ¼ teaspoon dill weed
- 10 slices whole wheat bread, toasted
- 5 lettuce leaves

In a large bowl, combine the first seven ingredients. For each sandwich, layer a slice of toast with a lettuce leaf and 1/2 cup tuna salad. Top with a second slice of toast.

PER SERVING *1 sandwich equals 289 cal., 4 g fat (1 g sat. fat), 34 mg chol., 907 mg sodium, 29 g carb., 5 g fiber, 34 g pro.*

294 CALORIES Garden Vegetable Wraps

My husband and I love these light, tasty wraps for lunch. I found the recipe years ago and it was an instant hit.

—BARBARA BLAKE WEST BRATTLEBORO, VERMONT

START TO FINISH: 25 MIN. • **MAKES:** 4 SERVINGS

- ½ cup reduced-fat garlic-herb spreadable cheese
- 4 flour tortillas (10 inches)
- 1¼ cups chopped seeded tomatoes
- 1¼ cups julienned fresh spinach
- ¾ cup chopped sweet red pepper
- 2 bacon strips, cooked and crumbled
- ¼ teaspoon coarsely ground pepper

Spread 2 tablespoons spreadable cheese over each tortilla. Top with tomatoes, spinach, red pepper, bacon and pepper. Roll up tightly.

PER SERVING *1 wrap equals 294 cal., 9 g fat (4 g sat. fat), 16 mg chol., 584 mg sodium, 36 g carb., 7 g fiber, 11 g pro.* **Diabetic Exchanges:** *2½ starch, 2 fat, 1 vegetable.*

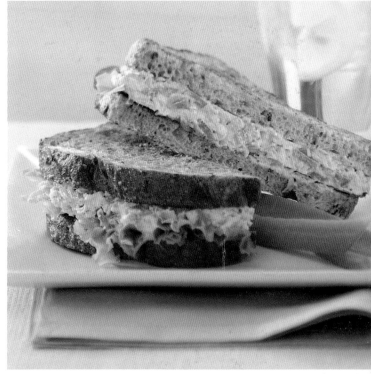

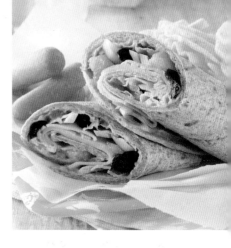

312 CALORIES

Buffalo Turkey Burgers

There's nothing bland about these juicy turkey burgers! Celery and blue cheese salad dressing help tame the hot sauce. For an even skinnier version, skip the bun and add some sliced onion and chopped tomato.

—MARY PAX-SHIPLEY BEND, OR

START TO FINISH: 25 MIN.
MAKES: 4 SERVINGS

- 2 tablespoons Louisiana-style hot sauce, divided
- 2 teaspoons ground cumin
- 2 teaspoons chili powder
- 2 garlic cloves, minced
- ½ teaspoon salt
- ⅛ teaspoon pepper
- 1 pound lean ground turkey
- 4 whole wheat hamburger buns, split
- 1 cup shredded lettuce
- 2 celery ribs, chopped
- 2 tablespoons fat-free blue cheese salad dressing

1. In a large bowl, combine 1 tablespoon hot sauce, cumin, chili powder, garlic, salt and pepper. Crumble turkey over mixture and mix well. Shape into four patties.
2. In a large nonstick skillet coated with cooking spray, cook patties over medium heat for 4-5 minutes on each side or until a thermometer reads 165° and juices run clear.
3. Serve on buns with lettuce, celery, blue cheese dressing and remaining hot sauce.
PER SERVING *1 burger equals 312 cal., 12 g fat (3 g sat. fat), 90 mg chol., 734 mg sodium, 28 g carb., 5 g fiber, 24 g pro.* **Diabetic Exchanges:** *3 lean meat, 2 starch, ½ fat.*

332 CALORIES

Fruited Turkey Wraps

This colorful wrap tastes great and is so good for you. It's packed with lean protein, fruit and veggies and wrapped in whole-grain goodness. And, surprise, it takes only a few minutes to put together!

—LISA RENSHAW KANSAS CITY, MO

START TO FINISH: 15 MIN.
MAKES: 4 SERVINGS

- ½ cup fat-free mayonnaise
- 1 tablespoon orange juice
- 1 teaspoon grated orange peel
- ¾ teaspoon curry powder
- 4 whole wheat tortillas (8 inches), room temperature
- 2 cups finely shredded Chinese or napa cabbage
- 1 small red onion, thinly sliced
- 1 can (11 ounces) mandarin oranges, drained
- ⅔ cup dried cranberries
- ½ pound thinly sliced deli smoked turkey

Combine mayonnaise, orange juice, peel and curry; spread over tortillas. Top with cabbage, onion, oranges, cranberries and turkey. Roll up.
PER SERVING *1 wrap equals 332 cal., 5 g fat (trace sat. fat), 23 mg chol., 845 mg sodium, 54 g carb., 5 g fiber, 17 g pro.*

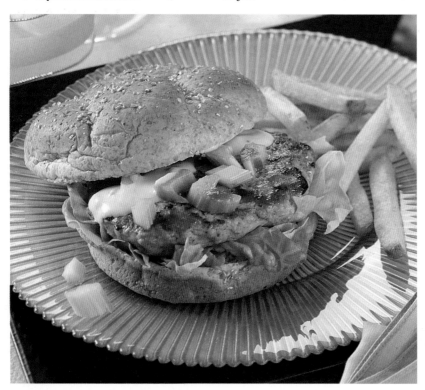

251 CALORIES Flavorful Crab Pasta Salad

After enjoying this recipe for years, I substituted fat-free mayonnaise and reduced-fat dressing one day. I was just delighted to find it kept all the same wonderful flavor!
—**HEATHER O'NEILL** DUDLEY, MA

PREP: 30 MIN. + CHILLING
MAKES: 6 SERVINGS

- 8 ounces uncooked spiral pasta
- 1 package (8 ounces) imitation crabmeat, chopped
- 1 cup frozen peas, thawed
- 1 cup fresh broccoli florets
- ½ cup chopped green pepper
- ¼ cup sliced green onions
- ¾ cup fat-free mayonnaise
- ⅓ cup reduced-fat Italian salad dressing
- 3 tablespoons grated Parmesan cheese

Cook pasta according to package directions; drain and rinse in cold water. In a large bowl, combine the pasta, crab, peas, broccoli, green pepper and onions. Combine the mayonnaise, salad dressing and Parmesan cheese; pour over pasta mixture and toss to coat. Cover and refrigerate for 2 hours or until chilled.
PER SERVING *1⅓ cups equals 251 cal., 5 g fat (1 g sat. fat), 10 mg chol., 746 mg sodium, 42 g carb., 3 g fiber, 12 g pro.* **Diabetic Exchanges:** *3 starch, 1 lean meat.*

274 CALORIES Best Sloppy Joes

Who isn't looking for quick healthy meal solutions during busy weekdays and jam-packed schedules? Here's a sophisticated twist on a kids' favorite. My daughter Tiffany came up with this lower-fat version of traditional sloppy joes—and we all love it!
—**SUZANNE MCKINLEY** LYONS, GA

START TO FINISH: 25 MIN.
MAKES: 6 SERVINGS

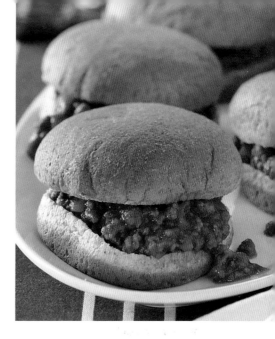

- 1 pound ground beef
- ⅓ cup chopped onion
- 1 garlic clove, minced
- 1 can (8 ounces) tomato sauce
- ½ cup ketchup
- 4 teaspoons Worcestershire sauce
- 1 teaspoon molasses
- 1 teaspoon prepared mustard
- ½ teaspoon ground mustard
  Pinch ground cloves
  Pinch cayenne pepper
- ¼ teaspoon grated orange peel, optional
- 6 whole wheat buns, split

In a saucepan, cook the beef, onion and garlic over medium heat until meat is no longer pink; drain. Stir in the tomato sauce, ketchup, Worcestershire sauce, molasses, prepared mustard, ground mustard, cloves, cayenne and orange peel if desired. Bring to a boil. Reduce heat; simmer, uncovered, for 5 minutes. Serve on buns.
PER SERVING *1 sandwich equals 274 cal., 9 g fat (3 g sat. fat), 37 mg chol., 713 mg sodium, 32 g carb., 4 g fiber, 18 g pro.*

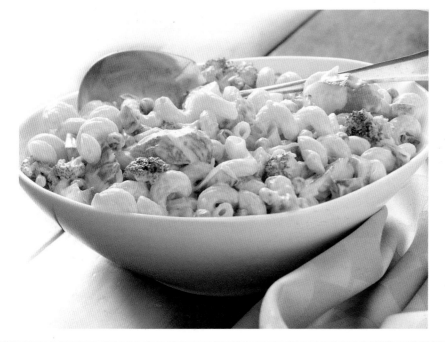

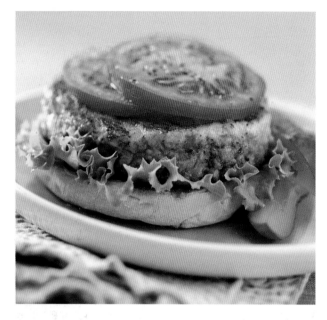

270 CALORIES

Open-Faced Salmon Sandwiches

I keep several cans of salmon in my pantry at all times so I never have to worry about unexpected drop-in guests. This recipe is so tasty and quick...and it doubles easily for company.

—KATNEE CABECEIRAS SOUTH PRAIRIE, WA

START TO FINISH: 25 MIN. • **MAKES:** 4 SERVINGS

- 1 egg, lightly beaten
- 1 small onion, finely chopped
- 1 small green pepper, finely chopped
- ⅓ cup soft bread crumbs
- 1 tablespoon lemon juice
- 1 teaspoon reduced-sodium teriyaki sauce
- ¼ teaspoon dried parsley flakes
- ¼ teaspoon dried basil
- ¼ teaspoon pepper
- 1 can (14¾ ounces) salmon, drained, bones and skin removed
- 2 English muffins, split and toasted
  Lettuce leaves and tomato slices, optional

1. In a small bowl, combine the first nine ingredients. Fold in salmon. Shape into four patties.

2. In a large nonstick skillet coated with cooking spray, cook patties over medium heat for 4-5 minutes on each side or until lightly browned. Serve on English muffin halves with lettuce and tomato if desired.

PER SERVING *1 sandwich equals 270 cal., 10 g fat (2 g sat. fat), 99 mg chol., 757 mg sodium, 19 g carb., 2 g fiber, 26 g pro.* **Diabetic Exchanges:** *3 lean meat, 1 starch.*

287 CALORIES

Hearty Chipotle Chicken Soup

Sweet corn and cool sour cream help tame the smoky hot flavors of chipotle pepper. This zesty soup is wonderful for chilly nights.

—SONALI RUDER NEW YORK, NY

PREP: 15 MIN. • **COOK:** 30 MIN. • **MAKES:** 8 SERVINGS (3¼ QUARTS)

- 1 large onion, chopped
- 1 tablespoon canola oil
- 4 garlic cloves, minced
- 4 cups reduced-sodium chicken broth
- 2 cans (15 ounces each) pinto beans, rinsed and drained
- 2 cans (14½ ounces each) fire-roasted diced tomatoes, undrained
- 3 cups frozen corn
- 2 chipotle peppers in adobo sauce, seeded and minced
- 2 teaspoons adobo sauce
- 1 teaspoon ground cumin
- ¼ teaspoon pepper
- 2 cups cubed cooked chicken breast
- ½ cup fat-free sour cream
- ¼ cup minced fresh cilantro

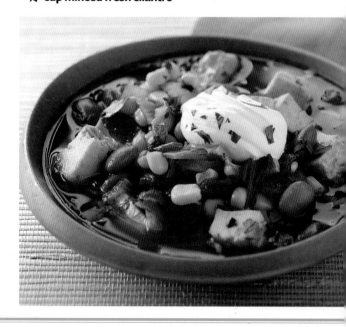

1. In a Dutch oven, saute onion in oil until tender. Add garlic; cook 1 minute longer. Add the broth, beans, tomatoes, corn, chipotle peppers, adobo sauce, cumin and pepper. Bring to a boil. Reduce heat; simmer, uncovered, for 20 minutes.
2. Stir in chicken; heat through. Garnish with sour cream; sprinkle with cilantro.

PER SERVING *1⅔ cups with 1 tablespoon sour cream equals 287 cal., 4 g fat (1 g sat. fat), 29 mg chol., 790 mg sodium, 42 g carb., 7 g fiber, 21 g pro. **Diabetic Exchanges:** 2 starch, 2 lean meat, 2 vegetable.*

291 CALORIES Beef Fajita Salad

This easy salad features colorful peppers, beans, tomato and tender strips of beef. The beef marinates for only 10 minutes, but it gets great flavor from the lime juice, cilantro and chili powder.
—**ARDEENA HARRIS** ROANOKE, AL

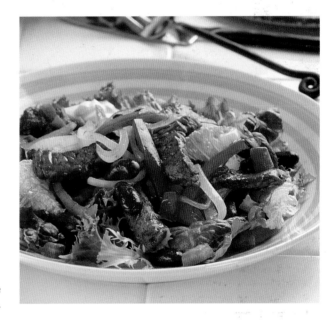

START TO FINISH: 30 MIN. • **MAKES:** 4 SERVINGS

- ¼ cup lime juice
- 2 tablespoons minced fresh cilantro
- 1 garlic clove, minced
- 1 teaspoon chili powder
- ¾ pound beef top sirloin steak, cut into thin strips
- 1 medium green pepper, julienned
- 1 medium sweet red pepper, julienned
- 1 medium onion, sliced and halved
- 1 teaspoon olive oil
- 1 can (16 ounces) kidney beans, rinsed and drained
- 4 cups torn mixed salad greens
- 1 medium tomato, chopped
- 4 tablespoons fat-free sour cream
- 2 tablespoons salsa

1. In a large resealable plastic bag, combine the lime juice, cilantro, garlic and chili powder; add beef. Seal bag and turn to coat; refrigerate for 10 minutes, turning once.
2. Meanwhile, in a nonstick skillet, cook the peppers and onion in oil over medium-high heat for 5 minutes or until tender. Remove and keep warm. Add beef with marinade to the skillet; cook and stir for 4-5 minutes or until meat is tender and mixture comes to a boil. Add beans and pepper mixture; heat through.
3. Divide the salad greens and tomato among four bowls; top each with 1¼ cups beef mixture, 1 tablespoon sour cream and 1½ teaspoons salsa.

PER SERVING *1 serving equals 291 cal., 6 g fat (2 g sat. fat), 50 mg chol., 291 mg sodium, 34 g carb., 9 g fiber, 27 g pro. **Diabetic Exchanges:** 2 lean meat, 2 vegetable, 1½ starch.*

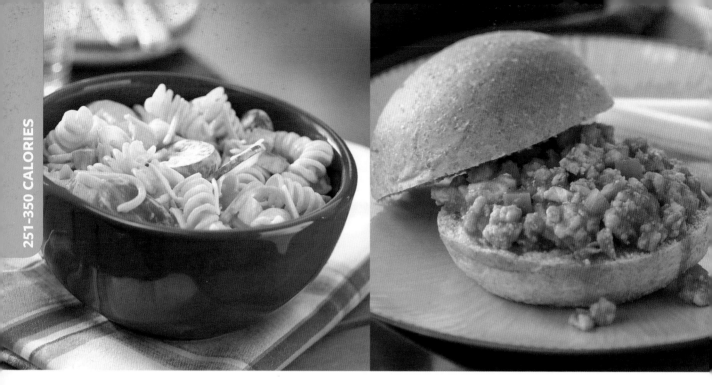

271 CALORIES

Creamy Pasta Salad

I love creating tasty new foods, including this garden-fresh pasta salad. I make it often for my husband and me, especially during summer. If you add some cubed cooked chicken breast, you can make it a hearty dinner.

—**LORRAINE MENARD** OMAHA, NE

PREP: 25 MIN. + CHILLING
MAKES: 2 SERVINGS

- 1 cup cooked spiral pasta
- ⅓ cup grape tomatoes, halved
- ¼ cup shredded cheddar cheese
- 3 tablespoons chopped onion
- 3 tablespoons chopped cucumber
- 3 tablespoons chopped green pepper
- 2 tablespoons shredded Parmesan cheese
- 2 tablespoons sliced pepperoncini
- 2 radishes, sliced
- ⅛ teaspoon pepper
- ¼ cup reduced-fat ranch salad dressing

In a small bowl, combine the first 10 ingredients. Drizzle with dressing and toss to coat. Cover and refrigerate for at least 1 hour before serving.

PER SERVING *1 cup equals 271 cal., 13 g fat (5 g sat. fat), 27 mg chol., 966 mg sodium, 28 g carb., 2 g fiber, 9 g pro.*

280 CALORIES

Barbecued Turkey on Buns

You'll feel good serving these luscious sandwiches that make the most of unsweetened pineapple juice. Folks never guess they're made with ground turkey.

—**CHRISTA NORWALK** LA VALLE, WI

PREP: 10 MIN. • **COOK:** 35 MIN.
MAKES: 6 SERVINGS

- 1 pound lean ground turkey
- ½ cup chopped onion
- ½ cup chopped green pepper
- 1 can (6 ounces) tomato paste
- 1 can (6 ounces) unsweetened pineapple juice
- ¼ cup water
- 2 teaspoons Dijon mustard
- ½ teaspoon garlic powder
- ½ teaspoon salt
- ⅛ teaspoon pepper
- 6 whole wheat hamburger buns, split and toasted

1. In a large saucepan coated with cooking spray, cook the turkey, onion and green pepper over medium heat until meat is no longer pink; drain.

2. Stir in tomato paste, pineapple juice, water, mustard, garlic powder, salt and pepper. Bring to a boil. Reduce heat; simmer, uncovered, for 20-30 minutes or until sauce is thickened. Spoon ⅓ cup onto each bun.

PER SERVING *1 sandwich equals 280 cal., 8 g fat (2 g sat. fat), 60 mg chol., 538 mg sodium, 34 g carb., 6 g fiber, 18 g pro.* **Diabetic Exchanges:** *2 starch, 2 lean meat, 1 vegetable.*

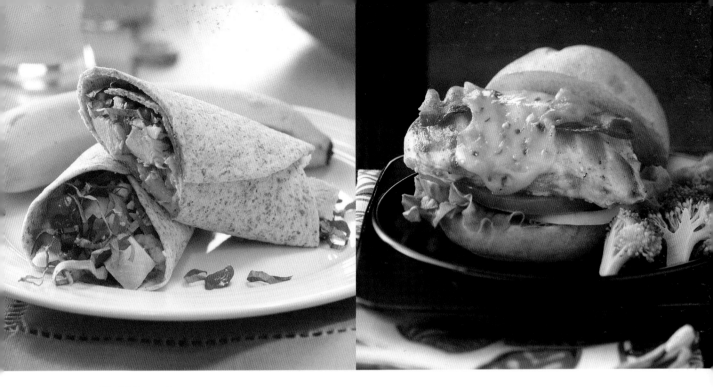

California Chicken Wraps

Hummus is a fantastic alternative to mayonnaise. The combination of hummus and feta gives these wraps unbeatable flavor.
—**DONNA MUNCH** EL PASO, TX

START TO FINISH: 15 MIN.
MAKES: 4 SERVINGS

- ⅓ **cup prepared hummus**
- 4 **whole wheat tortillas (8 inches)**
- 2 **cups cubed cooked chicken breast**
- ¼ **cup chopped roasted sweet red peppers**
- ¼ **cup crumbled feta cheese**
- ¼ **cup thinly sliced fresh basil leaves**

Spread hummus on tortillas; top with chicken, peppers, cheese and basil. Roll up.
PER SERVING *1 wrap equals 300 cal., 8 g fat (2 g sat. fat), 58 mg chol., 408 mg sodium, 26 g carb., 3 g fiber, 27 g pro.* **Diabetic Exchanges:** *3 lean meat, 2 starch.*

Grilled Pepper Jack Chicken Sandwiches

Zesty cheese, yummy bacon and grilled flavor will have you thinking this sandwich came from a restaurant. Use a grill pan if you don't want to venture outside.
—**LINDA FOREMAN**
LOCUST GROVE, OK

START TO FINISH: 25 MIN.
MAKES: 2 SERVINGS

- 2 **boneless skinless chicken breast halves (4 ounces each)**
- 1 **teaspoon poultry seasoning**
- 2 **center-cut bacon strips, cooked and halved**
- 2 **slices (½ ounce each) pepper jack cheese**
- 2 **hamburger buns, split**
- 2 **lettuce leaves**
- 1 **slice onion, separated into rings**
- 2 **slices tomato**
  Dill pickle slices, optional

1. Sprinkle chicken with poultry seasoning. Moisten a paper towel with cooking oil; using long-handled tongs, lightly coat the grill rack.
2. Grill chicken, covered, over medium heat or broil 4 in. from the heat for 4-7 minutes on each side or until a thermometer reads 170°. Top with bacon and cheese; cover and cook 1-2 minutes longer or until cheese is melted.
3. Serve on buns with lettuce, onion, tomato and pickles if desired.
PER SERVING *1 sandwich (calculated without pickles) equals 335 cal., 11 g fat (4 g sat. fat), 85 mg chol., 456 mg sodium, 25 g carb., 2 g fiber, 33 g pro.* **Diabetic Exchanges:** *4 lean meat, 1½ starch.*

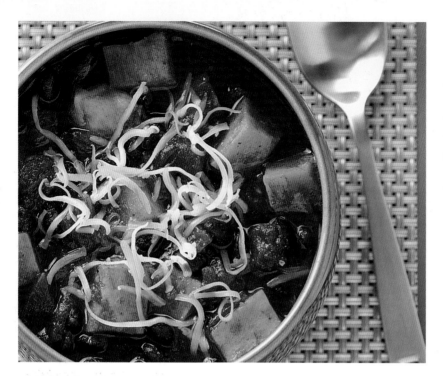

252 CALORIES Sweet Potato & Black Bean Chili

My whole family enjoys this vegetarian chili, but my daughter especially loves it. I like to make it because it's so easy and very flavorful. It's the perfect comfort food for the chilly months.

—**JOY PENDLEY** ORTONVILLE, MI

PREP: 25 MIN. • **COOK:** 35 MIN.
MAKES: 8 SERVINGS (2 QUARTS)

- **3** large sweet potatoes, peeled and cut into ½-inch cubes
- **1** large onion, chopped
- **1** tablespoon olive oil
- **2** tablespoons chili powder
- **3** garlic cloves, minced
- **1** teaspoon ground cumin
- **¼** teaspoon cayenne pepper
- **2** cans (15 ounces each) black beans, rinsed and drained
- **1** can (28 ounces) diced tomatoes, undrained
- **¼** cup brewed coffee
- **2** tablespoons honey
- **½** teaspoon salt
- **¼** teaspoon pepper
- **½** cup shredded reduced-fat Monterey Jack cheese or reduced-fat Mexican cheese blend

1. In a nonstick Dutch oven coated with cooking spray, saute sweet potatoes and onion in oil until crisp-tender. Add the chili powder, garlic, cumin and cayenne; cook mixture 1 minute longer. Stir in the beans, tomatoes, coffee, honey, salt and pepper.

2. Bring to a boil. Reduce heat; cover and simmer for 30-35 minutes or until sweet potatoes are tender. Sprinkle with cheese.

PER SERVING *1 cup chili with 1 tablespoon cheese equals 252 cal., 4 g fat (1 g sat. fat), 5 mg chol., 554 mg sodium, 47 g carb., 9 g fiber, 10 g pro.*

322 CALORIES Fruity Crab Pasta Salad

A sweet ginger dressing spices up this tasty medley of oranges, grapes, crabmeat and pasta. It's an ideal warm-weather entree.

—**DARLENE JUREK** FOLEY, MN

START TO FINISH: 30 MIN.
MAKES: 2 SERVINGS

- **¾** cup uncooked spiral pasta
- **1** package (8 ounces) imitation crabmeat
- **1** snack-size cup (4 ounces) mandarin oranges, drained
- **¼** cup halved seedless red grapes
- **¼** cup halved seedless green grapes
- **¼** cup reduced-fat plain yogurt
- **2** tablespoons fat-free mayonnaise
- **1½** teaspoons honey
- **¼** teaspoon ground ginger

1. Cook pasta according to package directions; drain and rinse in cold water. In a small bowl, combine the pasta, crab, oranges and grapes.

2. Combine the yogurt, mayonnaise, honey and ginger; pour over salad and toss to coat. Refrigerate until serving.

PER SERVING *1½ cups equals 322 cal., 2 g fat (1 g sat. fat), 59 mg chol., 215 mg sodium, 55 g carb., 2 g fiber, 21 g pro.*

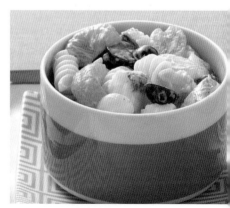

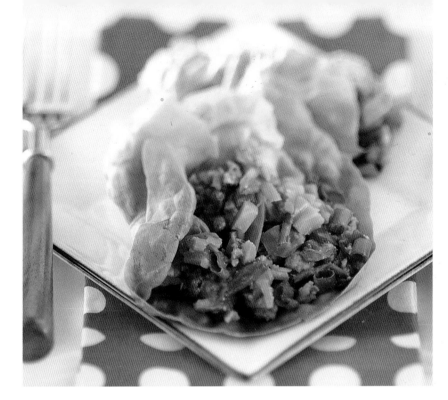

336 CALORIES

Tangy Tuna Bunwiches

Ketchup and Worcestershire sauce lend a tangy flavor to these quick tuna sandwiches. They're great for casual get-togethers, summer lunches or brown-bagging to work.

—BRENDA BIRON SYDNEY, NS

START TO FINISH: 10 MIN.
MAKES: 2 SERVINGS

- 1 can (5 ounces) light water-packed tuna
- 3 tablespoons fat-free mayonnaise
- 1 tablespoon ketchup
- ½ teaspoon lemon juice
- ½ teaspoon Worcestershire sauce
- 2 sandwich buns, split
- 2 lettuce leaves

In a large bowl, combine the tuna, mayonnaise, ketchup, lemon juice and Worcestershire sauce. Serve on buns with lettuce.

PER SERVING *1 sandwich equals 336 cal., 6 g fat (3 g sat. fat), 28 mg chol., 917 mg sodium, 41 g carb., 3 g fiber, 29 g pro.*

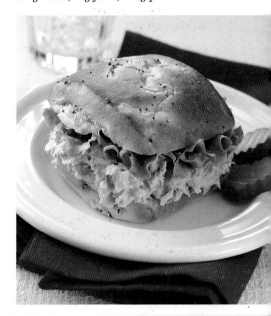

275 CALORIES ## Asian Turkey Lettuce Wraps

Chopped frozen vegetables make these wraps a snap. Add some Asian chili sauce if you want to spice it up a bit.

—SUSAN RILEY ALLEN, TX

START TO FINISH: 20 MIN.
MAKES: 5 SERVINGS

- 1¼ pounds extra-lean ground turkey
- 1 package (16 ounces) frozen stir-fry vegetable blend, thawed
- ⅓ cup reduced-sodium teriyaki sauce
- ¼ cup hoisin sauce
- 3 tablespoons reduced-fat creamy peanut butter
- 2 tablespoons minced fresh gingerroot
- 1 tablespoon rice vinegar
- 1 tablespoon sesame oil
- 3 garlic cloves, minced
- 4 green onions, chopped
- 10 Boston lettuce leaves
   Additional hoisin sauce, optional

1. In a large nonstick skillet coated with cooking spray, cook the ground turkey over medium heat until no longer pink.

2. Coarsely chop stir-fry vegetables; add to the pan. Stir in the teriyaki sauce, hoisin sauce, peanut butter, ginger, vinegar and oil. Stir-fry over medium-high heat for 5 minutes. Add garlic; cook 1 minute longer.

3. Remove from the heat; stir in onions. Place a scant ½ cup turkey mixture on each lettuce leaf; fold lettuce over filling. Serve with additional hoisin sauce if desired.

PER SERVING *2 wraps (calculated without additional hoisin sauce) equals 275 cal., 8 g fat (1 g sat. fat), 45 mg chol., 686 mg sodium, 19 g carb., 4 g fiber, 34 g pro.*
Diabetic Exchanges: 3 very lean meat, 1½ fat, 1 starch, 1 vegetable.

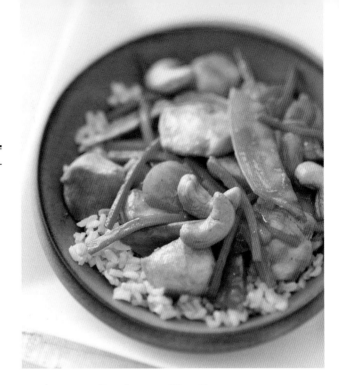

350 CALORIES Turkey a la King

I like to make this dish with our leftover turkey. It's a nice change from casseroles and so simple. Serve over rice, noodles, biscuits or even toast.

—**PAT LEMKE** BRANDON, WI

START TO FINISH: 30 MIN. • **MAKES:** 4 SERVINGS

- 1¾ cups sliced fresh mushrooms
- 1 celery rib, chopped
- ¼ cup chopped onion
- ¼ cup chopped green pepper
- 2 tablespoons butter
- ¼ cup all-purpose flour
- 1 cup reduced-sodium chicken broth
- 1 cup fat-free milk
- 2 cups cubed cooked turkey breast
- 1 cup frozen peas
- ½ teaspoon salt
- 2 cups hot cooked rice

1. In a large nonstick skillet, saute the mushrooms, celery, onion and pepper in butter until tender.

2. Combine flour and broth until smooth; stir into vegetable mixture. Stir in milk. Bring to a boil. Cook and stir for 2 minutes or until thickened. Add the turkey, peas and salt; heat through. Serve with rice.

PER SERVING *1¼ cups turkey mixture with ½ cup rice equals 350 cal., 7 g fat (4 g sat. fat), 76 mg chol., 594 mg sodium, 40 g carb., 3 g fiber, 30 g pro.* **Diabetic Exchanges:** *3 lean meat, 2 starch, 1½ fat, 1 vegetable.*

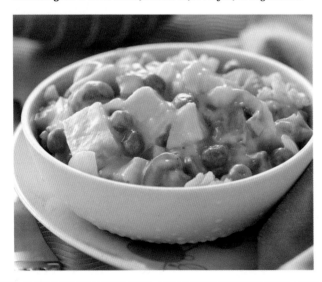

301 CALORIES Cashew Chicken

Whenever my friends and I get together for a potluck, they always ask me to bring this dish. The recipe came from my brother; it has a distinct Chinese flavor from all the spices.

—**LINDA AVILA** TOONE, TN

PREP: 20 MIN. + MARINATING • **COOK:** 15 MIN.
MAKES: 4 SERVINGS

- 3 tablespoons reduced-sodium soy sauce, divided
- 1 tablespoon sherry or reduced-sodium chicken broth
- ¾ teaspoon sesame oil, divided
- 1 pound boneless skinless chicken breasts, cut into 1-inch pieces
- 1 tablespoon cornstarch
- ⅓ cup reduced-sodium chicken broth
- 1 tablespoon sugar
- 1 tablespoon rice vinegar
- 1 tablespoon hoisin sauce
- ½ teaspoon minced fresh gingerroot
- ¼ teaspoon salt
- 2 teaspoons canola oil, divided
- 1½ cups fresh snow peas
- 2 medium carrots, julienned
- 1 can (8 ounces) sliced water chestnuts, drained
- ¼ cup unsalted cashews, toasted
  Hot cooked rice, optional

1. In a large resealable plastic bag, combine 2 tablespoons soy sauce, sherry and ½ teaspoon of sesame oil; add the chicken. Seal bag and turn to coat. Refrigerate for 30 minutes.

2. In a small bowl, combine cornstarch and broth until smooth. Stir in the sugar, vinegar, hoisin sauce, ginger, salt, and remaining soy sauce and sesame oil; set aside.

3. Drain chicken and discard marinade. In a large nonstick wok or skillet, stir-fry chicken in 1 teaspoon canola oil until no longer pink. Remove and keep warm.

4. In same pan, stir-fry peas and carrots in remaining canola oil until crisp-tender. Add water chestnuts.

5. Return chicken to the pan. Stir sauce mixture and add to chicken mixture. Bring to a boil; cook and stir for 1 minute or until thickened. Sprinkle with cashews. Serve with rice if desired.

PER SERVING *1 cup (calculated without rice) equals 301 cal., 10 g fat (2 g sat. fat), 63 mg chol., 590 mg sodium, 25 g carb., 4 g fiber, 28 g pro.*

350 CALORIES Pumpkin Sloppy Joes for 2

Here's a wonderful harvest version of an old standby—sloppy joes made with pumpkin! I add cloves, nutmeg and chili powder for extra zest. I suggest serving dill pickle slices on the side.

—DONNA MUSSER PEARL CITY, IL

START TO FINISH: 30 MIN. • **MAKES:** 2 SERVINGS

- ½ **pound lean ground beef (90% lean)**
- 3 **tablespoons finely chopped onion**
- ¼ **cup ketchup**
- 2 **tablespoons tomato juice**
- ¼ **teaspoon chili powder**
- **Dash each ground cloves and nutmeg**
- **Dash pepper**
- ⅔ **cup canned pumpkin**
- 2 **hamburger buns, split**

1. In a large skillet, cook beef and onion over medium heat until meat is no longer pink; drain.

2. Add the ketchup, tomato juice, chili powder, cloves, nutmeg and pepper. Bring to a boil. Stir in pumpkin. Reduce heat; cover and simmer for 15-20 minutes to allow flavors to blend. Serve on buns.

PER SERVING *1 sandwich equals 350 cal., 11 g fat (4 g sat. fat), 56 mg chol., 730 mg sodium, 36 g carb., 3 g fiber, 27 g pro.* **Diabetic Exchanges:** *3 lean meat, 2½ starch.*

301 CALORIES Honey-Dijon Chicken Salad

This delightful main-dish salad has an easy dressing that lends a sweet-tangy flavor to the mix. You can add or take away vegetables to suit your taste.

—JANELLE HENSLEY HARRISONBURG, VA

PREP: 15 MIN. • **BAKE:** 20 MIN. • **MAKES:** 2 SERVINGS

- ½ **pound chicken tenderloins, cut into 1½-inch pieces**
- 2 **tablespoons honey, divided**
- 2 **tablespoons Dijon mustard, divided**
- 3 **cups torn leaf lettuce**
- 2 **hard-cooked eggs, chopped**
- 2 **tablespoons each chopped green, sweet orange and yellow pepper**
- 1 **tablespoon chopped onion**
- 2 **teaspoons sesame seeds**

1. Place chicken in a 1½-qt. baking dish coated with cooking spray. Combine 1 tablespoon each of honey and mustard; pour over chicken. Cover and bake at 350° for 20-25 minutes or until meat is no longer pink.

2. In a large bowl, combine the lettuce, eggs, peppers, onion and sesame seeds; divide between two plates. Top with chicken. Combine remaining honey and mustard; drizzle over chicken.

PER SERVING *1 serving equals 301 cal., 9 g fat (2 g sat. fat), 279 mg chol., 498 mg sodium, 25 g carb., 2 g fiber, 35 g pro.* **Diabetic Exchanges:** *4 lean meat, 2 vegetable, 1 starch.*

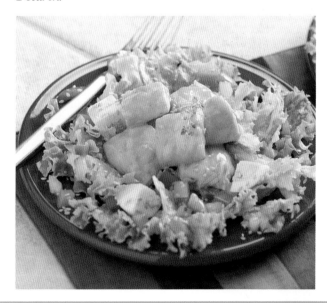

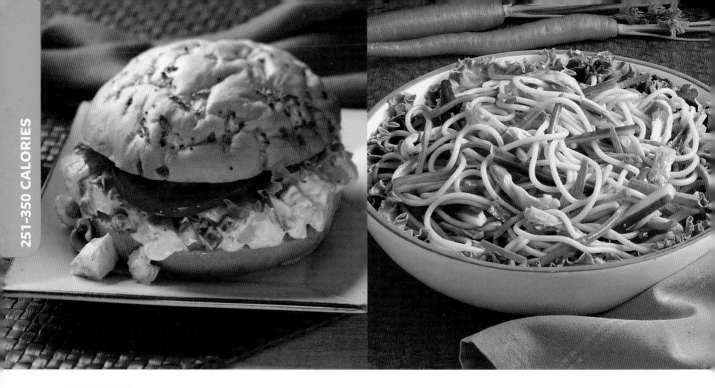

257 CALORIES

Ranch Chicken Salad Sandwiches

My husband, who is diabetic, takes lunch to work with him every day. We love chicken salad, and I created a low-fat version that we both feel good about.

—**BOBBIE SCROGGIE** SCOTT DEPOT, WV

START TO FINISH: 15 MIN.
MAKES: 6 SERVINGS

- ¼ cup reduced-fat mayonnaise
- 3 tablespoons fat-free ranch salad dressing
- 3 tablespoons fat-free sour cream
- 1 tablespoon lemon juice
- ⅛ teaspoon pepper
- 2 cups cubed cooked chicken breast
- ½ cup thinly sliced celery
- 2 tablespoons diced sweet red pepper
- 1 tablespoon chopped green onion
- 6 hamburger buns, split
- 6 lettuce leaves
- 6 slices tomato

In a small bowl, combine the mayonnaise, ranch dressing, sour cream, lemon juice and pepper. Stir in the chicken, celery, red pepper and onion until combined. Spoon ⅓ cup onto each bun bottom; top with lettuce and tomato. Replace bun tops.

PER SERVING *1 sandwich equals 257 cal., 7 g fat (1 g sat. fat), 41 mg chol., 456 mg sodium, 29 g carb., 2 g fiber, 18 g pro.* **Diabetic Exchanges:** *2 starch, 2 lean meat, ½ fat.*

282 CALORIES

Chicken Spaghetti Salad

I make this quick little dish when I'm in a hurry and don't want a huge meal.

—**HOLLY SIPHAVONG** EUREKA, CA

START TO FINISH: 20 MIN.
MAKES: 2 SERVINGS

- 3 ounces uncooked spaghetti
- ½ cup shredded cooked chicken breast
- ½ cup julienned cucumber
- ⅓ cup julienned carrot
- 1 tablespoon white vinegar
- 1 tablespoon reduced-sodium soy sauce
- 2 teaspoons canola oil
- 1 teaspoon minced fresh gingerroot
- ¾ teaspoon sugar
- ¼ teaspoon minced garlic

Cook spaghetti according to package directions; drain and rinse in cold water. Combine spaghetti, chicken, cucumber and carrot. In a small saucepan, combine the vinegar, soy sauce, oil, ginger, sugar and garlic. Bring to a boil; remove from the heat. Drizzle over spaghetti mixture and toss to coat.

PER SERVING *282 cal., 7 g fat (1 g sat. fat), 36 mg chol., 343 mg sodium, 34 g carb., 3 g fiber, 19 g pro.* **Diabetic Exchanges:** *2 starch, 2 lean meat, 1 vegetable.*

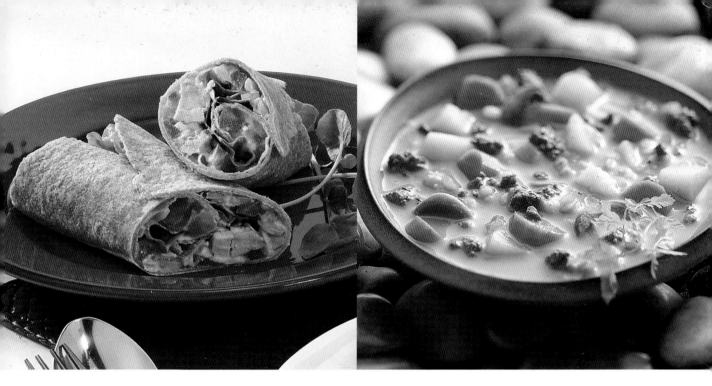

279 CALORIES Grecian
Gold Medal Wraps

For a healthy dish, I created these wraps with fat-free yogurt and whole wheat tortillas. Only a small quantity of the Greek olives is needed to give them loads of Mediterranean flavor.

—MARGEE BERRY WHITE SALMON, WA

START TO FINISH: 20 MIN.
MAKES: 4 SERVINGS

- ½ cup canned white kidney or cannellini beans, rinsed and drained
- ⅓ cup crumbled feta cheese
- ⅓ cup fat-free plain yogurt
- ¼ cup chopped red onion
- 2 teaspoons lemon juice
- 2 small tomatoes, chopped
- 4 whole wheat tortillas (8 inches), room temperature
- 1 package (6 ounces) ready-to-use grilled chicken breast strips
- ⅔ cup torn romaine
- 2 tablespoons chopped pitted Greek olives

In a bowl, mash beans with a fork. Stir in feta, yogurt, onion and lemon juice. Fold in tomatoes. Spread ¼ cup onto each tortilla. Top with chicken, romaine and olives; roll up.

PER SERVING *1 wrap equals 279 cal., 7 g fat (2 g sat. fat), 33 mg chol., 774 mg sodium, 33 g carb., 5 g fiber, 18 g pro.* **Diabetic Exchanges:** *2 starch, 2 lean meat, 1 fat.*

317 CALORIES
Easy Beef Barley Soup

This soup is really easy and takes very little time to put together. You can serve it alone for lunch or for supper with homemade bread, which I do on occasion.

—CAROLE LANTHIER COURTICE, ON

PREP: 15 MIN. • **COOK:** 55 MIN.
MAKES: 4 SERVINGS

- ½ pound lean ground beef (90% lean)
- 2 large fresh mushrooms, sliced
- 1 celery rib, chopped
- 1 small onion, chopped
- 2 teaspoons all-purpose flour
- 3 cans (14½ ounces each) reduced-sodium beef broth
- 2 medium carrots, sliced
- 1 large potato, peeled and cubed
- ½ teaspoon pepper
- ⅛ teaspoon salt
- ⅓ cup medium pearl barley
- 1 can (5 ounces) evaporated milk
- 2 tablespoons tomato paste

1. In a Dutch oven over medium heat, cook and stir the beef, mushrooms, celery and onion until meat is no longer pink; drain. Stir in flour until blended; gradually add broth. Stir in carrots, potato, pepper and salt. Bring to a boil. Stir in barley.
2. Reduce heat; cover and simmer for 45-50 minutes or until barley is tender. Whisk in milk and tomato paste; heat through.

PER SERVING *1¾ cups equals 317 cal., 7 g fat (3 g sat. fat), 45 mg chol., 753 mg sodium, 42 g carb., 6 g fiber, 21 g pro.* **Diabetic Exchanges:** *2½ starch, 2 lean meat, 1 vegetable.*

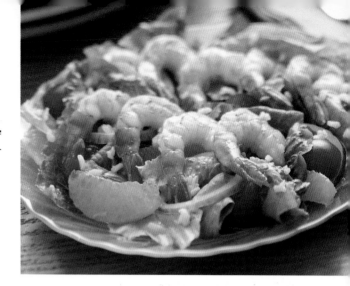

312 CALORIES ## Ham 'n' Chickpea Soup

Chock-full of ham, vegetables, chickpeas and orzo, my hearty soup is loaded with good-for-you flavor.

—LINDA ARNOLD EDMONTON, AB

PREP: 15 MIN. • **COOK:** 25 MIN. • **MAKES:** 4 SERVINGS

- ½ cup uncooked orzo pasta
- 1 small onion, chopped
- 2 teaspoons canola oil
- 1 cup cubed fully cooked lean ham
- 2 garlic cloves, minced
- 1 teaspoon dried rosemary, crushed
- 1 teaspoon rubbed sage
- 2 cups reduced-sodium beef broth
- 1 can (14½ ounces) diced tomatoes, undrained
- 1 can (15 ounces) chickpeas or garbanzo beans, rinsed and drained
- 4 tablespoons shredded Parmesan cheese
- 1 tablespoon minced fresh parsley

1. Cook orzo according to package directions. Meanwhile, in a large saucepan, saute onion in oil for 3 minutes. Add the ham, garlic, rosemary and sage; saute 1 minute longer. Stir in broth and tomatoes. Bring to a boil. Reduce heat; simmer, uncovered, for 10 minutes.
2. Drain orzo; stir into soup. Add chickpeas; heat through. Sprinkle each serving with cheese and parsley.
PER SERVING *1½ cups equals 312 cal., 8 g fat (2 g sat. fat), 19 mg chol., 1,015 mg sodium, 43 g carb., 7 g fiber, 18 g pro.*

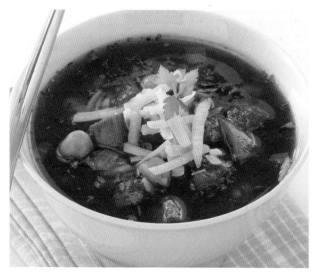

301 CALORIES ## Shrimp Romaine Salad

A refreshing lunch awaits when this shrimp-topped entree salad is on the menu. Brown rice boosts the nutrition, and citrus flavors make it a refreshing delight.

—TASTE OF HOME TEST KITCHEN

START TO FINISH: 25 MIN. • **MAKES:** 4 SERVINGS

- 2 cups cooked brown rice
- 2 cups torn romaine
- 1½ cups orange segments
- 1 cup halved cherry tomatoes
- ½ cup sliced red onion
- 3 tablespoons orange juice concentrate
- 2 tablespoons cider vinegar
- 1 tablespoon olive oil
- ¾ teaspoon dried tarragon
- ½ teaspoon garlic powder
- ½ teaspoon salt
- ¼ teaspoon pepper
- ¾ pound cooked medium shrimp, peeled and deveined

In a large bowl, combine the rice, romaine, oranges, tomatoes and onion. For dressing, in a small bowl, whisk the orange juice concentrate, vinegar, oil, tarragon, garlic powder, salt and pepper. Set aside 4 teaspoons. Pour remaining dressing over rice mixture and toss to coat. Divide among four plates; top with shrimp. Drizzle with reserved dressing.
PER SERVING *301 cal., 6 g fat (1 g sat. fat), 166 mg chol., 498 mg sodium, 41 g carb., 5 g fiber, 22 g pro.*
Diabetic Exchanges: *2 lean meat, 1½ starch, 1 vegetable, 1 fruit, ½ fat.*

273 CALORIES Southwest Black Bean Soup

A friend brought this recipe to a family gathering, and it's been a hit in my household ever since! I use instant brown rice for whole-grain goodness without a long cook time.
—**JILL HEATWOLE** PITTSVILLE, MD

PREP: 15 MIN. • **COOK:** 35 MIN. • **MAKES:** 6 SERVINGS

- 1 **medium sweet red pepper, chopped**
- 2 **celery ribs, chopped**
- 1 **small onion, chopped**
- 1 **tablespoon canola oil**
- 2 **cans (15 ounces each) black beans, rinsed and drained**
- 1 **can (14½ ounces) reduced-sodium chicken broth**
- 1 **can (14½ ounces) diced tomatoes, undrained**
- 1 **can (4 ounces) chopped green chilies**
- ¾ **teaspoon ground cumin**
- 1½ **cups cooked instant brown rice**
- 6 **tablespoons reduced-fat sour cream**

1. In a large nonstick saucepan, saute the pepper, celery and onion in oil until tender. Add the beans, broth, tomatoes, chilies and cumin. Bring to a boil. Reduce heat; simmer, uncovered, for 30 minutes or until soup is thickened.
2. Divide rice among six serving bowls; top with soup and sour cream.
PER SERVING *1 cup soup with ¼ cup rice and 1 tablespoon sour cream equals 273 cal., 5 g fat (1 g sat. fat), 5 mg chol., 655 mg sodium, 45 g carb., 9 g fiber, 12 g pro.* **Diabetic Exchanges:** *2½ starch, 1 lean meat, 1 vegetable, ½ fat.*

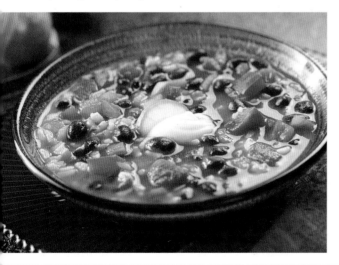

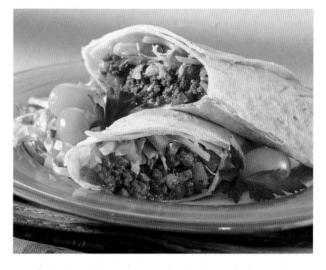

345 CALORIES Taco Salad Wraps

These fun and flavorful wraps will be a hit at lunch or dinner. You'll love the little bit of crunch from the taco chips inside.
—**MARLENE ROBERTS** MOORE, OK

START TO FINISH: 25 MIN. • **MAKES:** 2 SERVINGS

- ¼ **pound lean ground beef (90% lean)**
- ⅓ **cup plus 2 tablespoons salsa, divided**
- ¼ **cup chili beans, drained**
- 1½ **teaspoons Worcestershire sauce**
- 1 **teaspoon onion powder**
- 1 **teaspoon chili powder**
- ⅛ **teaspoon garlic powder**
  Pepper to taste
- 2 **flour tortillas (8 inches), warmed**
- ⅓ **cup shredded lettuce**
- 1 **plum tomato, chopped**
- 2 **tablespoons shredded cheddar cheese**
- 6 **baked tortilla chip scoops, coarsely crushed**

1. In a small nonstick skillet, cook beef over medium heat until no longer pink; drain. Stir in ⅓ cup salsa, beans, Worcestershire sauce, onion powder, chili powder, garlic powder and pepper. Bring to a boil; reduce heat and simmer, uncovered, for 5 minutes.
2. Spoon meat mixture onto each tortilla. Layer with lettuce, tomato, cheese, crushed tortilla chips and remaining salsa; roll up.
PER SERVING *1 wrap equals 345 cal., 10 g fat (4 g sat. fat), 35 mg chol., 764 mg sodium, 42 g carb., 5 g fiber, 20 g pro.*

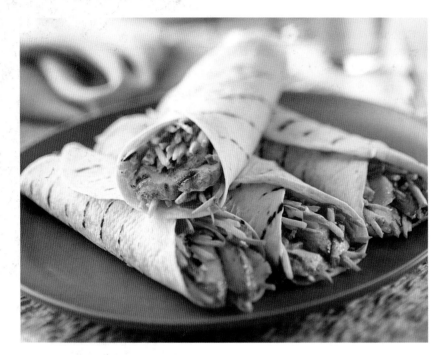

273 CALORIES Old-Fashioned Lamb Stew

This hearty stew is chock-full of tender lamb and vegetables. Sometimes, I prepare it in my slow cooker.

—MICHELLE WISE SPRING MILLS, PA

PREP: 20 MIN. • **COOK:** 3 HOURS
MAKES: 10-12 SERVINGS

- ¼ **cup all-purpose flour**
- 1 **teaspoon salt**
- ½ **teaspoon pepper**
- 3 **pounds boneless lamb, cut into 3-inch pieces**
- 2 **tablespoons canola oil**
- 1 **can (28 ounces) diced tomatoes, undrained**
- 1 **medium onion, cut into eighths**
- 1 **tablespoon dried parsley flakes**
- 2 **teaspoons dried rosemary, crushed**
- ¼ **teaspoon garlic powder**
- 4 **large carrots, cut into ½-inch pieces**
- 4 **medium potatoes, peeled and cut into 1-inch pieces**
- 1 **package (10 ounces) frozen peas**
- 1 **can (4 ounces) mushroom stems and pieces, drained**

1. In a large resealable plastic bag, combine flour, salt and pepper; add lamb, a few pieces at a time, and shake to coat. In a Dutch oven, brown the lamb in oil; drain. Add tomatoes, onion, parsley, rosemary and garlic powder. Cover and simmer for 2 hours.

2. Add carrots and potatoes; cover and cook 1 hour longer or until meat is tender. Add peas and mushrooms; heat through. Thicken if desired.

PER SERVING *1 cup equals 273 cal., 8 g fat (2 g sat. fat), 74 mg chol., 426 mg sodium, 22 g carb., 4 g fiber, 27 g pro.*

295 CALORIES Jamaican Jerk Turkey Wraps

After tasting these at a neighborhood block party, I got the recipe. The grilled turkey tenderloins along with the light jalapeno dressing make these spicy wraps tops with my gang!

—MARY ANN DELL PHOENIXVILLE, PA

PREP: 20 MIN. • **GRILL:** 20 MIN.
MAKES: 4 SERVINGS

- 2 **cups broccoli coleslaw mix**
- 1 **medium tomato, seeded and chopped**
- 3 **tablespoons reduced-fat coleslaw dressing**
- 1 **jalapeno pepper, seeded and chopped**
- 1 **tablespoon prepared mustard**
- 1½ **teaspoons Caribbean jerk seasoning**
- 2 **turkey breast tenderloins (8 ounces each)**
- 4 **fat-free flour tortillas (8 inches)**

1. In a large bowl, toss coleslaw mix, tomato, coleslaw dressing, jalapeno and mustard; set aside.

2. Rub seasoning over turkey. Moisten a paper towel with cooking oil; using long-handled tongs, lightly coat the grill rack. Grill turkey, covered, over medium heat or broil 4 in. from heat for 8-10 minutes on each side or until a thermometer reads 170°. Let stand 5 minutes.

3. Grill tortillas, uncovered, over medium heat 45-55 seconds on each side or until warmed. Thinly slice turkey; place down the center of tortillas. Top with coleslaw mixture and roll up.

NOTE *Wear disposable gloves when cutting hot peppers; the oils can burn skin. Avoid touching your face.*

PER SERVING *1 wrap equals 295 cal., 4 g fat (1 g sat. fat), 59 mg chol., 658 mg sodium, 34 g carb., 3 g fiber, 31 g pro.* **Diabetic Exchanges:** *3 lean meat, 2 starch, 1 vegetable, ½ fat.*

332 CALORIES Herbed Tuna Sandwiches

Give tuna salad an upgrade in a flash. Herbs and cheddar cheese make this simple sandwich really stand out! It's perfect for lunch or a no-fuss dinner.

—**MARIE CONNOR** VIRGINIA BEACH, VA

START TO FINISH: 20 MIN.
MAKES: 4 SERVINGS

- 2 **cans (6 ounces each) light water-packed tuna, drained and flaked**
- 2 **hard-cooked eggs, chopped**
- ⅓ **cup fat-free mayonnaise**
- ¼ **cup minced chives**
- 2 **teaspoons minced fresh parsley**
- ½ **teaspoon dried basil**
- ¼ **teaspoon onion powder**
- 8 **slices whole wheat bread, toasted**
- ½ **cup shredded reduced-fat cheddar cheese**

1. Combine the first seven ingredients. Place four slices of toast on an ungreased baking sheet; top with tuna mixture and sprinkle with cheese.

2. Broil 3-4 in. from the heat for 1-2 minutes or until cheese is melted. Top with remaining toast.

PER SERVING *1 sandwich equals 332 cal., 9 g fat (4 g sat. fat), 144 mg chol., 864 mg sodium, 30 g carb., 4 g fiber, 34 g pro.*

251 CALORIES Zesty Hamburger Soup

You won't face early afternoon hunger pangs when this wonderful soup is part of your lunch. Freeze leftovers in small batches so you can enjoy them anytime.

—**KELLY MILAN** LAKE JACKSON, TX

START TO FINISH: 30 MIN.
MAKES: 9 SERVINGS (ABOUT 4 QUARTS)

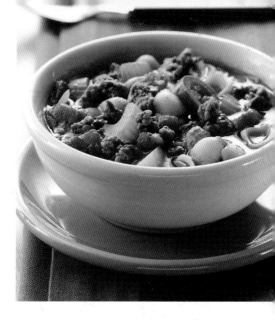

- 1 **pound lean ground beef (90% lean)**
- 2 **cups sliced celery**
- 1 **cup chopped onion**
- 2 **teaspoons minced garlic**
- 4 **cup water**
- 2 **medium red potatoes, peeled and cubed**
- 2 **cups frozen corn**
- 1½ **cups uncooked small shell pasta**
- 4 **pickled jalapeno slices, chopped**
- 4 **cups V8 juice**
- 2 **cans (10 ounces each) diced tomatoes with green chilies**
- 1 **to 2 tablespoons sugar**

1. In a Dutch oven, cook beef, celery and onion over medium heat until meat is no longer pink. Add garlic; cook 1 minute longer. Drain. Stir in the water, potatoes, corn, pasta and jalapeno.

2. Bring to a boil. Reduce heat; cover and simmer for 10-15 minutes or until pasta is tender. Add the remaining ingredients; cook and stir until heated through.

PER SERVING *1¾ cups equals 251 cal., 5 g fat (2 g sat. fat), 31 mg chol., 603 mg sodium, 36 g carb., 4 g fiber, 16 g pro.*

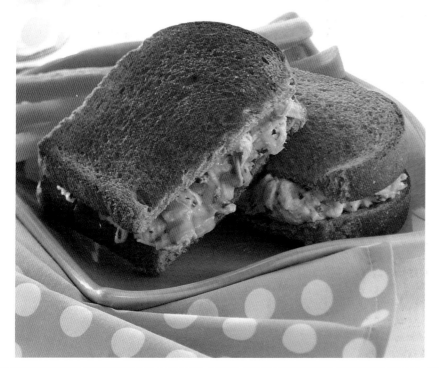

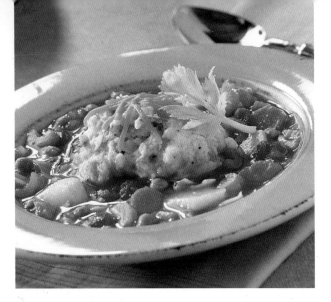

broth, potatoes, tomatoes, garlic, salt and pepper. Bring to a boil. Reduce heat; cover and simmer for 15-20 minutes or until vegetables are tender.

2. In a small bowl, combine flour and water until smooth; stir into vegetable mixture. Bring to a boil; cook and stir for 2 minutes or until thickened. Stir in cabbage and peas.

3. For dumplings, in a small bowl, combine baking mix, carrots and parsley. Stir in water until moistened. Drop in 10 mounds onto simmering soup. Cover and simmer for 15 minutes or until a toothpick inserted in a dumpling comes out clean (do not lift cover while simmering). Garnish with cheese.

PER SERVING *1¼ cups soup with 1 dumpling and 1 tablespoon cheese equals 258 cal., 7 g fat (2 g sat. fat), 5 mg chol., 826 mg sodium, 44 g carb., 5 g fiber, 8 g pro.* **Diabetic Exchanges:** *2 starch, 2 vegetable, 1 fat.*

---

258 CALORIES

Vegetable Soup with Dumplings

Not only is this hearty soup my family's favorite meatless recipe, but it's a complete meal and loaded with vegetables. The fluffy carrot dumplings are a great change of pace at dinnertime.

—**KAREN MAU** JACKSBORO, TN

PREP: 25 MIN. • **COOK:** 40 MIN. • **MAKES:** 10 SERVINGS

- 1½ cups chopped onions
- 4 medium carrots, sliced
- 3 celery ribs, sliced
- 2 tablespoons canola oil
- 3 cups vegetable broth
- 4 medium potatoes, peeled and sliced
- 4 medium tomatoes, chopped
- 2 garlic cloves, minced
- ½ teaspoon salt
- ½ teaspoon pepper
- ¼ cup all-purpose flour
- ½ cup water
- 1 cup chopped cabbage
- 1 cup frozen peas

CARROT DUMPLINGS

- 2¼ cups reduced-fat biscuit/baking mix
- 1 cup shredded carrots
- 1 tablespoon minced fresh parsley
- 1 cup cold water
- 10 tablespoons shredded reduced-fat cheddar cheese

1. In a Dutch oven, cook the onions, carrots and celery in oil for 6-8 minutes or until crisp-tender. Stir in the

---

317 CALORIES

Chicken Alfredo Veggie Pizza

I created this pizza myself, and it's become one of our favorites! The bright veggies make it so colorful and appealing.

—**NANCY LINDSAY** NEW MARKET, IA

PREP: 45 MIN. + RISING • **BAKE:** 25 MIN. • **MAKES:** 8 SERVINGS

- 1 package (¼ ounce) active dry yeast
- 1 cup warm water (110° to 115°)
- 1 tablespoon canola oil
- 2 teaspoons sugar
- ¾ teaspoon salt, divided
- ½ teaspoon garlic-herb seasoning blend
- ½ cup whole wheat flour
- 2¼ to 2½ cups bread flour
- 1 tablespoon cornmeal
- 4 teaspoons all-purpose flour
- 1¼ cups 2% milk
- 1½ cups cubed cooked chicken breast
- 1 cup fresh baby spinach
- ⅓ cup shredded Parmesan cheese
  Dash white pepper
- 1 cup sliced fresh mushrooms
- 1 plum tomato, seeded and chopped
- 1 small onion, diced
- ½ cup chopped green pepper
- ¼ cup sliced ripe olives
- 1 cup (4 ounces) shredded part-skim mozzarella cheese
- ½ cup shredded Colby-Monterey Jack cheese

1. In a large bowl, dissolve yeast in warm water. Add the oil, sugar, ½ teaspoon salt, seasoning blend, whole wheat flour and 2¼ cups bread flour. Beat until smooth. Stir in enough remaining flour to form a stiff dough.
2. Turn onto a lightly floured surface; knead until smooth and elastic, about 6-8 minutes. Place in a bowl coated with cooking spray, turning once to coat the top. Cover and let rise for 20 minutes.
3. Punch dough down; roll into a 15-in. circle. Sprinkle cornmeal over a 14-in. pizza pan coated with cooking spray. Transfer dough to prepared pan; build up edges slightly. Bake at 425° for 12-14 minutes or until edges are lightly browned.
4. Meanwhile, in a large saucepan, combine flour and milk until smooth. Bring to a boil; cook and stir for 2 minutes or until thickened. Add the chicken, spinach, Parmesan cheese, pepper and remaining salt. Cook and stir until spinach is wilted.
5. Spread sauce over crust; top with remaining ingredients. Bake 10-15 minutes longer or until cheeses are melted.

PER SERVING *1 slice equals 317 cal., 9 g fat (4 g sat. fat), 40 mg chol., 476 mg sodium, 38 g carb., 3 g fiber, 22 g pro.* **Diabetic Exchanges:** *2½ starch, 2 lean meat, ½ fat.*

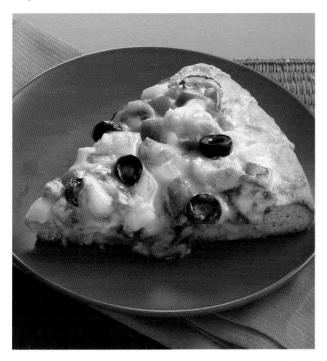

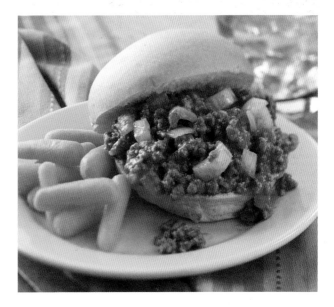

348 CALORIES Barbecue Beef Sandwiches

A tangy sauce gives family-pleasing sandwiches a bit of zip. I've had this recipe for years and have shared it many, many times.
—**SHARON ZAGAR** GARDNER, IL

START TO FINISH: 30 MIN. • **MAKES:** 6 SERVINGS

- 1½ **pounds lean ground beef (90% lean)**
- 2 **celery ribs, sliced**
- 1 **large onion, chopped**
- 1 **can (8 ounces) tomato sauce**
- ¼ **cup ketchup**
- 2 **tablespoons brown sugar**
- 2 **tablespoons barbecue sauce**
- 1 **tablespoon prepared mustard**
- 1 **tablespoon Worcestershire sauce**
- 6 **hamburger buns, split**

1. In a large nonstick skillet, cook beef, celery and onion over medium heat until the meat is no longer pink; drain.
2. Stir in the tomato sauce, ketchup, brown sugar, barbecue sauce, mustard and Worcestershire sauce. Bring to a boil. Reduce heat; simmer, uncovered, for 10-15 minutes to allow flavors to blend. Spoon ¾ cup onto each bun.

PER SERVING *1 sandwich equals 348 cal., 11 g fat (4 g sat. fat), 56 mg chol., 719 mg sodium, 35 g carb., 2 g fiber, 27 g pro.* **Diabetic Exchanges:** *3 lean meat, 2 starch.*

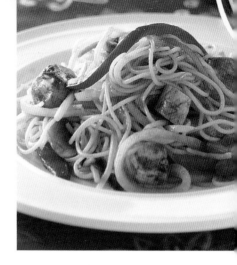

295 CALORIES
Potato-Lentil Stew

Jam-packed with nutritious veggies, my hearty soup makes a stick-to-your-ribs meatless meal the whole family will love. Serve with a crusty loaf of bread and dinner's done!

—KRISTA GOODWIN YPSILANTI, MI

PREP: 20 MIN. • **COOK:** 40 MIN.
MAKES: 6 SERVINGS (2½ QUARTS)

- 1 large onion, chopped
- 2 medium carrots, chopped
- 2 teaspoons olive oil
- 4 teaspoons chili powder
- 3 garlic cloves, minced
- 3 teaspoons ground cumin
- 1 teaspoon dried oregano
- 1 carton (32 ounces) vegetable broth
- ¾ cup dried lentils, rinsed
- 2 cans (10 ounces each) diced tomatoes and green chilies
- 3½ cups frozen cubed hash brown potatoes
- 1 can (16 ounces) kidney beans, rinsed and drained
- ½ teaspoon salt
- ¼ teaspoon pepper

1. In a Dutch oven, saute onion and carrots in oil for 3 minutes. Add the chili powder, garlic, cumin and oregano; cook 1 minute longer.
2. Stir in broth and lentils. Bring to a boil. Reduce heat; cover and simmer for 20-22 minutes or until lentils are tender. Stir in the tomatoes, potatoes, beans, salt and pepper. Return to a boil. Reduce heat; cover and simmer 10-15 minutes longer or until potatoes are tender.

PER SERVING *1⅔ cups equals 295 cal., 2 g fat (trace sat. fat), 0 chol., 1,478 mg sodium, 56 g carb., 16 g fiber, 15 g pro.*

320 CALORIES
Asian Chicken with Pasta

Mild flavors make this a dish even picky eaters will like. The coleslaw mix brings a pleasing crunch to the recipe.

—REBECCA SAMS OAK HARBOR, OH

START TO FINISH: 25 MIN.
MAKES: 6 SERVINGS

- ½ pound uncooked angel hair pasta
- 1 pound chicken tenderloins, cut into 1-inch cubes
- ⅓ cup prepared balsamic vinaigrette
- ⅓ cup prepared Italian salad dressing
- 1 package (12 ounces) broccoli coleslaw mix
- ½ pound sliced fresh mushrooms
- ¾ cup julienned sweet red pepper
- ½ cup sliced onion
- ½ teaspoon garlic powder
- ½ teaspoon ground ginger
- ¼ teaspoon salt
- ⅛ teaspoon pepper

1. Cook pasta according to package directions. Meanwhile, in a large skillet, saute chicken in vinaigrette and salad dressing until no longer pink. Remove and keep warm.
2. In the same skillet, saute the coleslaw mix, mushrooms, red

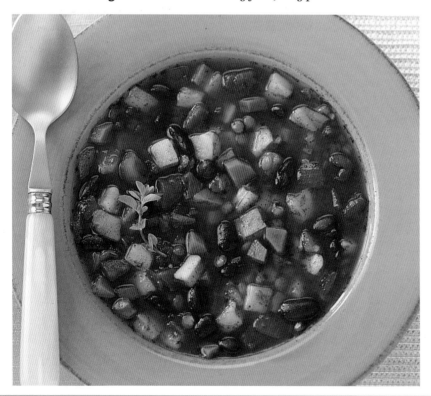

pepper and onion until tender. Add the seasonings. Stir in the chicken; heat through. Drain pasta. Add to chicken mixture; toss to coat.

PER SERVING *1½ cups equals 320 cal., 8 g fat (1 g sat. fat), 44 mg chol., 474 mg sodium, 38 g carb., 4 g fiber, 25 g pro.* **Diabetic Exchanges:** *3 lean meat, 2 starch, 1 vegetable, 1 fat.*

Grandma's French Tuna Salad Wraps

My French-Canadian grandmother always made tuna salad with chopped egg in it. I tried a version of it, added veggies for more nutrition and turned it into a wrap. I remember Grandmother with each delicious bite.

—JENNIFER MAGREY STERLING, CT

START TO FINISH: 15 MIN.
MAKES: 2 SERVINGS

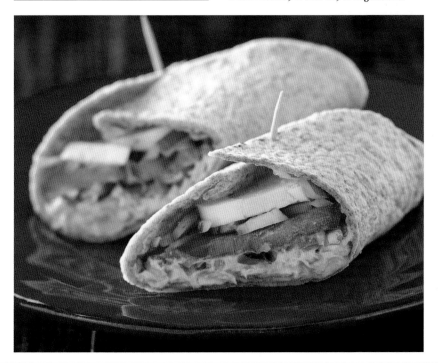

- 1 **can (5 ounces) light water-packed tuna, drained and flaked**
- 1 **celery rib, finely chopped**
- ¼ **cup fat-free mayonnaise**
- ¼ **teaspoon pepper**
- 2 **whole wheat tortillas (8 inches), room temperature**
- ½ **cup shredded lettuce**
- 1 **small carrot, shredded**
- 4 **slices tomato**
- 2 **slices red onion, separated into rings**
- 1 **hard-cooked egg, sliced**

In a bowl, combine tuna, celery, mayonnaise and pepper. Spoon tuna mixture down the center of each tortilla. Top with lettuce, carrot, tomato, onion and egg. Roll up tightly.

PER SERVING *1 wrap equals 328 cal., 7 g fat (1 g sat. fat), 135 mg chol., 770 mg sodium, 32 g carb., 4 g fiber, 30 g pro.* **Diabetic Exchanges:** *3 lean meat, 2 starch, 1 vegetable.*

Creamy Chicken Salad

I modified the original recipe for this chicken salad to make it healthier. The ingredients are so flavorful that my changes didn't take away from the taste. This refreshing salad never lasts long at our house. Even when I double the recipe, my husband says he wishes I'd made more!

—KRISTI ABERNATHY LEWISTOWN, MT

START TO FINISH: 15 MIN.
MAKES: 6 SERVINGS

- 2 **cups cubed cooked chicken breast**
- 1 **cup cooked small ring pasta**
- 1 **cup halved seedless red grapes**
- 1 **can (11 ounces) mandarin oranges, drained**
- 3 **celery ribs, chopped**
- ½ **cup sliced almonds**
- 1 **tablespoon grated onion**
- 1 **cup reduced-fat mayonnaise**
- 1 **cup reduced-fat whipped topping**
- ¼ **teaspoon salt**
  Lettuce leaves, optional

1. In a large bowl, combine the chicken, pasta, grapes, oranges, celery, almonds and onion.

2. In a small bowl, combine the mayonnaise, whipped topping and salt. Add to the chicken mixture; stir to coat. Serve in a lettuce-lined bowl if desired.

PER SERVING *1 cup equals 261 cal., 13 g fat (0 sat. fat), 38 mg chol., 307 mg sodium, 25 g carb., 2 g fiber, 11 g pro.* **Diabetic Exchanges:** *1½ fat, 1 starch, 1 meat, ½ fruit.*

> 66 I substitute whole-grain sandwich rounds and tortillas for bread and buns, and I drink only water. I swim laps in the community pool and get up hourly at work to briefly walk around. 99
> —JACKIE COBB WOODWARD

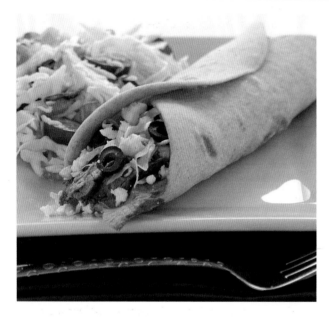

348 CALORIES Super Flatbread Wraps

These are my family's favorite! My kids will eat anything we roll up in the yummy homemade wraps. The original recipe called for all white flour and a lot of salt. I added whole wheat flour and cut back on the salt to make them healthier.
—**FAY STRAIT** WAUKEE, IA

PREP: 40 MIN. + RISING • **GRILL:** 15 MIN. • **MAKES:** 4 SERVINGS

- ½ teaspoon active dry yeast
- ½ cup warm water (110° to 115°)
- 1 teaspoon olive oil
- ½ teaspoon salt
- ⅓ cup whole wheat flour
- 1 cup all-purpose flour

FILLING
- 1 beef flank steak (1 pound)
- ½ teaspoon salt
- ¼ teaspoon pepper
- 1 cup shredded lettuce
- ¼ cup sliced ripe olives
- 2 tablespoons crumbled feta cheese

1. In a small bowl, dissolve yeast in warm water. Add the oil, salt, whole wheat flour and ¾ cup all-purpose flour; beat on medium speed for 3 minutes. Stir in enough remaining flour to form a firm dough.
2. Turn onto a lightly floured surface; knead until smooth and elastic, about 6-8 minutes. Place in a large bowl coated with cooking spray, turning once to coat the top. Cover and let rise in a warm place until doubled, about 45 minutes.
3. Punch dough down. Turn onto a lightly floured surface; divide into four portions. Roll each into an 8-in. circle.
4. Heat a large nonstick skillet coated with cooking spray over medium heat; add a portion of dough. Cook for 30-60 seconds or until bubbles form on top. Turn and cook until the second side is golden brown. Remove and keep warm. Repeat with remaining dough, adding cooking spray as needed.
5. Moisten a paper towel with cooking oil; using long-handled tongs, lightly coat the grill rack. Sprinkle steak with salt and pepper. Grill, covered, over medium-high heat or broil 4 in. from the heat for 6-8 minutes on each side or until meat reaches desired doneness (for medium-rare, a thermometer should read 145°; medium, 160°; well-done, 170°).
6. Let stand for 5 minutes before cutting steak thinly across the grain. Serve on warm flatbreads with lettuce, olives and cheese.

PER SERVING *1 wrap equals 348 cal., 11 g fat (4 g sat. fat), 56 mg chol., 770 mg sodium, 32 g carb., 3 g fiber, 28 g pro.* **Diabetic Exchanges:** *3 lean meat, 2 starch, ½ fat.*

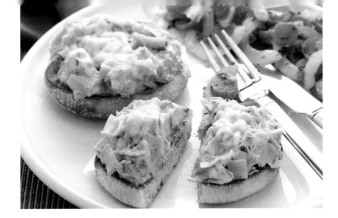

335 CALORIES Tuna Artichoke Melts

After sampling a similar open-faced sandwich at a restaurant, I created my own version of lemon-seasoned tuna salad with artichoke hearts. Serve it on the patio for lunch with a friend.
—**EVELYN BASINGER** LINVILLE, VA

START TO FINISH: 15 MIN. • **MAKES:** 2 SERVINGS

- 1 can (6 ounces) light water-packed tuna, drained and flaked
- ⅓ cup coarsely chopped water-packed artichoke hearts, rinsed and drained
- 2 tablespoons fat-free mayonnaise
- ½ cup shredded reduced-fat Mexican cheese blend, divided
- ¼ teaspoon salt-free lemon-pepper seasoning
- ⅛ teaspoon dried oregano
- 2 English muffins, split and toasted

1. In a small bowl, combine the tuna, artichokes, mayonnaise, ¼ cup cheese, lemon-pepper and oregano. Spread over English muffin halves.
2. Place on a baking sheet. Broil 4-6 in. from the heat for 3-5 minutes or until heated through. Sprinkle with remaining cheese; broil 1-2 minutes longer or until cheese is melted.
PER SERVING *1 serving equals 335 cal., 8 g fat (4 g sat. fat), 47 mg chol., 989 mg sodium, 31 g carb., 2 g fiber, 34 g pro.* **Diabetic Exchanges:** *4 lean meat, 2 starch, 1 fat.*

258 CALORIES Turkey Meatball Soup

Every Italian-American family I know seems to have their own version of meatball soup. This recipe is my family's version.
—**CHRISTIE LADD** MECHANICSBURG, PA

PREP: 30 MIN. • **COOK:** 40 MIN. • **MAKES:** 6 SERVINGS

- 2 egg whites, lightly beaten
- ½ cup seasoned bread crumbs
- 1 tablespoon grated Parmesan cheese
- 4 teaspoons Italian seasoning, divided
- 1 pound lean ground turkey
- 3 medium carrots, sliced
- 3 celery ribs, finely chopped
- 1 tablespoon olive oil
- 4 garlic cloves, minced
- 3 cans (14½ ounces each) reduced-sodium chicken broth
- ¼ teaspoon pepper
- ½ cup ditalini or other small pasta

1. In a bowl, combine egg whites, bread crumbs, cheese and 2 teaspoons Italian seasoning. Crumble turkey over mixture and mix well. Shape into ¾-in. balls.
2. Place in a 15-in. x 10-in. x 1-in. baking pan coated with cooking spray. Bake, uncovered, at 350° for 10-15 minutes or until no longer pink.
3. Meanwhile, in a Dutch oven, saute carrots and celery in oil for 5 minutes. Add garlic; cook 1 minute longer. Add the broth, pepper and remaining Italian seasoning. Bring to a boil. Reduce heat; cover and simmer for 15 minutes.
4. Stir in pasta; cook 10-12 minutes longer or until vegetables and pasta are tender. Add meatballs and heat through.
PER SERVING *1 cup equals 258 cal., 10 g fat (2 g sat. fat), 60 mg chol., 783 mg sodium, 21 g carb., 2 g fiber, 21 g pro.* **Diabetic Exchanges:** *2 lean meat, 1½ starch, ½ fat.*

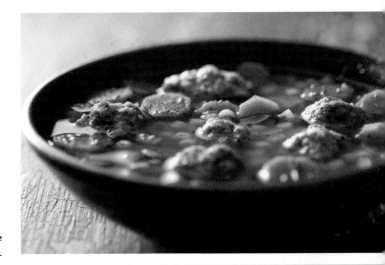

285 CALORIES Jamaican-Style Beef Stew

This delicious stew makes a hearty supper with a lighter touch. It's so flavorful, you won't want to stop at just one bowlful!

—JAMES HAYES RIDGECREST, CA

PREP: 25 MIN. • **COOK:** 1¼ HOURS
MAKES: 5 SERVINGS

- 1 tablespoon canola oil
- 1 tablespoon sugar
- 1½ pounds beef top sirloin steak, cut into ¾-inch cubes
- 5 plum tomatoes, finely chopped
- 3 large carrots, sliced
- 3 celery ribs, sliced
- 4 green onions, chopped
- ¾ cup reduced-sodium beef broth
- ¼ cup barbecue sauce
- ¼ cup reduced-sodium soy sauce
- 2 tablespoons steak sauce
- 1 tablespoon garlic powder
- 1 teaspoon dried thyme
- ¼ teaspoon ground allspice
- ¼ teaspoon pepper
- ⅛ teaspoon hot pepper sauce
- 1 tablespoon cornstarch
- 2 tablespoons cold water
  Hot cooked rice or mashed potatoes, optional

1. In a Dutch oven, heat oil over medium-high heat. Add sugar; cook and stir for 1 minute or until lightly browned. Add beef and brown on all sides.

2. Stir in the vegetables, broth, barbecue sauce, soy sauce, steak sauce and seasonings. Bring to a boil. Reduce heat; cover and simmer for 1 to 1¼ hours or until meat and vegetables are tender.

3. Combine cornstarch and water until smooth; stir into stew. Bring to a boil; cook and stir for 2 minutes or until thickened. Serve with rice or potatoes if desired.

PER SERVING *1 cup (calculated without rice or potatoes) equals 285 cal., 9 g fat (2 g sat. fat), 56 mg chol., 892 mg sodium, 18 g carb., 3 g fiber, 32 g pro.*

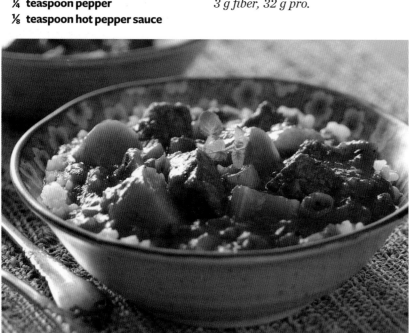

274 CALORIES Hominy Taco Chili

Made with hominy, seasonings and two kinds of beans, my chili offers an exciting change of pace.

—BARBARA WHELESS SHELDON, SC

PREP: 15 MIN. • **COOK:** 30 MIN.
MAKES: 2 BATCHES (5 SERVINGS EACH)

- 1 pound ground beef
- 1 large onion, chopped
- 2 cans (15½ ounces each) hominy, drained
- 2 cans (14½ ounces each) stewed tomatoes, undrained
- 1 can (15¼ ounces) whole kernel corn, drained
- 1 can (15 ounces) pinto beans, rinsed and drained
- 1 can (15 ounces) black beans, rinsed and drained
- 1 cup water
- 1 envelope taco seasoning
- 1 envelope ranch salad dressing mix
- 2 teaspoons ground cumin
- ½ teaspoon garlic salt
- ½ teaspoon pepper
  Corn chips, optional

1. In a Dutch oven, cook beef and onion until meat is no longer pink; drain. Stir in next 11 ingredients. Bring to a boil. Reduce heat; cover and simmer for 30 minutes.

2. Serve half of the chili with corn chips if desired. Freeze remaining chili in a freezer container for up to 3 months.

TO USE FROZEN CHILI *Thaw in the refrigerator. Transfer to a large saucepan; heat through, adding water if desired.*

PER SERVING *1 cup (calculated without chips) equals 274 cal., 6 g fat (2 g sat. fat), 28 mg chol., 1,439 mg sodium, 39 g carb., 7 g fiber, 14 g pro.*

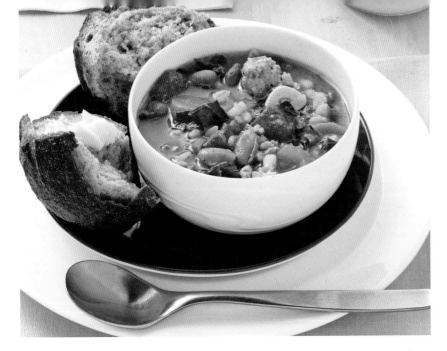

Italian Sausage Bean Soup

339 CALORIES

In the cold months, I like to put on a big pot of this comforting soup. It cooks away while I do other things like baking bread, crafting or even cleaning the house.
—**GLENNA REIMER** GIG HARBOR, WA

PREP: 20 MIN. • **COOK:** 1½ HOURS
MAKES: 8 SERVINGS (3 QUARTS)

- 1 **pound bulk Italian sausage**
- 1 **medium onion, finely chopped**
- 3 **garlic cloves, sliced**
- 4 **cans (14½ ounces each) reduced-sodium chicken broth**
- 2 **cans (15 ounces each) pinto beans, rinsed and drained**
- 1 **can (14½ ounces) diced tomatoes, undrained**
- 1 **cup medium pearl barley**
- 1 **large carrot, sliced**
- 1 **celery rib, sliced**
- 1 **teaspoon minced fresh sage**
- ½ **teaspoon minced fresh rosemary or ⅛ teaspoon dried rosemary, crushed**
- 6 **cups chopped fresh kale**

1. In a Dutch oven, cook sausage and onion over medium heat until meat is no longer pink. Add garlic; cook 1 minute longer. Drain.
2. Stir in the broth, beans, tomatoes, barley, carrot, celery, sage and rosemary. Bring to a boil. Reduce heat; cover and simmer for 45 minutes.
3. Stir in kale; return to a boil. Reduce heat; cover and simmer for 25-30 minutes or until vegetables are tender.
PER SERVING *1½ cups equals 339 cal., 9 g fat (3 g sat. fat), 23 mg chol., 1,100 mg sodium, 48 g carb., 11 g fiber, 19 g pro.*

Lasagna Soup

280 CALORIES

All the traditional flavors of lasagna come together in an irresistible and heartwarming meal in a bowl.
—**SHERYL OLENICK** DEMAREST, NJ

START TO FINISH: 30 MIN.
MAKES: 8 SERVINGS (2¾ QUARTS)

- 1 **pound lean ground beef (90% lean)**
- 1 **large green pepper, chopped**
- 1 **medium onion, chopped**
- 2 **garlic cloves, minced**
- 2 **cans (14½ ounces each) diced tomatoes, undrained**
- 2 **cans (14½ ounces each) reduced-sodium beef broth**
- 1 **can (8 ounces) tomato sauce**
- 1 **cup frozen corn**
- ¼ **cup tomato paste**
- 2 **teaspoons Italian seasoning**
- ¼ **teaspoon pepper**
- 2½ **cups uncooked spiral pasta**
- ½ **cup shredded Parmesan cheese**

1. In a large saucepan, cook beef, green pepper and onion over medium heat 6-8 minutes or until meat is no longer pink, breaking up beef into crumbles. Add garlic; cook 1 minute longer. Drain.
2. Stir in tomatoes, broth, tomato sauce, corn, tomato paste, Italian seasoning and pepper. Bring to a boil. Stir in pasta. Return to a boil. Reduce heat; simmer, covered, 10-12 minutes or until pasta is tender. Sprinkle with cheese.
PER SERVING *1⅓ cups equals 280 cal., 7 g fat (3 g sat. fat), 41 mg chol., 572 mg sodium, 35 g carb., 4 g fiber, 20 g pro.* **Diabetic Exchanges:** *2 lean meat, 2 vegetable, 1½ starch.*

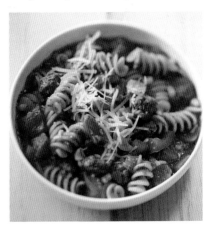

273 CALORIES

Spicy Buffalo Chicken Wraps

This recipe has a real kick and is one of my husband's favorites. It's ready in a flash, is easily doubled and the closest thing to restaurant Buffalo wings I've ever tasted in a light version.

—JENNIFER BECK MERIDIAN, ID

START TO FINISH: 25 MIN. • **MAKES:** 2 SERVINGS

- ½ **pound boneless skinless chicken breast, cubed**
- ½ **teaspoon canola oil**
- 2 **tablespoons Louisiana-style hot sauce**
- 1 **cup shredded lettuce**
- 2 **flour tortillas (6 inches), warmed**
- 2 **teaspoons reduced-fat ranch salad dressing**
- 2 **tablespoons crumbled blue cheese**

1. In a large nonstick skillet coated with cooking spray, cook chicken in oil over medium heat for 6 minutes; drain. Stir in hot sauce. Bring to a boil. Reduce heat;

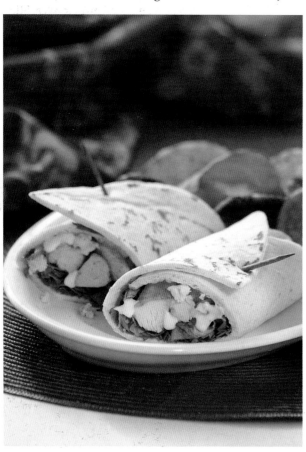

simmer, uncovered, for 3-5 minutes or until sauce is thickened and chicken is no longer pink.

2. Place lettuce on tortillas; drizzle with ranch dressing. Top with chicken mixture and blue cheese; roll up.

PER SERVING *1 wrap equals 273 cal., 11 g fat (3 g sat. fat), 70 mg chol., 453 mg sodium, 15 g carb., 1 g fiber, 28 g pro.* **Diabetic Exchanges:** *3 lean meat, 1½ fat, 1 starch.*

269 CALORIES Italian Lentil Soup

Lentils are part of the legume family and add plenty of cholesterol-reducing fiber to this tasty soup. Adjust the amount of red pepper flakes according to how much heat you like.

—MARYBETH GESSELE GASTON, OR

PREP: 15 MIN. • **COOK:** 40 MIN. • **MAKES:** 6 SERVINGS (2 QUARTS)

- 1 **medium onion, chopped**
- 1 **tablespoon olive oil**
- 2 **garlic cloves, minced**
- 3¾ **cups water**
- 1 **can (14½ ounces) vegetable broth**
- 1 **cup dried lentils, rinsed**
- 1 **medium carrot, shredded**
- 1 **small green pepper, finely chopped**
- 1 **teaspoon dried oregano**
- ½ **teaspoon dried basil**
- ¼ **teaspoon crushed red pepper flakes, optional**
- 1 **can (14½ ounces) no-salt-added diced tomatoes**
- 1 **can (6 ounces) tomato paste**
- 1 **tablespoon lemon juice**
- 2 **cups cooked brown rice**

1. In a Dutch oven, saute onion in oil until tender. Add garlic; cook 1 minute longer. Add the water, broth, lentils, carrot, green pepper, oregano, basil and pepper flakes if desired. Bring to a boil. Reduce heat; cover and simmer for 20-25 minutes or until lentils are almost tender.

2. Stir in the tomatoes, tomato paste and lemon juice. Bring to a boil. Reduce heat; cover and simmer 10 minutes longer or until lentils are tender. Serve with rice.

PER SERVING *1⅓ cups with ⅓ cup rice equals 269 cal., 3 g fat (trace sat. fat), 0 chol., 383 mg sodium, 48 g carb., 14 g fiber, 13 g pro.*

351-450 CALORIES

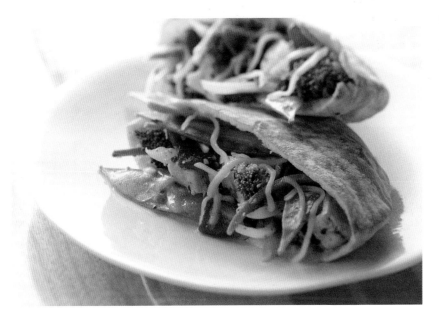

Veggie Chicken Pitas

These delicious pita pockets are literally stuffed with veggies, chicken and cheese. They make for great on-the-go dinners.
—**BILL PARKIS** WILMINGTON, NC

START TO FINISH: 30 MIN.
MAKES: 5 SERVINGS

- 1 **medium red onion, sliced**
- 1 **cup julienned carrots**
- 1 **cup chopped fresh broccoli**
- 1 **cup fresh snow peas**
- 2 **tablespoons olive oil**
- ½ **teaspoon minced garlic**
- 1 **cup cubed cooked chicken**
- 1 **jar (7 ounces) roasted sweet red peppers, drained and chopped**
- ¼ **cup white wine or chicken broth**
- ½ **teaspoon dried oregano**
- ½ **teaspoon cayenne pepper**
- 10 **pita pocket halves**
- ⅓ **cup shredded part-skim mozzarella cheese**
- ⅓ **cup shredded cheddar cheese**

1. In a large skillet, saute the onion, carrots, broccoli and peas in oil for 4-5 minutes or until tender. Add garlic; cook 1 minute longer.
2. Stir in the chicken, red peppers, wine, oregano and cayenne; heat through. Spoon mixture into pita breads; sprinkle with mozzarella and cheddar cheeses.
PER SERVING *2 stuffed pita halves equals 373 cal., 12 g fat (4 g sat. fat), 37 mg chol., 595 mg sodium, 43 g carb., 4 g fiber, 19 g pro.*
Diabetic Exchanges: *2 starch, 2 lean meat, 2 vegetable, 1 fat.*

Chicken Fried Rice

I use leftover chicken and rice to make this classic Chinese recipe, enhanced with soy sauce and green onions.
—**DAVID TIREN** CATONSVILLE, MD

START TO FINISH: 20 MIN.
MAKES: 2 SERVINGS

- ¼ **cup chopped fresh mushrooms**
- 1 **tablespoon canola oil**
- 1½ **cups cold cooked long grain rice**
- ¾ **cup cubed cooked chicken**
- 2 **tablespoons reduced-sodium soy sauce**
- 1 **egg, lightly beaten**
- 1 **green onion, sliced**

1. In a large skillet or wok, stir-fry mushrooms in oil until tender. Stir in the rice, chicken and soy sauce. Cook over low heat for 8-10 minutes, stirring occasionally.
2. Add egg and onion; cook and stir for 1-2 minutes or until egg is set.
PER SERVING *1 cup equals 368 cal., 14 g fat (2 g sat. fat), 153 mg chol., 684 mg sodium, 36 g carb., 1 g fiber, 23 g pro.*

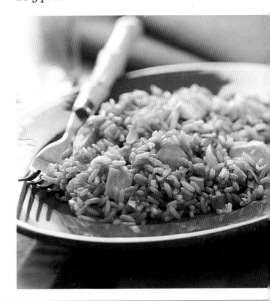

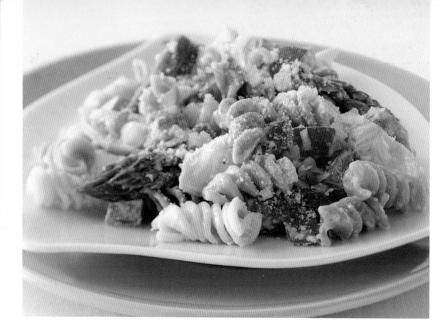

363 CALORIES Chicken Caesar Pasta Toss

Here's a no-hassle dinner to serve your family. Caesar salad dressing and Parmesan cheese give the pasta an authentic taste without added work.
—JOY BILBEY HOLT, MI

START TO FINISH: 30 MIN.
MAKES: 6 SERVINGS

- 3 quarts water
- 2½ cups uncooked tricolor spiral pasta
- 1½ cups cut fresh asparagus (1-inch pieces)
- 1½ pounds boneless skinless chicken breasts, cut into 1-inch pieces
- 2 teaspoons olive oil
- 2 large tomatoes, chopped
- ⅔ cup reduced-fat Caesar vinaigrette
- 3 green onions, chopped
- 3 tablespoons grated Parmesan cheese

1. In a Dutch oven, bring water to a boil. Add pasta. Return to a boil; cook for 4 minutes. Add asparagus; cook 6-8 minutes longer or until pasta and asparagus are tender.
2. Meanwhile, in a large nonstick skillet, saute chicken in oil until no longer pink. Remove from the heat.
3. Drain pasta mixture. Add the chicken, tomatoes and vinaigrette; cook over low heat until heated through. Sprinkle with onions and cheese.
PER SERVING *1⅓ cups equals 363 cal., 10 g fat (2 g sat. fat), 67 mg chol., 609 mg sodium, 35 g carb., 2 g fiber, 31 g pro.* **Diabetic Exchanges:** *3 lean meat, 2 starch, 1 vegetable, 1 fat.*

367 CALORIES Chicken Gyros

These yummy Greek specialties are a cinch to prepare at home. Just take tender chicken strips, coat them with a creamy cucumber-yogurt sauce, and tuck into pita breads.
—TASTE OF HOME TEST KITCHEN

PREP: 20 MIN. + MARINATING
COOK: 10 MIN. • **MAKES:** 2 SERVINGS

- ¼ cup lemon juice
- 2 tablespoons olive oil
- ¾ teaspoon minced garlic, divided
- ½ teaspoon ground mustard
- ½ teaspoon dried oregano
- ½ pound boneless skinless chicken breasts, cut into ½-inch strips
- ½ cup chopped peeled cucumber
- ⅓ cup plain yogurt
- ¼ teaspoon dill weed
- 2 whole pita breads
- ½ small red onion, thinly sliced

1. In a large resealable plastic bag, combine the lemon juice, oil, ½ teaspoon garlic, mustard and oregano; add chicken. Seal bag and turn to coat; refrigerate for at least 1 hour. In a small bowl, combine the cucumber, yogurt, dill and remaining garlic; cover and refrigerate until serving.
2. Drain and discard marinade. In a large nonstick skillet, cook and stir the chicken for 7-8 minutes or until no longer pink. Spoon onto pita breads. Top with yogurt mixture and onion; fold in half.
PER SERVING *1 gyro equals 367 cal., 9 g fat (2 g sat. fat), 68 mg chol., 397 mg sodium, 39 g carb., 2 g fiber, 30 g pro.*

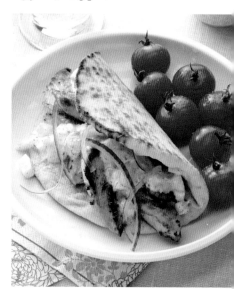

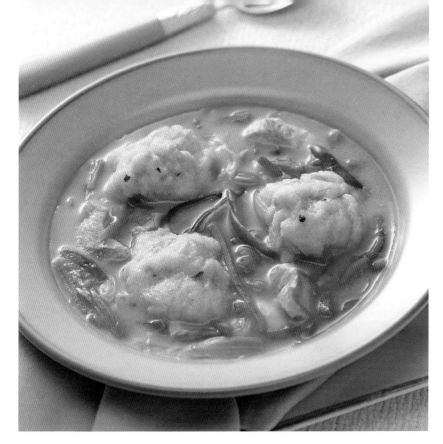

3. Meanwhile, in a small bowl, mix biscuit mix, cornmeal and cheese. Stir in milk just until moistened. Drop batter in 12 portions on top of the simmering soup.

4. Reduce heat to low; cover and cook 15 minutes or until a toothpick inserted in center of dumpling comes out clean.

PER SERVING *1¼ cups soup with 3 dumplings equals 353 cal., 8 g fat (2 g sat. fat), 52 mg chol., 1,111 mg sodium, 44 g carb., 5 g fiber, 28 g pro.* **Diabetic Exchanges:** *3 lean meat, 2 starch, 2 vegetable, 1 fat.*

356 CALORIES Berry Turkey Sandwiches

Sliced fresh strawberries, Swiss cheese and a nutty cream cheese spread make this turkey sandwich different. Try it on whole wheat, oatmeal or sunflower seed bread. It's tasty and easy to put together.
—**EDWARD MEYER** ARNOLD, MO

START TO FINISH: 5 MIN.
MAKES: 2 SERVINGS

- 4 slices whole wheat bread
- 2 lettuce leaves
- 2 slices reduced-fat Swiss cheese
- ¼ pound thinly sliced deli turkey breast
- 4 fresh strawberries, sliced
- 2 tablespoons reduced-fat spreadable cream cheese
- 2 teaspoons finely chopped pecans

On two bread slices, layer the lettuce, cheese, turkey and strawberries. Combine cream cheese and pecans; spread over the remaining bread. Place over strawberries.

PER SERVING *1 sandwich equals 356 cal., 10 g fat (3 g sat. fat), 39 mg chol., 932 mg sodium, 39 g carb., 5 g fiber, 28 g pro.*

353 CALORIES Chicken and Dumpling Soup

Looking for a true classic to serve for dinner? Give my chicken and dumpling soup a try. My husband loves it so much, he says he could eat it every day of the week. This is true comfort food!
—**MORGAN BYERS** BERKLEY, MI

PREP: 25 MIN. • **COOK:** 40 MIN.
MAKES: 4 SERVINGS

- ¾ pound boneless skinless chicken breasts, cut into 1-inch cubes
- ¼ teaspoon salt
- ⅛ teaspoon pepper
- 2 teaspoons olive oil
- ¼ cup all-purpose flour
- 4 cups reduced-sodium chicken broth, divided
- 1 cup water
- 2 cups frozen French-cut green beans
- 1½ cups sliced onions
- 1 cup shredded carrots
- ¼ teaspoon dried marjoram
- ⅔ cup reduced-fat biscuit/baking mix
- ⅓ cup cornmeal
- ¼ cup shredded reduced-fat cheddar cheese
- ⅓ cup fat-free milk

1. Sprinkle chicken with salt and pepper. In a large nonstick skillet, heat oil over medium-high heat. Add chicken; cook and stir until no longer pink. Remove from heat.

2. In a large saucepan, whisk flour and ½ cup broth until smooth. Stir in water and remaining broth. Add beans, onions, carrots and marjoram. Bring to a boil. Reduce heat; simmer, uncovered, 10 minutes. Add chicken; return to a simmer.

353 CALORIES Chili Beef Quesadillas

Served in whole wheat tortillas, these scrumptious beef-and-veggie quesadillas pack a healthy dose of fiber. They're spicy enough to suit my husband, but mild enough to please our son.

—ROBYN LARABEE LUCKNOW, ON

PREP: 30 MIN. • **BAKE:** 10 MIN. • **MAKES:** 4 SERVINGS

- ¾ **pound lean ground beef (90% lean)**
- 1 **medium onion, chopped**
- ¾ **cup finely chopped fresh mushrooms**
- 1 **medium zucchini, shredded**
- 1 **medium carrot, shredded**
- 2 **garlic cloves, minced**
- 2 **teaspoons chili powder**
- ¼ **teaspoon salt**
- ¼ **teaspoon hot pepper sauce**
- 2 **medium tomatoes, seeded and chopped**
- ¼ **cup minced fresh cilantro**
- 4 **whole wheat tortillas (8 inches), warmed**
  Cooking spray
- ½ **cup shredded part-skim mozzarella cheese**

1. In a large nonstick skillet over medium heat, cook beef and onion until meat is no longer pink; drain. Remove and keep warm. In the same skillet, cook and stir the mushrooms, zucchini, carrot, garlic, chili powder, salt and pepper sauce until vegetables are tender. Stir in the tomatoes, cilantro and beef mixture.

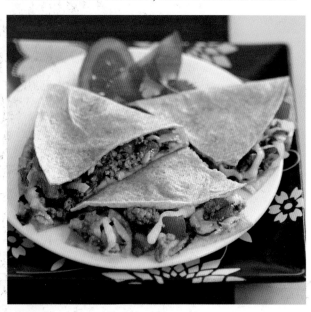

2. Spritz one side of each tortilla with cooking spray; place plain side up in a 15-in. x 10-in. x 1-in. baking pan coated with cooking spray. Spoon beef mixture over half of each tortilla; sprinkle with cheese. Fold tortillas over filling.

3. Bake at 400° for 5 minutes. Carefully turn over; bake 5-6 minutes longer or until cheese is melted. Cut into wedges.

PER SERVING *1 quesadilla equals 353 cal., 12 g fat (4 g sat. fat), 50 mg chol., 475 mg sodium, 33 g carb., 5 g fiber, 26 g pro.* **Diabetic Exchanges:** *3 lean meat, 2 vegetable, 1½ starch.*

382 CALORIES Grilled Pork Tenderloin Sandwiches

I got the recipe for these quick-fixing pork sandwiches from a friend at work years ago. I'm always asked for it when I serve the sandwiches to someone new.

—GERI BIERSCHBACH WEIDMAN, MI

PREP: 15 MIN. + MARINATING • **GRILL:** 25 MIN.
MAKES: 6 SERVINGS

- 2 **tablespoons canola oil**
- 2 **tablespoons reduced-sodium soy sauce**
- 2 **tablespoons steak sauce**
- 2 **garlic cloves, minced**
- 1½ **teaspoons brown sugar**
- ½ **teaspoon ground mustard**
- ½ **teaspoon minced fresh gingerroot**
- 2 **pork tenderloins (1 pound each)**

MUSTARD HORSERADISH SAUCE

- ¼ **cup fat-free mayonnaise**
- ¼ **cup reduced-fat sour cream**
- 1½ **teaspoons lemon juice**
- 1 **teaspoon sugar**
- ½ **teaspoon ground mustard**
- ½ **teaspoon Dijon mustard**
- ½ **teaspoon prepared horseradish**
- 6 **kaiser rolls, split**
- 6 **lettuce leaves**

1. In a large resealable plastic bag, combine the first seven ingredients; add pork. Seal bag and turn to coat; refrigerate for 8 hours or overnight.

2. Drain and discard marinade. Prepare grill for indirect heat. Moisten a paper towel with cooking oil; using long-handled tongs, lightly coat the grill rack.

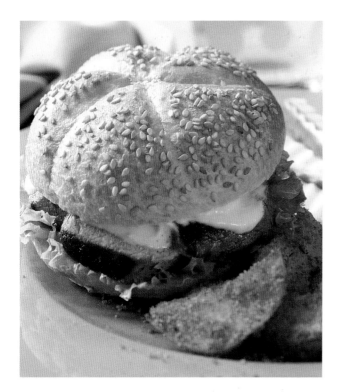

Grill pork, covered, over indirect medium-hot heat for 25-40 minutes or until a thermometer reads 160°. Let stand for 5 minutes before slicing.

3. In a small bowl, combine the mayonnaise, sour cream, lemon juice, sugar, ground mustard, Dijon mustard and horseradish. Serve pork on rolls with lettuce and mustard horseradish sauce.

PER SERVING *1 sandwich equals 382 cal., 10 g fat (3 g sat. fat), 89 mg chol., 528 mg sodium, 34 g carb., 2 g fiber, 37 g pro.* **Diabetic Exchanges:** *4 lean meat, 2 starch.*

351 CALORIES Fully Loaded Chili

With lean ground beef, four types of beans and lots of seasonings and toppings, this chili really is fully loaded!
—CYNTHIA BACA CRANBERRY TOWNSHIP, PA

PREP: 20 MIN. • **COOK:** 40 MIN. • **MAKES:** 8 SERVINGS (2 QUARTS)

- 1 **pound lean ground beef (90% lean)**
- 1 **medium onion, chopped**
- 1 **medium green pepper, chopped**
- 1¾ **cups water**
- 2 **cans (8 ounces each) tomato sauce**
- 1 **can (16 ounces) kidney beans, rinsed and drained**
- 1 **can (15½ ounces) great northern beans, rinsed and drained**
- 1 **can (15 ounces) garbanzo beans or chickpeas, rinsed and drained**
- 1 **can (15 ounces) black beans, rinsed and drained**
- 1 **tablespoon baking cocoa**
- 2 **teaspoons Louisiana-style hot sauce**
- ½ **teaspoon pepper**
- ½ **teaspoon chili powder**
- ¼ **teaspoon garlic powder**
- ⅛ **teaspoon cayenne pepper**

GARNISHES

- ½ **cup reduced-fat sour cream**
- ½ **cup crushed baked tortilla chip scoops**
- ½ **cup shredded reduced-fat cheddar cheese**

1. In a Dutch oven over medium heat, cook the beef, onion and pepper until meat is no longer pink; drain.
2. Stir in the water, tomato sauce, beans, cocoa, hot sauce and seasonings. Bring to a boil. Reduce heat; cover and simmer for 30 minutes.
3. Garnish each serving with 1 tablespoon each of sour cream, crushed chips and cheese.

PER SERVING *1 cup equals 351 cal., 9 g fat (4 g sat. fat), 38 mg chol., 762 mg sodium, 42 g carb., 11 g fiber, 26 g pro.*

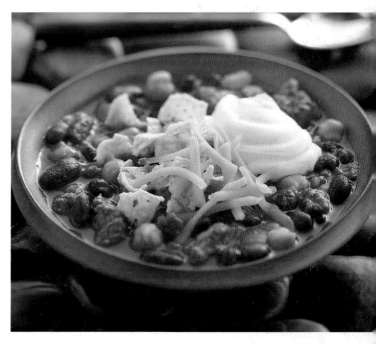

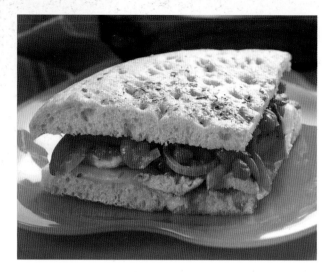

404 CALORIES

Roasted Pepper Chicken Sandwiches

This is a wonderful, flavorful sandwich perfect for a casual dinner or special luncheon. It's sure to get rave reviews.
—**LAURA MERKLE** DOVER, DE

PREP: 30 MIN. + MARINATING • **GRILL:** 10 MIN. • **MAKES:** 4 SERVINGS

- 1 tablespoon lemon juice
- 1 tablespoon Dijon mustard
- 2 teaspoons olive oil
- 1 garlic clove, minced
- ¼ teaspoon dried thyme
- ¼ teaspoon dried marjoram
- 4 boneless skinless chicken breast halves (4 ounces each)

PEPPER MIXTURE
- 1 large onion, thinly sliced
- 1 teaspoon sugar
- 4 garlic cloves, minced
- ¾ teaspoon fennel seed, crushed
- ¼ teaspoon crushed red pepper flakes
- ⅛ teaspoon salt
- ⅛ teaspoon pepper
- 1 jar (7 ounces) roasted sweet red peppers, drained and sliced
- 1 tablespoon red wine vinegar

SANDWICHES
- 1 loaf (8 ounces) focaccia bread
- 4 teaspoons fat-free mayonnaise
- 4 slices reduced-fat Swiss cheese

1. In a large resealable plastic bag, combine the first six ingredients; add chicken. Seal bag and turn to coat; refrigerate for 1 hour.

2. In a large nonstick skillet coated with cooking spray, cook and stir onion and sugar over medium heat until tender. Add garlic and seasonings; cook for 1 minute. Stir in roasted peppers and vinegar; cook 2 minutes longer. Remove from the heat; keep warm.

3. Drain chicken if necessary, discarding any excess marinade. Moisten a paper towel with cooking oil; using long-handled tongs, lightly coat the grill rack.

4. Grill chicken, covered, over medium heat or broil 4 in. from the heat for 4-7 minutes on each side or until a thermometer reads 170°. Cut into ½-in. strips.

5. Cut focaccia in half lengthwise; spread mayonnaise over cut side of bread bottom. Layer with cheese, chicken strips and pepper mixture. Replace bread top; lightly press down. Grill, covered, for 2-3 minutes or until cheese is melted. Cut into four sandwiches.

PER SERVING *1 sandwich equals 404 cal., 11 g fat (3 g sat. fat), 73 mg chol., 795 mg sodium, 41 g carb., 2 g fiber, 35 g pro.* **Diabetic Exchanges:** *4 lean meat, 2 starch, 1 vegetable.*

358 CALORIES

Makeover Gourmet Enchiladas

The *Taste of Home* kitchen pros created a healthier version of my enchiladas by tweaking the original. With this better-for-you recipe, now we can enjoy their great flavor without the guilt!
—**BETH DAUENHAUER** PUEBLO, CO

PREP: 35 MIN. • **BAKE:** 35 MIN.
MAKES: 2 DISHES (6 SERVINGS EACH)

- 1 pound lean ground beef (90% lean)
- 1 pound extra-lean ground turkey
- 1 large onion, chopped
- 1½ cups (12 ounces) 2% cottage cheese
- 1½ cups (12 ounces) reduced-fat sour cream
- 2 cans (4 ounces each) chopped green chilies
- ½ teaspoon ground cumin
- ½ teaspoon ground coriander

SAUCE
- 1 medium onion, chopped
- 2 cans (8 ounces each) tomato sauce
- 1 cup salsa
- 1 tablespoon chili powder
- 1 teaspoon dried oregano

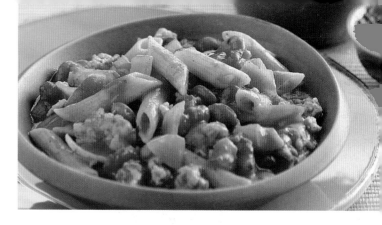

- ½ teaspoon garlic powder
- ½ teaspoon dried thyme
- 12 whole wheat tortillas (8 inches), warmed
- ¾ cup shredded cheddar cheese, divided

1. In a large skillet, cook the beef, turkey and onion over medium heat until meat is no longer pink; drain. Stir in the cottage cheese, sour cream, chilies, cumin and coriander; set aside.
2. For sauce, in a large nonstick skillet coated with cooking spray, saute onion until tender. Stir in the tomato sauce, salsa, chili powder, oregano, garlic powder and thyme. Bring to a boil. Reduce heat; simmer, uncovered, for 15-20 minutes or until slightly thickened.
3. Place a heaping ½ cup meat mixture down the center of each tortilla. Roll up and place seam side down in two 13-in. x 9-in. baking dishes coated with cooking spray. Pour sauce over top.
4. Sprinkle one dish with 6 tablespoons cheese; cover and freeze for up to 3 months. Bake the remaining dish, uncovered, at 350° for 30-35 minutes or until heated through. Sprinkle with remaining cheese; bake 5 minutes longer or until cheese is melted.

TO USE FROZEN ENCHILADAS *Thaw in refrigerator overnight. Remove from the refrigerator 30 minutes before baking. Bake, covered, at 350° for 35-40 minutes or until heated through..*

PER SERVING *1 enchilada equals 358 cal., 12 g fat (5 g sat. fat), 55 mg chol., 715 mg sodium, 33 g carb., 3 g fiber, 28 g pro.* **Diabetic Exchanges:** *3 lean meat, 2 starch, 1 vegetable, 1 fat.*

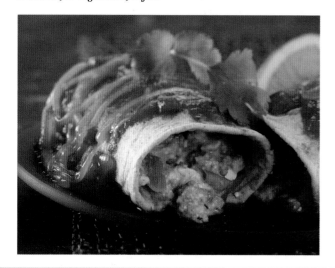

384 CALORIES One-Pot Chili

This hearty entree is low in fat and full of flavor. I love that you can cook the dried pasta right in the chili. One less pot to wash! This also reheats perfectly in the microwave.
—**DAWN FORSBERG** SAINT JOSEPH, MO

PREP: 25 MIN. • **COOK:** 15 MIN. • **MAKES:** 6 SERVINGS (2 QUARTS)

- 1 pound lean ground turkey
- 1 small onion, chopped
- ¼ cup chopped green pepper
- 1 teaspoon olive oil
- 2 cups water
- 1 can (15 ounces) pinto beans, rinsed and drained
- 1 can (14½ ounces) reduced-sodium beef broth
- 1 can (14½ ounces) diced tomatoes with mild green chilies, undrained
- 1 can (8 ounces) no-salt-added tomato sauce
- 2 teaspoons chili powder
- 1 teaspoon ground cumin
- ½ teaspoon dried oregano
- 2 cups uncooked multigrain penne pasta
- ¼ cup reduced-fat sour cream
- ¼ cup minced fresh cilantro

1. In a large saucepan coated with cooking spray, cook the turkey, onion and pepper in oil over medium heat until meat is no longer pink; drain.
2. Stir in the water, beans, broth, tomatoes, tomato sauce, chili powder, cumin and oregano. Bring to a boil. Add pasta; cook for 15-20 minutes or until tender, stirring occasionally. Serve with sour cream; sprinkle with cilantro.

PER SERVING *1⅓ cups with 2 teaspoons sour cream equals 384 cal., 10 g fat (2 g sat. fat), 64 mg chol., 598 mg sodium, 47 g carb., 8 g fiber, 25 g pro.* **Diabetic Exchanges:** *3 starch, 2 lean meat, 1 vegetable.*

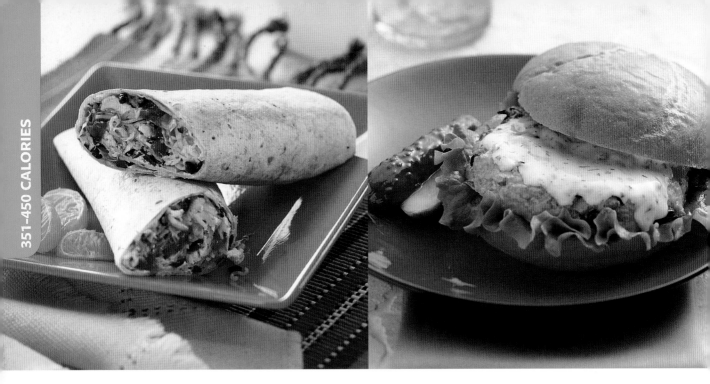

353 CALORIES Turkey Tortilla Roll-Ups

To keep lunches new and exciting for my family, I like to make these roll-ups. They can be prepared ahead, so they're perfect for brown-bag lunches.

—DARLENE BRENDEN SALEM, OR

START TO FINISH: 10 MIN.
MAKES: 6 SERVINGS

- ¾ cup sour cream
- 6 spinach tortillas or flour tortillas of your choice (8 inches)
- 1½ cups cubed cooked turkey or ready-to-use grilled chicken breast strips
- 1 cup (4 ounces) finely shredded cheddar cheese
- 1 cup shredded lettuce
- ½ cup chopped ripe olives
- ½ cup chunky salsa

Spread 2 tablespoons sour cream over each tortilla. Top with turkey, cheese, lettuce, olives and salsa. Roll up each tortilla tightly; wrap in plastic wrap. Refrigerate until serving.

PER SERVING *1 roll-up equals 353 cal., 16 g fat (9 g sat. fat), 67 mg chol., 577 mg sodium, 29 g carb., trace fiber, 20 g pro.*

357 CALORIES Fiesta Ranch Burgers

Depending on how spicy you and your family like your burgers, add more or less chipotle pepper, which also gives a nice smoky flavor.

—CAROL BREWER FAIRBORN, OH

START TO FINISH: 30 MIN.
MAKES: 5 SERVINGS

- 2 egg whites, lightly beaten
- ½ cup canned diced tomatoes, drained
- ½ cup canned black beans, rinsed and drained
- 1 small onion, chopped
- 1 tablespoon lime juice
- 1 to 2 tablespoons chopped chipotle peppers in adobo sauce
- 1 garlic clove, minced
- ¼ teaspoon salt
- 1¼ pounds lean ground turkey
- ⅓ cup fat-free ranch salad dressing
- 1 tablespoon minced fresh cilantro
- 5 lettuce leaves
- 5 hamburger buns, split

1. In a large bowl, combine the first eight ingredients. Crumble turkey over mixture and mix well. Shape into five burgers.

2. Broil 4 in. from the heat for 7-9 minutes on each side or until a thermometer reads 165° and the juices run clear.

3. In a small bowl, combine the salad dressing and cilantro. Serve burgers with dressing on lettuce-lined buns.

PER SERVING *1 burger equals 357 cal., 12 g fat (3 g sat. fat), 90 mg chol., 745 mg sodium, 34 g carb., 3 g fiber, 27 g pro.* **Diabetic Exchanges:** *3 lean meat, 2 starch.*

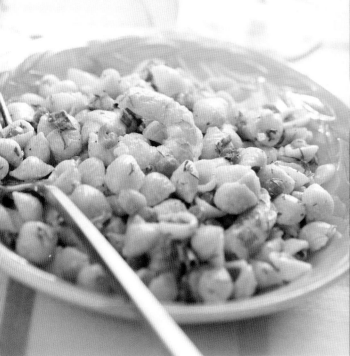
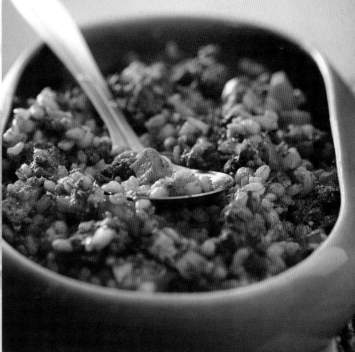

Shrimp Pasta Salad

This salad combines two of my favorite foods: pasta and shrimp. It makes a wonderfully satisfying summertime lunch. The salad is also great alongside grilled steak, hamburgers and hot dogs.

—**TRACI WYNNE** DENVER, PA

PREP: 30 MIN. + CHILLING
MAKES: 6 SERVINGS

- 4 **cups uncooked small pasta shells**
- 1 **pound cooked small shrimp, peeled and deveined**
- 1½ **cups frozen peas, thawed**
- ½ **cup thinly sliced green onions**
- ¼ **cup minced fresh parsley**
- ⅓ **cup reduced-fat mayonnaise**
- ⅓ **cup reduced-fat plain yogurt**
- 2 **tablespoons lemon juice**
- 1 **tablespoon minced fresh dill**
- ¼ **teaspoon salt**
- ¼ **teaspoon pepper**

1. Cook pasta according to package directions; drain and rinse in cold water. In a large bowl, combine the shrimp, peas, onions and parsley. Stir in the pasta.

2. In a small bowl, combine the remaining ingredients. Pour over pasta mixture and toss to coat. Cover and refrigerate for at least 1 hour.

PER SERVING *1½ cups equals 391 cal., 7 g fat (1 g sat. fat), 153 mg chol., 430 mg sodium, 55 g carb., 4 g fiber, 27 g pro.*

Barley Beef Skillet

Even my 3-year-old loves this family favorite. It's very filling, inexpensive and full of veggies. You can spice it up with chili powder, cayenne or a few dashes of Tabasco.

—**KIT TUNSTALL** BOISE, ID

PREP: 20 MIN. • **COOK:** 1 HOUR
MAKES: 4 SERVINGS

- 1 **pound lean ground beef (90% lean)**
- ¼ **cup chopped onion**
- 1 **garlic clove, minced**
- 1 **can (14½ ounces) reduced-sodium beef broth**
- 1 **can (8 ounces) tomato sauce**
- 1 **cup water**
- 2 **small carrots, chopped**
- 1 **small tomato, seeded and chopped**
- 1 **small zucchini, chopped**
- 1 **cup medium pearl barley**
- 2 **teaspoons Italian seasoning**
- ¼ **teaspoon salt**
- ⅛ **teaspoon pepper**

In a large skillet, cook beef and onion over medium heat until meat is no longer pink. Add garlic; cook 1 minute longer. Drain. Add the broth, tomato sauce and water; bring to a boil. Stir in remaining ingredients. Reduce the heat; cover and simmer for 45-50 minutes or until the barley is tender.

PER SERVING *1½ cups equals 400 cal., 10 g fat (4 g sat. fat), 73 mg chol., 682 mg sodium, 48 g carb., 10 g fiber, 30 g pro.*

391 CALORIES

Family-Favorite Cheeseburger Pasta

I created this recipe to satisfy a cheeseburger craving. What a delicious, healthy take on a classic!

—**RAQUEL HAGGARD** EDMOND, OK

START TO FINISH: 30 MIN.
MAKES: 4 SERVINGS

- 1½ cups uncooked whole wheat penne pasta
- ¾ pound lean ground beef (90% lean)
- 2 tablespoons finely chopped onion
- 1 can (14½ ounces) no-salt-added diced tomatoes
- 2 tablespoons dill pickle relish
- 2 tablespoons prepared mustard
- 2 tablespoons ketchup
- 1 teaspoon steak seasoning
- ¼ teaspoon seasoned salt
- ¾ cup shredded reduced-fat cheddar cheese
   Chopped green onions, optional

1. Cook pasta according to package directions. Meanwhile, in a large skillet, cook beef and onion over medium heat until meat is no longer pink; drain. Drain pasta; add to meat mixture.

2. Stir in the tomatoes, relish, mustard, ketchup, steak seasoning and seasoned salt. Bring to a boil. Reduce heat; simmer, uncovered, for 5 minutes.

3. Sprinkle with cheese. Remove from the heat; cover and let stand until cheese is melted. Garnish with green onions if desired.

NOTE *This recipe was tested with McCormick's Montreal Steak Seasoning. Look for it in the spice aisle at your grocery store.*

PER SERVING *1½ cups equals 391 cal., 12 g fat (6 g sat. fat), 57 mg chol., 759 mg sodium, 43 g carb., 4 g fiber, 28 g pro.* **Diabetic Exchanges:** *3 lean meat, 2 starch, 1 vegetable, ½ fat.*

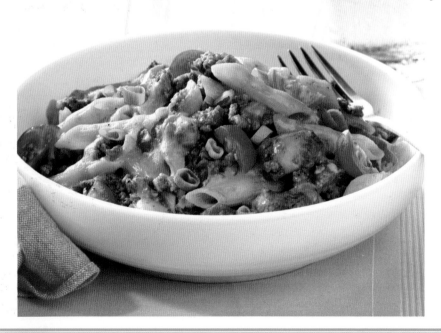

399 CALORIES Turkey Avocado Sandwiches

Hearty and delicious, these satisfying turkey sandwiches have just the right amount of heat!

—**DAVE BREMSON** PLANTATION, FL

START TO FINISH: 10 MIN.
MAKES: 2 SERVINGS

- 3 ounces fat-free cream cheese
- 2 teaspoons taco sauce
- 4 drops hot pepper sauce
- 4 slices whole wheat bread
- 4 ounces sliced cooked turkey
- ½ medium ripe avocado, peeled and sliced
- 1 medium tomato, sliced
- 2 to 4 tablespoons minced fresh cilantro
- 2 lettuce leaves

1. In a large bowl, beat cream cheese until smooth. Beat in taco sauce and pepper sauce; spread over the bread.

2. Layer the turkey, avocado and tomato on two bread slices; sprinkle with cilantro. Top with lettuce and remaining bread.

PER SERVING *1 sandwich equals 399 cal., 11 g fat (2 g sat. fat), 52 mg chol., 617 mg sodium, 40 g carb., 7 g fiber, 33 g pro.* **Diabetic Exchanges:** *3 lean meat, 2 starch, 1 vegetable, 1 fat.*

358 CALORIES

Asian Vegetable Pasta

A little peanut butter and a sprinkling of peanuts give this dish plenty of flavor. While red pepper flakes offer a little kick, brown sugar balances it out with a hint of sweetness.

—**MITZI SENTIFF** ANNAPOLIS, MD

START TO FINISH: 20 MIN.
MAKES: 5 SERVINGS

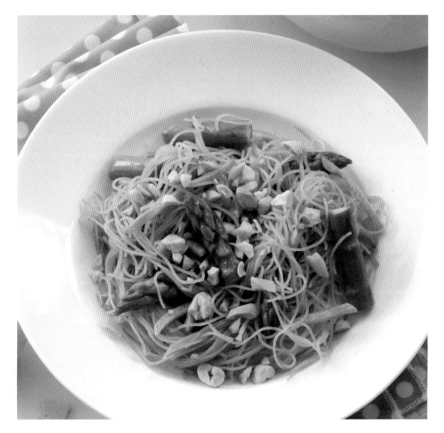

1 pound lean ground turkey
½ cup chopped onion
2 garlic cloves, minced
1 tablespoon sugar
1 tablespoon all-purpose flour
¼ teaspoon pepper
1 cup ketchup
1 tablespoon prepared mustard
1 tablespoon barbecue sauce
1 tablespoon Worcestershire sauce
6 sandwich buns, split

1. In a large nonstick skillet, cook the turkey and onion over medium heat until turkey is no longer pink; drain if necessary. Add garlic; cook for 1-2 minutes or until tender.

2. Stir in the sugar, flour and pepper. Add the ketchup, mustard, barbecue sauce and Worcestershire sauce. Bring to a boil. Reduce heat; cover and simmer for 5-10 minutes or until heated through. Serve on buns.

PER SERVING *1 sandwich equals 388 cal., 11 g fat (4 g sat. fat), 60 mg chol., 969 mg sodium, 52 g carb., 3 g fiber, 22 g pro.* **Diabetic Exchanges:** *3½ starch, 2 lean meat.*

4 quarts water
1 pound fresh asparagus, cut into 1-inch pieces
8 ounces uncooked angel hair pasta
¾ cup julienned carrots
⅓ cup reduced-fat creamy peanut butter
3 tablespoons rice vinegar
3 tablespoons reduced-sodium soy sauce
2 tablespoons brown sugar
½ teaspoon crushed red pepper flakes
¼ cup unsalted peanuts, chopped

1. In a Dutch oven, bring the water to a boil. Add asparagus and pasta; cook for 3 minutes. Stir in carrots; cook for 1 minute or until pasta is tender. Drain and keep warm.

2. In a small saucepan, combine the peanut butter, vinegar, soy sauce, brown sugar and pepper flakes. Bring to a boil over medium heat, stirring constantly. Pour over pasta mixture; toss to coat. Sprinkle with peanuts.

PER SERVING *1 cup equals 358 cal., 10 g fat (2 g sat. fat), 0 chol., 472 mg sodium, 54 g carb., 5 g fiber, 15 g pro.*

388 CALORIES Family-Pleasing Sloppy Joes
My grandma gave me this recipe long ago. I made changes over the years to give the yummy meal even more pizzazz.
—**JILL ZOSEL** SEATTLE, WA

START TO FINISH: 30 MIN.
MAKES: 6 SERVINGS

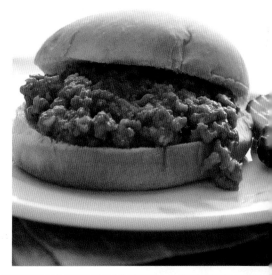

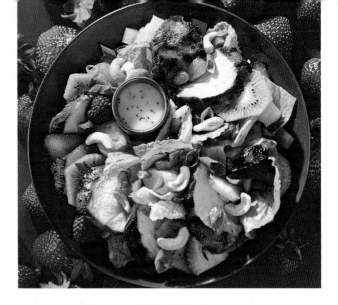

353 CALORIES Santa Fe Rice Salad

A warm rice and bean salad served with crunchy tortilla chips turns lunch into a fiesta! My whole family enjoys it. Occasionally, I add other ingredients, depending on what I have on hand, but this combination is most popular at our house.
—**MARILYN SHERWOOD** FREMONT, NE

START TO FINISH: 20 MIN. • **MAKES:** 6 SERVINGS

- 1 **medium green pepper, julienned**
- 1 **medium sweet red pepper, julienned**
- 1 **small onion, thinly sliced**
- 2 **teaspoons canola oil**
- 2 **cups cooked rice**
- 1 **can (16 ounces) kidney beans, rinsed and drained**
- 1 **can (11 ounces) Mexicorn, drained**
- 1 **jar (8 ounces) picante sauce**
- 6 **cups shredded lettuce**
- ¾ **cup shredded reduced-fat cheddar cheese**
- 6 **tablespoons reduced-fat sour cream**
  Tortilla chips

In a nonstick skillet, saute peppers and onion in oil for 6-7 minutes or until tender. Stir in the rice, beans, corn and picante sauce until heated through. Place 1 cup of lettuce on each of six salad plates. Top with 1 cup rice mixture, 2 tablespoons cheese and 1 tablespoon sour cream. Serve with tortilla chips.

PER SERVING *1 cup salad with 10 tortilla chips equals 353 cal., 7 g fat (3 g sat. fat), 15 mg chol., 800 mg sodium, 59 g carb., 9 g fiber, 15 g pro. **Diabetic Exchanges:** 3 starch, 2 vegetable, 1 lean meat.*

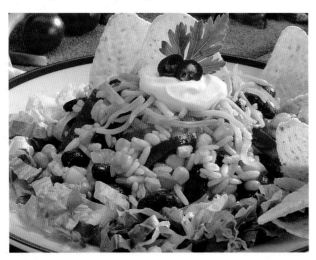

361 CALORIES Teriyaki Chicken Salad with Poppy Seed Dressing

I've made this salad so often and shared it with many people. It's originally from my friend's daughter, and we always receive compliments on how wonderfully the light fruit flavors come alive with the poppy seed dressing.
—**CATHLEEN LEONARD** WOODBRIDGE, CA

PREP: 30 MIN. + MARINATING • **GRILL:** 10 MIN. • **MAKES:** 6 SERVINGS

- 1 **cup honey teriyaki marinade**
- 1 **pound boneless skinless chicken breasts**
- 6 **cups torn romaine**
- 3 **medium kiwifruit, peeled and sliced**
- 1 **can (20 ounces) unsweetened pineapple chunks, drained**
- 1 **can (11 ounces) mandarin oranges, drained**
- 2 **celery ribs, chopped**
- 1 **medium sweet red pepper, chopped**
- 1 **medium green pepper, chopped**
- 1 **cup fresh raspberries**
- 1 **cup sliced fresh strawberries**
- 3 **green onions, chopped**
- ½ **cup salted cashews**
- ⅓ **cup reduced-fat poppy seed salad dressing**

1. Place marinade in a large resealable plastic bag; add the chicken. Seal bag and turn to coat; refrigerate for 8 hours or overnight. Drain and discard marinade.
2. Grill chicken, covered, over medium heat or broil 4 in. from the heat for 5-7 minutes on each side or until a thermometer reads 170°.

3. Slice chicken. Divide the romaine, kiwi, pineapple, oranges, celery, peppers, raspberries and strawberries among six plates; top with chicken. Sprinkle with green onions and cashews. Drizzle with salad dressing.

PER SERVING *1 serving equals 361 cal., 11 g fat (2 g sat. fat), 42 mg chol., 761 mg sodium, 49 g carb., 7 g fiber, 20 g pro.* **Diabetic Exchanges:** *2 lean meat, 1½ starch, 1½ fat, 1 vegetable, 1 fruit.*

353 CALORIES Floribbean Fish Burgers with Tropical Sauce

I like to make fish burgers because they're lower in saturated fat and cholesterol than other ones. And because there's not a lot of other fat in the burgers, I figure I can add some avocado!

—VIRGINIA ANTHONY JACKSONVILLE, FL

PREP: 35 MIN. • **GRILL:** 10 MIN. • **MAKES:** 6 SERVINGS

- ½ cup fat-free mayonnaise
- 1 tablespoon minced fresh cilantro
- 1 tablespoon minced chives
- 1 tablespoon sweet pickle relish
- 1 tablespoon lime juice
- 1 teaspoon grated lime peel
- 1½ teaspoons Caribbean jerk seasoning
- ⅛ teaspoon hot pepper sauce

BURGERS

- 1 egg white, lightly beaten
- 4 green onions, chopped
- ⅓ cup soft bread crumbs
- 2 tablespoons minced fresh cilantro
- 2 teaspoons Caribbean jerk seasoning
- 1 garlic clove, minced
- ⅛ teaspoon salt
- 1½ pounds grouper or red snapper fillets
- 6 kaiser rolls, split
- 6 lettuce leaves
- 1 medium ripe avocado, peeled and cut into 12 slices

1. In a small bowl, combine the first eight ingredients; cover and refrigerate until serving.
2. In a large bowl, combine the egg white, onions, bread crumbs, cilantro, jerk seasoning, garlic and salt. Place fish in a food processor; cover and process until finely chopped. Add to egg white mixture and mix well. Shape into six burgers.
3. Spray both sides of burgers with cooking spray. Moisten a paper towel with cooking oil; using long-handled tongs, lightly coat the grill rack. Grill burgers, covered, over medium heat or broil 4 in. from the heat for 4-5 minutes on each side or until a thermometer reads 160°.
4. Serve each on a roll with lettuce, avocado and 5 teaspoons sauce.

PER SERVING *1 burger equals 353 cal., 9 g fat (1 g sat. fat), 44 mg chol., 797 mg sodium, 39 g carb., 4 g fiber, 29 g pro.* **Diabetic Exchanges:** *3 lean meat, 2½ starch, 1 fat.*

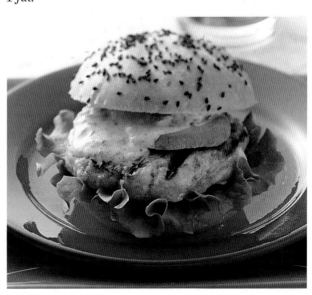

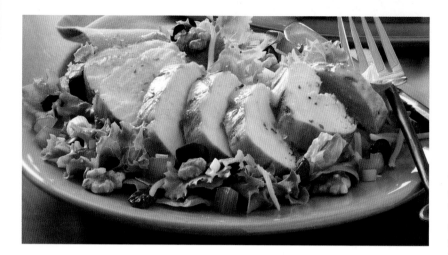

383 CALORIES
Grilled Chicken Salad

Perfect for two, this pretty entree salad features strips of hearty grilled chicken. Tomatoes, dried cranberries, olives and crunchy walnuts add wonderful flavor to each forkful.

—MARY CAMPE LAKEWOOD, CO

START TO FINISH: 30 MIN.
MAKES: 2 SERVINGS

- 2 **boneless skinless chicken breast halves (6 ounces each)**
- 3 **cups torn mixed salad greens**
- 1 **small tomato, chopped**
- ¼ **cup dried cranberries**
- ¼ **cup shredded reduced-fat cheddar cheese**
- ¼ **cup sliced ripe olives**
- 2 **green onions, chopped**
- 2 **tablespoons chopped walnuts**
- ¼ **cup fat-free Italian salad dressing**

1. Moisten a paper towel with cooking oil; using long-handled tongs, lightly coat the grill rack. Grill chicken, covered, over medium heat or broil 4 in. from the heat for 8-10 minutes on each side or until a thermometer reads 170°.
2. Divide salad greens between two serving plates; top with tomato, cranberries, cheese, olives, onions and walnuts. Slice chicken; arrange over salads. Serve with Italian dressing.

PER SERVING *1 serving equals 383 cal., 14 g fat (4 g sat. fat), 105 mg chol., 776 mg sodium, 24 g carb., 5 g fiber, 42 g pro.* **Diabetic Exchanges:** *5 lean meat, 1½ starch, 1 vegetable, 1 fat.*

357 CALORIES
Summer Veggie Subs

Every Sunday night during the summer, a local park near our home holds free outdoor concerts. We've been going for years. These subs are perfect for picnics, and I've taken them to the concerts several times.

—JENNIE TODD LANCASTER, PA

PREP: 30 MIN. + STANDING
MAKES: 12 SERVINGS

- 4 **medium sweet red peppers**
- ½ **cup fat-free mayonnaise**
- 2 **tablespoons minced fresh basil**
- 1 **tablespoon minced fresh parsley**
- 1 **tablespoon minced fresh tarragon**
- 2 **loaves French bread (1 pound each), halved lengthwise**
- 2 **cups fresh baby spinach**
- 2 **cups thinly sliced cucumbers**
- 2 **cups alfalfa sprouts**
- 4 **medium tomatoes, sliced**
- 2 **medium ripe avocados, peeled and sliced**
- ¾ **pound thinly sliced deli turkey**
- 6 **slices reduced-fat Swiss cheese, halved**

1. Broil peppers 4 in. from the heat until skins blister, about 5 minutes. With tongs, rotate peppers a quarter turn. Broil and rotate until all sides are blistered and blackened. Immediately place peppers in a large bowl; cover and let stand for 15-20 minutes.
2. Peel off and discard charred skin. Remove stems and seeds. Julienne peppers.
3. Combine the mayonnaise, basil, parsley and tarragon; spread over bread bottoms. Top with spinach, cucumbers, sprouts, roasted peppers, tomatoes, avocados, turkey and cheese. Replace tops. Cut each loaf into six slices.

PER SERVING *1 slice equals 357 cal., 9 g fat (2 g sat. fat), 19 mg chol., 894 mg sodium, 53 g carb., 6 g fiber, 20 g pro.*

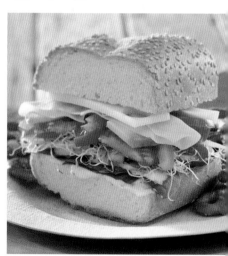

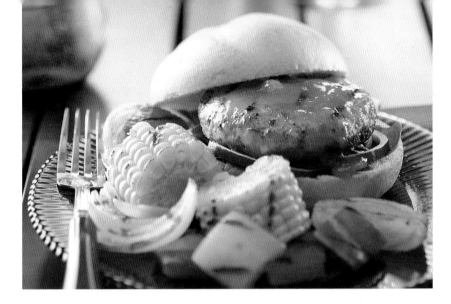

359 CALORIES Chutney
Turkey Burgers

Arugula adds a special wow to these saucy, slightly sweet burgers. I get lots of compliments whenever I serve them. The burgers are great for summer or fall cookouts.

—**JEANNE LUEDERS** WATERLOO, IA

START TO FINISH: 20 MIN.
MAKES: 4 SERVINGS

- ½ cup chutney, divided
- 1 tablespoon Dijon mustard
- 2 teaspoons lime juice
- ¼ cup minced fresh parsley
- 2 green onions, chopped
- ½ teaspoon salt
- ¼ teaspoon pepper
- 1 pound lean ground turkey
- 4 hamburger buns, split
- 16 fresh arugula or baby spinach leaves
- 4 slices red onion

1. Combine ¼ cup chutney, mustard and lime juice; set aside. In a large bowl, combine the parsley, onions, salt, pepper and remaining chutney. Crumble turkey over mixture and mix well. Shape into four patties.

2. Moisten a paper towel with cooking oil; using long-handled tongs, lightly coat the grill rack. Grill burgers, covered, over medium heat or broil 4 in. from the heat for 5-7 minutes on each side or until a thermometer reads 165° and juices run clear.

3. Serve on buns with arugula, onion and reserved chutney mixture.

PER SERVING *1 burger equals 359 cal., 12 g fat (3 g sat. fat), 90 mg chol., 749 mg sodium, 38 g carb., 3 g fiber, 25 g pro.* **Diabetic Exchanges:** *3 lean meat, 2½ starch.*

402 CALORIES Pineapple
Chicken Fajitas

Honey and pineapple add a sweet twist to these fajitas that my family requests often. I like to serve them with coleslaw and potatoes. Just add fresh fruit for dessert and you have a great meal.

—**RAYMONDE BOURGEOIS**
SWASTIKA, ON

PREP: 25 MIN. • **COOK:** 15 MIN.
MAKES: 8 SERVINGS

- 2 pounds boneless skinless chicken breasts, cut into strips
- 1 tablespoon olive oil
- 1 each medium green, sweet red and yellow pepper, julienned
- 1 medium onion, cut into thin wedges
- 2 tablespoons fajita seasoning mix
- ¼ cup water
- 2 tablespoons honey
- 1 tablespoon dried parsley flakes
- 1 teaspoon garlic powder
- ½ teaspoon salt
- ½ cup unsweetened pineapple chunks, drained
- 8 flour tortillas (10 inches), warmed

1. In a large nonstick skillet, cook chicken in oil for 4-5 minutes. Add peppers and onion; cook and stir 4-5 minutes longer.

2. Combine seasoning mix and water; stir in honey, parsley, garlic powder and salt. Stir into the pan. Add pineapple; cook and stir for 1-2 minutes or until chicken is no longer pink and vegetables are tender. Place chicken mixture on one side of each tortilla; fold tortillas over filling.

PER SERVING *1 fajita equals 402 cal., 8 g fat (2 g sat. fat), 63 mg chol., 839 mg sodium, 44 g carb., 7 g fiber, 30 g pro.*

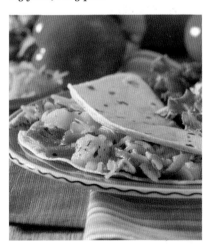

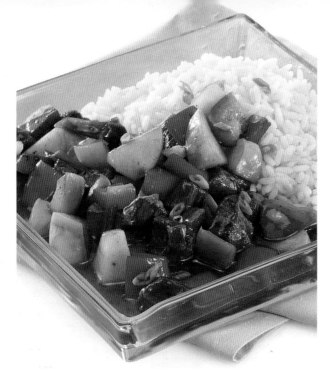

2. In the same pan, stir-fry peppers and apples in remaining oil for 3 minutes. Add ½ cup green onions. Stir-fry 2-3 minutes longer or until peppers are crisp-tender. Remove and keep warm.

3. Add brown sugar and vinegar to pan; bring to a boil. Combine cornstarch and water until smooth; stir into brown sugar mixture. Return to a boil; cook and stir for 2 minutes or until thickened and bubbly.

4. Return beef and vegetable mixture to pan; heat through. Garnish with remaining onions. Serve with rice if desired.

PER SERVING *1½ cups (calculated without rice) equals 389 cal., 8 g fat (2 g sat. fat), 46 mg chol., 663 mg sodium, 53 g carb., 4 g fiber, 25 g pro.*

351 CALORIES
Red, White and Blue Pita Pockets

Completely packed with delicious fillings, these pockets get their patriotic name from red peppers, white sour cream and tangy blue cheese. But don't wait for the Fourth of July to serve them; they're fantastic any night of the year!
—CHARLENE CHAMBERS ORMOND BEACH, FL

PREP: 15 MIN. + MARINATING • **COOK:** 5 MIN.
MAKES: 4 SERVINGS

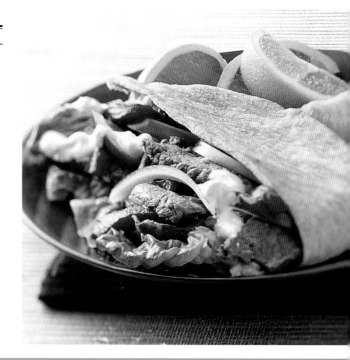

389 CALORIES Sweet-and-Sour Beef

This healthful stir-fry recipe is a family favorite. I've used a variety of meats and apples and sometimes replace the green onion with yellow onion. It always tastes great!
—BRITTANY MCCLOUD KENYON, MN

START TO FINISH: 30 MIN. • **MAKES:** 4 SERVINGS

- 1 **pound beef top sirloin steak, cut into ½-inch cubes**
- 1 **teaspoon salt**
- ½ **teaspoon pepper**
- 3 **teaspoons canola oil, divided**
- 1 **large green pepper, cut into ½-inch pieces**
- 1 **large sweet red pepper, cut into ½-inch pieces**
- 2 **medium tart apples, chopped**
- ½ **cup plus 2 tablespoons thinly sliced green onions, divided**
- ⅔ **cup packed brown sugar**
- ½ **cup cider vinegar**
- 1 **tablespoon cornstarch**
- 2 **tablespoons cold water**
  Hot cooked rice, optional

1. Sprinkle beef with salt and pepper. In a large nonstick skillet or wok coated with cooking spray, stir-fry beef in 2 teaspoons oil until no longer pink. Remove and keep warm.

2 tablespoons red wine vinegar
4 teaspoons olive oil
2 garlic cloves, minced
1 pound beef top sirloin steak, thinly sliced
½ cup fat-free sour cream
⅓ cup crumbled blue cheese
4 whole wheat pita pocket halves
2 cups torn red leaf lettuce
½ cup roasted sweet red peppers, drained and cut into strips
¼ cup sliced red onion

1. In a large resealable plastic bag, combine vinegar, oil and garlic; add the beef. Seal bag and turn to coat; refrigerate for 8 hours or overnight.
2. In a small bowl, combine sour cream and blue cheese; set aside. Drain and discard marinade.
3. In a large nonstick skillet or wok coated with cooking spray, stir-fry beef for 2-3 minutes or until no longer pink. Line pita halves with lettuce, red peppers and onion; fill each with ⅓ cup beef. Serve with sour cream mixture.

PER SERVING *1 filled pita half equals 351 cal., 12 g fat (4 g sat. fat), 59 mg chol., 522 mg sodium, 26 g carb., 3 g fiber, 32 g pro.* **Diabetic Exchanges:** *4 lean meat, 1½ fat, 1 starch, 1 vegetable.*

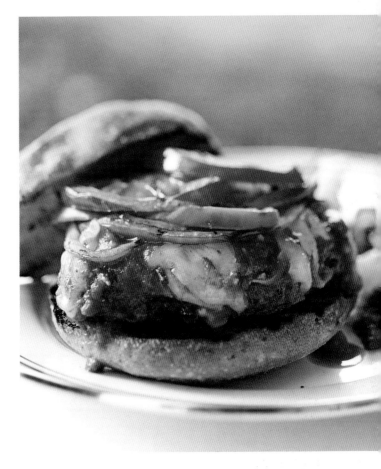

399 CALORIES
Grilled Italian Meatball Burgers

I just love these burgers! They're a big hit with both kids and adults. I serve them with sliced green peppers, tomatoes and onions—and a jar of crushed red pepper flakes on the side for adults. Kids enjoy them best as is.
—**PRISCILLA GILBERT** INDIAN HARBOUR BEACH, FL

PREP: 25 MIN. • **GRILL:** 15 MIN. • **MAKES:** 8 SERVINGS

1 egg, lightly beaten
⅓ cup seasoned bread crumbs
3 garlic cloves, minced
1 teaspoon dried oregano
1 teaspoon dried basil
¼ teaspoon salt
¼ teaspoon dried thyme
1½ pounds lean ground beef (90% lean)
½ pound Italian turkey sausage links, casings removed
¾ cup shredded part-skim mozzarella cheese
8 kaiser rolls, split
1 cup roasted garlic Parmesan spaghetti sauce, warmed

1. In a large bowl, combine the first seven ingredients. Crumble beef and sausage over mixture and mix well. Shape into eight burgers.
2. Moisten a paper towel with cooking oil; using long-handled tongs, lightly coat the grill rack. Grill burgers, covered, over medium heat or broil 4 in. from the heat for 5-7 minutes on each side or until a thermometer reads 165° and juices run clear.
3. Sprinkle burgers with cheese; cook 2-3 minutes longer or until cheese is melted. Remove burgers and keep warm.
4. Grill or broil rolls for 1-2 minutes or until toasted. Serve burgers on rolls with spaghetti sauce.

PER SERVING *1 burger equals 399 cal., 14 g fat (5 g sat. fat), 102 mg chol., 743 mg sodium, 35 g carb., 2 g fiber, 30 g pro.*

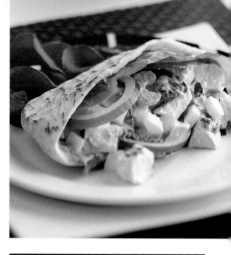

Italian Beef and Shells

A hearty entree comes easy with a simple veggie-and-pasta combo. Wine lends a special touch to the sauce and makes this pasta dish a winner.

—MIKE TCHOU PEPPER PIKE, OH

START TO FINISH: 30 MIN.
MAKES: 4 SERVINGS

- 1½ cups uncooked medium pasta shells
- 1 pound lean ground beef (90% lean)
- 1 small onion, chopped
- 1 garlic clove, minced
- 1 jar (23 ounces) marinara sauce
- 1 small yellow summer squash, quartered and sliced
- 1 small zucchini, quartered and sliced
- ¼ cup dry red wine or reduced-sodium beef broth
- ½ teaspoon salt
- ½ teaspoon Italian seasoning
- ½ teaspoon pepper

1. Cook pasta according to package directions.
2. Meanwhile, in a Dutch oven, cook the beef, onion and garlic over medium heat until meat is no longer pink; drain. Stir in the marinara sauce, squash, zucchini, wine and seasonings. Bring to a boil. Reduce heat; simmer, uncovered, for 10-15 minutes or until thickened. Drain pasta; stir into beef mixture and heat through.

PER SERVING *1¾ cups equals 396 cal., 10 g fat (4 g sat. fat), 71 mg chol., 644 mg sodium, 45 g carb., 5 g fiber, 29 g pro.* **Diabetic Exchanges:** *3 starch, 3 lean meat.*

Fruited Turkey Salad Pitas

Leftover turkey gets a great makeover in these tasty sandwiches that feed a crowd. Apples, pecans and celery give the salad filling a nice crunch.

—DONNA NOEL GRAY, ME

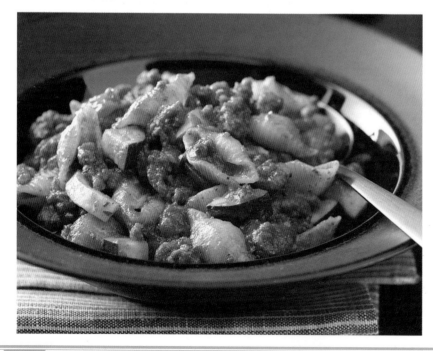

PREP: 30 MIN. + CHILLING
MAKES: 8 SERVINGS

- ½ cup reduced-fat plain yogurt
- ½ cup reduced-fat mayonnaise
- 2 tablespoons lemon juice
- ½ teaspoon pepper
- 4 cups cubed cooked turkey breast
- 2 celery ribs, thinly sliced
- 1 medium apple, peeled and chopped
- ½ cup finely chopped fresh spinach
- ⅓ cup dried cranberries
- ⅓ cup chopped pecans
- 8 pita breads (6 inches), halved
- 16 romaine leaves
- 8 slices red onion, separated into rings

1. In a small bowl, combine the yogurt, mayonnaise, lemon juice and pepper. In a large bowl, combine the turkey, celery, apple, spinach, cranberries and pecans. Add yogurt mixture and stir to coat. Cover and refrigerate until chilled.
2. Line pita halves with lettuce and onion; fill each with ½ cup turkey mixture.

PER SERVING *2 filled pita halves equals 393 cal., 11 g fat (2 g sat. fat), 66 mg chol., 501 mg sodium, 45 g carb., 3 g fiber, 29 g pro.* **Diabetic Exchanges:** *3 starch, 3 lean meat, 1 fat.*

Black Bean Burgers

My son asked me to create a good veggie burger for him, and he gave this recipe an A+! The burgers are moist, flavorful and easy to freeze. Now, like my son, I prefer them over meat burgers.

—CLARA HONEYAGER
NORTH PRAIRIE, WI

START TO FINISH: 25 MIN.
MAKES: 6 SERVINGS

- 1 cup frozen mixed vegetables, thawed
- 1 small onion, chopped
- ½ cup chopped sweet red pepper
- 1 can (15 ounces) black beans, rinsed and drained, divided
- 1 tablespoon cornstarch
- 2 tablespoons cold water
- 1 cup mashed potato flakes
- ¼ cup quick-cooking oats
- 3 tablespoons whole wheat flour
- 2 tablespoons nonfat dry milk powder
- 1 egg, lightly beaten
- ½ teaspoon salt
- ¼ teaspoon pepper
- 4 teaspoons canola oil
- 6 kaiser rolls, split
- 2 cups shredded lettuce
- ¾ cup salsa

1. In a large microwave-safe bowl, combine the mixed vegetables, onion and red pepper. Cover and microwave on high for 2 minutes or until crisp-tender.
2. Coarsely mash ¾ cup black beans. In a bowl, combine the cornstarch and water until smooth; stir in the mashed beans, potato flakes, oats, flour, milk powder, egg, salt and pepper. Stir in vegetable mixture and remaining black beans. Shape into six ⅝-in.-thick patties.
3. In a large nonstick skillet, cook patties in oil for 4-5 minutes on each side or until lightly browned. Serve on rolls with lettuce and salsa.
NOTE *This recipe was tested in a 1,100-watt microwave.*
PER SERVING *1 burger equals 381 cal., 7 g fat (1 g sat. fat), 36 mg chol., 841 mg sodium, 64 g carb., 9 g fiber, 14 g pro.*

 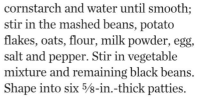 Turkey 'n' Swiss Sandwiches

Perfect for two, these toasted sandwiches turn boring lunches into exciting meals. They offer a wonderful combination of flavors.

—LEAH STARNES BEDFORD, TX

START TO FINISH: 15 MIN.
MAKES: 2 SERVINGS

- 4 slices sourdough bread, lightly toasted
- 2 teaspoons Dijon mustard
- 4 slices jellied cranberry sauce (¼ inch thick)
- 6 ounces thinly sliced deli smoked turkey
- 2 slices reduced-fat Swiss cheese

Spread two slices of bread with mustard. Top with cranberry sauce, turkey and cheese. Broil 3-4 in. from the heat for 1-2 minutes or until cheese is melted. Top with remaining bread.
PER SERVING *1 sandwich equals 384 cal., 8 g fat (2 g sat. fat), 43 mg chol., 1,315 mg sodium, 54 g carb., 3 g fiber, 27 g pro.*

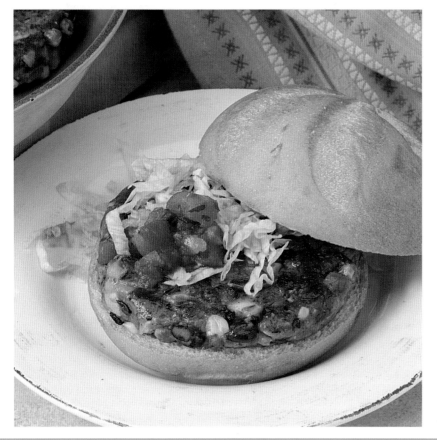

Dinners

Dig into classic **comfort foods** such as cheesy **pizzas**, bubbling **casseroles** and tempting **pasta** dishes...and still lose weight! Aim for **500 calories** for your entire meal. When planning the menu, be sure to **reserve some calories for a side dish and dessert**.

CONTENTS

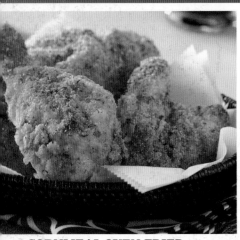

CORNMEAL OVEN-FRIED CHICKEN *PAGE 209*

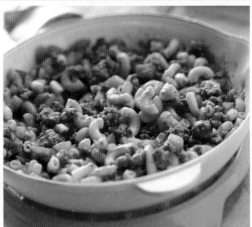

BEEF MACARONI SKILLET *PAGE 249*

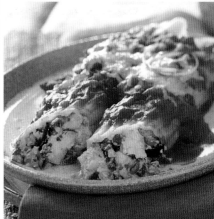

MEXICAN MANICOTTI *PAGE 318*

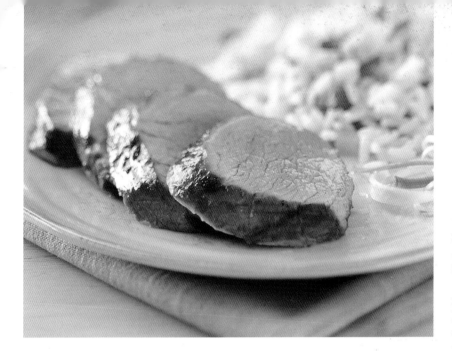

214 CALORIES Gingered Pork Tenderloin

Here's a pork tenderloin recipe that's absolutely delicious and great for entertaining. The quick prep is done ahead of time, and the grilling is so simple. This dish is foolproof!

—MICHELLE SANDERS FRASER LAKE, BC

PREP: 10 MIN. + MARINATING
GRILL: 25 MIN. • **MAKES:** 6 SERVINGS

- 2 tablespoons reduced-sodium soy sauce
- ¼ cup sherry or reduced-sodium chicken broth
- 2 tablespoons canola oil
- 2 tablespoons minced fresh gingerroot
- 2 teaspoons sugar
- 2 garlic cloves, minced
- 2 pork tenderloins (1 pound each)

1. In a large resealable plastic bag, combine the first six ingredients; add pork. Seal bag and turn to coat; refrigerate for 8 hours or overnight.
2. Drain pork and discard marinade. Prepare grill for indirect heat.

Moisten a paper towel with cooking oil; using long-handled tongs, lightly coat the grill rack.
3. Grill the pork, covered, over indirect medium-hot heat for 25-40 minutes or until a thermometer reads 160°.
4. Let pork stand for 5 minutes before slicing.

PER SERVING *4 ounces cooked pork equals 214 cal., 8 g fat (2 g sat. fat), 84 mg chol., 194 mg sodium, 2 g carb., trace fiber, 30 g pro.* **Diabetic Exchanges:** *4 lean meat, ½ fat.*

187 CALORIES

Broiled Sirloin Steaks

A butcher gave me some great advice on cooking different types of meat. Marinating and broiling work well on very lean cuts like this. Let the steaks rest for a couple of minutes before serving to keep them juicy.

—KAROL CHANDLER-EZELL
NACOGDOCHES, TX

START TO FINISH: 20 MIN.
MAKES: 4 SERVINGS

- 2 tablespoons lime juice
- 1 teaspoon onion powder
- 1 teaspoon garlic powder
- ¼ teaspoon ground mustard
- ¼ teaspoon dried oregano
- ¼ teaspoon dried thyme
- 4 beef top sirloin steaks (5 ounces each)
- 1 cup sliced fresh mushrooms

1. In a small bowl, combine the first six ingredients; rub over both sides of steaks.
2. Broil 4 in. from the heat for 7 minutes. Turn steaks; top with mushrooms. Broil 7-8 minutes longer or until meat reaches desired doneness (for medium-rare, a thermometer should read 145°; medium, 160°; well-done, 170°) and mushrooms are tender.

PER SERVING *1 steak with 3 tablespoons mushrooms equals 187 cal., 7 g fat (3 g sat. fat), 80 mg chol., 60 mg sodium, 3 g carb., trace fiber, 28 g pro.* **Diabetic Exchange:** *4 lean meat.*

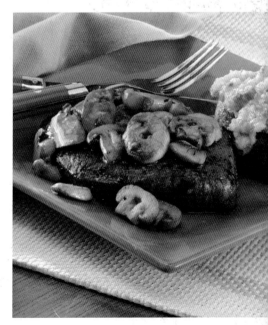

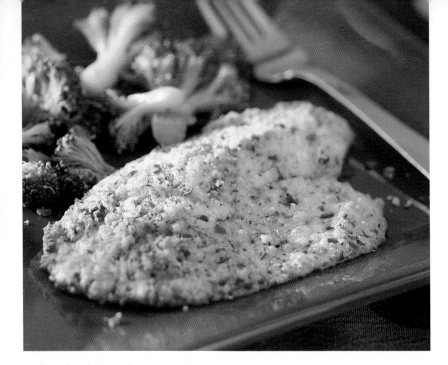

1 cup water
½ cup chopped zucchini
½ cup fat-free ricotta cheese
2 tablespoons grated Parmesan cheese
1 tablespoon minced fresh parsley or 1 teaspoon dried parsley flakes
½ cup shredded part-skim mozzarella cheese

1. In a large nonstick skillet, cook sausage and onion over medium heat until no longer pink; drain. Stir in the spaghetti sauce, egg noodles, water and zucchini. Bring to a boil. Reduce heat; cover and simmer for 8-10 minutes or until noodles are tender, stirring occasionally.

2. Combine the ricotta, Parmesan cheese and parsley. Drop by tablespoonfuls over pasta mixture. Sprinkle with mozzarella cheese; cover and cook 3-5 minutes longer or until cheese is melted.

PER SERVING *1 cup equals 250 cal., 10 g fat (3 g sat. fat), 41 mg chol., 783 mg sodium, 24 g carb., 3 g fiber, 17 g pro.* **Diabetic Exchanges:** *2 lean meat, 1½ starch, 1 fat.*

179 CALORIES Red Pepper & Parmesan Tilapia

My husband and I are always looking for light fish recipes because of their health benefits. This one's a hit with him, and we've served it at dinner parties, too. It's a staple at our house.

—MICHELLE MARTIN DURHAM, NC

START TO FINISH: 20 MIN.
MAKES: 4 SERVINGS

¼ cup egg substitute
½ cup grated Parmesan cheese
1 teaspoon Italian seasoning
½ to 1 teaspoon crushed red pepper flakes
½ teaspoon pepper
4 tilapia fillets (6 ounces each)

1. Place egg substitute in a shallow bowl. In another shallow bowl, combine the cheese, Italian seasoning, pepper flakes and pepper. Dip fillets in egg substitute, then cheese mixture.

2. Place in a 15-in. x 10-in. x 1-in. baking pan coated with cooking spray. Bake at 425° for 10-15 minutes or until fish flakes easily with a fork.

PER SERVING *1 fillet equals 179 cal., 4 g fat (2 g sat. fat), 89 mg chol., 191 mg sodium, 1 g carb., trace fiber, 35 g pro.* **Diabetic Exchanges:** *5 lean meat, ½ fat.*

250 CALORIES Favorite Skillet Lasagna

Whole wheat noodles and zucchini pump up nutrition in this delicious, family-friendly dinner. Topped with dollops of ricotta cheese, it has an extra touch of decadence. No one will guess this one's lighter!

—LORIE MINER KAMAS, UTAH

START TO FINISH: 30 MIN.
MAKES: 5 SERVINGS

½ pound Italian turkey sausage links, casings removed
1 small onion, chopped
1 jar (14 ounces) spaghetti sauce
2 cups uncooked whole wheat egg noodles

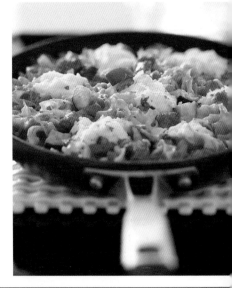

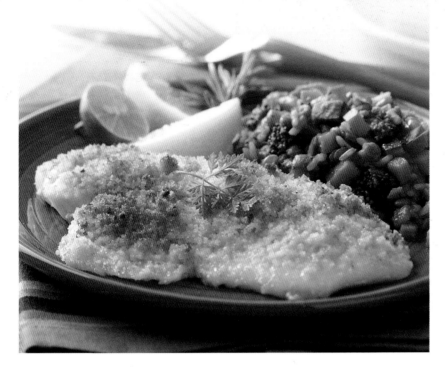

214 CALORIES

Dijon-Crusted Fish

Dijon, Parmesan and horseradish give this toasty, golden-brown fish lots of flavor. And it takes only a few minutes to get it ready for the oven.

—**SCOTT SCHMIDTKE** CHICAGO, IL

START TO FINISH: 25 MIN.
MAKES: 4 SERVINGS

- 3 **tablespoons reduced-fat mayonnaise**
- 2 **tablespoons grated Parmesan cheese, divided**
- 1 **tablespoon lemon juice**
- 2 **teaspoons Dijon mustard**
- 1 **teaspoon horseradish**
- 4 **tilapia fillets (5 ounces each)**
- ¼ **cup dry bread crumbs**
- 2 **teaspoons butter, melted**

1. Combine mayonnaise, 1 tablespoon cheese, lemon juice, mustard and horseradish. Place fish on a greased baking sheet; spread with mayonnaise mixture.

2. In a small bowl, combine the bread crumbs, butter and the remaining cheese; sprinkle mixture over the fillets.

3. Bake at 425° for 13-18 minutes or until fish flakes easily with a fork.

PER SERVING *1 fillet equals 214 cal., 8 g fat (3 g sat. fat), 80 mg chol., 327 mg sodium, 7 g carb., trace fiber, 29 g pro.* **Diabetic Exchanges:** *4 lean meat, 1½ fat, ½ starch.*

244 CALORIES Cornmeal Oven-Fried Chicken

This dish really perks up the dinner table! A flavorful cornmeal and bread crumb coating bakes up golden and crispy, yet it's still a sensible dinner choice.

—**DEB WILLIAMS** PEORIA, AZ

PREP: 20 MIN. • **BAKE:** 40 MIN.
MAKES: 6 SERVINGS

- ½ **cup dry bread crumbs**
- ½ **cup cornmeal**
- ⅓ **cup grated Parmesan cheese**
- ¼ **cup minced fresh parsley or 4 teaspoons dried parsley flakes**
- ¾ **teaspoon garlic powder**
- ½ **teaspoon salt**
- ½ **teaspoon onion powder**
- ½ **teaspoon dried thyme**
- ½ **teaspoon pepper**
- ½ **cup buttermilk**
- 1 **broiler/fryer chicken (3 to 4 pounds), cut up and skin removed**
- 1 **tablespoon butter, melted**

1. In a large resealable plastic bag, combine the first nine ingredients. Place the buttermilk in a shallow bowl. Dip chicken in buttermilk, then add to bag, a few pieces at a time, and shake to coat.

2. Place in a 13-in. x 9-in. baking pan coated with cooking spray. Bake at 375° for 10 minutes; drizzle with butter. Bake 30-40 minutes longer or until juices run clear.

PER SERVING *1 serving equals 244 cal., 9 g fat (3 g sat. fat), 82 mg chol., 303 mg sodium, 11 g carb., 1 g fiber, 27 g pro.* **Diabetic Exchanges:** *3 lean meat, 1 starch, ½ fat.*

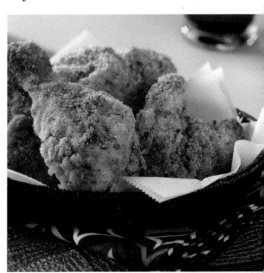

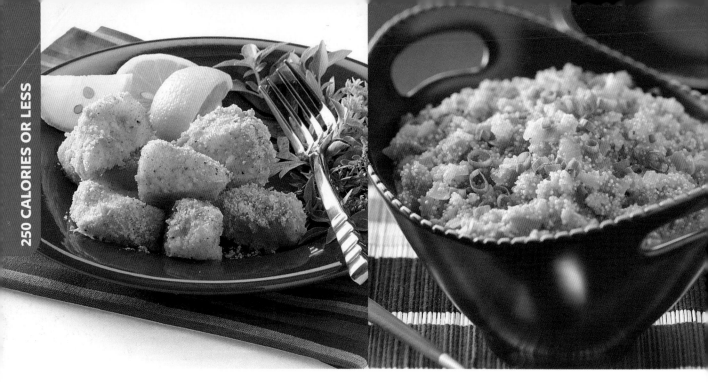

171 CALORIES

Oven-Fried Fish Nuggets

These buttery-tasting fish bites don't taste light at all. My husband and I love fried fish, but we're both trying to cut back on fats. So I made up this recipe and it was a hit. He likes it as much as deep-fried fish—and that's saying a lot!

—**LADONNA REED** PONCA CITY, OK

START TO FINISH: 25 MIN.
MAKES: 4 SERVINGS

- ⅓ **cup seasoned bread crumbs**
- ⅓ **cup crushed cornflakes**
- 3 **tablespoons grated Parmesan cheese**
- ½ **teaspoon salt**
- ¼ **teaspoon pepper**
- 1½ **pounds cod fillets, cut into 1-inch cubes**
  Butter-flavored cooking spray

1. In a shallow bowl, combine the bread crumbs, cornflakes, Parmesan cheese, salt and pepper. Coat fish with butter-flavored spray, then roll in crumb mixture.

2. Place on a baking sheet coated with cooking spray. Bake at 375° for 15-20 minutes or until fish flakes easily with a fork.

PER SERVING *1 serving equals 171 cal., 2 g fat (1 g sat. fat), 66 mg chol., 415 mg sodium, 7 g carb., trace fiber, 29 g pro.* ***Diabetic Exchanges:*** *5 lean meat, ½ starch.*

250 CALORIES ## Quinoa Pilaf

I created this recipe after tasting quinoa at a local restaurant. I really enjoy rice pilaf, but don't often have time to make it. This quick-cooking side is a tasty and quick alternative.

—**SONYA FOX** PEYTON, CO

START TO FINISH: 30 MIN.
MAKES: 3 SERVINGS

- 1 **medium onion, chopped**
- 1 **medium carrot, finely chopped**
- 1 **teaspoon olive oil**
- 1 **garlic clove, minced**
- 1 **can (14½ ounces) reduced-sodium chicken broth or vegetable broth**
- ¼ **cup water**
- ¼ **teaspoon salt**
- 1 **cup quinoa, rinsed**

1. In a small nonstick saucepan coated with cooking spray, cook onion and carrot in oil until crisp-tender. Add garlic; cook 1 minute longer. Stir in the broth, water and salt; bring mixture to a boil.

2. Add quinoa. Reduce heat; cover and simmer for 12-15 minutes or until liquid is absorbed. Remove from the heat. Fluff with a fork.

NOTE *If using vegetable broth, omit the salt.*

NOTE *Look for quinoa in the cereal, rice or organic food aisle.*

PER SERVING *1 cup equals 250 cal., 4 g fat (1 g sat. fat), 0 chol., 579 mg sodium, 45 g carb., 5 g fiber, 10 g pro.*

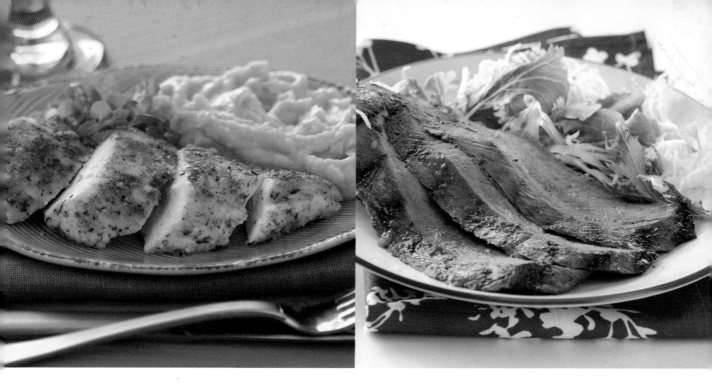

169 CALORIES Dijon-Crusted Chicken Breasts

If you're craving fried chicken, here's a dish sure to hit the spot! A crisp and flavorful coating makes the easy entree feel special and indulgent.

—JACQUELINE CORREA LANDING, NJ

START TO FINISH: 25 MIN.
MAKES: 4 SERVINGS

- ⅓ cup dry bread crumbs
- 1 tablespoon grated Parmesan cheese
- 1 teaspoon Italian seasoning
- ½ teaspoon dried thyme
- ¼ teaspoon salt
- ¼ teaspoon pepper
- 4 boneless skinless chicken breast halves (4 ounces each)
- 2 tablespoons Dijon mustard
- 1 teaspoon olive oil
- 1 teaspoon reduced-fat margarine

1. Place the first six ingredients in a shallow bowl. Brush chicken with mustard; roll in crumb mixture.

2. In a large nonstick skillet, cook chicken in oil and margarine over medium heat for 5-6 minutes on each side or until a thermometer reads 170°.
PER SERVING *1 chicken breast half equals 169 cal., 5 g fat (1 g sat. fat), 63 mg chol., 380 mg sodium, 6 g carb., trace fiber, 24 g pro.* **Diabetic Exchanges:** *3 lean meat, ½ starch, ½ fat.*

196 CALORIES Savory Marinated Flank Steak

It takes just a few ingredients to whip up a flavorful marinade for tender grilled flank steak. Try placing the sliced meat on a green salad with your favorite dressing.

—LISA RUEHLOW BLAINE, MN

PREP: 10 MIN. + MARINATING
GRILL: 15 MIN. • **MAKES:** 6 SERVINGS

- 3 tablespoons canola oil
- 2 tablespoons lemon juice
- 2 tablespoons Worcestershire sauce
- 1 tablespoon dried minced garlic
- 1 tablespoon Greek seasoning
- 1 tablespoon brown sugar
- 1 teaspoon onion powder
- 1 beef flank steak (1½ pounds)

1. In a large resealable plastic bag, combine the first seven ingredients; add steak. Seal bag and turn to coat; refrigerate for 6 hours or overnight.
2. Drain and discard marinade. Moisten a paper towel with cooking oil; using long-handled tongs, lightly coat the grill rack. Grill the steak, covered, over medium heat or broil 4 in. from heat for 6-8 minutes on each side or until steak reaches desired doneness (for medium-rare, a thermometer should read 145°; medium, 160°; well-done, 170°).
3. To serve, thinly slice across grain.
PER SERVING *3 ounces cooked beef equals 196 cal., 11 g fat (4 g sat. fat), 54 mg chol., 269 mg sodium, 2 g carb., trace fiber, 22 g pro.* **Diabetic Exchanges:** *3 lean meat, 1 fat.*

> " I lost weight by including more fiber and protein in my diet. Choosing the right snacks, like nuts and veggies with hummus, helps keep my hunger at bay between meals and helps me make better choices for lunch and dinner. "

—RENEE MCDANIEL

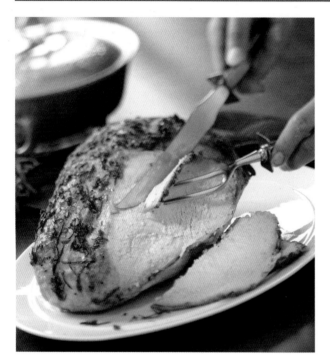

148 CALORIES Rosemary Turkey Breast

I like to season turkey with a blend of rosemary, garlic and paprika. Because I rub the mixture directly on the meat under the skin, I can remove the skin before serving and not lose any of the flavor.

—**DOROTHY PRITCHETT** WILLS POINT, TX

PREP: 10 MIN. • **BAKE:** 1½ HOURS + STANDING
MAKES: 15 SERVINGS

- 2 tablespoons olive oil
- 8 to 10 garlic cloves, peeled
- 3 tablespoons chopped fresh rosemary or 3 teaspoons dried rosemary, crushed
- 1 teaspoon salt
- 1 teaspoon paprika
- ½ teaspoon coarsely ground pepper
- 1 bone-in turkey breast (5 pounds)

1. In a food processor, combine the oil, garlic, rosemary, salt, paprika and pepper; cover and process until garlic is coarsely chopped.

2. With your fingers, carefully loosen the skin from both sides of turkey breast. Spread half of the garlic mixture over the meat under the skin. Smooth skin over meat and secure to underside of breast with toothpicks. Spread remaining garlic mixture over the turkey skin.

3. Place turkey breast on a rack in a shallow roasting pan. Bake, uncovered, at 325° for 1½ to 2 hours or until a thermometer reads 170°. Let stand for 15 minutes before slicing. Discard toothpicks.

PER SERVING *4 ounces cooked turkey (calculated without skin) equals 148 cal., 3 g fat (trace sat. fat), 78 mg chol., 207 mg sodium, 1 g carb., trace fiber, 29 g pro.* **Diabetic Exchange:** *4 lean meat.*

223 CALORIES Italian Cabbage Casserole

If your gang likes stuffed cabbage, they'll love this beefy and satisfying recipe. And you'll love that it has all the flavor of stuffed cabbage—but with a lot less work!

—**DEBRA SANDERS** BREVARD, NC

PREP: 35 MIN. • **BAKE:** 15 MIN. • **MAKES:** 6 SERVINGS

- 1 medium head cabbage, coarsely shredded
- 1 pound lean ground beef (90% lean)
- 1 large green pepper, chopped
- 1 medium onion, chopped
- 1 can (14½ ounces) diced tomatoes, undrained
- 1 can (8 ounces) tomato sauce
- 3 tablespoons tomato paste
- 1½ teaspoons dried oregano
- ½ teaspoon garlic powder

½ teaspoon pepper
⅛ teaspoon salt
½ cup shredded part-skim mozzarella cheese

1. Place the cabbage in a steamer basket; place in a large saucepan over 1 in. of water. Bring to a boil; cover and steam for 6-8 minutes or until tender. Drain and set aside.
2. In a large nonstick skillet over medium heat, cook and stir the beef, green pepper and onion until meat is no longer pink; drain. Stir in the tomatoes, tomato sauce, tomato paste and seasonings. Bring to a boil. Reduce heat; simmer, uncovered, for 10 minutes.
3. Place half of the cabbage in an 11-in. x 7-in. baking dish coated with cooking spray; top with half of beef mixture. Repeat layers (dish will be full). Sprinkle with cheese. Bake, uncovered, at 350° for 15-20 minutes or until heated through. Serve immediately or before baking, cover and freeze casserole for up to 3 months.
TO USE FROZEN CASSEROLE *Remove from the freezer 30 minutes before baking (do not thaw). Cover and bake at 350° for 45-50 minutes. Uncover; bake 15-20 minutes longer or until heated through.*
PER SERVING *1⅓ cups equals 223 cal., 7 g fat (3 g sat. fat), 42 mg chol., 438 mg sodium, 20 g carb., 7 g fiber, 21 g pro.* **Diabetic Exchanges:** *2 lean meat, 1 starch, 1 vegetable.*

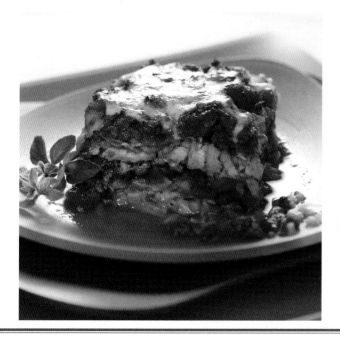

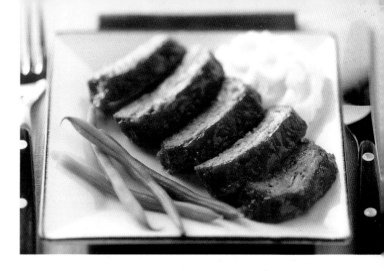

187 CALORIES
Makeover Li'l Cheddar Meat Loaves
My husband adores my meat loaf recipe. Thanks to the *Taste of Home* staff, it's now lower in calories and fat and makes a healthier dinner option than it ever did before. We both love it!
—**JODIE MITCHELL** DENVER, PA

PREP: 15 MIN. • **BAKE:** 25 MIN. • **MAKES:** 8 SERVINGS

2 egg whites, beaten
¾ cup fat-free milk
1 cup (4 ounces) shredded reduced-fat cheddar cheese
¾ cup quick-cooking oats
1 medium onion, chopped
1 medium carrot, shredded
½ teaspoon salt
¾ pound lean ground beef (90% lean)
⅔ cup ketchup
2 tablespoons brown sugar
1½ teaspoons prepared mustard

1. In a large bowl, whisk egg whites and milk. Stir in the cheese, oats, onion, carrot and salt. Crumble beef over mixture and mix well.
2. Shape into eight loaves; place in a 13-in. x 9-in. baking dish coated with cooking spray. In a small bowl, combine the ketchup, brown sugar and mustard; spoon over loaves.
3. Bake, uncovered, at 350° for 25-30 minutes or until no pink remains and a thermometer reads 160°.
PER SERVING *1 meat loaf equals 187 cal., 7 g fat (3 g sat. fat), 36 mg chol., 550 mg sodium, 18 g carb., 1 g fiber, 15 g pro.* **Diabetic Exchanges:** *2 lean meat, 1 starch.*

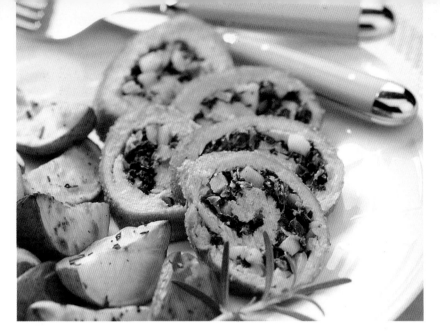

Garlic Lemon Shrimp

You'll be amazed that you can make this elegant pasta in mere minutes. Serve it with crusty bread to soak up every last drop of the garlic lemon sauce!

—ATHENA RUSSELL FLORENCE, SC

START TO FINISH: 20 MIN.
MAKES: 4 SERVINGS

- 1 **pound uncooked large shrimp, peeled and deveined**
- 2 **tablespoons olive oil**
- 3 **garlic cloves, sliced**
- 1 **tablespoon lemon juice**
- 1 **teaspoon ground cumin**
- ¼ **teaspoon salt**
- 2 **tablespoons minced fresh parsley**
   Hot cooked pasta or rice

In a large skillet, saute shrimp in oil for 3 minutes. Add the garlic, lemon juice, cumin and salt; cook and stir until shrimp turn pink. Stir in parsley. Serve with pasta or rice.
PER SERVING *¾ cup (calculated without rice or pasta) equals 163 cal., 8 g fat (1 g sat. fat), 138 mg chol., 284 mg sodium, 2 g carb., trace fiber, 19 g pro.* **Diabetic Exchanges:** *3 lean meat, 1½ fat.*

Turkey Roulades

The filling in this recipe goes so well with turkey! I love the hint of lemon, the savory combo of apples, mushrooms and spinach...and the bread-crumb coating adds a nice crunch.

—KARI WHEATON SOUTH BELOIT, IL

PREP: 40 MIN. • **BAKE:** 40 MIN.
MAKES: 8 SERVINGS

- 1 **cup diced peeled tart apple**
- 1 **cup chopped fresh mushrooms**
- ½ **cup finely chopped onion**
- 2 **teaspoons olive oil**
- 5 **ounces frozen chopped spinach, thawed and squeezed dry**
- 2 **tablespoons lemon juice**
- 2 **teaspoons grated lemon peel**
- ¾ **teaspoon salt, divided**
   Pinch ground nutmeg
- 4 **turkey breast tenderloins (8 ounces each)**
- ¼ **teaspoon pepper**
- 1 **egg, lightly beaten**
- ½ **cup seasoned bread crumbs**

1. In a large nonstick skillet coated with cooking spray, saute the apple, mushrooms and onion in oil until tender. Remove from the heat; stir in the spinach, lemon juice, lemon peel, ¼ teaspoon salt and nutmeg.
2. Make a lengthwise slit down the center of each tenderloin to within ½ in. of bottom. Open tenderloins so they lie flat; cover with plastic wrap. Flatten to ¼-in. thickness. Remove plastic; sprinkle turkey with pepper and remaining salt.
3. Spread spinach mixture over tenderloins to within 1 in. of edges. Roll up jelly-roll style, starting with a short side; tie with kitchen string. Place egg and bread crumbs in separate shallow bowls. Dip roulades in egg, then roll in crumbs.
4. Place in an 11-in. x 7-in. baking pan coated with cooking spray. Bake, uncovered, at 375° for 40-45 minutes or until a thermometer reads 170°. Let stand for 5 minutes before slicing.
PER SERVING *½ roulade equals 184 cal., 4 g fat (1 g sat. fat), 82 mg chol., 405 mg sodium, 9 g carb., 1 g fiber, 29 g pro.* **Diabetic Exchanges:** *3 lean meat, ½ starch.*

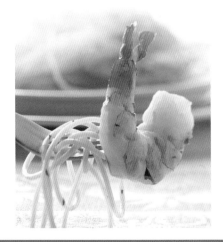

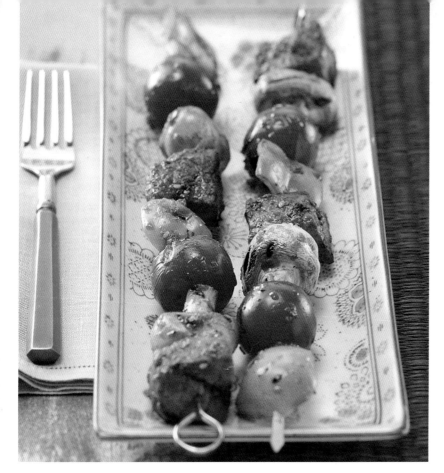

alternately thread the beef, mushrooms, tomatoes and remaining peppers. Brush lightly with oil.

4. Moisten a paper towel with cooking oil; using long-handled tongs, lightly coat the grill rack. Grill kabobs, covered, over medium heat or broil 4 in. from the heat for 10-15 minutes or until beef reaches desired doneness, turning occasionally and basting with reserved marinade.

PER SERVING *2 kabobs equals 216 cal., 7 g fat (2 g sat. fat), 46 mg chol., 364 mg sodium, 10 g carb., 3 g fiber, 28 g pro.* **Diabetic Exchanges:** *3 lean meat, 2 vegetable.*

143 CALORIES Baked Tilapia

Tilapia brings the health benefits of fish into my diet in a delicious and easy way. Just add a side of vegetables for a nutritious, delicious meal.

—**BRANDI CASTILLO** SANTA MARIA, CA

START TO FINISH: 20 MIN.
MAKES: 4 SERVINGS

- ¾ cup soft bread crumbs
- ⅓ cup grated Parmesan cheese
- 1 teaspoon garlic salt
- 1 teaspoon dried oregano
- 4 tilapia fillets (5 ounces each)

1. Preheat oven to 425°. In a shallow bowl, combine bread crumbs, cheese, garlic salt and oregano. Coat fillets in crumb mixture. Place on a baking sheet coated with cooking spray.

2. Bake 8-12 minutes or until fish flakes easily with a fork.

PER SERVING *1 fillet equals 143 cal., 2 g fat (1 g sat. fat), 72 mg chol., 356 mg sodium, 2 g carb., trace fiber, 28 g pro.* **Diabetic Exchange:** *4 lean meat.*

216 CALORIES
Sesame Beef 'n' Veggie Kabobs

This is a favorite meal with my family. Chalk it up to the fact that it delivers great flavor, tender chunks of meat and a presentation as pretty as a picture!

—**FRANCES KLINGEMANN** OMAHA, NE

PREP: 25 MIN. + MARINATING
GRILL: 10 MIN. • **MAKES:** 8 SERVINGS

- ½ cup reduced-sodium soy sauce
- ¼ cup white wine or unsweetened apple juice
- 3 medium green peppers, cut into 1-inch pieces, divided
- 1 medium onion, cut into wedges
- 1 garlic clove, peeled
- ½ teaspoon ground ginger
- 1 tablespoon sesame seeds
- 2 pounds beef top sirloin steak, cut into 1-inch pieces
- 32 medium fresh mushrooms
- 32 cherry tomatoes
- 1 tablespoon canola oil

1. In a blender, combine the soy sauce, wine, ½ cup green pepper, onion, garlic and ginger; cover and process until smooth. Stir in sesame seeds.

2. Cover and refrigerate ⅓ cup mixture for basting. Pour remaining mixture into a large resealable plastic bag; add the beef. Seal the bag and turn to coat; refrigerate overnight. Refrigerate the remaining peppers.

3. Drain and discard marinade. On 16 metal or soaked wooden skewers,

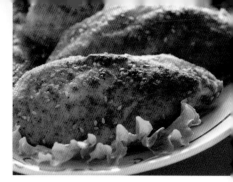

238 CALORIES · Shrimp & Shiitake Stir-Fry with Crispy Noodles

We love the crispy noodles on top of this time-saving Thai dish, but roasted cashews make a wonderful complement as well. It's excellent for parties.

—WOLFGANG HANAU
WEST PALM BEACH, FL

PREP: 20 MIN. • **COOK:** 15 MIN.
MAKES: 4 SERVINGS

- 1½ teaspoons cornstarch
- ½ cup chicken broth
- 2 tablespoons reduced-sodium soy sauce
- 1 small head bok choy
- 1 pound uncooked medium shrimp, peeled and deveined
- 2 tablespoons canola oil, divided
- 2 tablespoons minced fresh gingerroot
- 1 garlic clove, thinly sliced
- ½ teaspoon crushed red pepper flakes
- 1 large onion, halved and thinly sliced
- 2 cups sliced fresh shiitake mushrooms
- ¼ cup chow mein noodles
  Hot cooked brown rice, optional

1. In a small bowl, combine the cornstarch, broth and soy sauce until smooth; set aside. Cut off and discard root end of bok choy, leaving stalks with leaves. Cut leaves from stalks. Slice leaves; set aside. Slice stalks.

2. In a large skillet or wok, stir-fry shrimp in 1 tablespoon oil until shrimp turn pink. Remove and keep warm.

3. Stir-fry the ginger, garlic and pepper flakes in remaining oil for 1 minute. Add the onion, mushrooms and bok choy stalks; stir-fry for 4 minutes. Add bok choy leaves; stir-fry for 2-4 minutes more or until vegetables are crisp-tender.

4. Stir the cornstarch mixture and add to the pan. Bring to a boil; cook and stir for 2 minutes or until thickened. Stir in shrimp and heat through. Sprinkle with chow mein noodles. Serve with rice if desired.

PER SERVING *1 cup stir-fry with 1 tablespoon noodles (calculated without rice) equals 238 cal., 10 g fat (1 g sat. fat), 139 mg chol., 710 mg sodium, 15 g carb., 3 g fiber, 24 g pro.* **Diabetic Exchanges:** *3 lean meat, 2 vegetable, 1 fat.*

214 CALORIES · Pecan-Crusted Chicken

These moist, tender chicken breasts have a crunchy coating of pecans and sesame seeds. They're wonderful served alone or with chicken gravy.

—MOLLY LLOYD BOURNEVILLE, OH

PREP: 25 MIN. • **BAKE:** 15 MIN.
MAKES: 8 SERVINGS

- ¼ cup milk
- ½ cup all-purpose flour
- ½ cup finely chopped pecans
- 2 tablespoons sesame seeds
- 1½ teaspoons paprika
- 1½ teaspoons pepper
- 1 teaspoon salt
- 8 boneless skinless chicken breast halves (4 ounces each), partially flattened
- 2 tablespoons canola oil

1. Place milk in a shallow bowl. In another shallow bowl, combine flour, pecans, sesame seeds, paprika, pepper and salt. Dip chicken in milk, then coat in flour mixture.

2. In a large nonstick skillet, brown chicken in oil on both sides. Transfer to a 15-in. x 10-in. x 1-in. baking pan coated with cooking spray. Bake, uncovered, at 350° for 15-20 minutes or until no longer pink.

PER SERVING *1 chicken breast half equals 214 cal., 10 g fat (2 g sat. fat), 63 mg chol., 252 mg sodium, 5 g carb., 1 g fiber, 24 g pro.* **Diabetic Exchanges:** *3 lean meat, 1½ fat.*

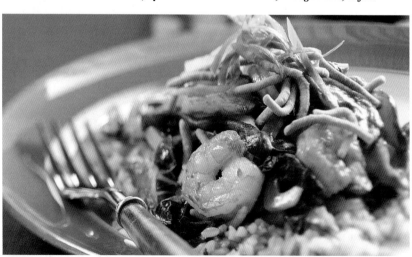

Basil Tuna Steaks

One of my favorite creations is this five-ingredient recipe. I think tuna is delicious, and it can be grilled in no time.
—LINDA MCLYMAN SYRACUSE, NY

START TO FINISH: 20 MIN.
MAKES: 6 SERVINGS

- 6 **tuna steaks (6 ounces each)**
- 4½ **teaspoons olive oil**
- 3 **tablespoons minced fresh basil**
- ¾ **teaspoon salt**
- ¼ **teaspoon pepper**

1. Drizzle both sides of tuna steaks with oil. Sprinkle with the basil, salt and pepper.
2. Moisten a paper towel with cooking oil; using long-handled tongs, lightly coat the grill rack. Grill tuna, covered, over medium heat or broil 4 in. from the heat for 4-5 minutes on each side for medium-rare or until tuna is slightly pink in the center.
PER SERVING *1 tuna steak equals 214 cal., 5 g fat (1 g sat. fat), 77 mg chol., 358 mg sodium, trace carb., trace fiber, 40 g pro.* **Diabetic Exchanges:** *5 lean meat, 1 fat.*

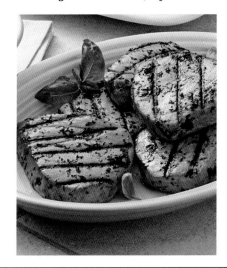

Consider these typical **dinner foods** and their calorie counts to help you stay within a **500-calorie meal**.

- 4 oz. ground sirloin beef patty, **175 CALORIES**

- 4 oz. beef tenderloin, **200 CALORIES**

- 2 skinless chicken drumsticks, **154 CALORIES**

- 4 oz. boneless, skinless chicken breast, **130 CALORIES**

- 4 oz. boneless, skinless turkey breast, **118 CALORIES**

- 4 oz. ground turkey (93% lean), **169 CALORIES**

- 4 oz. turkey Italian sausage, **175 CALORIES**

- 4 oz. boneless pork loin chop, **154 CALORIES**

- 4 oz. pork tenderloin, **136 CALORIES**

- 4 oz. ham, **145 CALORIES**

- 4 oz. fresh salmon, **184 CALORIES**

- 4 oz. tilapia, **134 CALORIES**

- 4 oz. cod, **80 CALORIES**

- 4 oz. halibut, **125 CALORIES**

- 4 oz. fresh tuna, **124 CALORIES**

- 4 oz. orange roughy, **87 CALORIES**

- 4 oz. scallops, **111 CALORIES**

- 4 oz. shell-on shrimp, **90 CALORIES**

- 4 oz. imitation crab, **108 CALORIES**

- 4 oz. portobello mushroom cap, **25 CALORIES**

- 1 Morningstar Farms® Garden Veggie Patties™ veggie burger, **110 CALORIES**

- ½ cup cooked black beans, **114 CALORIES**

- ½ cup cooked pinto beans, **103 CALORIES**

- ½ cup spaghetti/marinara sauce, **111 CALORIES**

- 1 cup cooked whole wheat spaghetti, **176 CALORIES**

- ½ cup cooked brown rice, **108 CALORIES**

Weights listed are before cooking. Also see the Side Dishes Calorie List on page 367 and check the Nutrition Facts labels on packaged foods.

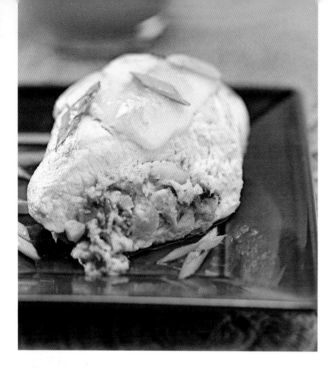

2. Chop one cheese slice; stir into crab mixture. Spread over chicken; roll up and secure with toothpicks.

3. In a large nonstick skillet coated with cooking spray, brown chicken on all sides. Place seam side down in a shallow 3-qt. baking dish coated with cooking spray. Brush with remaining marinade for chicken.

4. Bake, uncovered, at 350° for 25 minutes. Cut each remaining cheese slice into six strips; place two cheese strips over each chicken breast. Bake 5-10 minutes longer or until a thermometer reads 170°. Discard toothpicks. Sprinkle remaining onions over chicken.

NOTE *This recipe was tested with Lea & Perrins Marinade for Chicken.*

PER SERVING *1 stuffed chicken breast half equals 225 cal., 7 g fat (2 g sat. fat), 95 mg chol., 469 mg sodium, 5 g carb., trace fiber, 35 g pro.* **Diabetic Exchange:** *5 lean meat.*

227 CALORIES Sizzling Beef Kabobs

A mild soy sauce marinade lends an appealing flavor to these tender beef and veggie kabobs. With colorful chunks of yellow squash and sweet red and green peppers, they're perfect for parties.

—KATHY SPANG MANHEIM, PA

PREP: 20 MIN. + MARINATING • **GRILL:** 10 MIN.
MAKES: 8 SERVINGS

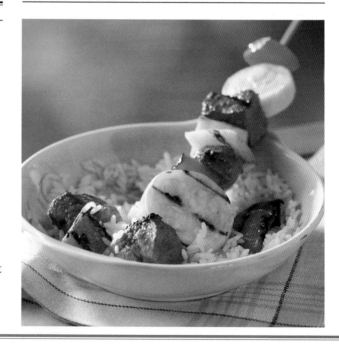

225 CALORIES

Elegant Crab-Stuffed Chicken Breasts

Here's a delicious chicken dish that's special enough for dinner guests. Imitation crabmeat works just as well as regular crab. Even my husband, who isn't especially fond of seafood, likes it!

—MARY PLUMMER DE SOTO, KS

PREP: 45 MIN. • **BAKE:** 30 MIN. • **MAKES:** 6 SERVINGS

- 6 **boneless skinless chicken breast halves (5 ounces each)**
- ½ **teaspoon salt**
- ¼ **teaspoon pepper**
- ½ **cup canned crabmeat, drained, flaked and cartilage removed**
- ¼ **cup sliced water chestnuts, drained and chopped**
- 2 **tablespoons dry bread crumbs**
- 2 **tablespoons reduced-fat mayonnaise**
- 1 **tablespoon minced fresh parsley**
- 1 **teaspoon Dijon mustard**
- 6 **teaspoons marinade for chicken, divided**
- 2 **green onions, thinly sliced, divided**
- 3 **slices reduced-fat Swiss cheese, divided**

1. Flatten chicken to ¼-in. thickness; sprinkle with salt and pepper. Combine the crab, water chestnuts, bread crumbs, mayonnaise, parsley, mustard, 2 teaspoons marinade for chicken and half of the onions.

- ⅓ cup canola oil
- ¼ cup soy sauce
- 2 tablespoons red wine vinegar
- 2 teaspoons garlic powder
- 2 pounds beef top sirloin steak, cut into 1-inch pieces
- 2 medium yellow summer squash, cut into ½-inch slices
- 1 large onion, cut into 1-inch chunks
- 1 large green pepper, cut into 1-inch pieces
- 1 large sweet red pepper, cut into 1-inch pieces

1. In a large resealable plastic bag, combine the oil, soy sauce, vinegar and garlic powder; add beef. Seal bag and turn to coat; refrigerate for at least 1 hour.

2. Drain and discard marinade. On eight metal or soaked wooden skewers, alternately thread beef and vegetables. Grill, covered, over medium-hot heat or broil 4-6 in. from the heat for 8-10 minutes or until meat reaches desired doneness, turning occasionally.

PER SERVING *1 kabob equals 227 cal., 12 g fat 3 g sat. fat), 63 mg chol., 326 mg sodium, 6 g carb., 2 g fiber, 23 g pro.* **Diabetic Exchanges:** *3 lean meat, 1 vegetable, 1 fat.*

216 CALORIES

Spinach-Tomato Phyllo Bake

My flaky phyllo pie is a lightened-up version of that beloved Greek classic, spanakopita. No one will miss the meat when this tasty vegetarian recipe is on the table.

—SHIRLEY KACMARIK GLASGOW, SCOTLAND

PREP: 25 MIN. • **BAKE:** 55 MIN. + STANDING • **MAKES:** 6 SERVINGS

- 4 eggs, lightly beaten
- 2 packages (10 ounces each) frozen chopped spinach, thawed and squeezed dry
- 1 cup (4 ounces) crumbled feta cheese
- ½ cup 1% cottage cheese
- 3 green onions, sliced
- 1 teaspoon dill weed
- ½ teaspoon salt
- ¼ teaspoon pepper
- ¼ teaspoon ground nutmeg
- 10 sheets phyllo dough (14 inches x 9 inches) Butter-flavored cooking spray
- 3 large tomatoes, sliced

1. Preheat oven to 350°. In a large bowl, combine first nine ingredients; set aside.

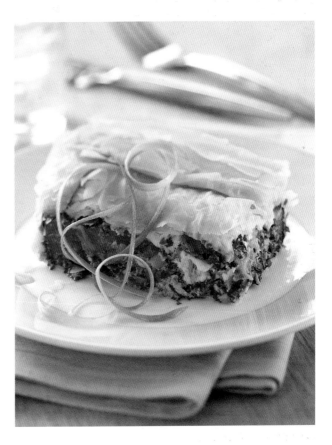

2. Spritz one sheet of phyllo dough with butter-flavored cooking spray. Place in an 8-in. square baking dish coated with cooking spray, allowing one end of dough to hang over edge of dish. Repeat with four more phyllo sheets, staggering the overhanging phyllo around edges of dish. (Keep remaining phyllo covered with plastic wrap and a damp towel to prevent it from drying out.)

3. Spoon a third of the spinach mixture into crust. Layer with half of the tomatoes, another third of the spinach mixture, remaining tomatoes and remaining spinach mixture. Spritz and layer remaining phyllo dough as before.

4. Gently fold ends of dough over filling and toward center of baking dish; spritz with butter-flavored spray. Cover edges with foil. Bake 55-60 minutes or until a thermometer reads 160°. Let stand for 15 minutes before cutting.

PER SERVING *1 piece equals 216 cal., 9 g fat (3 g sat. fat), 153 mg chol., 652 mg sodium, 21 g carb., 5 g fiber, 15 g pro.* **Diabetic Exchanges:** *2 medium-fat meat, 2 vegetable, 1 starch.*

214 CALORIES Stuffed Steak Spirals

When I want an extra-special entree for guests, I rely on this appealing recipe. Tender and swirled with tomato stuffing, it's a sensational way to serve flank steak.
—MARGARET PACHE MESA, AZ

PREP: 35 MIN. • **BAKE:** 30 MIN. + STANDING • **MAKES:** 6 SERVINGS

- ¼ cup chopped sun-dried tomatoes (not packed in oil)
- ½ cup boiling water
- ½ cup grated Parmesan cheese
- ¼ cup minced fresh parsley
- 1 tablespoon prepared horseradish, drained
- 1 to 1½ teaspoons coarsely ground pepper
- 1 beef flank steak (1½ pounds)
- 2 teaspoons canola oil

1. Place tomatoes in a small bowl; add water. Cover and let stand for 5 minutes; drain. Stir in the cheese, parsley, horseradish and pepper; set aside.
2. Cut steak horizontally from a long side to within ½ in. of opposite side. Open meat so it lies flat; cover with plastic wrap. Flatten to ¼-in. thickness. Remove plastic; spoon tomato mixture over meat to within ½ in. of edges. Roll up tightly jelly-roll style, starting with a long side. Tie with kitchen string.
3. Line a shallow roasting pan with heavy-duty foil; coat the foil with cooking spray. In a large nonstick skillet coated with cooking spray, brown meat in oil on all sides. Place in prepared pan.

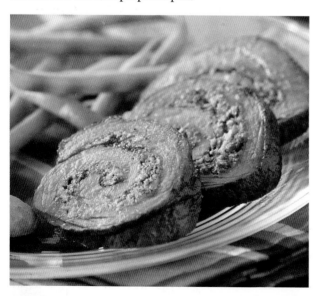

4. Bake, uncovered, at 400° for 30-40 minutes or until meat reaches desired doneness (for medium-rare, a thermometer should read 145°; medium, 160°; well-done, 170°). Let stand for 10-15 minutes. Remove string and cut into slices.
PER SERVING *1 serving equals 214 cal., 12 g fat (5 g sat. fat), 53 mg chol., 229 mg sodium, 2 g carb., 1 g fiber, 22 g pro.* **Diabetic Exchanges:** *3 lean meat, 1 fat.*

242 CALORIES
Beef Tenderloin with Balsamic Sauce

Roasted beef tenderloin is quick and easy to fix—but a rich port wine sauce makes this recipe elegant enough for the holidays.
—TASTE OF HOME TEST KITCHEN

PREP: 10 MIN. + CHILLING • **BAKE:** 50 MIN. + STANDING
MAKES: 8 SERVINGS

- 2 tablespoons minced fresh rosemary or 2 teaspoons dried rosemary, crushed
- 2 tablespoons minced garlic
- 1½ teaspoons salt
- 1 teaspoon coarsely ground pepper
- 1 beef tenderloin roast (2 pounds)

SAUCE

- 2 cups port wine or 1 cup grape juice and 1 cup reduced-sodium beef broth
- 2 tablespoons balsamic vinegar
- 1 teaspoon butter
- ¼ teaspoon salt
- ⅛ teaspoon pepper

1. Combine the rosemary, garlic, salt and pepper; rub evenly over tenderloin. Cover and refrigerate for 2 hours. Place meat on a rack in shallow roasting pan. Bake, uncovered, at 400° for 50-70 minutes or until meat reaches desired doneness (for medium-rare, a thermometer should read 145°; medium, 160°; well-done, 170°). Let stand for 10 minutes before slicing.
2. In a saucepan, bring wine to a boil; cook until reduced to ¾ cup. Add vinegar; cook for 3-4 minutes or until reduced to a sauce consistency. Stir in butter, salt and pepper. Serve with tenderloin.
PER SERVING *3 ounces cooked beef with 3½ teaspoons sauce equals 242 cal., 9 g fat (3 g sat. fat), 72 mg chol., 576 mg sodium, 6 g carb., 0 fiber, 24 g pro.* **Diabetic Exchanges:** *3 lean meat, 1 fat.*

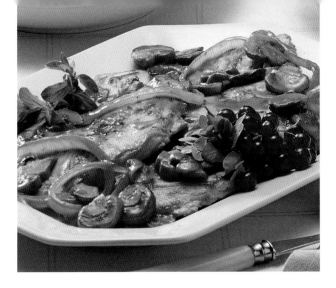

Chicken with Mushroom Sauce

212 CALORIES

It looks impressive, but this mouthwatering dish comes together in no time. I think its flavor rivals that of many full-fat entrees found in fancy restaurants.

—**JENNIFER PEMBERTON** MUNCIE, IN

START TO FINISH: 25 MIN. • **MAKES:** 4 SERVINGS

- 2 **teaspoons cornstarch**
- ½ **cup fat-free milk**
- 4 **boneless skinless chicken breast halves (4 ounces each)**
- 1 **tablespoon olive oil**
- ½ **pound fresh mushrooms, sliced**
- ½ **medium onion, sliced and separated into rings**
- 1 **tablespoon reduced-fat butter**
- ¼ **cup sherry or chicken broth**
- ½ **teaspoon salt**
- ⅛ **teaspoon pepper**

1. In a small bowl, combine cornstarch and milk until smooth; set aside. Flatten chicken to ¼-in. thickness. In a large nonstick skillet, cook chicken in oil over medium heat for 5-6 minutes on each side or until juices run clear. Remove and keep warm.

2. In the same skillet, saute mushrooms and onion in butter until tender. Stir in the sherry, salt and pepper; bring to a boil. Stir cornstarch mixture, add to the pan. Bring to a boil; cook and stir for 2 minutes or until thickened. Serve with chicken.

NOTE *This recipe was tested with Land O'Lakes light stick butter.*

PER SERVING *1 chicken breast half with ⅓ cup sauce equals 212 cal., 8 g fat (2 g sat. fat), 68 mg chol., 387 mg sodium, 7 g carb., 1 g fiber, 26 g pro.* **Diabetic Exchanges:** *3 lean meat, 1 vegetable, 1 fat, ½ starch.*

200 CALORIES Glazed Pork Medallions

When my husband was told to lower his cholesterol, he was worried that would mean foods with less flavor on the menu. This lean entree proves that fish isn't the only option when it comes to keeping fat in check.

—**MICHELE FLAGEL** SHELLSBURG, IA

START TO FINISH: 30 MIN. • **MAKES:** 4 SERVINGS

- 1 **pork tenderloin (1¼ pounds)**
- ¼ **teaspoon salt**
- ⅓ **cup reduced-sugar orange marmalade**
- 2 **teaspoons cider vinegar**
- 2 **teaspoons Worcestershire sauce**
- ½ **teaspoon minced fresh gingerroot**
- ⅛ **teaspoon crushed red pepper flakes**

Cut pork into 1-in. slices and flatten to ¼-in. thickness; sprinkle with salt. Cook pork in batches over medium-high heat in a large nonstick skillet coated with cooking spray until tender. Reduce heat to low; return all meat to the pan. Combine the remaining ingredients; pour over pork and turn to coat. Heat through.

PER SERVING *4 ounces cooked pork equals 200 cal., 5 g fat (2 g sat. fat), 79 mg chol., 231 mg sodium, 9 g carb., trace fiber, 28 g pro.* **Diabetic Exchanges:** *4 lean meat, ½ fruit, ½ fat.*

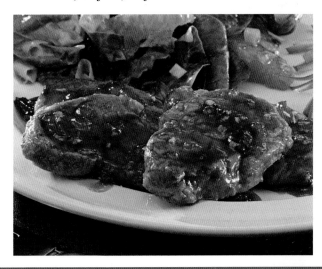

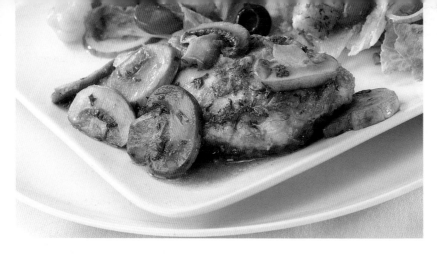

Tuscan Pork Roast

A handful of ingredients are all you need for this memorable entree. I've had so many compliments on how moist and tender this pork is.

—DIANE TOOMEY METHUEN, MA

PREP: 10 MIN. + CHILLING
BAKE: 1 HOUR + STANDING
MAKES: 10 SERVINGS

- 3 garlic cloves, minced
- 2 tablespoons olive oil
- 1 tablespoon fennel seed, crushed
- 1 tablespoon dried rosemary, crushed
- 1 teaspoon salt
- ¼ teaspoon pepper
- 1 boneless pork loin roast (3 pounds)

1. In a small bowl, combine first six ingredients; rub over pork roast. Cover and refrigerate overnight.
2. Place roast on a rack in a shallow roasting pan. Bake, uncovered, at 350° for 1 hour or until a thermometer reads 145°, basting occasionally with pan juices. Let meat stand for 10-15 minutes before slicing.
PER SERVING *4 ounces cooked pork equals 229 cal., 10 g fat (3 g sat. fat), 80 mg chol., 282 mg sodium, 1 g carb., 1 g fiber, 31 g pro.*

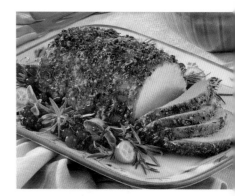

Chicken Marsala

Chicken Marsala is usually high in fat and calories. But this version gets so much flavor from deglazing the skillet with broth and wine. Even though I cut back on fat, the taste is fabulous!

—NANCY GRANAMAN
BURLINGTON, IA

PREP: 25 MIN. + MARINATING
BAKE: 25 MIN. • **MAKES:** 6 SERVINGS

- 6 boneless skinless chicken breast halves (4 ounces each)
- 1 cup fat-free Italian salad dressing
- 1 tablespoon all-purpose flour
- 1 teaspoon Italian seasoning
- ½ teaspoon garlic powder
- ¼ teaspoon paprika
- ¼ teaspoon pepper
- 2 tablespoons olive oil, divided
- 1 tablespoon butter
- ½ cup reduced-sodium chicken broth
- ½ cup Marsala wine or 3 tablespoons unsweetened apple juice plus 5 tablespoons additional reduced-sodium chicken broth
- 1 pound sliced fresh mushrooms
- ½ cup minced fresh parsley

1. Flatten chicken to ½-in. thickness. Place in a large resealable plastic bag; add salad dressing. Seal bag and turn to coat; refrigerate for 8 hours or overnight.
2. Drain and discard marinade. Combine the flour, Italian seasoning, garlic powder, paprika and pepper; sprinkle over both sides of chicken. In a large nonstick skillet coated with cooking spray, cook chicken in 1 tablespoon oil and butter for 2 minutes on each side or until browned. Transfer to a 13-in. x 9-in. baking dish coated with cooking spray.
3. Gradually add broth and wine to skillet, stirring to loosen browned bits. Bring to a boil; cook and stir for 2 minutes. Strain sauce; set aside. In the same skillet, cook mushrooms in remaining oil for 2 minutes; drain. Stir sauce into mushrooms; heat through. Pour over chicken; sprinkle with parsley. Bake, uncovered, at 350° for 25-30 minutes or until chicken juices run clear.
PER SERVING *1 chicken breast half with ⅓ cup mushroom mixture equals 247 cal., 9 g fat (3 g sat. fat), 68 mg chol., 348 mg sodium, 9 g carb., 1 g fiber, 26 g pro.*
Diabetic Exchanges: *3 lean meat, 1½ fat, ½ starch.*

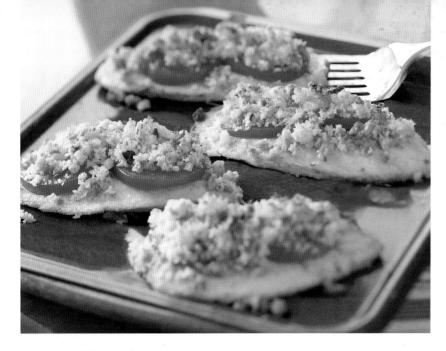

Tomato Walnut Tilapia

205 CALORIES

Fresh tomato, bread crumbs and crunchy walnuts dress up tilapia fillets in this delightful main dish. I often serve it with cooked green beans and julienned carrots.

—PHYL BROICH-WESSLING GARNER, IA

START TO FINISH: 20 MIN.
MAKES: 4 SERVINGS

- 4 tilapia fillets (4 ounces each)
- ¼ teaspoon salt
- ¼ teaspoon pepper
- 1 tablespoon butter
- 1 medium tomato, thinly sliced

TOPPING

- ½ cup soft bread crumbs
- ¼ cup chopped walnuts
- 2 tablespoons lemon juice
- 1½ teaspoons butter, melted

1. Sprinkle fillets with salt and pepper. In a large skillet coated with cooking spray, cook fillets in butter over medium-high heat for 2-3 minutes on each side or until lightly browned.

2. Transfer fish to a broiler pan or baking sheet; top with tomato. Combine the topping ingredients; spoon over the tops.

3. Broil 3-4 in. from the heat for 2-3 minutes or until topping is lightly browned and fish flakes easily with a fork.

PER SERVING *1 fillet equals 205 cal., 10 g fat (3 g sat. fat), 67 mg chol., 265 mg sodium, 7 g carb., 1 g fiber, 24 g pro.* **Diabetic Exchanges:** *3 lean meat, 2 fat, ½ starch.*

Beef 'n' Turkey Meat Loaf

240 CALORIES

Shredded potato makes a delicous, low-calorie meat loaf even more satisfying. This one is perfectly seasoned with garlic and thyme.

—FERN NEAD FLORENCE, KY

PREP: 15 MIN. • **BAKE:** 50 MIN. + STANDING
MAKES: 6 SERVINGS

- 2 egg whites, beaten
- ⅔ cup ketchup, divided
- 1 medium potato, peeled and finely shredded
- 1 medium green pepper, finely chopped
- 1 small onion, grated
- 3 garlic cloves, minced
- 1 teaspoon salt
- 1 teaspoon dried thyme
- ½ teaspoon pepper
- ¾ pound lean ground beef (90% lean)
- ¾ pound lean ground turkey

1. In a large bowl, combine egg whites and ⅓ cup ketchup. Stir in the potato, green pepper, onion, garlic, salt, thyme and pepper. Crumble beef and turkey over mixture and mix well. Shape into a 10-in. x 4-in. loaf.

2. Line a 15-in. x 10-in. x 1-in. baking pan with heavy-duty foil and coat the foil with cooking spray. Place loaf in pan. Bake, uncovered, at 375° for 45 minutes; drain. Brush with remaining ketchup. Bake 5-10 minutes longer or until no pink remains and a thermometer reads 165°. Let stand 10 minutes before slicing.

PER SERVING *1 slice equals 240 cal., 9 g fat (3 g sat. fat), 79 mg chol., 808 mg sodium, 16 g carb., 2 g fiber, 23 g pro.*

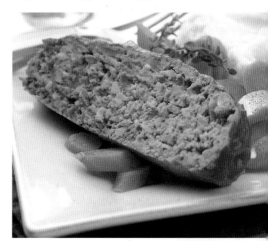

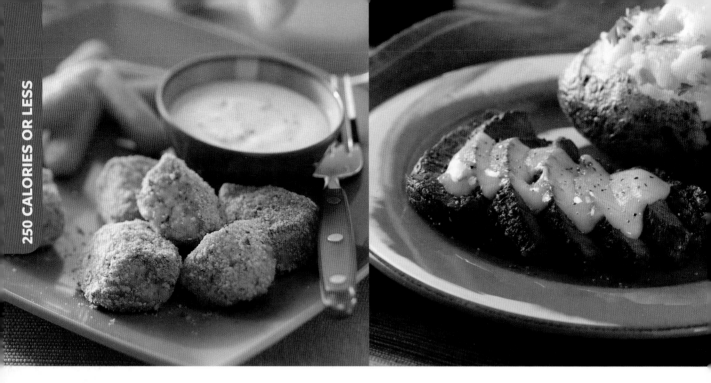

194 CALORIES

Tender Chicken Nuggets

Four ingredients are all it takes to create these moist golden bites that are healthier than the fast-food variety. I serve them with ranch dressing and barbecue sauce for dipping.

—LYNNE HAHN WINCHESTER, CA

START TO FINISH: 25 MIN.
MAKES: 4 SERVINGS

- ½ cup seasoned bread crumbs
- 2 tablespoons grated Parmesan cheese
- 1 egg white
- 1 pound boneless skinless chicken breasts, cut into 1-inch cubes

1. In a large resealable plastic bag, combine bread crumbs and cheese. In a shallow bowl, beat egg white. Dip chicken pieces in egg white, then place in bag and shake to coat.
2. Place in a 15-in. x 10-in. x 1-in. baking pan coated with cooking spray. Bake, uncovered, at 400° for 12-15 minutes or until no longer pink, turning once.

PER SERVING *3 ounces cooked chicken equals 194 cal., 3 g fat (1 g sat. fat), 68 mg chol., 250 mg sodium, 10 g carb., trace fiber, 30 g pro.* **Diabetic Exchanges:** *3 lean meat, ½ starch.*

188 CALORIES

Balsamic-Seasoned Steak

A two-ingredient sauce makes this sirloin so delicious! You'll love its simple preparation—and the scrumptious Swiss cheese topping.

—TASTE OF HOME TEST KITCHEN

START TO FINISH: 25 MIN.
MAKES: 4 SERVINGS

- 2 tablespoons balsamic vinegar
- 2 teaspoons steak sauce
- 1 beef top sirloin steak (1 pound)
- ¼ teaspoon coarsely ground pepper
- 2 ounces reduced-fat Swiss cheese, cut into thin strips

1. In a small bowl, combine vinegar and steak sauce; set aside. Rub steak with pepper. Place on a broiler pan. Broil 4 in. from heat for 7 minutes.
2. Turn; spoon half of the steak sauce mixture over steak. Broil 5-7 minutes longer or until meat reaches desired doneness (for medium-rare, a thermometer should read 145°; medium, 160°; well-done, 170°).
3. Remove steak to a cutting board; cut across the grain into ¼-in. slices. Place on a foil-lined baking sheet; drizzle with juices from cutting board and remaining steak sauce mixture. Top with cheese. Broil for 1 minute or until cheese is melted.

PER SERVING *3 ounces cooked beef with ½ ounce cheese equals 188 cal., 8 g fat (3 g sat. fat), 70 mg chol., 116 mg sodium, 2 g carb., trace fiber, 26 g pro.*

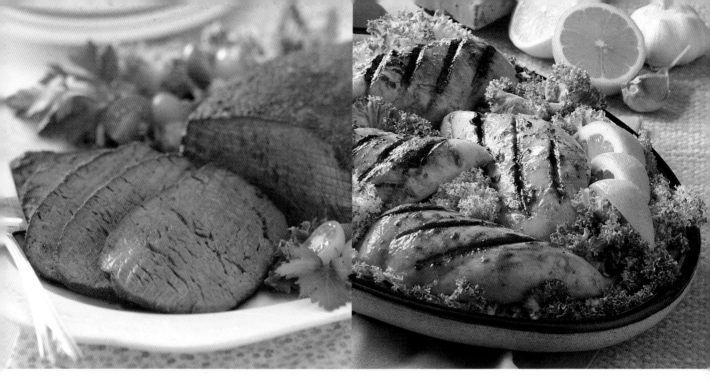

Chipotle-Rubbed Beef Tenderloin

Go ahead, rub it in! Coating beef tenderloin with lively, peppery flavors gives it a south-of-the-border twist. Your dinner guests will be impressed.
—TASTE OF HOME TEST KITCHEN

PREP: 10 MIN. + CHILLING
BAKE: 45 MIN. + STANDING
MAKES: 8 SERVINGS

- 1 **beef tenderloin roast (2 pounds)**
- 2 **teaspoons canola oil**
- 3 **teaspoons coarsely ground pepper**
- 3 **garlic cloves, minced**
- 2½ **teaspoons brown sugar**
- 1 **teaspoon salt**
- 1 **teaspoon ground coriander**
- ½ **teaspoon ground chipotle pepper**
- ¼ **teaspoon cayenne pepper**

1. Brush beef with oil. Combine the remaining ingredients; rub over meat. Cover and refrigerate for 2 hours.

2. Place on a rack coated with cooking spray in a shallow roasting pan. Bake, uncovered, at 400° for 45-55 minutes or until meat reaches desired doneness (for medium-rare, a thermometer should read 145°; medium, 160°; well-done, 170°). Let stand for 10 minutes before slicing.

PER SERVING *3 ounces cooked beef equals 195 cal., 9 g fat (3 g sat. fat), 71 mg chol., 351 mg sodium, 2 g carb., trace fiber, 24 g pro.* **Diabetic Exchange:** *3 lean meat.*

Mustard-Herb Chicken Breasts

Dijon mayonnaise makes my grilled chicken moist and flavorful. Even though I learned to cook when I was young, I didn't really enjoy it until lately. My husband appreciates my new interest in finding and trying new recipes!
—TERRI WEME SMITHERS, BC

PREP: 10 MIN. + MARINATING
GRILL: 15 MIN. • **MAKES:** 4 SERVINGS

- ¼ **cup chopped green onions**
- ¼ **cup Dijon-mayonnaise blend**
- 2 **tablespoons lemon juice**
- 1 **garlic clove, minced**
- ½ **teaspoon salt**
- ½ **teaspoon dried thyme**
- ¼ **teaspoon pepper**
- 4 **boneless skinless chicken breast halves (4 ounces each)**

1. In a large resealable plastic bag, combine the first seven ingredients; add chicken. Seal bag and turn to coat. Refrigerate for 2 hours, turning once.

2. Grill chicken, covered, over medium heat for 6-8 minutes on each side or until a thermometer reads 170°.

PER SERVING *1 chicken breast half equals 163 cal., 3 g fat (1 g sat. fat), 73 mg chol., 720 mg sodium, 2 g carb., trace fiber, 27 g pro.* **Diabetic Exchanges:** *3 lean meat, ½ fat.*

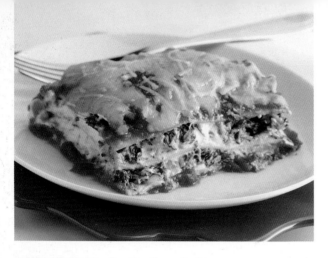

227 CALORIES Tofu Spinach Lasagna

With a similar texture to cheese, tofu is a simple way to add protein to meatless lasagna. Most people don't even realize it's buried between the saucy, cheesy layers.
—**CHRISTINE LABA** ARLINGTON, VA

PREP: 45 MIN. • **BAKE:** 30 MIN. + STANDING
MAKES: 12 SERVINGS

- 9 lasagna noodles
- 1 medium onion, chopped
- 3 garlic cloves, minced
- 1 tablespoon olive oil
- 2 cups sliced fresh mushrooms
- 1 package (14 ounces) firm tofu
- 1 carton (15 ounces) part-skim ricotta cheese
- ½ cup minced fresh parsley
- 1 teaspoon salt, divided
- 2 packages (10 ounces each) frozen chopped spinach, thawed and squeezed dry
- 1¾ cups marinara or meatless spaghetti sauce
- 1 cup (4 ounces) shredded part-skim mozzarella cheese
- ⅓ cup shredded Parmesan cheese

1. Cook noodles according to package directions. Meanwhile, in a large nonstick skillet, saute onion and garlic in oil for 1 minute. Add mushrooms; saute until tender. Set aside.
2. Drain tofu, reserving 2 tablespoons liquid. Place tofu and reserved liquid in a food processor; cover and process until blended. Add ricotta cheese; cover and process for 1-2 minutes or until smooth. Transfer to a large bowl; stir in the parsley, ½ teaspoon salt and mushroom mixture. Combine spinach and remaining salt; set aside.
3. Drain noodles. Spread half of the marinara sauce into a 13-in. x 9-in. baking dish coated with cooking spray. Layer with three noodles, half of the tofu mixture and half of the spinach mixture. Repeat layers of noodles, tofu and spinach. Top with remaining noodles and marinara sauce. Sprinkle with cheeses.
4. Bake, uncovered, at 350° for 30-35 minutes or until heated through and cheese is melted. Let stand for 10 minutes before cutting.
PER SERVING *1 piece equals 227 cal., 8 g fat (4 g sat. fat), 18 mg chol., 429 mg sodium, 25 g carb., 3 g fiber, 15 g pro.* **Diabetic Exchanges:** *1½ starch, 1 lean meat, 1 vegetable, ½ fat.*

240 CALORIES

Orange-Maple Glazed Chicken

Use a fresh orange for the zest and juice in this tasty recipe that combines citrus with maple syrup and balsamic vinegar.
—**LILY JULOW** GAINESVILLE, FL

PREP: 25 MIN. • **GRILL:** 10 MIN. • **MAKES:** 6 SERVINGS

- ⅓ cup orange juice
- ⅓ cup maple syrup
- 2 tablespoons balsamic vinegar
- 1½ teaspoons Dijon mustard
- 1 teaspoon salt, divided
- ¾ teaspoon pepper, divided
- 1 tablespoon minced fresh basil or 1 teaspoon dried basil
- ½ teaspoon grated orange peel
- 6 boneless skinless chicken breast halves (6 ounces each)

1. In a small saucepan, combine the orange juice, syrup, vinegar, mustard, ½ teaspoon salt and ¼ teaspoon pepper. Bring to a boil; cook until liquid is reduced to ½ cup, about 5 minutes. Stir in basil and orange peel. Remove from the heat; set aside.
2. Sprinkle chicken with remaining salt and pepper. Grill chicken, covered, over medium heat for 5-7 minutes on each side or until a thermometer reads 170°, basting frequently with orange juice mixture.
PER SERVING *1 chicken breast half equals 240 cal., 4 g fat (1 g sat. fat), 94 mg chol., 508 mg sodium, 15 g carb., trace fiber, 34 g pro.* **Diabetic Exchanges:** *5 lean meat, 1 starch.*

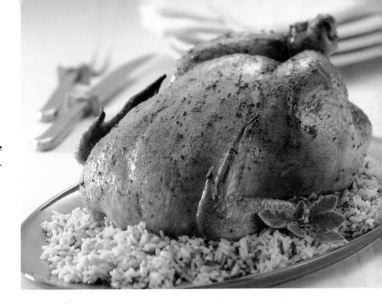

Sweet and Sour Turkey Meat Loaf

I've made this meat loaf many times, and everyone raves about it. One bite, and I promise you will, too!

—DOROTHY HAVNER SAN RAFAEL, CA

PREP: 15 MIN. • **BAKE:** 45 MIN. + STANDING • **MAKES:** 2 SERVINGS

- ¼ **cup tomato sauce**
- 1 **tablespoon brown sugar**
- 1 **tablespoon cider vinegar**
- ¼ **teaspoon prepared mustard**
- 1 **tablespoon beaten egg or egg substitute**
- 2 **tablespoons finely chopped onion**
- 1 **tablespoon crushed butter-flavored crackers**
- 1 **tablespoon minced fresh parsley**
- ¼ **teaspoon salt**
  Dash pepper
- ½ **pound lean ground turkey**

1. In a small bowl, combine the tomato sauce, brown sugar, vinegar and mustard; set aside. In another bowl, combine the egg, onion, crackers, parsley, salt, pepper and 2 tablespoons reserved tomato mixture. Crumble turkey over mixture and mix well. Shape into a 4-in. x 3-in. oval.

2. Place in an 8-in. square baking dish coated with cooking spray; top with remaining tomato mixture. Bake, uncovered, at 350° for 45-50 minutes or until meat is no longer pink and a thermometer reads 165°. Let stand for 10 minutes before slicing.

PER SERVING *½ meat loaf equals 235 cal., 11 g fat (3 g sat. fat), 122 mg chol., 587 mg sodium, 11 g carb., 1 g fiber, 22 g pro.* **Diabetic Exchanges:** *3 lean meat, 1 starch.*

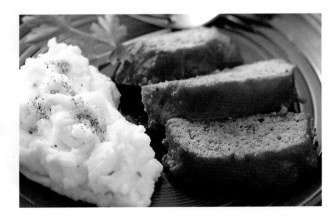

Honey-Lime Roasted Chicken

It's hard to believe this finger-licking main course starts with only five ingredients. The chicken is easy, light and so good! It's just as tasty prepared outside on the grill.

—LORI CARBONELL SPRINGFIELD, VERMONT

PREP: 10 MIN. • **BAKE:** 2½ HOURS + STANDING
MAKES: 10 SERVINGS

- 1 **whole roasting chicken (5 to 6 pounds)**
- ½ **cup lime juice**
- ¼ **cup honey**
- 1 **tablespoon stone-ground mustard or spicy brown mustard**
- 1 **teaspoon ground cumin**

1. Carefully loosen skin from the entire chicken. Place breast side up on a rack in a roasting pan. In a small bowl, whisk the lime juice, honey, mustard and cumin.

2. Using a turkey baster, baste under the chicken skin with ⅓ cup lime juice mixture. Tie drumsticks together. Pour remaining lime juice mixture over chicken.

3. Bake, uncovered, at 350° for 2½ to 3 hours or until a thermometer reads 180°, basting every 30 minutes with drippings (cover loosely with foil after 1 to 1½ hours or when golden brown). Let stand for 10 minutes before carving.

PER SERVING *3 ounces cooked chicken (calculated without skin) equals 197 cal., 7 g fat (2 g sat. fat), 77 mg chol., 95 mg sodium, 8 g carb., trace fiber, 25 g pro.* **Diabetic Exchanges:** *3 lean meat, ½ starch.*

201 CALORIES

Hot 'n' Spicy Flank Steak

With its flavorful marinade, this flank steak makes a succulent meal. I received the recipe from a friend, and it's been a family favorite since I first prepared it.

—JULEE WALLBERG SALT LAKE CITY, UT

PREP: 15 MIN. + MARINATING
GRILL: 15 MIN. • **MAKES:** 6 SERVINGS

- 3 **tablespoons brown sugar**
- 3 **tablespoons red wine vinegar**
- 3 **tablespoons sherry or reduced-sodium chicken broth**
- 3 **tablespoons reduced-sodium soy sauce**
- 1 **tablespoon canola oil**
- 1½ **teaspoons crushed red pepper flakes**
- 1½ **teaspoons paprika**
- 1½ **teaspoons chili powder**
- 1½ **teaspoons Worcestershire sauce**
- ¾ **teaspoon seasoned salt**
- ¾ **teaspoon garlic powder**
- ¾ **teaspoon dried parsley flakes**
- 1 **beef flank steak (1½ pounds)**

1. In a small bowl, combine the first 12 ingredients. Pour ⅓ cup marinade into a large resealable plastic bag; add steak. Seal bag and turn to coat; refrigerate for 1-3 hours. Cover and refrigerate remaining marinade for basting.

2. Moisten a paper towel with cooking oil; using long-handled tongs, lightly coat the grill rack. Grill steak, covered, over medium heat or broil 4 in. from the heat for 6-8 minutes on each side or until meat reaches desired doneness (for medium-rare, a thermometer should read 145°; medium, 160°; well-done, 170°), basting frequently with remaining marinade. Let stand 5 minutes before slicing. Thinly slice steak across the grain.

PER SERVING *3 ounces cooked beef equals 201 cal., 9 g fat (4 g sat. fat), 54 mg chol., 326 mg sodium, 5 g carb., trace fiber, 22 g pro.* **Diabetic Exchange:** *3 lean meat.*

157 CALORIES

Best-Ever Lamb Chops

My mom just loved a good lamb chop, and this easy recipe was her favorite way to enjoy them. I've also grilled the chops with great results.

—KIM MUNDY VISALIA, CA

PREP: 10 MIN. + CHILLING
BROIL: 10 MIN. • **MAKES:** 4 SERVINGS

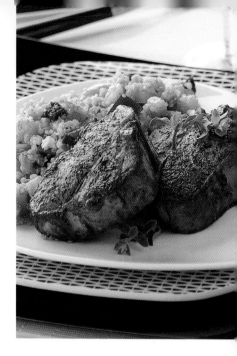

- 1 **teaspoon each dried basil, marjoram and thyme**
- ½ **teaspoon salt**
- 8 **lamb loin chops (3 ounces each)**
  Mint jelly, optional

1. Combine herbs and salt; rub over lamb chops. Cover and refrigerate for 1 hour.

2. Broil 4-6 in. from the heat for 5-8 minutes on each side or until meat reaches desired doneness (for medium-rare, a meat thermometer should read 145°; medium, 160°; well-done, 170°). Serve with mint jelly if desired.

PER SERVING *2 lamb chops (calculated without jelly) equals 157 cal., 7 g fat (2 g sat. fat), 68 mg chol., 355 mg sodium, trace carb., trace fiber, 22 g pro.* **Diabetic Exchange:** *3 lean meat.*

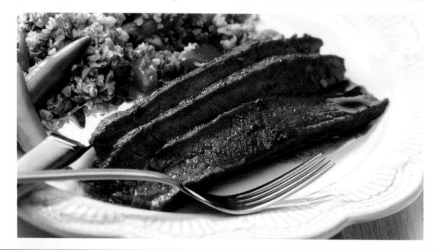

184 CALORIES Green Tea Teriyaki Chicken

Tender chicken in an Asian-inspired sauce flavored with green tea makes a low-fat entree that really stands out. Serve it with jasmine rice for a restaurant-quality meal.

—TASTE OF HOME TEST KITCHEN

START TO FINISH: 25 MIN.
MAKES: 4 SERVINGS

- 3½ teaspoons green tea leaves, divided
- 1 cup boiling water
- 4 green onions, chopped, divided
- 3 tablespoons honey
- 2 tablespoons cider vinegar
- 2 tablespoons reduced-sodium soy sauce
- 4 garlic cloves, minced
- ½ teaspoon minced fresh gingerroot
- ⅛ teaspoon sesame oil
- 4 boneless skinless chicken breast halves (4 ounces each)

1. Place 2½ teaspoons tea leaves in a small bowl; add boiling water. Cover and steep for 5-6 minutes.
2. Strain and discard leaves; pour tea into a large skillet. Add half of the onions. Stir in the honey, vinegar, soy sauce, garlic, ginger and sesame oil. Bring to a boil. Reduce heat; simmer, uncovered, until sauce is reduced to about ¾ cup.
3. Add chicken and remaining tea leaves; cover and cook over medium heat for 4-5 minutes on each side or until a thermometer reads 170°. Cut chicken into thin slices; serve with sauce. Garnish with the remaining onions.

PER SERVING *1 chicken breast half with 3 tablespoons sauce equals 184 cal., 3 g fat (1 g sat. fat), 63 mg chol., 359 mg sodium, 16 g carb., trace fiber, 24 g pro.* **Diabetic Exchanges:** *3 lean meat, 1 starch.*

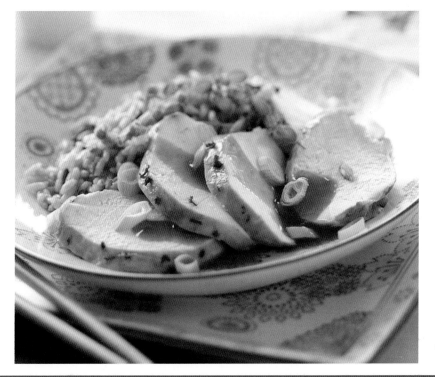

243 CALORIES Honey Chicken Stir-Fry

I'm a new mom, and my schedule is very dependent upon our young son. So I like meals that can be ready in as little time as possible. This stir-fry with a hint of sweetness is a big time-saver.

—CAROLINE SPERRY ALLENTOWN, MI

START TO FINISH: 30 MIN.
MAKES: 4 SERVINGS

- 1 pound boneless skinless chicken breasts, cut into 1-inch pieces
- 1 garlic clove, minced
- 3 teaspoons olive oil, divided
- 3 tablespoons honey
- 2 tablespoons reduced-sodium soy sauce
- ⅛ teaspoon salt
- ⅛ teaspoon pepper
- 1 package (16 ounces) frozen broccoli stir-fry vegetable blend
- 2 teaspoons cornstarch
- 1 tablespoon cold water
  Hot cooked rice

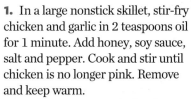

1. In a large nonstick skillet, stir-fry chicken and garlic in 2 teaspoons oil for 1 minute. Add honey, soy sauce, salt and pepper. Cook and stir until chicken is no longer pink. Remove and keep warm.
2. In the same pan, stir-fry the vegetables in remaining oil for 4-5 minutes or until tender. Return chicken to pan; stir to coat. Combine cornstarch and cold water until smooth; gradually stir into chicken mixture. Bring to a boil; cook and stir for 1 minute or until thickened. Serve with rice.

PER SERVING *1 cup stir-fry mixture (calculated without rice) equals 243 cal., 5 g fat (1 g sat. fat), 66 mg chol., 470 mg sodium, 19 g carb., 3 g fiber, 28 g pro.* **Diabetic Exchanges:** *3 lean meat, 3 vegetable..*

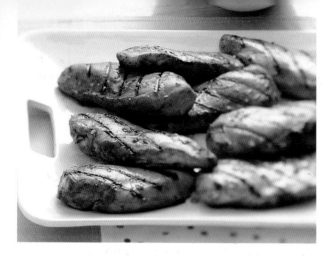

221 CALORIES

Honey-Grilled Chicken Breasts

Orange juice and soy sauce make such a tasty combination in this recipe from my mother-in-law. And the longer this chicken marinates, the fuller the flavor!

—JENNIFER PETERSEN MURRAY, UTAH

PREP: 15 MIN. + MARINATING • **GRILL:** 10 MIN. • **MAKES:** 8 SERVINGS

- ½ **cup orange juice**
- ⅓ **cup honey**
- ¼ **cup lemon juice**
- ¼ **cup reduced-sodium soy sauce**
- 2 **tablespoons minced fresh gingerroot**
- 12 **garlic cloves, minced**
- ½ **teaspoon pepper**
- ¼ **teaspoon salt**
- 8 **boneless skinless chicken breast halves (6 ounces each)**

1. In a small bowl, combine the first eight ingredients. Pour ½ cup marinade into a large resealable plastic bag; add chicken. Seal bag and turn to coat; refrigerate for 8 hours or overnight. Cover and refrigerate the remaining marinade.

2. Drain and discard marinade. Moisten a paper towel with cooking oil; using long-handled tongs, lightly coat the grill rack. Grill chicken, covered, over medium heat or broil 4 in. from the heat for 5-7 minutes on each side or until a thermometer reads 170°, basting frequently with reserved marinade.

PER SERVING *1 chicken breast half equals 221 cal., 4 g fat (1 g sat. fat), 94 mg chol., 331 mg sodium, 10 g carb., trace fiber, 35 g pro.* **Diabetic Exchanges:** *5 lean meat, ½ starch.*

---

240 CALORIES Grilled Pork Chops with Cilantro Salsa

These quick, easy chops create a colorful and appetizing statement when they hit the table. Your guests will rave!

—LISA RUEHLOW BLAINE, MN

START TO FINISH: 25 MIN. • **MAKES:** 6 SERVINGS

- 1½ **cups cubed cantaloupe**
- 1 **cup chopped tomatoes**
- ½ **cup chopped green pepper**
- 2 **tablespoons thawed limeade concentrate**
- 2 **tablespoons chopped green onion**
- 2 **tablespoons minced fresh cilantro**
- ¼ **teaspoon salt**
- 6 **bone-in pork loin chops (7 ounces each)**
  Pepper to taste

1. In a large bowl combine the cantaloupe, tomatoes, green pepper, limeade, onion, cilantro and salt. Cover and refrigerate until serving.

2. Season pork with pepper. Moisten a paper towel with cooking oil; using long-handled tongs, lightly coat the grill rack. Grill chops, covered, over medium heat or broil 4-5 in. from the heat for 4-5 minutes on each side or until a thermometer reads 145°. Let meat stand for 5 minutes before serving.

PER SERVING *1 pork chop with ⅓ cup salsa equals 240 cal., 9 g fat (3 g sat. fat), 86 mg chol., 168 mg sodium, 9 g carb., 1 g fiber, 31 g pro.* **Diabetic Exchanges:** *4 lean meat, ½ starch.*

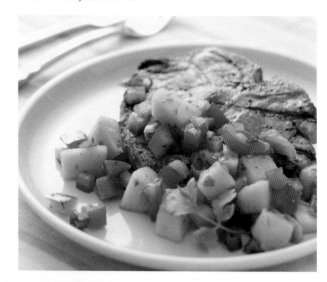

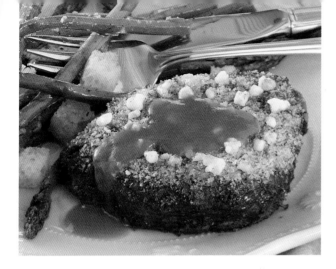

228 CALORIES Blue Cheese-Topped Steaks

Juicy tenderloin steaks, lightly crusted with blue cheese and bread crumbs, are special enough for holiday dining. Drizzled with wine sauce, this beef melts in your mouth.
—**TIFFANY VANCIL** SAN DIEGO, CA

START TO FINISH: 30 MIN. • **MAKES:** 4 SERVINGS

- 2 tablespoons crumbled blue cheese
- 4½ teaspoons dry bread crumbs
- 4½ teaspoons minced fresh parsley
- 4½ teaspoons minced chives
  Dash pepper
- 4 beef tenderloin steaks (4 ounces each)
- 1½ teaspoons butter
- 1 tablespoon all-purpose flour
- ½ cup reduced-sodium beef broth
- 1 tablespoon Madeira wine
- ⅛ teaspoon browning sauce, optional

1. Combine blue cheese, bread crumbs, parsley, chives and pepper. Press onto one side of each steak.
2. In a large nonstick skillet coated with cooking spray, cook steaks over medium-high heat for 2 minutes on each side. Transfer to a 15-in. x 10-in. x 1-in. baking pan coated with cooking spray.
3. Bake at 350° for 6-8 minutes or until meat reaches desired doneness (for medium-rare, a thermometer should read 145°; medium, 160°; well-done, 170°).
4. Meanwhile, in a small saucepan, melt butter. Whisk in flour until smooth. Gradually whisk in broth and wine. Bring to a boil; cook and stir for 2 minutes or until thickened. Stir in browning sauce if desired. Serve with steaks.

PER SERVING *1 steak equals 228 cal., 11 g fat (5 g sat. fat), 78 mg chol., 197 mg sodium, 4 g carb., trace fiber, 26 g pro.* **Diabetic Exchange:** *3 lean meat, 1½ fat, ½ fat-free milk.*

244 CALORIES Chili Sauce Meat Loaf

Here's a meat loaf with zesty chili sauce that's sure to please the entire family. My son-in-law just loves when I serve it. And I never have leftovers!
—**AVERLEEN RESSIE** RICE LAKE, WI

PREP: 20 MIN. • **BAKE:** 55 MIN. + STANDING • **MAKES:** 6 SERVINGS

- ⅓ cup plus 2 tablespoons chili sauce, divided
- 1 egg white
- 1 tablespoon Worcestershire sauce
- ¾ cup quick-cooking oats
- ¾ cup finely chopped onion
- 2 garlic cloves, minced
- 1 teaspoon dried thyme
- ½ teaspoon salt
- ½ teaspoon pepper
- 1½ pounds lean ground beef (90% lean)

1. In a large bowl, combine ⅓ cup chili sauce, egg white, Worcestershire sauce, oats, onion, garlic, thyme, salt and pepper. Crumble beef over mixture and mix well.
2. Shape into a 9-in. x 4-in. loaf; place in an 11x7-in. baking dish coated with cooking spray.
3. Bake, uncovered, at 350° for 50 minutes. Brush with remaining chili sauce. Bake 5-10 minutes longer or until no pink remains and a thermometer reads 160°. Let stand for 10 minutes before slicing.

PER SERVING *1 serving equals 244 cal., 10 g fat (4 g sat. fat), 69 mg chol., 565 mg sodium, 14 g carb., 2 g fiber, 24 g pro.* **Diabetic Exchanges:** *3 lean meat, 1 starch.*

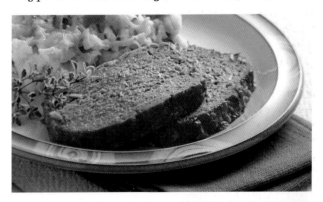

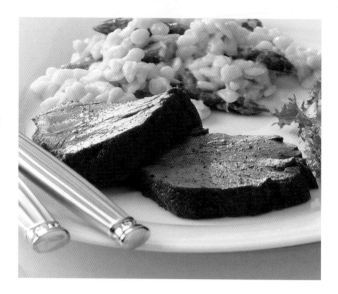

198 CALORIES Sweet 'n' Sour Pork Chops

My best friend gave me the recipe for these delightful pork chops years ago. It's become one of my family's favorites, and I prepare them often for us.
—GINA YOUNG LAMAR, CO

START TO FINISH: 25 MIN. • **MAKES:** 6 SERVINGS

- 6 **boneless pork loin chops (4 ounces each)**
- ¾ **teaspoon pepper**
- ½ **cup water**
- ⅓ **cup cider vinegar**
- ¼ **cup packed brown sugar**
- 2 **tablespoons reduced-sodium soy sauce**
- 1 **tablespoon Worcestershire sauce**
- 1 **tablespoon cornstarch**
- 2 **tablespoons cold water**

1. Sprinkle pork chops with pepper. In a large nonstick skillet coated with cooking spray, cook pork over medium heat for 4-6 minutes on each side or until lightly browned. Remove and keep warm.

2. Add the water, vinegar, brown sugar, soy sauce and Worcestershire sauce to skillet; stir to loosen browned bits. Bring to a boil. Combine cornstarch and cold water until smooth; stir into skillet. Bring to a boil; cook and stir for 2 minutes or until thickened.

3. Return chops to the pan. Reduce heat; cover and simmer for 4-5 minutes or until meat is tender.

PER SERVING *1 pork chop with 3 tablespoons sauce equals 198 cal., 6 g fat (2 g sat. fat), 55 mg chol., 265 mg sodium, 12 g carb., trace fiber, 22 g pro.* **Diabetic Exchanges:** *3 lean meat, 1 starch.*

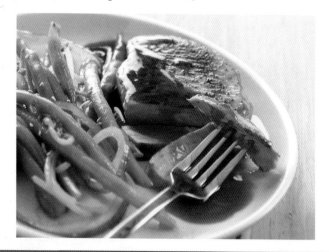

172 CALORIES Cajun Beef Tenderloin

Spice up tenderloin with this flavorful blend of salt, spices and herbs. If you like a milder beef, just use less of the cayenne.
—SUE DANNAHOWER FORT PIERCE, FL

PREP: 15 MIN. • **GRILL:** 50 MIN. + STANDING • **MAKES:** 12 SERVINGS

- 1 **beef tenderloin roast (3 pounds)**
- 4 **teaspoons salt**
- 1 **tablespoon paprika**
- 2¼ **teaspoons onion powder**
- 1½ **teaspoons garlic powder**
- 1½ **teaspoons white pepper**
- 1½ **teaspoons pepper**
- 1 **to 3 teaspoons cayenne pepper**
- 1 **teaspoon dried basil**
- ½ **teaspoon chili powder**
- ⅛ **teaspoon dried thyme**
- ⅛ **teaspoon ground mustard**
  Dash ground cloves

1. Tie tenderloin at 2-in. intervals with kitchen string. Combine the seasonings; rub over beef. Moisten a paper towel with cooking oil; using long-handled tongs, lightly coat the grill rack.

2. Prepare grill for indirect heat. Grill beef, covered, over indirect medium heat for 50-60 minutes, or until meat reaches desired doneness (for medium-rare, a thermometer should read 145°; medium, 160°; well-done, 170°), turning occasionally. Let stand for 10 minutes before slicing.

> "I jump on my treadmill while I watch the evening news. That way, I kill two birds with one stone."

— **ELAINE VINDAS BERBERIAN**

3. To roast the tenderloin, bake on a rack in a shallow roasting pan at 425° for 45-60 minutes or until meat reaches desired doneness.

PER SERVING *3 ounces cooked beef equals 172 cal., 7 g fat (3 g sat. fat), 50 mg chol., 788 mg sodium, 2 g carb., 1 g fiber, 25 g pro.* **Diabetic Exchange:** *3 lean meat.*

248 CALORIES Italian Skillet Supper

Romano cheese, sliced vegetables and pine nuts help to jazz up this easy chicken-and-veggie dish. This one's a keeper!

—BARBARA LENTO HOUSTON, PA

START TO FINISH: 30 MIN. • **MAKES:** 2 SERVINGS

- 2 **boneless skinless chicken breast halves (4 ounces each)**
- ¼ **teaspoon garlic salt**
- ¼ **teaspoon pepper**
- 2 **teaspoons reduced-fat butter**
- 1 **teaspoon olive oil**
- ¼ **pound small fresh mushrooms**
- ½ **medium onion, chopped**
- ¼ **cup chopped sweet red pepper**
- 1 **tablespoon pine nuts**
- 2 **cups fresh baby spinach**
- 1 **tablespoon all-purpose flour**
- ½ **cup reduced-sodium chicken broth**
- 1½ **teaspoons spicy brown mustard**
- 2 **teaspoons shredded Romano cheese**

1. Flatten chicken slightly; sprinkle with garlic salt and pepper. In a large nonstick skillet, cook chicken in butter and oil over medium heat for 3-4 minutes on each side or until a thermometer reads 170°. Remove and keep warm.

2. In the same skillet, saute the mushrooms, onion, red pepper and pine nuts until vegetables are tender. Add spinach; cook and stir for 2-3 minutes or until wilted. Stir in flour. Gradually stir in broth and mustard. Bring to a boil. Reduce heat; cook and stir for 2 minutes or until thickened.

3. Return chicken to the pan; heat through. Sprinkle with cheese.

NOTE *This recipe was tested with Land O'Lakes light stick butter.*

PER SERVING *1 chicken breast half with ½ cup vegetable mixture equals 248 cal., 10 g fat (3 g sat. fat), 70 mg chol., 548 mg sodium, 12 g carb., 3 g fiber, 29 g pro.* **Diabetic Exchanges:** *3 lean meat, 2 vegetable, 1½ fat.*

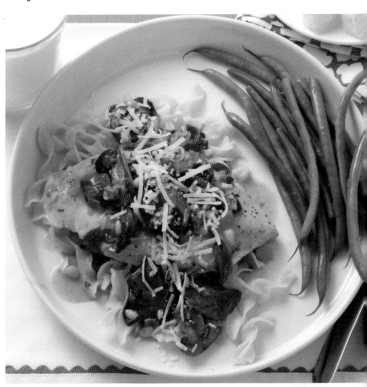

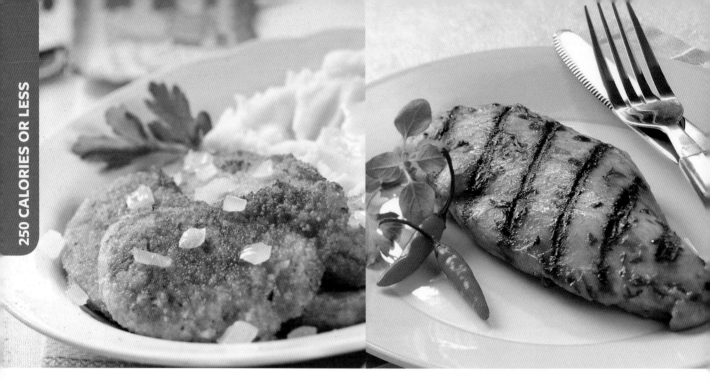

220 CALORIES Parmesan Pork Medallions

I have served this recipe countless times to family and friends. I like that it takes very little prep time.

—ANGELA CIOCCA SALTSBURG, PA

START TO FINISH: 20 MIN.
MAKES: 2 SERVINGS

- ½ **pound pork tenderloin**
- 2 **tablespoons seasoned bread crumbs**
- 1 **tablespoon grated Parmesan cheese**
- ¼ **teaspoon salt**
  Dash pepper
- 2 **teaspoons canola oil**
- ¼ **cup chopped onion**
- 1 **garlic clove, minced**

1. Cut pork into four slices; flatten to ¼-in. thickness.
2. In a large resealable plastic bag, combine the bread crumbs, cheese, salt and pepper. Add the pork, one slice at a time, and shake to coat.
3. In a large skillet over medium heat, cook pork in oil for 2-3 minutes on each side or until no longer pink. Remove and keep warm.
4. Add onion to the pan; cook and stir until tender. Add garlic, cook 1 minute longer. Serve with pork.
PER SERVING *2 medallions equals 220 cal., 9 g fat (2 g sat. fat), 65 mg chol., 487 mg sodium, 8 g carb., 1 g fiber, 25 g pro.* **Diabetic Exchanges:** *3 lean meat, 1 fat, ½ starch.*

208 CALORIES
Quick Marinated Grilled Chicken

On hot summer days, this yummy chicken is a cinch to throw together without heating up the kitchen. Just add grilled potatoes or corn on the cob.

—MISSY HERR QUARRYVILLE, PA

PREP: 10 MIN. + MARINATING
GRILL: 15 MIN. • **MAKES:** 4 SERVINGS

- 6 **tablespoons white vinegar**
- 3 **tablespoons canola oil**
- 2 **tablespoons ketchup**
- 2 **teaspoons dried parsley flakes**
- 1½ **teaspoons garlic salt**
- ½ **teaspoon paprika**
- ¼ **teaspoon dried oregano**
- ⅛ **teaspoon hot pepper sauce**
- ⅛ **teaspoon Worcestershire sauce**
- 1 **bay leaf**
- 4 **boneless skinless chicken breast halves (6 ounces each)**

1. In a large resealable plastic bag, combine the first 10 ingredients; add chicken. Seal bag and turn to coat; refrigerate for 4-8 hours, turning occasionally.
2. Drain and discard marinade. Grill chicken, covered, over medium heat for 6-8 minutes on each side or until juices run clear.
PER SERVING *1 chicken breast half equals 208 cal., 7 g fat (1 g sat. fat), 94 mg chol., 275 mg sodium, 1 g carb., trace fiber, 34 g pro.* **Diabetic Exchanges:** *5 lean meat, ½ fat.*

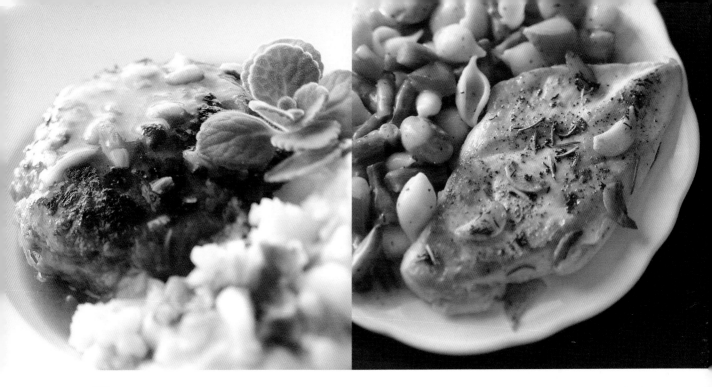

Hearty Salisbury Steaks

With its down-home taste, this always disappears fast! I love to serve it with mashed potatoes and vegetables.
—DOROTHY BAYES SARDIS, OH

START TO FINISH: 30 MIN.
MAKES: 5 SERVINGS

- ¼ cup egg substitute
- 1 medium onion, finely chopped
- ½ cup crushed saltines (about 15 crackers)
- ½ teaspoon pepper
- 1 pound lean ground beef (90% lean)
- 1 tablespoon canola oil
- 1 envelope reduced-sodium onion soup mix
- 2 tablespoons all-purpose flour
- 2 cups water

1. In a bowl, combine egg substitute, onion, saltines and pepper. Crumble beef over mixture and mix well. Shape into five patties.
2. In a large skillet, cook patties in oil over medium heat for 3 minutes on each side or until lightly browned. Remove patties and keep warm; discard drippings.
3. Combine soup mix, flour and water; stir into skillet. Bring to a boil. Return patties to skillet. Reduce heat; cover and simmer for 5-7 minutes or until meat is no longer pink.
PER SERVING *1 patty with ¼ cup gravy equals 233 cal., 10 g fat (3 g sat. fat), 45 mg chol., 418 mg sodium, 14 g carb., 1 g fiber, 20 g pro.* **Diabetic Exchanges:** *2 lean meat, 1 starch, 1 fat.*

Tuscan Chicken for Two

Have dinner on the table in no time flat! This chicken entree comes together in just 15 minutes. Really!
—DEBRA LEGRAND PORT ORCHARD, WA

START TO FINISH: 15 MIN.
MAKES: 2 SERVINGS

- 2 boneless skinless chicken breast halves (5 ounces each)
- ¼ teaspoon salt
- ¼ teaspoon pepper
- 1 garlic clove, sliced
- 1 teaspoon dried rosemary, crushed
- ¼ teaspoon rubbed sage
- ¼ teaspoon dried thyme
- 1 tablespoon olive oil

1. Flatten the chicken to ½-in. thickness; sprinkle with salt and pepper.
2. In a large skillet over medium heat, cook and stir the garlic, rosemary, sage and thyme in oil for 1 minute. Add chicken; cook for 5-7 minutes on each side or until juices run clear.
PER SERVING *1 chicken breast half equals 217 cal., 10 g fat (2 g sat. fat), 78 mg chol., 364 mg sodium, 1 g carb., 1 g fiber, 29 g pro.* **Diabetic Exchanges:** *4 lean meat, 1 fat.*

242 CALORIES

Chive Crab Cakes

These tasty crab cakes are wonderful as appetizers or served alongside a salad to make a light meal.

—CINDY WORTH LAPWAI, ID

PREP: 20 MIN. + CHILLING
COOK: 10 MIN./BATCH • **MAKES:** 6 SERVINGS

- 4 **egg whites**
- 1 **egg**
- 6 **tablespoons minced chives**
- 3 **tablespoons all-purpose flour**
- 1 **to 2 teaspoons hot pepper sauce**
- 1 **teaspoon baking powder**
- ½ **teaspoon salt**
- ¼ **teaspoon pepper**
- 4 **cans (6 ounces each) crabmeat, drained, flaked and cartilage removed**
- 2 **cups panko (Japanese) bread crumbs**
- 2 **tablespoons canola oil**

1. In a large bowl, lightly beat the egg whites and egg. Add the chives, flour, pepper sauce, baking powder, salt and pepper; mix well. Fold in crab. Cover and refrigerate for at least 2 hours.

2. Place bread crumbs in a shallow bowl. Drop crab mixture by ¼ cupfuls into crumbs. Gently coat and shape into ¾-in.-thick patties.

3. In a large nonstick skillet, cook crab cakes in oil in batches over medium-high heat for 3-4 minutes on each side or until golden brown.
PER SERVING *2 crab cakes equals 242 cal., 7 g fat (1 g sat. fat), 136 mg chol., 731 mg sodium, 12 g carb., 1 g fiber, 29 g pro. Diabetic Exchanges: 3 lean meat, 1 starch, ½ fat.*

247 CALORIES # Mahi Mahi with Nectarine Salsa

A ripe nectarine inspired me to put together a fruity salsa to serve with fish fillets. I received six small thumbs up from our three young children for this easy and nutritious meal.

—MICHELLE AUGUSTINE
CINCINNATI, OH

START TO FINISH: 25 MIN.
MAKES: 2 SERVINGS

- 1 **medium nectarine, peeled and chopped**
- ¼ **cup chopped onion**

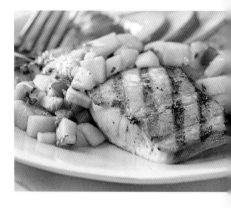

- 2 **tablespoons chopped cucumber**
- 1 **tablespoon minced fresh cilantro**
- 2 **teaspoons chopped seeded jalapeno pepper**
- 2 **teaspoons lime juice**
- ¼ **teaspoon salt**
- ¼ **teaspoon pepper**
- ¼ **teaspoon Louisiana-style hot sauce**

FISH FILLETS

- 2 **mahi mahi fillets (6 ounces each)**
- 1 **tablespoon olive oil**
  Dash salt

1. For salsa, in a small bowl, combine the first nine ingredients. Cover and refrigerate until serving.

2. Drizzle fillets with oil; sprinkle with salt. Moisten a paper towel with cooking oil; using long-handled tongs, lightly coat the grill rack. Grill fillets, covered, over medium heat or broil 4 in. from the heat for 3-5 minutes on each side or until fish just turns opaque. Serve with the salsa.
NOTE *Wear disposable gloves when cutting hot peppers; the oils can burn skin. Avoid touching your face.*
PER SERVING *1 fillet with ½ cup salsa equals 247 cal., 8 g fat (1 g sat. fat), 124 mg chol., 520 mg sodium, 10 g carb., 2 g fiber, 33 g pro. Diabetic Exchanges: 5 lean meat, 1½ fat, ½ fruit.*

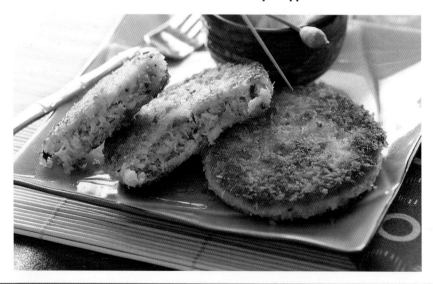

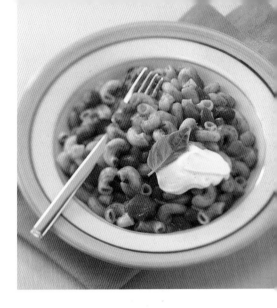

247 CALORIES Chicken with Rosemary-Onion Sauce

Is there anything more flavorful or aromatic than chicken with rosemary?
—**DONNA ROBERTS** MANHATTAN, KS

PREP: 15 MIN. • **BAKE:** 20 MIN.
MAKES: 4 SERVINGS

4 **boneless skinless chicken breast halves (6 ounces each)**
½ **teaspoon salt**
¼ **teaspoon pepper**
3 **teaspoons butter, divided**
1 **medium onion, chopped**
1 **garlic clove, minced**
4 **teaspoons all-purpose flour**
½ **cup reduced-sodium chicken broth**
½ **cup fat-free milk**
1 **teaspoon dried rosemary, crushed**

1. Sprinkle chicken with salt and pepper. In a large nonstick skillet, brown chicken in 1 teaspoon butter. Transfer to an 11-in. x 7-in. baking dish coated with cooking spray.
2. In the same skillet, saute onion and garlic in remaining butter until tender. Stir in flour until blended. Gradually stir in broth and milk. Add rosemary. Bring to a boil; cook and stir for 2 minutes or until thickened.
3. Pour sauce over chicken. Cover and bake at 350° for 20-25 minutes or until a thermometer reads 170°.
PER SERVING *1 chicken breast half with ¼ cup sauce equals 247 cal., 7 g fat (3 g sat. fat), 102 mg chol., 501 mg sodium, 8 g carb., 1 g fiber, 37 g pro.* **Diabetic Exchanges:** *5 lean meat, ½ starch, ½ fat.*

214 CALORIES Meatless Chili Mac

I came across this recipe in a newspaper years ago, and it's been a real hit at our house ever since. Try this one!
—**CINDY RAGAN**
NORTH HUNTINGDON, PA

PREP: 15 MIN. • **COOK:** 25 MIN.
MAKES: 8 SERVINGS

1 **large onion, chopped**
1 **medium green pepper, chopped**
1 **tablespoon olive oil**
1 **garlic clove, minced**
2 **cups water**
1½ **cups uncooked elbow macaroni**
1 **can (16 ounces) mild chili beans, undrained**
1 **can (15½ ounces) great northern beans, rinsed and drained**
1 **can (14½ ounces) diced tomatoes, undrained**
1 **can (8 ounces) tomato sauce**
4 **teaspoons chili powder**
1 **teaspoon salt**
1 **teaspoon ground cumin**
½ **cup fat-free sour cream**

1. In a Dutch oven, saute onion and green pepper in oil until tender. Add garlic; cook 1 minute longer. Stir in the water, macaroni, beans, tomatoes, tomato sauce, chili powder, salt and cumin.
2. Bring to a boil. Reduce heat; cover and simmer for 15-20 minutes or until macaroni is tender. Top each serving with 1 tablespoon of sour cream.
PER SERVING *1¼ cups equals 214 cal., 3 g fat (1 g sat. fat), 3 mg chol., 857 mg sodium, 37 g carb., 8 g fiber, 10 g pro.* **Diabetic Exchanges:** *2 starch, 1 lean meat, 1 vegetable.*

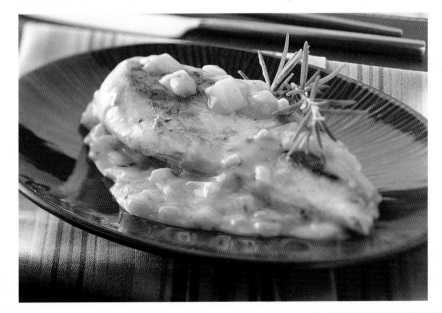

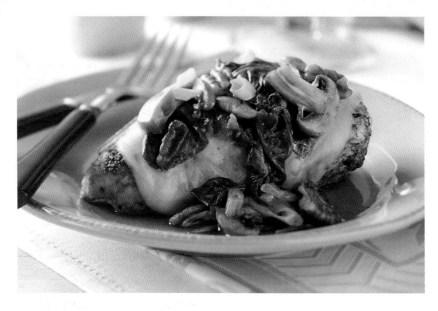

203 CALORIES
Spinach and Mushroom Smothered Chicken

Chicken with a mushroom and spinach topping is tucked under a blanket of melted cheese. It's extra-special to serve but not at all tricky to make.

—KATRINA WAGNER GRAIN VALLEY, MO

START TO FINISH: 30 MIN.
MAKES: 4 SERVINGS

- 3 **cups fresh baby spinach**
- 1¾ **cups sliced fresh mushrooms**
- 3 **green onions, sliced**
- 2 **tablespoons chopped pecans**
- 1½ **teaspoons olive oil**
- 4 **boneless skinless chicken breast halves (4 ounces each)**
- ½ **teaspoon rotisserie chicken seasoning**
- 2 **slices reduced-fat provolone cheese, halved**

1. In a large skillet, saute the spinach, mushrooms, onions and pecans in oil until mushrooms are tender. Set aside and keep warm.
2. Sprinkle chicken with seasoning. Moisten a paper towel with cooking oil; using long-handled tongs, lightly coat the grill rack. Grill chicken, covered, over medium heat or broil 4 in. from the heat for 4-5 minutes on each side or until a thermometer reads 170°.
3. Top with cheese. Cover and grill 2-3 minutes longer or until cheese is melted. To serve, top each chicken breast with reserved spinach mixture.

PER SERVING *1 chicken breast half equals 203 cal., 9 g fat (2 g sat. fat), 68 mg chol., 210 mg sodium, 3 g carb., 2 g fiber, 27 g pro. Diabetic Exchanges: 3 lean meat, 1 vegetable, 1 fat.*

171 CALORIES
Grilled Pork Tenderloin

We've been making this dish for years, and everyone who tastes it requests the recipe. I often double it and serve the leftovers on salad next day. Just add your favorite dressing and dinner's ready.

—DEBBIE WIGLE WILLIAMSON, NY

PREP: 10 MIN. + MARINATING
GRILL: 25 MIN. • **MAKES:** 4 SERVINGS

- ½ **cup Italian salad dressing**
- ¼ **cup reduced-sodium soy sauce**
- 1 **pork tenderloin (1 pound)**
- ½ **teaspoon steak seasoning**

1. In a large resealable plastic bag, combine salad dressing and soy sauce; add pork. Seal the bag and turn to coat; refrigerate for up to 4 hours.
2. Drain and discard marinade. Rub pork with steak seasoning. Moisten a paper towel with cooking oil; using long-handled tongs, lightly coat the grill rack. Prepare grill for indirect heat.
3. Grill pork, covered, over indirect medium-hot heat for 25-40 minutes or until a thermometer reads 160°. Let stand 5 minutes before slicing.

NOTE *This recipe was tested with McCormick's Montreal Steak Seasoning. Look for it in the spice aisle of your grocery store.*

PER SERVING *3 ounces cooked pork equals 171 cal., 8 g fat (2 g sat. fat), 63 mg chol., 500 mg sodium, 1 g carb., trace fiber, 23 g pro. Diabetic Exchanges: 3 lean meat, ½ fat.*

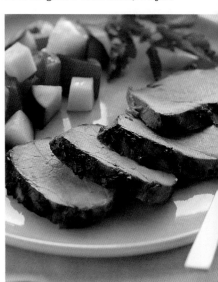

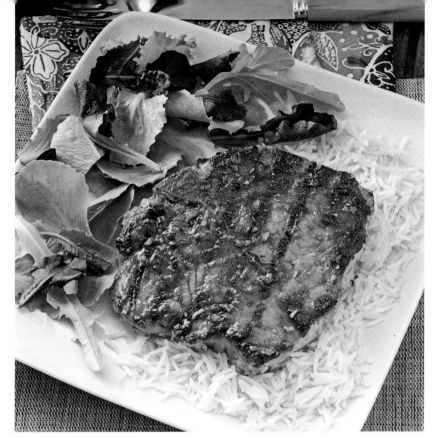

208 CALORIES
Garlic Chicken 'n' Gravy

Here's a classic family favorite you can prepare in less than 30 minutes—using just a skillet!

—TASTE OF HOME TEST KITCHEN

START TO FINISH: 25 MIN.
MAKES: 4 SERVINGS

- 4 **boneless skinless chicken breast halves (4 ounces each)**
- ¼ **teaspoon salt**
- ¼ **teaspoon pepper**
- 5 **garlic cloves, peeled and chopped**
- 2 **tablespoons butter**
- ½ **cup plus 2 tablespoons chicken broth, divided**
- ½ **cup white wine or additional chicken broth**
- ½ **teaspoon dried basil**
- ¼ **teaspoon dried oregano**
- 1 **tablespoon all-purpose flour**

1. Sprinkle chicken with salt and pepper. In a large skillet, cook chicken and garlic in butter over medium-high heat for 5 minutes or until browned. Add ½ cup broth, wine or additional broth, basil and oregano. Bring to a boil. Reduce heat; cover and simmer for 7-9 minutes or until chicken is no longer pink.
2. Remove the chicken and keep warm. In a small bowl, combine the flour and remaining broth until smooth; stir into the pan juices.
3. Bring to a boil; cook and stir for 1-2 minutes or until thickened. Serve over chicken.
PER SERVING *1 chicken breast half with 3 tablespoons gravy equals 208 cal., 8 g fat (4 g sat. fat), 78 mg chol., 407 mg sodium, 3 g carb., trace fiber, 24 g pro.* ***Diabetic Exchanges:*** *3 lean meat, 1½ fat.*

234 CALORIES Southwest Summer Pork Chops

These ribs get their zesty appeal from a simple combination of herbs and seasonings. We love the seasoning blend on pork, but you can also use it on chicken. It gives foods terrific flavor without added salt.

—SANDY SHORTT CEDARVILLE, OH

PREP: 15 MIN. + MARINATING
GRILL: 10 MIN. • **MAKES:** 6 SERVINGS

- 4 **teaspoons dried minced onion**
- 2 **teaspoons ground cumin**
- 1 **teaspoon cornstarch**
- 1 **teaspoon chili powder**
- 1 **teaspoon dried minced garlic**
- ½ **teaspoon dried oregano**
- ½ **teaspoon paprika**
- ¼ **teaspoon cayenne pepper**
- 6 **bone-in pork loin chops (about ¾ inch thick and 7 ounces each)**
- ¼ **cup barbecue sauce**
- 2 **tablespoons lemon juice**

1. In a bowl, combine first eight ingredients; rub over pork chops. In a large resealable plastic bag, combine barbecue sauce and lemon juice; add pork chops. Seal bag and turn to coat; refrigerate for 1-2 hours.
2. Discard marinade. Moisten a paper towel with cooking oil; using long-handled tongs, lightly coat grill rack. Grill chops, covered, over medium heat or broil 4 in. from heat for 4-5 minutes on each side or until a thermometer reads 145°. Let stand for 5 minutes before serving.
PER SERVING *1 pork chop equals 234 cal., 8 g fat (3 g sat. fat), 81 mg chol., 202 mg sodium, 8 g carb., 1 g fiber, 30 g pro.* ***Diabetic Exchanges:*** *4 lean meat, ½ starch.*

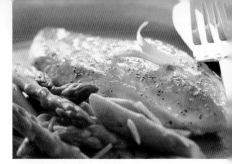

241 CALORIES Mushroom Pepper Steak

A fast marinade tenderizes the sirloin steak in this colorful stir-fry. Garlic and ginger round out the taste.

—BILLIE MOSS WALNUT CREEK, CA

PREP: 15 MIN. + MARINATING
COOK: 15 MIN. • **MAKES:** 4 SERVINGS

- 6 **tablespoons reduced-sodium soy sauce, divided**
- ⅛ **teaspoon pepper**
- 1 **pound beef top sirloin steak, cut into thin strips**
- 1 **tablespoon cornstarch**
- ½ **cup reduced-sodium beef broth**
- 1 **garlic clove, minced**
- ½ **teaspoon minced fresh gingerroot**
- 3 **teaspoons canola oil, divided**
- 1 **cup julienned sweet red pepper**
- 1 **cup julienned green pepper**
- 2 **cups sliced fresh mushrooms**
- 2 **medium tomatoes, cut into wedges**
- 6 **green onions, sliced**
  Hot cooked rice, optional

1. In a large resealable plastic bag, combine 3 tablespoons soy sauce and pepper; add beef. Seal bag and turn to coat; refrigerate for 30-60 minutes. In a small bowl, combine cornstarch, broth and remaining soy sauce until smooth; set aside.

2. Drain and discard marinade from beef. In a large nonstick skillet or wok, stir-fry the garlic and ginger in 2 teaspoons oil for 1 minute. Add the beef; stir-fry for 4-6 minutes or until no longer pink. Remove beef and keep warm.

3. Stir-fry the peppers in remaining oil for 1 minute. Add mushrooms; stir-fry 2 minutes longer or until peppers are crisp-tender. Stir broth mixture and add to the pan. Bring to a boil; cook and stir for 2 minutes or until thickened. Return beef to the pan; add tomatoes and onions. Cook for 2 minutes or until heated through. Serve over rice if desired.

PER SERVING *1¼ cups beef mixture (calculated without rice) equals 241 cal., 10 g fat (3 g sat. fat), 64 mg chol., 841 mg sodium, 13 g carb., 3 g fiber, 25 g pro.* **Diabetic Exchanges** *3 lean meat, 2 vegetable, 1 fat.*

226 CALORIES Maple-Glazed Chicken

This chicken recipe offers sweet and savory flavors and a pleasant maple sauce. Tender and loaded with appeal, it will please everyone at the table.

—TARYN KUEBELBECK PLYMOUTH, MN

START TO FINISH: 20 MIN.
MAKES: 4 SERVINGS

- 4 **boneless skinless chicken breast halves (5 ounces each)**
- ¼ **teaspoon salt**
- ⅛ **teaspoon pepper**
- 1 **tablespoon canola oil**
- ½ **teaspoon cornstarch**
- ½ **cup apple cider or unsweetened apple juice**
- 2 **tablespoons maple syrup**
- ½ **teaspoon onion powder**

1. Flatten chicken to ½-in. thickness. Sprinkle with salt and pepper. In a large skillet, cook chicken in oil for 5-6 minutes on each side or until no longer pink. Remove and keep warm.

2. Meanwhile, in a bowl, combine cornstarch and cider until smooth. Stir in syrup and onion powder; add to skillet. Bring to a boil; cook and stir for 2 minutes or until thickened. Add chicken and turn to coat.

PER SERVING *1 chicken breast half with 2 tablespoons glaze equals 226 cal., 7 g fat (1 g sat. fat), 78 mg chol., 220 mg sodium, 11 g carb., trace fiber, 29 g pro.* **Diabetic Exchange:** *4 lean meat, 1 starch, ½ fat.*

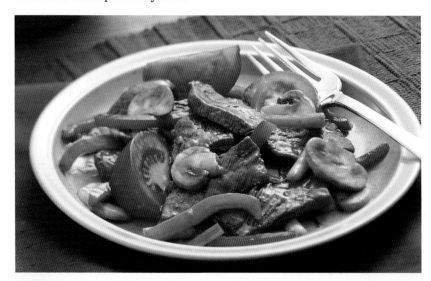

Southwestern Goulash

I had some extra cilantro in the fridge and didn't want to throw it away. So instead, I came up with a Southwest-inspired soup using ingredients I had on hand. The whole family loved it!
—**VIKKI REBHOLZ** WEST CHESTER, OH

START TO FINISH: 30 MIN.
MAKES: 6 SERVINGS

- 1 cup uncooked elbow macaroni
- 1 pound lean ground beef (90% lean)
- 1 medium onion, chopped
- 1 can (28 ounces) diced tomatoes, undrained
- ⅔ cup frozen corn
- 1 can (8 ounces) tomato sauce
- 1 can (4 ounces) chopped green chilies
- ½ teaspoon ground cumin
- ½ teaspoon pepper
- ¼ teaspoon salt
- ¼ cup minced fresh cilantro

1. Cook macaroni according to package directions. Meanwhile, in a Dutch oven over medium heat, cook beef and onion until meat is no longer pink; drain. Stir in the tomatoes, corn, tomato sauce, chilies, cumin, pepper and salt. Bring to a boil. Reduce the heat; simmer, uncovered, for 3-5 minutes to allow flavors to blend.
2. Drain macaroni; add to meat mixture. Stir in the cilantro and heat through.
PER SERVING *1⅓ cups equals 224 cal., 6 g fat (2 g sat. fat), 37 mg chol., 567 mg sodium, 24 g carb., 4 g fiber, 19 g pro. Diabetic Exchanges: 2 lean meat, 2 vegetable, 1 starch.*

Braised Pork Chops

I'm always looking for recipes that are low-calorie and sugar- and salt-free to fix for my husband—he's diabetic and prone to high blood pressure. These tender chops are healthy without sacrificing flavor.
—**SHIRLEY ANTAYA** ARAB, AL

PREP: 5 MIN. • **COOK:** 55 MIN.
MAKES: 4 SERVINGS

- ½ teaspoon dried marjoram
- ⅛ teaspoon onion powder
- ⅛ teaspoon garlic powder
- ⅛ teaspoon pepper
- 4 bone-in pork loin chops (6 ounces each)
- 1 teaspoon olive oil
- ½ cup water
- 2 teaspoons cornstarch
- ¼ cup reduced-sodium chicken broth

1. Combine seasonings; sprinkle over pork chops. In a nonstick skillet, cook chops in oil until browned on both sides. Add water. Bring to a boil. Reduce heat; cover and simmer for 45-60 minutes or until tender.
2. Remove meat and keep warm. Combine cornstarch and broth until smooth; stir into cooking juices. Bring to a boil; cook and stir for 2 minutes or until thickened. Serve over pork chops.
PER SERVING *1 pork chop with 2 tablespoons gravy equals 180 cal., 9 g fat (3 g sat. fat), 67 mg chol., 83 mg sodium, 1 g carb., trace fiber, 23 g pro. Diabetic Exchange: 3 lean meat.*

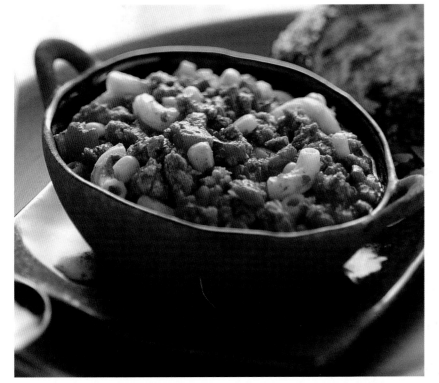

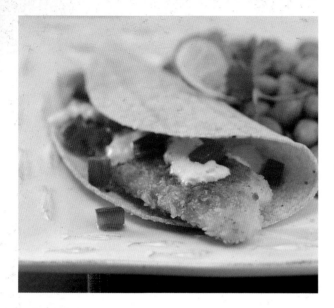

3. In a large skillet over medium heat, cook tilapia in oil in batches for 4-5 minutes on each side or until the fish flakes easily with a fork. Combine the seasonings; sprinkle over fish.

4. Place a portion of fish on each tortilla; top with about 2 tablespoons of sour cream mixture. Sprinkle with chopped tomato.

PER SERVING *1 taco equals 196 cal., 3 g fat (trace sat. fat), 31 mg chol., 303 mg sodium, 26 g carb., 2 g fiber, 16 g pro.* **Diabetic Exchanges:** *2 lean meat, 1½ starch, ½ fat.*

196 CALORIES Fish Tacos

A cool sauce with just a bit of zing tops these crisp and spicy fish tacos. They make a great, guilt-free meal and don't break the bank...always a good thing when you're a college kid!

—LENA LIM SEATTLE, WA

PREP: 30 MIN. • **COOK:** 20 MIN. • **MAKES:** 8 SERVINGS

- ¾ **cup fat-free sour cream**
- 1 **can (4 ounces) chopped green chilies**
- 1 **tablespoon fresh cilantro leaves**
- 1 **tablespoon lime juice**
- 4 **tilapia fillets (4 ounces each)**
- ½ **cup all-purpose flour**
- 1 **egg white, beaten**
- ½ **cup panko (Japanese) bread crumbs**
- 1 **tablespoon canola oil**
- ½ **teaspoon salt**
- ½ **teaspoon each white pepper, cayenne pepper and paprika**
- 8 **corn tortillas (6 inches), warmed**
- 1 **large tomato, finely chopped**

1. Place the sour cream, chilies, cilantro and lime juice in a food processor; cover and process until blended. Set aside.

2. Cut each tilapia fillet lengthwise into two portions. Place the flour, egg white and bread crumbs in separate shallow bowls. Dip tilapia in flour, then egg white, then in crumbs.

212 CALORIES
Garlic-Ginger Turkey Tenderloins

This healthier-for-you entree can be on your family's plates quicker than Chinese takeout...and for a lot less money! It has a ginger- and brown sugar-flavored sauce that spices up the turkey as it bakes.

—TASTE OF HOME TEST KITCHEN

START TO FINISH: 30 MIN. • **MAKES:** 4 SERVINGS

- 1 **package (20 ounces) turkey breast tenderloins**
- 3 **tablespoons brown sugar, divided**
- 8 **teaspoons reduced-sodium soy sauce, divided**
- 2 **tablespoons minced fresh gingerroot**
- 6 **garlic cloves, minced**
- ½ **teaspoon pepper**
- 1 **tablespoon cornstarch**
- 1 **cup reduced-sodium chicken broth**

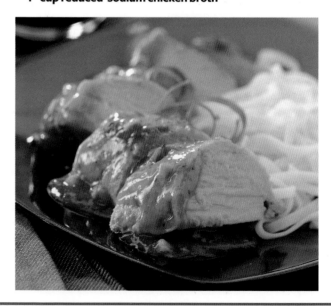

1. Place turkey in a shallow 3-qt. baking dish coated with cooking spray. In a small bowl, combine 2 tablespoons brown sugar, 6 teaspoons soy sauce, ginger, garlic and pepper. Set half aside; sprinkle remaining mixture over turkey.

2. Bake, uncovered, at 375° for 25-30 minutes or until a thermometer reads 170°. Let stand for in 5 minutes before slicing.

3. Meanwhile, in a small saucepan, combine the cornstarch and broth until smooth. Stir in reserved soy sauce mixture and remaining brown sugar and soy sauce. Bring to a boil; cook and stir for 2 minutes or until thickened. Serve with turkey.

PER SERVING *4 ounces cooked turkey equals 212 cal., 2 g fat (1 g sat. fat), 69 mg chol., 639 mg sodium, 14 g carb., trace fiber, 35 g pro.* **Diabetic Exchanges**: *4 lean meat, 1 starch.*

190 CALORIES Chicken and Shrimp Satay

I lightened up a recipe that I found in a cookbook, and these grilled kabobs were the tasty result. The scrumptious dipping sauce is always a hit.

—HANNAH BARRINGER LOUDON, TN

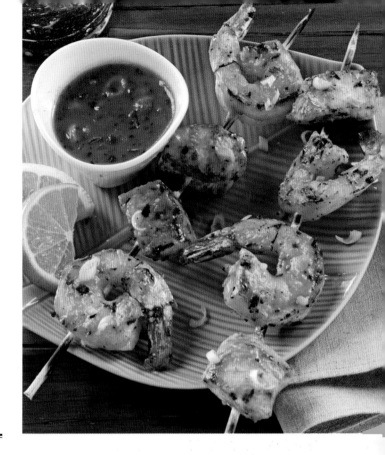

PREP: 20 MIN. + MARINATING • **GRILL:** 10 MIN.
MAKES: 6 SERVINGS

- ¾ **pound uncooked medium shrimp, peeled and deveined**
- ¾ **pound chicken tenderloins, cut into 1-inch cubes**
- 4 **green onions, chopped**
- 1 **tablespoon butter**
- 2 **garlic cloves, minced**
- 1 **tablespoon minced fresh parsley**
- ½ **cup white wine or chicken broth**
- 1 **tablespoon lemon juice**
- 1 **tablespoon lime juice**

SAUCE

- ¼ **cup chopped onion**
- 1 **tablespoon butter**
- ⅔ **cup reduced-sodium chicken broth**
- ¼ **cup reduced-fat chunky peanut butter**
- 2¼ **teaspoons brown sugar**
- ¾ **teaspoon lemon juice**
- ¾ **teaspoon lime juice**
- ¼ **teaspoon salt**
- ¼ **teaspoon each dried basil, thyme and rosemary, crushed**
- ⅛ **teaspoon cayenne pepper**

1. On 12 metal or soaked wooden skewers, alternately thread shrimp and chicken. Place in a large shallow dish; set aside.

2. In a small skillet, saute green onions in butter until crisp-tender. Add garlic; cook 1 minute longer. Stir in parsley, wine, lemon juice and lime juice. Remove from heat; cool slightly. Pour over skewers and turn to coat. Cover and refrigerate for 4 hours, turning occasionally.

3. In a small saucepan, saute onion in butter. Add the remaining sauce ingredients; cook and stir until blended. Remove from the heat; set aside.

4. Drain and discard marinade. Moisten a paper towel with cooking oil; using long-handled tongs, lightly coat the grill rack. Prepare grill for indirect heat. Grill skewers, covered, over indirect medium heat or broil 4 in. from the heat for 7 to 8 minutes, turning often. Brush with ¼ cup sauce during the last minute of grilling. Serve with remaining sauce.

PER SERVING *2 kabobs with 2 tablespoons sauce equals 190 cal., 7 g fat (3 g sat. fat), 126 mg chol., 339 mg sodium, 7 g carb., 1 g fiber, 25 g pro.* **Diabetic Exchanges:** *3 lean meat, 1 fat, ½ starch.*

207 CALORIES

Zesty Horseradish Meat Loaf

You'll love the bit of heat in this savory meat loaf. Make sandwiches out of the leftovers and get double duty from this comfort-food classic.

—**NANCY ZIMMERMAN** CAPE MAY COURT HOUSE, NJ

PREP: 15 MIN. • **BAKE:** 45 MIN. + STANDING • **MAKES:** 8 SERVINGS

- 4 **slices whole wheat bread, crumbled**
- ¼ **cup fat-free milk**
- ½ **cup finely chopped celery**
- ¼ **cup finely chopped onion**
- ¼ **cup prepared horseradish**
- 2 **tablespoons Dijon mustard**
- 2 **tablespoons chili sauce**
- 1 **egg, lightly beaten**
- 1½ **teaspoons Worcestershire sauce**
- ½ **teaspoon salt**
- ¼ **teaspoon pepper**
- 1½ **pounds lean ground beef (90% lean)**
- ½ **cup ketchup**

1. In a large bowl, soak bread in milk for 5 minutes. Drain and discard milk. Stir in the celery, onion, horseradish, mustard, chili sauce, egg, Worcestershire sauce, salt and pepper. Crumble beef over mixture and mix well.

2. Shape into a loaf in an 11-in. x 7-in. baking dish coated with cooking spray. Spread top with ketchup. Bake at 350° for 45-55 minutes or until no pink remains and a thermometer reads 160°. Let stand for 10 minutes before cutting.

PER SERVING *1 slice equals 207 cal., 8 g fat (3 g sat. fat), 79 mg chol., 640 mg sodium, 14 g carb., 1 g fiber, 19 g pro.* **Diabetic Exchanges:** *2 lean meat, 1 starch, ½ fat.*

246 CALORIES # Glazed Pork Chops

Rosemary adds special flavor to these beautifully glazed chops that are ideal for a busy weeknight meal.

—**LOUISE GILBERT** QUESNEL, BC

PREP: 10 MIN. + MARINATING • **GRILL:** 10 MIN.
MAKES: 8 SERVINGS

- ½ **cup ketchup**
- ¼ **cup packed brown sugar**
- ¼ **cup white vinegar**
- ¼ **cup orange juice**
- ¼ **cup Worcestershire sauce**
- 2 **garlic cloves, minced**
- ½ **teaspoon dried rosemary, crushed**
- 8 **bone-in pork loin chops (7 ounces each)**

1. In a small bowl, combine the first seven ingredients. Pour ¾ cup into a large resealable plastic bag; add the pork chops. Seal bag and turn to coat; refrigerate for 8 hours or overnight. Cover and refrigerate remaining marinade for basting.

2. Drain and discard marinade. Moisten a paper towel with cooking oil; using long-handled tongs, lightly coat the grill rack.

3. Grill pork, covered, over medium heat or broil 4-5 in. from heat for 4-5 minutes on each side or until a thermometer reads 145°, basting occasionally with reserved marinade. Let the chops stand for 5 minutes before serving.

PER SERVING *1 pork chop equals 246 cal., 8 g fat (3 g sat. fat), 86 mg chol., 284 mg sodium, 11 g carb., trace fiber, 30 g pro.* **Diabetic Exchanges:** *4 lean meat, 1 starch.*

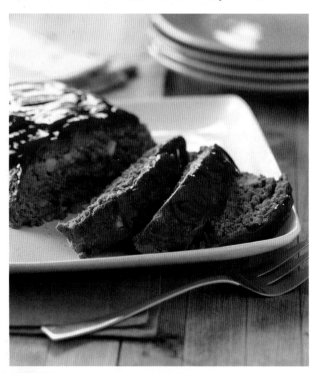

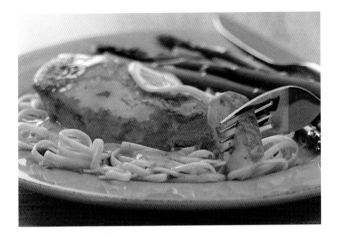

Chicken in Creamy Gravy

This lightened-up meal idea uses convenient canned soup as the base for a savory gravy. It comes together in a snap.
—**JEAN LITTLE** CHARLOTTE, NC

START TO FINISH: 25 MIN. • **MAKES:** 4 SERVINGS

- 4 boneless skinless chicken breast halves (4 ounces each)
- 1 tablespoon canola oil
- 1 can (10¾ ounces) condensed cream of broccoli soup, undiluted
- ¼ cup fat-free milk
- 1 tablespoon minced fresh parsley
- 2 teaspoons lemon juice
- ⅛ teaspoon pepper
- ⅛ teaspoon Worcestershire sauce
- 4 lemon slices
  Hot cooked spaghetti, optional
  Additional minced fresh parsley, optional

1. In a nonstick skillet, cook chicken in oil until golden brown on both sides.
2. In a large bowl, combine the soup, milk, parsley, lemon juice, pepper and Worcestershire sauce. Pour over chicken. Top each chicken breast with a lemon slice. Reduce heat; cover and cook for 5 minutes or until a thermometer reads 170°. Serve with spaghetti if desired. Sprinkle with additional parsley if desired.
PER SERVING *1 serving (calculated without spaghetti) equals 242 cal., 12 g fat (3 g sat. fat), 73 mg chol., 643 mg sodium, 8 g carb., 1 g fiber, 26 g pro. **Diabetic Exchanges:** 3 lean meat, 1 fat, ½ starch.*

198 CALORIES Herbed Beef Tenderloin

It doesn't take a lot of seasoning to flavor this tender beef roast. A mild blend of rosemary, basil and garlic does the trick in this simple but sensational recipe.
—**RUTH ANDREWSON** LEAVENWORTH, WA

PREP: 5 MIN. • **BAKE:** 40 MIN. + STANDING • **MAKES:** 12 SERVINGS

- 1 beef tenderloin roast (3 pounds)
- 2 teaspoons olive oil
- 2 garlic cloves, minced
- 1½ teaspoons dried basil
- 1½ teaspoons dried rosemary, crushed
- 1 teaspoon salt
- 1 teaspoon pepper

1. Tie tenderloin at 2-in. intervals with kitchen string. Combine oil and garlic; brush over the meat. Combine the basil, rosemary, salt and pepper; sprinkle evenly over meat. Place beef roast on a rack in a shallow roasting pan.
2. Bake, uncovered, at 425° for 40-50 minutes or until meat reaches desired doneness (for medium-rare, a thermometer should read 145°; medium, 160°; well-done, 170°). Let stand for 10 minutes before slicing.
PER SERVING *3 ounces cooked beef equals 198 cal., 10 g fat (4 g sat. fat), 78 mg chol., 249 mg sodium, 1 g carb., trace fiber, 25 g pro. **Diabetic Exchange:** 3 lean meat.*

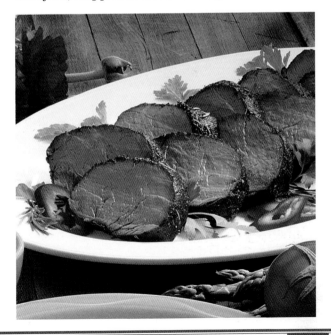

251-350 CALORIES

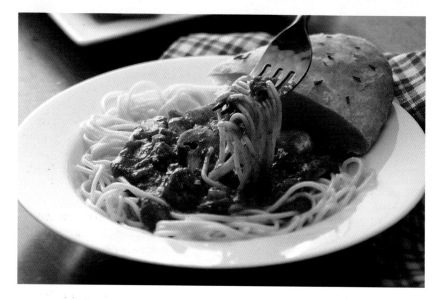

315 CALORIES
Hearty Spaghetti Sauce

My mom's easy sauce requires just minutes of preparation. Then it gently simmers until dinnertime.

—KIMBERLY ROCKWELL
CHARLOTTE, NC

PREP: 15 MIN. • **COOK:** 2 HOURS
MAKES: 12 SERVINGS

- 1½ pounds lean ground beef (90% lean)
- 1 large onion, chopped
- 1 large green pepper, chopped
- ½ pound sliced fresh mushrooms
- 3 cans (15 ounces each) crushed tomatoes
- 1 can (6 ounces) tomato paste
- ½ cup ketchup
- 1 tablespoon sugar
- 1 tablespoon chili powder
- 1 teaspoon salt
- 1 teaspoon garlic powder
- 1 teaspoon dried basil
- 1 teaspoon dried oregano
- 1 teaspoon Italian seasoning
- 1 teaspoon Worcestershire sauce
- ½ teaspoon pepper

In a large saucepan coated with cooking spray, cook beef, onion and green pepper over medium heat until meat is no longer pink; drain. Add the mushrooms; cook and stir for 2 minutes. Stir in the remaining ingredients. Bring to a boil. Reduce heat; cover and simmer for 1½ hours.
PER SERVING *⅔ cup sauce with ¾ cup cooked multigrain spaghetti equals 315 cal., 6 g fat (2 g sat. fat), 28 mg chol., 535 mg sodium, 47 g carb., 7 g fiber, 22 g pro.*

334 CALORIES
Tasty Tuna Casserole

This is not your usual tuna casserole. The macaroni and tuna are coated in a creamy sauce made from reduced-fat cream cheese, tomato sauce and a dash of oregano.

—ELSIE EPP NEWTON, KS

PREP: 20 MIN. • **BAKE:** 20 MIN.
MAKES: 4 SERVINGS

- 2 cups uncooked elbow macaroni
- 1 can (12 ounces) albacore white tuna in water
- 1 can (8 ounces) tomato sauce
- 4 ounces reduced-fat cream cheese, cubed
- 1 small onion, finely chopped
- ¼ teaspoon salt
- ½ teaspoon dried oregano

1. Cook macaroni according to package directions. Meanwhile, in a large bowl, combine the remaining ingredients. Drain macaroni; stir into tuna mixture.
2. Transfer to a 2-qt. baking dish coated with cooking spray. Cover and bake at 350° for 20-25 minutes or until heated through.
PER SERVING *1½ cups equals 334 cal., 9 g fat (5 g sat. fat), 56 mg chol., 851 mg sodium, 33 g carb., 2 g fiber, 29 g pro.* **Diabetic Exchanges:** *3 lean meat, 2 starch, 1 fat.*

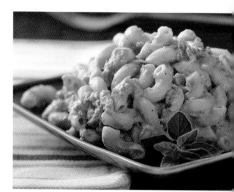

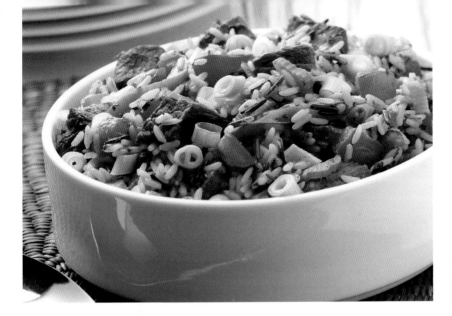

327 CALORIES Beef and Wild Rice Medley

A packaged rice mix speeds up the preparation of this meal-in-one entree. Cayenne pepper gives the beef a little kick, and an assortment of veggies add color and crunch.

—JANELLE CHRISTENSEN
BIG LAKE, MN

PREP: 5 MIN. • **COOK:** 40 MIN.
MAKES: 4 SERVINGS

- ½ **teaspoon garlic powder**
- ½ **teaspoon dried thyme**
- ⅛ **teaspoon cayenne pepper**
- 1 **pound beef top sirloin steak, cut into ¾-inch cubes**
- 1 **tablespoon canola oil**
- ¼ **cup sliced celery**
- ¼ **cup julienned green pepper**
- 2¼ **cups water**
- 1 **package (6 ounces) long grain and wild rice mix**
- 1 **small tomato, chopped**
- 2 **tablespoons chopped green onion**

1. In a small bowl, combine the garlic powder, thyme and cayenne. Sprinkle over beef.

2. In a large saucepan coated with cooking spray, cook beef in oil until no longer pink; drain. Stir in celery and green pepper; cook 2 minutes longer or until vegetables are crisp-tender. Stir in the water and rice mix with the contents of seasoning packet.

3. Bring to a boil. Reduce heat; cover and simmer for 23-28 minutes or until rice is tender. Stir in tomato; heat through. Sprinkle with onion.

PER SERVING *1 cup equals 327 cal., 10 g fat (2 g sat. fat), 63 mg chol., 626 mg sodium, 33 g carb., 1 g fiber, 26 g pro.* **Diabetic Exchanges:** *3 lean meat, 2 starch, ½ fat.*

350 CALORIES Apple-Cherry Pork Chops

You'll never want pork chops any other way once you try this recipe! I season the juicy chops with a fragrant herb rub and serve them with a scrumptious apple and cherry sauce.

—DORIS HEATH FRANKLIN, NC

START TO FINISH: 30 MIN.
MAKES: 2 SERVINGS

- 2 **boneless pork loin chops (½ inch thick and 5 ounces each)**
- ¼ **teaspoon dried thyme**
- ⅛ **teaspoon salt**
- 1 **tablespoon olive oil**
- ⅔ **cup apple juice**
- 1 **small red apple, sliced**
- 2 **tablespoons dried cherries or cranberries**
- 2 **tablespoons chopped onion**
- 1 **teaspoon cornstarch**
- 1 **tablespoon cold water**

1. Sprinkle pork chops with thyme and salt. In a large skillet, cook pork in oil for 3-4 minutes on each side or until a thermometer reads 145°. Remove and let meat stand for 5 minutes.

2. Meanwhile, in the same skillet, combine the apple juice, apple, cherries and onion. Bring to a boil. In a small bowl, combine the cornstarch and water until smooth; stir into skillet. Cook and stir for 1-2 minutes or until thickened. Spoon over pork chops.

PER SERVING *1 pork chop equals 350 cal., 15 g fat (4 g sat. fat), 68 mg chol., 191 mg sodium, 25 g carb., 2 g fiber, 28 g pro.*

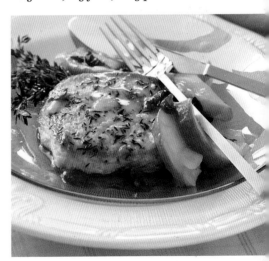

269 CALORIES

Baked Chicken Chimichangas

I developed this quick and easy recipe through trial and error. My friends all love it when I cook these because they're much healthier than the deep-fried chimichangas.
—**RICKEY MADDEN** CLINTON, SC

PREP: 20 MIN. • **BAKE:** 20 MIN. • **MAKES:** 6 SERVINGS

- 1½ cups cubed cooked chicken breast
- 1½ cups picante sauce, divided
- ½ cup shredded reduced-fat cheddar cheese
- ⅔ cup chopped green onions, divided
- 1 teaspoon ground cumin
- 1 teaspoon dried oregano
- 6 flour tortillas (8 inches), warmed
- 1 tablespoon butter, melted

1. In a small bowl, combine the chicken, ¾ cup picante sauce, cheese, ¼ cup onions, cumin and oregano.
2. Spoon ½ cup mixture down the center of each tortilla. Fold sides and ends over filling and roll up. Place seam side down in a 15-in. x 10-in. x 1-in. baking pan coated with cooking spray. Brush with butter.
3. Bake, uncovered, at 375° for 20-25 minutes or until heated through. Top with the remaining picante sauce and onions.

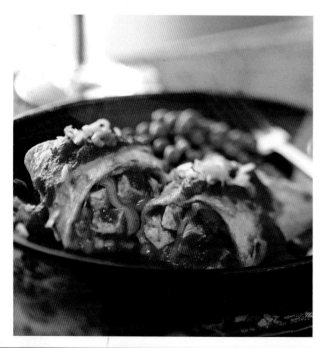

4. To freeze any extras, wrap chimichangas individually in foil. Transfer to a resealable plastic bag and freeze for up to 3 months.
PER SERVING *1 chimichanga equals 269 cal., 8 g fat (3 g sat. fat), 39 mg chol., 613 mg sodium, 31 g carb., 1 g fiber, 17 g pro.* **Diabetic Exchanges:** *2 lean meat, 1½ starch, 1 vegetable, ½ fat.*

255 CALORIES

Braised Southwest Beef Roast

Seasoned with Southwest zest, my slowly simmered beef roast is fork-tender and gets a little kick from salsa. It's one of our favorite ways to eat beef. Enjoy!
—**CATHY SESTAK** FREEBURG, MO

PREP: 20 MIN. • **COOK:** 2½ HOURS • **MAKES:** 5 SERVINGS

- 1½ teaspoons chili powder
- 1 teaspoon ground cumin
- ½ teaspoon garlic powder
- ½ teaspoon dried oregano
- 1 beef eye of round roast (2 pounds)
- 1 tablespoon canola oil
- 1 cup reduced-sodium beef broth
- 1¼ cups salsa
- ¼ cup water
- 1 bay leaf

1. In a small bowl, combine the chili powder, cumin, garlic powder and oregano; rub over roast. In a Dutch oven, brown meat in oil. Remove from the pan.
2. Gradually add the broth, stirring to loosen any browned bits from pan. Stir in salsa, water and bay leaf; return meat to pan. Bring to a boil. Reduce heat; cover and simmer for 2¼ to 2½ hours or until meat is fork-tender.
3. Set meat aside and keep warm. Bring pan juices to a boil. Cook, uncovered, for 10-15 minutes or until sauce is reduced to about 1⅓ cups; skim fat. Discard bay leaf. Serve sauce with meat.
PER SERVING *5 ounces cooked beef with ¼ cup sauce equals 255 cal., 9 g fat (2 g sat. fat), 84 mg chol., 451 mg sodium, 3 g carb., 2 g fiber, 35 g pro.* **Diabetic Exchanges:** *5 lean meat, ½ fat.*

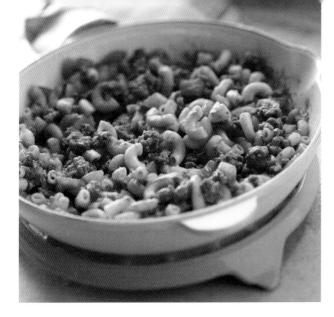

291 CALORIES Beef Macaroni Skillet

Here's a stovetop favorite that's tasty and filling. It's easy to prepare, even after a long day at work.
—**CARMEN EDWARDS** MIDLAND, TX

PREP: 15 MIN. • **COOK:** 30 MIN. • **MAKES:** 2 SERVINGS

- ½ pound lean ground beef (90% lean)
- ⅓ cup chopped onion
- ¼ cup chopped green pepper
- 1½ cups spicy hot V8 juice
- ½ cup uncooked elbow macaroni
- 1 teaspoon Worcestershire sauce
- ¼ teaspoon pepper

In a large skillet, cook the beef, onion and green pepper over medium heat until meat is no longer pink; drain. Stir in the remaining ingredients. Bring to a boil. Reduce heat; cover and simmer for 18-20 minutes or until macaroni is tender.
PER SERVING *1¼ cups equals 291 cal., 9 g fat (4 g sat. fat), 56 mg chol., 689 mg sodium, 25 g carb., 2 g fiber, 26 g pro.* **Diabetic Exchanges:** *3 lean meat, 2 vegetable, 1 starch.*

264 CALORIES Black Bean Taco Pizza

My husband absolutely loves this pizza. I make it several times a month, both for us and for our family and friends.
—**SHERIE NELSON** DULUTH, MN

PREP: 25 MIN. • **BAKE:** 10 MIN. • **MAKES:** 6 SERVINGS

- 1 tablespoon cornmeal
- 1 package (6½ ounces) pizza crust mix
- 1 bottle (8 ounces) taco sauce
- 2 medium tomatoes, seeded and chopped
- ¾ cup canned black beans
- ½ cup frozen corn
- 1 can (4 ounces) chopped green chilies
- 2 green onions, chopped
- 1½ cups (6 ounces) shredded reduced-fat Colby-Monterey Jack cheese
  Reduced-fat sour cream, optional

1. Coat a 12-in. pizza pan with cooking spray; sprinkle with cornmeal. Prepare pizza dough according to package directions. With floured hands, press dough onto prepared pan. Bake at 450° for 7-10 minutes or until lightly browned.
2. Spread taco sauce over crust to within 1 in. of edges. Top with tomatoes, beans, corn, chilies, onions and cheese.
3. Bake for 10-15 minutes or until cheese is melted and crust is golden brown. Serve with sour cream if desired.
PER SERVING *1 slice (calculated without sour cream) equals 264 cal., 6 g fat (4 g sat. fat), 15 mg chol., 783 mg sodium, 38 g carb., 4 g fiber, 14 g pro.* **Diabetic Exchanges:** *2½ starch, 1 medium-fat meat.*

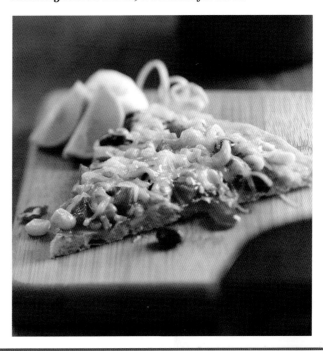

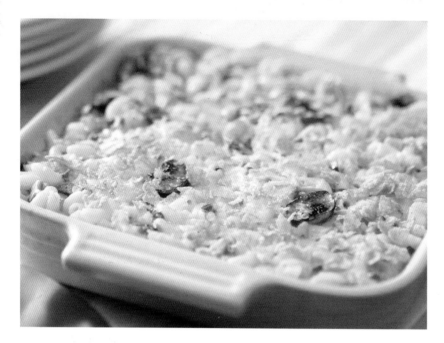

329 CALORIES

De-Lightful Tuna Casserole

This homemade tuna casserole will truly satisfy your family's craving for comfort food without all the fat!

—**COLLEEN WILLEY** HAMBURG, NY

PREP: 15 MIN. • **BAKE:** 25 MIN.
MAKES: 5 SERVINGS

- 1 **package (7 ounces) elbow macaroni**
- 1 **can (10¾ ounces) reduced-fat reduced-sodium condensed cream of mushroom soup, undiluted**
- 1 **cup sliced fresh mushrooms**
- 1 **cup (4 ounces) shredded reduced-fat cheddar cheese**
- 1 **cup fat-free milk**
- 1 **can (6 ounces) light water-packed tuna, drained and flaked**
- 2 **tablespoons diced pimientos**
- 3 **teaspoons dried minced onion**
- 1 **teaspoon ground mustard**
- ¼ **teaspoon salt**
- ⅓ **cup crushed cornflakes**

1. Cook macaroni according to package directions. Meanwhile, in a large bowl, combine the soup, mushrooms, cheese, milk, tuna, pimientos, onion, mustard and salt. Drain macaroni; add to tuna mixture and mix well.
2. Transfer to a 2-qt. baking dish coated with cooking spray. Sprinkle with cornflakes. Bake, uncovered, at 350° for 25-30 minutes or until bubbly.

PER SERVING *1¼ cups equals 329 cal., 8 g fat (4 g sat. fat), 32 mg chol., 684 mg sodium, 43 g carb., 2 g fiber, 23 g pro.* **Diabetic Exchanges:** *3 starch, 2 lean meat.*

282 CALORIES # Easy Chicken and Dumplings

Perfect for autumn nights, my main course is speedy, comforting and makes a delicious one-dish meal.

—**NANCY TUCK** ELK FALLS, KS

START TO FINISH: 30 MIN.
MAKES: 6 SERVINGS

- 3 **celery ribs, chopped**
- 1 **cup sliced fresh carrots**
- 3 **cans (14½ ounces each) reduced-sodium chicken broth**
- 3 **cups cubed cooked chicken breast**
- ½ **teaspoon poultry seasoning**
- ⅛ **teaspoon pepper**
- 1⅓ **cups reduced-fat biscuit/baking mix**
- ⅔ **cup fat-free milk**

1. In a Dutch oven coated with cooking spray, saute celery and carrots for 5 minutes. Stir in the broth, chicken, poultry seasoning and pepper. Bring to a boil; reduce heat to a gentle simmer.
2. For dumplings, combine biscuit mix and milk. Drop batter by tablespoonfuls onto simmering broth. Cover and simmer for 10-15 minutes or until a toothpick inserted in a dumpling comes out clean (do not lift the cover while simmering).

PER SERVING *1 cup chicken mixture with 3 dumplings equals 282 cal., 5 g fat (1 g sat. fat), 60 mg chol., 1,022 mg sodium, 29 g carb., 1 g fiber, 28 g pro.* **Diabetic Exchanges:** *3 lean meat, 1½ starch, 1 vegetable, ½ fat.*

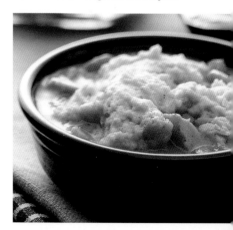

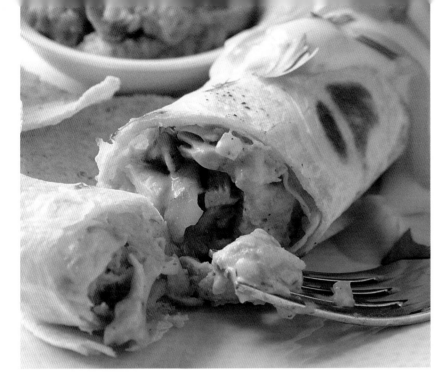

until heated through and cheese is melted. Sprinkle with cilantro.

PER SERVING *1 enchilada equals 263 cal., 10 g fat (4 g sat. fat), 59 mg chol., 472 mg sodium, 20 g carb., 1 g fiber, 22 g pro.* **Diabetic Exchanges:** *2 lean meat, 1½ starch, ½ fat.*

304 CALORIES Snapper with Spicy Pineapple Glaze

Ginger and cayenne bring spice to this tangy treatment for red snapper fillets. Sweet pineapple preserves round out the delectable combination of flavors.

—TASTE OF HOME TEST KITCHEN

START TO FINISH: 30 MIN.
MAKES: 4 SERVINGS

- ½ cup pineapple preserves
- 2 tablespoons rice vinegar
- 2 teaspoons minced fresh gingerroot
- 2 garlic cloves, minced
- ¾ teaspoon salt, divided
- ¼ teaspoon cayenne pepper
- 4 red snapper fillets (6 ounces each)
- 3 teaspoons olive oil

1. In a small bowl, combine the preserves, vinegar, ginger, garlic, ½ teaspoon salt and cayenne; set aside. Place fillets on a broiler pan coated with cooking spray. Rub fillets with oil; sprinkle with remaining salt.

2. Broil 4-6 in. from the heat for 5 minutes. Baste with half of the glaze. Broil 5-7 minutes longer or until fish flakes easily with a fork. Baste with remaining glaze.

PER SERVING *1 fillet equals 304 cal., 6 g fat (1 g sat. fat), 63 mg chol., 552 mg sodium, 27 g carb., trace fiber, 35 g pro.* **Diabetic Exchanges:** *5 lean meat, 2 starch.*

263 CALORIES

Turkey Pecan Enchiladas

A friend passed along this recipe, and I've served it at church potlucks many times since. It's nice because it's creamy, just a little spicy and different from the norm.

—CATHY HUPPE GEORGETOWN, MA

PREP: 25 MIN. • **BAKE:** 45 MIN.
MAKES: 12 SERVINGS

- 1 medium onion, chopped
- 4 ounces reduced-fat cream cheese
- 1 tablespoon water
- 1 teaspoon ground cumin
- ¼ teaspoon pepper
- ⅛ teaspoon salt
- 4 cups cubed cooked turkey breast
- ¼ cup chopped pecans, toasted
- 12 flour tortillas (6 inches), warmed
- 1 can (10¾ ounces) reduced-fat reduced-sodium condensed cream of chicken soup, undiluted
- 1 cup (8 ounces) reduced-fat sour cream
- 1 cup fat-free milk
- 2 tablespoons canned chopped green chilies
- ½ cup shredded reduced-fat cheddar cheese
- 2 tablespoons minced fresh cilantro

1. In a small nonstick skillet coated with cooking spray, cook and stir onion over medium heat until tender. Set aside.

2. In a large bowl, beat the cream cheese, water, cumin, pepper and salt until smooth. Stir in the onion, turkey and pecans.

3. Spoon ⅓ cup turkey mixture down the center of each tortilla. Roll up and place seam side down in a 13-in. x 9-in. baking dish coated with cooking spray. Combine the soup, sour cream, milk and chilies; pour over enchiladas.

4. Cover and bake at 350° for 40 minutes. Uncover; sprinkle with cheese. Bake 5 minutes longer or

318 CALORIES Colorful Beef Stir-Fry

This recipe is similar to beef stir-fries that I've had before. I really like the easy sesame-ginger marinade and the vibrant mix of vegetables.

—DEB BLENDERMANN BOULDER, CO

PREP: 35 MIN. + MARINATING • **COOK:** 15 MIN. • **MAKES:** 4 CUPS

- ¼ cup reduced-sodium soy sauce
- 1 tablespoon honey
- 2 teaspoons sesame oil
- 3 garlic cloves, minced
- ⅛ teaspoon ground ginger
- ½ pound boneless beef sirloin steak, thinly sliced
- 4½ teaspoons cornstarch
- ½ cup reduced-sodium beef broth
- 1½ teaspoons canola oil, divided
- 1 small green pepper, cut into chunks
- 1 small onion, cut into chunks
- 1 medium carrot, julienned
- ¼ cup sliced celery
- 1 small zucchini, julienned
- ½ cup fresh snow peas
- ½ cup canned bean sprouts, rinsed and drained
  Hot cooked rice or linguine, optional

1. In a small bowl, combine the first five ingredients. Place beef in a large resealable plastic bag; add half of the marinade. Seal bag and turn to coat; refrigerate for at least 2 hours. Cover and refrigerate the remaining marinade.

2. In a small bowl, combine cornstarch and broth until smooth. Stir in reserved marinade; set aside. Drain and discard marinade from beef. In a large nonstick skillet or wok coated with cooking spray, cook beef in 1 teaspoon oil until no longer pink; drain. Remove and keep warm.

3. In the same pan, stir-fry green pepper and onion in remaining oil for 2 minutes. Add carrot and celery; cook 2-3 minutes longer. Add zucchini and snow peas; stir-fry for 1 minute. Stir in bean sprouts and heat through.

4. Stir broth mixture and stir into vegetable mixture. Bring to a boil; cook and stir for 1-2 minutes or until thickened. Return beef to the pan; heat through. Serve over rice or linguine if desired.

PER SERVING *1 cup (calculated without rice) equals 318 cal., 8 g fat (2 g sat. fat), 43 mg chol., 542 mg sodium, 41 g carb., 4 g fiber, 21 g pro.* **Diabetic Exchanges:** *2 lean meat, 1 starch, ½ fat.*

314 CALORIES Fantastic Fish Tacos

Searching for a lighter substitute to traditional fried fish tacos, I came up with this entree. It's been a hit with friends and family. Cutting calories doesn't have to mean cutting flavor!

—JENNIFER PALMER RANCHO CUCAMONGA, CA

START TO FINISH: 25 MIN. • **MAKES:** 4 SERVINGS

- ½ cup fat-free mayonnaise
- 1 tablespoon lime juice
- 2 teaspoons fat-free milk
- ⅓ cup dry bread crumbs
- 2 tablespoons salt-free lemon-pepper seasoning
- 1 egg, lightly beaten
- 1 teaspoon water
- 1 pound tilapia fillets, cut into 1-inch strips
- 4 corn tortillas (6 inches), warmed
- 1 cup coleslaw mix
- 2 medium tomatoes, diced
- 1 cup (4 ounces) shredded reduced-fat Mexican cheese blend
- 1 tablespoon minced fresh cilantro

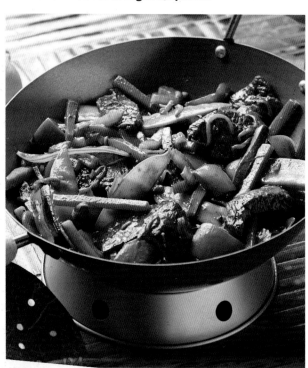

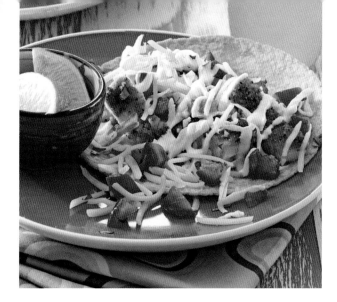

1. In a small bowl, combine the mayonnaise, lime juice and milk; cover and refrigerate until serving.
2. In a shallow bowl, combine bread crumbs and lemon-pepper. In another shallow bowl, combine egg and water. Dip fish in egg mixture, then roll in crumbs.
3. In a large nonstick skillet coated with cooking spray, cook fish over medium-high heat for 3-4 minutes on each side or until it flakes easily with a fork. Spoon onto tortillas; top with coleslaw mix, tomatoes, cheese and cilantro. Drizzle with mayonnaise mixture.

PER SERVING *1 taco equals 314 cal., 10 g fat (4 g sat. fat), 99 mg chol., 659 mg sodium, 32 g carb., 3 g fiber, 30 g pro.* **Diabetic Exchanges:** *4 lean meat, 2 starch.*

271 CALORIES Favorite Irish Stew

Lamb is a great source of protein and adds delicious taste to this classic stew. If it's not at your grocery store, try using beef stew meat instead.
—**TASTE OF HOME TEST KITCHEN**

PREP: 20 MIN. • **COOK:** 1¾ HOURS
MAKES: 8 SERVINGS (2½ QUARTS)

- ⅓ cup plus 1 tablespoon all-purpose flour, divided
- 1½ pounds lamb stew meat, cut into 1-inch cubes
- 3 tablespoons olive oil, divided
- 3 medium onions, chopped
- 3 garlic cloves, minced
- 4 cups reduced-sodium beef broth
- 2 medium potatoes, peeled and cubed
- 4 medium carrots, cut into 1-inch pieces
- 1 cup frozen peas
- 1 teaspoon salt
- 1 teaspoon dried thyme
- ½ teaspoon pepper
- ½ teaspoon Worcestershire sauce
- 2 tablespoons water

1. Place ⅓ cup flour in a large resealable plastic bag. Add lamb, a few pieces at a time, and shake to coat.
2. In a Dutch oven, brown lamb in batches in 2 tablespoons oil. Remove and set aside. In the same pan, saute onions in remaining oil until tender. Add garlic; cook 1 minute longer.
3. Add broth, stirring to loosen browned bits from pan. Return lamb to the pan. Bring to a boil. Reduce heat; cover and simmer for 1 hour or until meat is tender.
4. Add potatoes and carrots; cover and cook for 20 minutes. Stir in peas; cook 5-10 minutes longer or until vegetables are tender.
5. Add seasonings and Worcestershire sauce. Combine remaining flour with water until smooth; stir into stew. Bring to a boil; cook and stir for 2 minutes or until thickened.

PER SERVING *1¼ cup equals 271 cal., 10 g fat (2 g sat. fat), 58 mg chol., 618 mg sodium, 24 g carb., 4 g fiber, 22 g pro.* **Diabetic Exchanges:** *2 lean meat, 1 starch, 1 vegetable, 1 fat.*

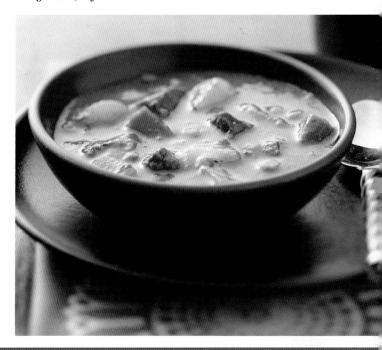

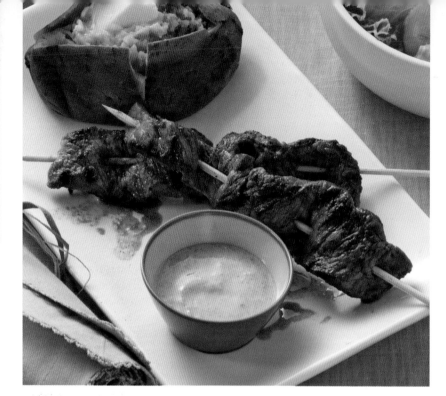

258 CALORIES Beef Kabobs with Chutney Sauce

I created this speedy grilled entree for our daughter, a fan of Indian food. The mango chutney and subtle curry give the beef a sweet and spicy flavor.

—JUDY THOMPSON ANKENY, IA

PREP: 15 MIN. + MARINATING
GRILL: 5 MIN.
MAKES: 8 KABOBS (ABOUT ½ CUP SAUCE)

- ¼ cup mango chutney
- 1 tablespoon water
- 1 tablespoon cider vinegar
- 1 teaspoon curry powder
- ¼ teaspoon cayenne pepper
- 1 pound beef top sirloin steak, cut into ¼-inch strips

CHUTNEY SAUCE

- ½ cup plain yogurt
- 3 tablespoons mango chutney
- 1 teaspoon lemon juice
- ½ teaspoon curry powder
- ¼ teaspoon ground cumin
- ⅛ teaspoon cayenne pepper

1. In a large resealable plastic bag, combine the first five ingredients; add the beef. Seal bag and turn to coat; refrigerate overnight.

2. In a small bowl, combine the sauce ingredients. Cover and refrigerate until serving.

3. Drain and discard marinade. Thread beef onto eight metal or soaked wooden skewers.

4. Moisten a paper towel with cooking oil; using long-handled tongs, lightly coat the grill rack. Grill kabobs, covered, over medium heat or broil 4 in. from the heat for 4-6 minutes or until meat reaches desired doneness, turning occasionally. Serve with sauce.

PER SERVING *2 skewers with 2 tablespoons sauce equals 258 cal., 6 g fat (2 g sat. fat), 50 mg chol., 321 mg sodium, 23 g carb., trace fiber, 25 g pro.* **Diabetic Exchanges:** *3 lean meat, 1½ starch.*

282 CALORIES
Enchilada Lasagna

The whole family will love the familiar Southwestern flavors in this marvelous and fun lasagna.

—JULIE CACKLER
WEST DES MOINES, IA

PREP: 25 MIN. • **BAKE:** 20 MIN. + STANDING
MAKES: 8 SERVINGS

- 1 pound lean ground turkey
- 1 large onion, chopped
- 1 large green pepper, chopped
- 1 small sweet red pepper, chopped
- 1 package (8 ounces) fat-free cream cheese
- 1 teaspoon chili powder
- 1 can (10 ounces) enchilada sauce
- 6 whole wheat flour tortillas (8 inches)
- 1 cup (4 ounces) shredded reduced-fat Mexican cheese blend
  Salsa and sour cream, optional

1. In a large skillet, cook the turkey, onion and peppers over medium heat until meat is no longer pink; drain. Stir in the cream cheese and chili powder.

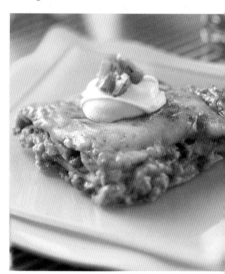

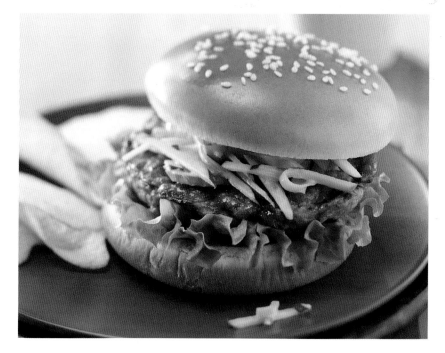

2. Pour enchilada sauce in a shallow bowl. Dip tortillas in sauce to coat. Place two tortillas in a 13-in. x 9-in. baking dish coated with cooking spray; spread with half of the turkey mixture. Sprinkle with 1/3 cup cheese. Repeat layers. Top with remaining tortillas and cheese.

3. Cover and freeze for up to 3 months or bake, uncovered, at 400° for 20-25 minutes or until heated through and cheese is melted. Let stand for 10 minutes before serving. Serve with salsa and sour cream if desired.

TO USE FROZEN LASAGNA *Thaw in the refrigerator overnight. Remove from refrigerator 30 minutes before baking. Bake as directed.*

PER SERVING *1 piece (calculated without salsa and sour cream) equals 282 cal., 11 g fat (3 g sat. fat), 57 mg chol., 697 mg sodium, 27 g carb., 2 g fiber, 22 g pro.* ***Diabetic Exchanges:*** *2 lean meat, 1½ starch, 1 fat.*

---

312 CALORIES

Buffalo Chicken Burgers with Tangy Slaw

Here's my way of enjoying the flavor of Buffalo wings while limiting fat and calories. These juicy chicken burgers will be the talk of the table. No one will guess they're lightened up!

—JEANNE HOLT
MENDOTA HEIGHTS, MN

PREP: 25 MIN. • **BROIL:** 10 MIN.
MAKES: 4 SERVINGS

SLAW
- ¼ **cup thinly sliced celery**
- ¼ **cup shredded peeled apple**
- 2 **tablespoons fat-free blue cheese salad dressing**
- 1 **teaspoon finely chopped walnuts**

SAUCE
- 3 **tablespoons Louisiana-style hot sauce**
- 2 **teaspoons ketchup**
- 2 **teaspoons reduced-fat butter, melted**

BURGERS
- 2 **tablespoons chopped sweet red pepper**
- 2 **tablespoons plus 4 teaspoons thinly sliced green onions, divided**
- 1 **tablespoon unsweetened applesauce**
- ¼ **teaspoon salt**
- ¼ **teaspoon garlic salt**
- ¼ **teaspoon pepper**
- 1 **pound ground chicken**
- 4 **lettuce leaves**
- 4 **hamburger buns, split**

1. In a small bowl, combine the celery, apple, salad dressing and walnuts. In another small bowl, combine the hot sauce, ketchup and butter; set aside.

2. In a large bowl, combine the red pepper, 2 tablespoons green onion, applesauce, salt, garlic salt and pepper. Crumble chicken over mixture and mix well. Shape into four burgers.

3. Broil 6 in. from the heat for 5-7 minutes on each side or until a thermometer reads 165° and juices run clear, basting occasionally with reserved sauce.

4. Serve on lettuce-lined buns; top each with 2 tablespoons slaw and sprinkle with the remaining green onion.

NOTE *This recipe was tested with Land O'Lakes light stick butter.*

PER SERVING *1 burger equals 312 cal., 12 g fat (4 g sat. fat), 78 mg chol., 682 mg sodium, 29 g carb., 2 g fiber, 23 g pro.* ***Diabetic Exchanges:*** *3 lean meat, 2 starch.*

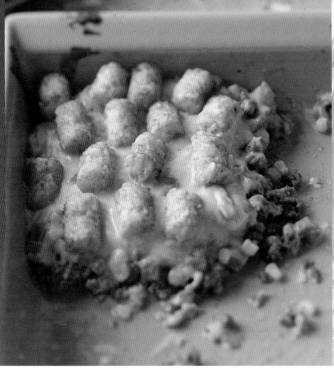

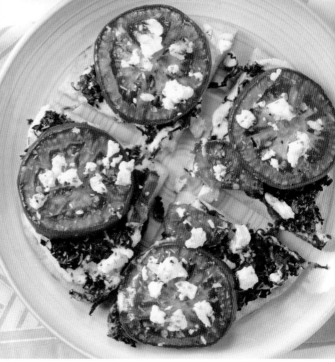

340 CALORIES
Makeover Tater-Topped Casserole

I love Tater Tots and my delicious casserole recipe, but I wanted it to be healthier. This lighter dish tastes great and keeps all the tots—and taste!

—SCOTT WOODWARD ELKHORN, WI

PREP: 15 MIN. • **BAKE:** 55 MIN.
MAKES: 8 SERVINGS

- 1 pound lean ground beef (90% lean)
- ½ pound extra-lean ground turkey
- 1 package (16 ounces) frozen mixed vegetables, thawed and drained
- ¾ cup French-fried onions
- 1 can (10¾ ounces) reduced-fat reduced-sodium condensed cream of celery soup, undiluted
- 1 can (10¾ ounces) reduced-fat reduced-sodium condensed cream of chicken soup, undiluted
- ½ cup fat-free milk
- 4 cups frozen Tater Tots, thawed

1. In a large skillet, cook beef and turkey over medium heat until no longer pink. In a 13-in. x 9-in. baking dish coated with cooking spray, layer the meat mixture, vegetables and onions.

2. In a small bowl, combine soups and milk; spread over onions. Top with Tater Tots. Bake, uncovered, at 350° for 55-60 minutes or until golden brown.

PER SERVING *1 cup equals 340 cal., 14 g fat (4 g sat. fat), 44 mg chol., 657 mg sodium, 33 g carb., 4 g fiber, 22 g pro.*

320 CALORIES Greek Pizzas

Customizable pita pizzas are a great way to please the whole family for lunch or dinner. Try using different vegetable-and-cheese blends to change things up. Sliced zucchini works well instead of tomato.

—DORIS ALLERS PORTAGE, MI

START TO FINISH: 30 MIN.
MAKES: 4 SERVINGS

- 4 pita breads (6 inches)
- 1 cup reduced-fat ricotta cheese
- ½ teaspoon garlic powder
- 1 package (10 ounces) frozen chopped spinach, thawed and squeezed dry
- 3 medium tomatoes, sliced
- ¾ cup crumbled feta cheese
- ¾ teaspoon dried basil

1. Place pita breads on a baking sheet. Combine ricotta cheese and garlic powder; spread over pitas. Top with spinach, tomatoes, feta cheese and basil.

2. Bake at 400° for 12-15 minutes or until bread is lightly browned.

PER SERVING *1 pizza equals 320 cal., 7 g fat (4 g sat. fat), 26 mg chol., 642 mg sodium, 46 g carb., 6 g fiber, 17 g pro.* **Diabetic Exchanges:** *2 starch, 2 vegetable, 1 lean meat, 1 fat.*

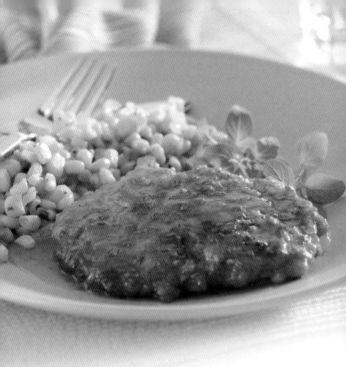

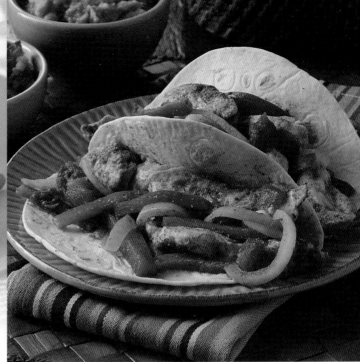

298 CALORIES Honey Lemon Schnitzel

These pork cutlets are coated in a sweet sauce with honey, lemon juice and butter. Good enough for company, they make a quick weeknight meal, too.
—**CAROLE FRASER** NORTH YORK, ON

START TO FINISH: 25 MIN.
MAKES: 4 SERVINGS

- 2 **tablespoons all-purpose flour**
- ½ **teaspoon salt**
- ½ **teaspoon pepper**
- 4 **pork sirloin cutlets (4 ounces each)**
- 2 **tablespoons butter**
- ¼ **cup lemon juice**
- ¼ **cup honey**

1. In a large resealable plastic bag, combine flour, salt and pepper. Add pork, two pieces at a time, and shake to coat. In a large skillet, cook the pork in butter over medium heat for 3-4 minutes on each side or until juices run clear. Remove; keep warm.

2. Add lemon juice and honey to the skillet; cook and stir for 3 minutes or until thickened. Return pork to pan; cook for 2-3 minutes longer or until heated through.

PER SERVING *1 cutlet equals 298 cal., 13 g fat (6 g sat. fat), 88 mg chol., 393 mg sodium, 22 g carb., trace fiber, 24 g pro.*

340 CALORIES
Baked Chicken Fajitas

I can't remember when or where I found this recipe, but I've used it nearly every week since. We like it with hot sauce for added spice.
—**AMY TRINKLE** MILWAUKEE, WI

PREP: 15 MIN. • **BAKE:** 20 MIN.
MAKES: 6 SERVINGS

- 1 **pound boneless skinless chicken breasts, cut into thin strips**
- 1 **can (14½ ounces) diced tomatoes and green chilies, drained**
- 1 **medium onion, cut into thin strips**
- 1 **each medium green and sweet red peppers, cut into thin strips**
- 2 **tablespoons canola oil**
- 2 **teaspoons chili powder**
- 2 **teaspoons ground cumin**
- ¼ **teaspoon salt**
- 12 **flour tortillas (6 inches), warmed**

1. In a 13-in. x 9-in. baking dish coated with cooking spray, combine the chicken, tomatoes, onion and peppers. Combine the oil, chili powder, cumin and salt. Drizzle over chicken mixture; toss to coat.

2. Bake, uncovered, at 400° for 20-25 minutes or until chicken is no longer pink and vegetables are tender. Spoon onto tortillas; fold in sides.

PER SERVING *2 fajitas equals 340 cal., 8 g fat (1 g sat. fat), 44 mg chol., 330 mg sodium, 41 g carb., 5 g fiber, 27 g pro.* **Diabetic Exchanges:** *2 starch, 2 lean meat, 2 vegetable, 1 fat.*

66 I lost significant weight over the last year by counting calories and watching portion sizes. For dinner, I fix what I normally would for my family, but I limit my intake. If I get hungry between meals, I eat a 100-calorie snack. If I can lose weight by doing this, anyone can. 99

—MICHELLE NICHOLS

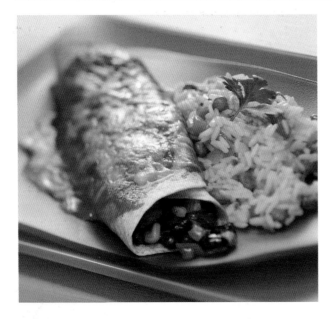

292 CALORIES

Black Bean Veggie Enchiladas

I created this tasty dish one night when we were in the mood for enchiladas, but didn't want all the fat and calories of the traditional ones. I used ingredients that I had on hand, and now the recipe is a family favorite!

—**NICOLE BARNETT** CENTENNIAL, CO

PREP: 30 MIN. • **BAKE:** 25 MIN. • **MAKES:** 6 ENCHILADAS

- 1 small onion, chopped
- 1 small green pepper, chopped
- ½ cup sliced fresh mushrooms
- 2 teaspoons olive oil
- 1 garlic clove, minced
- 1 can (15 ounces) black beans, rinsed and drained
- ¾ cup frozen corn, thawed

- 1 can (4 ounces) chopped green chilies
- 2 tablespoons reduced-sodium taco seasoning
- 1 teaspoon dried cilantro flakes
- 6 whole wheat tortillas (8 inches), warmed
- ½ cup enchilada sauce
- ¾ cup shredded reduced-fat Mexican cheese blend

1. In a large skillet, saute the onion, green pepper and mushrooms in oil until crisp-tender. Add garlic; cook 1 minute longer. Add the beans, corn, chilies, taco seasoning and cilantro; cook for 2-3 minutes or until heated through.

2. Spoon ½ cup bean mixture down the center of each tortilla. Roll up and place seam side down in a greased 13-in. x 9-in. baking dish. Top with enchilada sauce and cheese.

3. Bake, uncovered, at 350° for 25-30 minutes or until heated through.

PER SERVING *1 enchilada equals 292 cal., 8 g fat (2 g sat. fat), 10 mg chol., 759 mg sodium, 43 g carb., 6 g fiber, 13 g pro.*

278 CALORIES ## Baked Mostaccioli

This is my signature baked pasta that I often serve for dinner parties. It always gets tons of compliments!

—**DONNA EBERT** RICHFIELD, WI

PREP: 35 MIN. • **BAKE:** 30 MIN. • **MAKES:** 6 SERVINGS

- 8 ounces uncooked mostaccioli
- ½ pound lean ground turkey
- 1 small onion, chopped
- 1 can (14½ ounces) diced tomatoes, undrained
- 1 can (6 ounces) tomato paste
- ⅓ cup water
- 1 teaspoon dried oregano

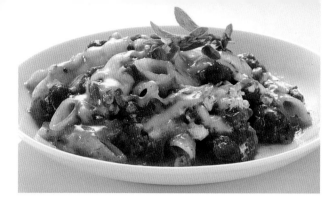

½ teaspoon salt
⅛ teaspoon pepper
2 cups (16 ounces) fat-free cottage cheese
1 teaspoon dried marjoram
1½ cups (6 ounces) shredded part-skim mozzarella
cheese
¼ cup grated Parmesan cheese

1. Cook mostaccioli according to package directions. Meanwhile, in a large saucepan, cook turkey and onion over medium heat until meat is no longer pink; drain if necessary.
2. Stir in the tomatoes, tomato paste, water, oregano, salt and pepper. Bring to a boil. Reduce heat; cover and simmer for 15 minutes.
3. In a small bowl, combine cottage cheese and marjoram; set aside. Drain mostaccioli.
4. Spread ½ cup meat sauce into an 11-in. x 7-in. baking dish coated with cooking spray. Layer with half of the mostaccioli, meat sauce and mozzarella cheese. Top with cottage cheese mixture. Layer with remaining mostaccioli, meat sauce and mozzarella cheese. Sprinkle with Parmesan cheese (dish will be full).
5. Bake, uncovered, at 350° for 30-40 minutes or until bubbly and heated through.
PER SERVING *1⅓ cups equals 278 cal., 7 g fat (3 g sat. fat), 39 mg chol., 607 mg sodium, 32 g carb., 3 g fiber, 23 g pro.* ***Diabetic Exchanges:*** *3 medium-fat meat, 2 vegetable, 1½ starch.*

303 CALORIES Broccoli-Turkey Casserole

I have a lot of company at Thanksgiving, and I enjoy making new things for them. I came up with this recipe as a great way to use up the leftover turkey.
—KELLIE MULLEAVY LAMBERTVILLE, MI

PREP: 20 MIN. • **BAKE:** 45 MIN. • **MAKES:** 6 SERVINGS

1½ cups fat-free milk
1 can (10¾ ounces) reduced-fat reduced-sodium condensed cream of chicken soup, undiluted
1 carton (8 ounces) egg substitute
¼ cup reduced-fat sour cream
½ teaspoon pepper
¼ teaspoon poultry seasoning
⅛ teaspoon salt
2½ cups cubed cooked turkey breast
1 package (16 ounces) frozen chopped broccoli, thawed and drained
2 cups seasoned stuffing cubes
1 cup (4 ounces) shredded reduced-fat cheddar cheese, divided

1. In a large bowl, combine the milk, soup, egg substitute, sour cream, pepper, poultry seasoning and salt. Stir in the turkey, broccoli, stuffing cubes and ¾ cup cheese. Transfer to a 13-in. x 9-in. baking dish coated with cooking spray.
2. Bake, uncovered, at 350° for 40 minutes. Sprinkle with remaining cheese. Bake 5-10 minutes longer or until a knife inserted near the center comes out clean. Let stand for 5 minutes before serving.
PER SERVING *1 serving equals 303 cal., 7 g fat (4 g sat. fat), 72 mg chol., 762 mg sodium, 26 g carb., 3 g fiber, 33 g pro.* ***Diabetic Exchanges:*** *3 lean meat, 1½ starch, 1 vegetable, 1 fat.*

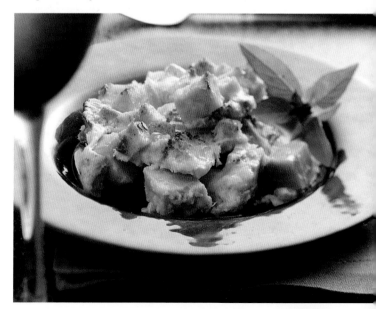

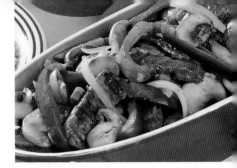

254 CALORIES "Little Kick" Jalapeno Burgers

I lightened up one of my husband's favorite burger recipes, and although the original was good, we actually like this version better!

—DAWN DHOOGHE CONCORD, NC

START TO FINISH: 25 MIN.
MAKES: 6 SERVINGS

- 2 **jalapeno peppers, seeded and finely chopped**
- 2 **tablespoons minced fresh cilantro**
- 2 **tablespoons light beer or water**
- 2 **dashes hot pepper sauce**
- 2 **garlic cloves, minced**
- ½ **teaspoon pepper**
- ¼ **teaspoon salt**
- ¼ **teaspoon cayenne pepper**
- 1 **pound extra-lean ground turkey**
- 3 **slices pepper jack cheese, cut in half**
- 6 **dinner rolls, split**
- 6 **tablespoons salsa**
- 6 **tablespoons fat-free sour cream**
- 6 **tablespoons shredded lettuce**

1. In a large bowl, combine the first eight ingredients. Crumble turkey over mixture and mix well. Shape into six patties.

2. Moisten a paper towel with cooking oil; using long-handled tongs, lightly coat the grill rack. Grill burgers, covered, over medium heat or broil 4 in. from the heat for 2-3 minutes on each side or until a thermometer reads 165° and juices run clear.

3. Top with cheese; cover and grill 1-2 minutes longer or until cheese is melted. Serve on rolls with salsa, sour cream and lettuce.

NOTE *Wear disposable gloves when cutting hot peppers; the oils can burn skin. Avoid touching your face.*

PER SERVING *1 burger equals 254 cal., 7 g fat (2 g sat. fat), 61 mg chol., 471 mg sodium, 23 g carb., 2 g fiber, 26 g pro.* **Diabetic Exchanges:** *3 lean meat, 1½ starch.*

254 CALORIES Beef Vegetable Stir-Fry

This simple stir-fry is often requested. You can replace the beef with chicken, fish or even tofu. It's delicious served over brown rice that's been seasoned with soy sauce, basil and ginger.

—BETSY LARIMER SOMERSET, PA

START TO FINISH: 25 MIN.
MAKES: 4 SERVINGS

- 4½ **teaspoons cornstarch**
- 4 **tablespoons reduced–sodium soy sauce, divided**
- 1 **pound boneless beef sirloin steak, cut into 2-inch strips**
- 2 **medium green pepper, cut into strips**
- 2 **medium onions, halved and thinly sliced**
- 1 **tablespoon canola oil**
- ½ **pound sliced fresh mushrooms**

1. In a bowl, combine cornstarch and 2 tablespoons soy sauce until smooth. Add beef; stir to coat.

2. In a large skillet or wok, stir-fry the green peppers and onions in oil for 3 minutes; add beef. Cook and stir for 3 minutes. Add mushrooms. Cook and stir for 3-5 minutes or until vegetables are tender and meat is no longer pink. Stir in remaining soy sauce.

PER SERVING *1 cup equals 254 cal., 9 g fat (3 g sat. fat), 63 mg chol., 658 mg sodium, 17 g carb., 3 g fiber, 26 g pro.* **Diabetic Exchanges:** *3 lean meat, 3 vegetable, ½ fat.*

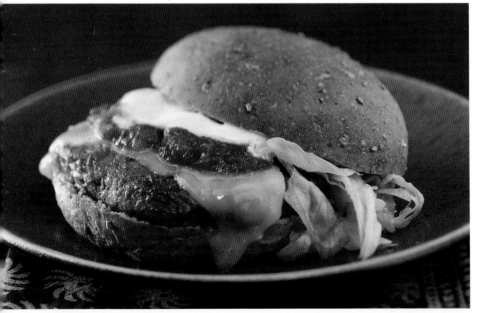

350 CALORIES Fettuccine
with Black Bean Sauce

When my husband needed to go on a
heart-smart diet, I had to come up with
new ways to get more vegetables into
our daily menus. This meatless
spaghetti sauce is especially good with
spinach fettuccine.
—**MARIANNE NEUMAN** EAST TROY, WI

START TO FINISH: 30 MIN.
MAKES: 5 SERVINGS

- 6 ounces uncooked fettuccine
- 1 small green pepper, chopped
- 1 small onion, chopped
- 1 tablespoon olive oil
- 2 cups garden-style pasta sauce
- 1 can (15 ounces) black beans,
  rinsed and drained
- 2 tablespoons minced fresh basil or
  2 teaspoons dried basil
- 1 teaspoon dried oregano
- ½ teaspoon fennel seed
- ¼ teaspoon garlic salt
- 1 cup (4 ounces) shredded
  part-skim mozzarella cheese

1. Cook fettuccine according to
package directions. Meanwhile, in
a saucepan, saute green pepper and
onion in oil until tender. Stir in pasta
sauce, black beans and seasonings.
2. Bring to a boil. Reduce heat;
simmer, uncovered, for 5 minutes.
Drain fettuccine. Top with sauce
and sprinkle with cheese.
NOTE *This recipe was tested with
Ragu Super Vegetable Primavera
pasta sauce.*
PER SERVING *¾ cup pasta with ¾
cup sauce and 3 tablespoons cheese
equals 350 cal., 10 g fat (3 g sat.
fat), 17 mg chol., 761 mg sodium,
51 g carb., 8 g fiber, 16 g pro.
Diabetic Exchanges: 2½ starch,
2 vegetable, 1 lean meat, 1 fat.*

262 CALORIES Chicken
with Mustard Gravy

Rich gravy made with honey mustard
and sour cream drapes nicely over these
golden-brown chicken breasts. The
dish is sure to please the whole family.
—**TASTE OF HOME TEST KITCHEN**

START TO FINISH: 25 MIN.
MAKES: 4 SERVINGS

- 4 boneless skinless chicken breast
  halves (6 ounces each)
- ½ teaspoon salt, divided
- ¼ teaspoon pepper, divided
- 2 tablespoons reduced-fat butter
- 4 teaspoons honey mustard
- 1 tablespoon milk
- ½ teaspoon dried basil
- ½ teaspoon dried parsley flakes
- ½ cup reduced-fat sour cream

1. Rub chicken with ¼ teaspoon
salt and ⅛ teaspoon pepper. In a
large skillet over medium heat, cook
chicken in butter for 6-8 minutes
on each side or until a thermometer
reads 170°. Remove chicken and
keep warm.
2. In the same skillet, combine the
mustard, milk, basil, parsley, and
remaining salt and pepper. Cook
and stir over low heat until heated
through. Remove from the heat; stir
in sour cream. Serve with chicken.
PER SERVING *1 chicken breast half
with 2 tablespoons gravy equals 262
cal., 10 g fat (5 g sat. fat), 115 mg
chol., 476 mg sodium, 5 g carb.,
trace fiber, 37 g pro. Diabetic
Exchanges: 4 lean meat, 2½ fat.*

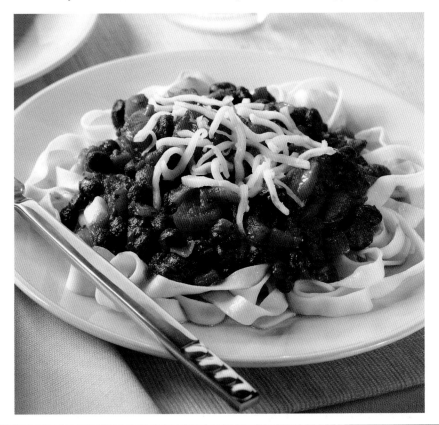

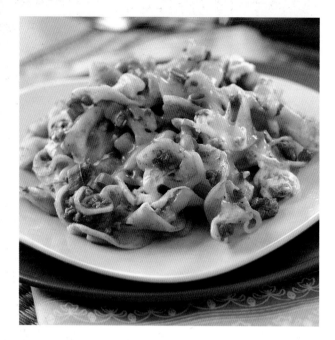

2. In a small bowl, beat the cream cheese, ricotta cheese and sour cream until blended. Stir in half of the onions.

3. Spoon half of the noodle mixture into a 13-in. x 9-in. baking dish coated with cooking spray. Top with cheese mixture and remaining noodle mixture.

4. Cover and bake at 350° for 30 minutes. Uncover; sprinkle with cheddar cheese. Bake 5-10 minutes longer or until heated through and cheese is melted. Sprinkle with remaining onions.

PER SERVING *1 cup equals 319 cal., 14 g fat (8 g sat. fat), 92 mg chol., 635 mg sodium, 23 g carb., 1 g fiber, 24 g pro.*

335 CALORIES Maple-Orange Pot Roast

This easy-to-prepare roast is a wonderful reminder of New England's autumn flavors. It always brings back memories of a friend's maple sap house in New Hampshire, where we're originally from.

—CHRISTINA MARQUIS ORLANDO, FL

PREP: 25 MIN. • **BAKE:** 3 HOURS
MAKES: 8 SERVINGS

- 1 **beef rump roast or bottom round roast (3 pounds)**
- ½ **cup orange juice**
- ¼ **cup sugar-free maple-flavored syrup**

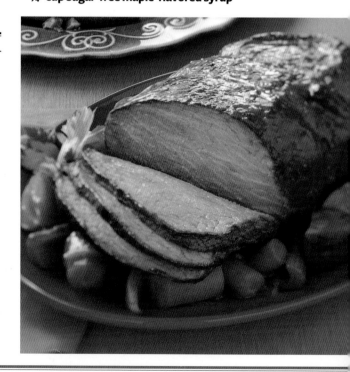

319 CALORIES
Hamburger Noodle Casserole

People have a hard time believing this homey and hearty casserole uses lighter ingredients. The taste is so rich and creamy...it's an ideal weeknight family entree!

—MARTHA HENSON WINNSBORO, TX

PREP: 30 MIN. • **BAKE:** 35 MIN. • **MAKES:** 10 SERVINGS

- 5 **cups uncooked egg noodles**
- 1½ **pounds lean ground beef (90% lean)**
- 2 **garlic cloves, minced**
- 3 **cans (8 ounces each) tomato sauce**
- ½ **teaspoon sugar**
- ½ **teaspoon salt**
- ⅛ **teaspoon pepper**
- 1 **package (8 ounces) reduced-fat cream cheese**
- 1 **cup reduced-fat ricotta cheese**
- ¼ **cup reduced-fat sour cream**
- 3 **green onions, thinly sliced, divided**
- ⅔ **cup shredded reduced-fat cheddar cheese**

1. Cook noodles according to package directions. Meanwhile, in a large nonstick skillet over medium heat, cook beef until no longer pink. Add garlic; cook 1 minute longer. Drain. Stir in the tomato sauce, sugar, salt and pepper; heat through. Drain noodles; stir into beef mixture.

¼ cup white wine or chicken broth
2 tablespoons balsamic vinegar
1 tablespoon Worcestershire sauce
1 teaspoon grated orange peel
1 bay leaf
½ teaspoon salt
¼ teaspoon pepper
1½ pounds red potatoes, cut into large chunks
5 medium carrots, cut into 2-inch pieces
2 celery ribs, cut into 2-inch pieces
2 medium onions, cut into wedges
4 teaspoons cornstarch
¼ cup cold water

1. In a large nonstick skillet coated with cooking spray, brown roast on all sides. Place in a roasting pan coated with cooking spray.

2. In the same skillet, combine the orange juice, syrup, wine, vinegar, Worcestershire sauce, orange peel, bay leaf, salt and pepper. Bring to a boil, stirring frequently; pour over meat. Place potatoes, carrots, celery and onions around roast. Cover and bake at 325° for 3 hours or until meat is tender.

3. Remove meat and vegetables and keep warm. Pour pan juices into a measuring cup. Discard bay leaf and skim fat. Return to roasting pan.

4. In a small bowl, combine cornstarch and water until smooth. Gradually stir into juices. Bring to a boil; cook and stir for 2 minutes or until thickened. Serve with pot roast and vegetables.

PER SERVING *3 ounces cooked beef with ¾ cup vegetables and 2 tablespoons gravy equals 335 cal., 8 g fat (3 g sat. fat), 102 mg chol., 264 mg sodium, 27 g carb., 4 g fiber, 36 g pro.* **Diabetic Exchanges:** *3 lean meat, 2 vegetable, 1 starch.*

263 CALORIES Spicy Chicken
Breasts with Pepper Peach Relish
My summery entree is packed with the good-for-you vitamins found in both peaches and peppers. Best of all, it's delicious!
—ROXANNE CHAN ALBANY, CA

PREP: 20 MIN. • **GRILL:** 15 MIN. • **MAKES:** 4 SERVINGS

½ teaspoon salt
¼ teaspoon each ground cinnamon, cloves and nutmeg
4 boneless skinless chicken breast halves
 (6 ounces each)

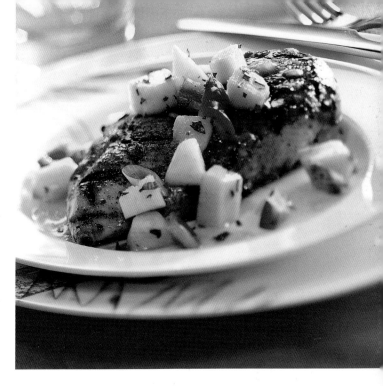

GLAZE
¼ cup peach preserves
2 tablespoons lemon juice
¼ teaspoon crushed red pepper flakes
RELISH
2 medium peaches, peeled and finely chopped
⅓ cup finely chopped sweet red pepper
⅓ cup finely chopped green pepper
1 green onion, finely chopped
2 tablespoons minced fresh mint

1. Combine the salt, cinnamon, cloves and nutmeg; rub over chicken. In a small bowl, combine the glaze ingredients; set aside. In another bowl, combine the peaches, peppers, onion, mint and 2 tablespoons glaze; set aside.

2. Moisten a paper towel with cooking oil; using long-handled tongs, lightly coat the grill rack. Grill chicken, covered, over medium heat or broil 4 in. from the heat for 6-8 minutes on each side or until a thermometer reads 170°, basting frequently with glaze. Serve with relish.

PER SERVING *1 chicken breast half with ½ cup relish equals 263 cal., 4 g fat (1 g sat. fat), 94 mg chol., 379 mg sodium, 20 g carb., 2 g fiber, 35 g pro.* **Diabetic Exchanges:** *5 lean meat, 1 starch, ½ fruit.*

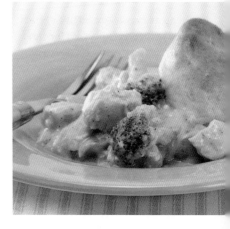

292 CALORIES

Vermont Turkey Loaf

The maple glaze on this turkey loaf makes it deliciously different from other meat loaves. I can easily double it for company, or bake an extra loaf and freeze it for a busy night in the future.

—KARI CAVEN COEUR D'ALENE, ID

PREP: 20 MIN. • **BAKE:** 20 MIN.
MAKES: 2 SERVINGS

- ⅓ **cup coarsely chopped onion**
- ⅓ **cup coarsely chopped fresh mushrooms**
- ⅓ **cup coarsely chopped carrot**
- ⅓ **cup dry bread crumbs**
- ¼ **teaspoon salt**
- ¼ **teaspoon pepper**
- ½ **pound lean ground turkey**
- 1 **tablespoon maple syrup**
- 1 **teaspoon Dijon mustard**

1. In a small skillet coated with cooking spray, saute the onion, mushrooms and carrot until tender; cool slightly.

2. In a small bowl, combine the vegetables, bread crumbs, salt and pepper. Crumble turkey over mixture and mix well. Shape into a 6-in. x 3-in. loaf.

3. Place in an 8-in. square baking dish coated with cooking spray. Bake, uncovered, at 375° for 15 minutes.

4. In a small bowl, combine syrup and mustard; pour half over the turkey loaf. Bake 5-10 minutes longer or until no pink remains and a thermometer reads 165°. Serve with remaining syrup mixture.

PER SERVING *½ meat loaf equals 292 cal., 11 g fat (3 g sat. fat), 90 mg chol., 629 mg sodium, 25 g carb., 2 g fiber, 23 g pro.* **Diabetic Exchanges:** *3 lean meat, 1 starch, 1 vegetable.*

326 CALORIES Weeknight Chicken Potpie

I have long days at work, so I really appreciate quick recipes. My husband enjoys this casserole and often makes it himself while I'm working.

LISA SJURSEN-DARLING
ROCHESTER, NY

PREP: 25 MIN. • **BAKE:** 25 MIN.
MAKES: 8 SERVINGS

- 1 **small onion, chopped**
- 1 **teaspoon canola oil**
- 1½ **cups fat-free milk, divided**
- ½ **cup reduced-sodium chicken broth**
- ¾ **teaspoon rubbed sage**
- ⅛ **teaspoon pepper**
- ¼ **cup all-purpose flour**
- 4 **cups cubed cooked chicken breast**
- 3 **cups frozen chopped broccoli, thawed and drained**
- 1½ **cups (6 ounces) shredded reduced-fat cheddar cheese**
- 1 **tube (11.3 ounces) refrigerated dinner rolls**

1. In a large nonstick saucepan, saute onion in oil until tender. Stir in ¾ cup milk, broth, sage and pepper. In a small bowl, combine flour and remaining milk until

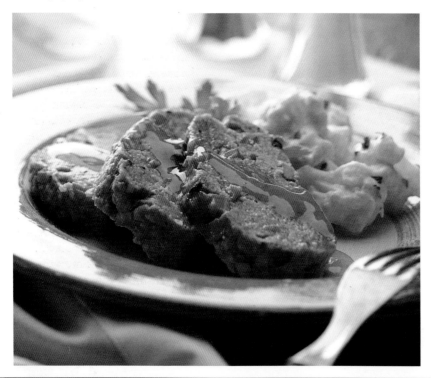

smooth; gradually stir into onion mixture. Bring to a boil; cook and stir for 1-2 minutes or until thickened. Stir in the chicken, broccoli and cheese; heat through.

2. Transfer to a 2-qt. baking dish coated with cooking spray. Separate rolls; arrange over chicken mixture. Bake, uncovered, at 350° for 25-30 minutes or until filling is bubbly and rolls are golden brown.

PER SERVING *¾ cup chicken mixture with 1 roll equals 326 cal., 9 g fat (4 g sat. fat), 70 mg chol., 511 mg sodium, 28 g carb., 2 g fiber, 33 g pro.* **Diabetic Exchanges:** *4 lean meat, 2 starch.*

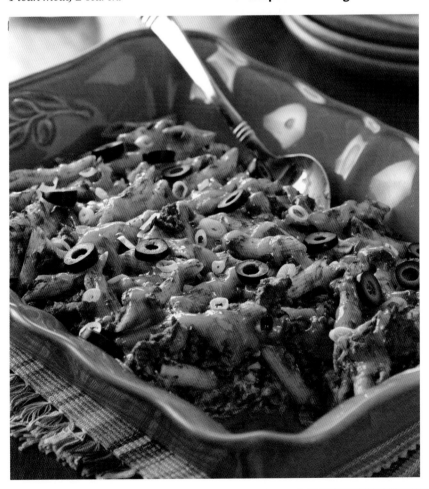

Southwest Pasta Bake

Fat-free cream cheese and reduced-fat cheddar make my creamy casserole lower in fat and calories. It's a good way to get our kids to eat spinach in disguise!
—**CAROL LEPAK** SHEBOYGAN, WI

PREP: 20 MIN. • **BAKE:** 35 MIN. + STANDING • **MAKES:** 8 SERVINGS

- **8** ounces uncooked penne pasta
- **1** package (8 ounces) fat-free cream cheese, cubed
- **½** cup fat-free milk
- **1** package (10 ounces) frozen chopped spinach, thawed and squeezed dry
- **1** teaspoon dried oregano
- **1** pound lean ground beef (90% lean)
- **2** garlic cloves, minced
- **1** jar (16 ounces) picante sauce
- **1** can (8 ounces) no-salt-added tomato sauce
- **1** can (6 ounces) no-salt-added tomato paste
- **2** teaspoons chili powder
- **1** teaspoon ground cumin
- **1** cup (4 ounces) shredded reduced-fat cheddar cheese
- **1** can (2¼ ounces) sliced ripe olives, drained
- **¼** cup sliced green onions

1. Cook pasta according to package directions. Meanwhile, in a small bowl, beat cream cheese until smooth. Beat in milk. Stir in spinach and oregano; set aside.

2. In a nonstick skillet, cook beef over medium heat until no longer pink. Add garlic; cook 1 minute longer. Drain. Stir in the picante sauce, tomato sauce, tomato paste, chili powder and cumin; bring to a boil. Reduce heat; simmer, uncovered, for 5 minutes. Drain pasta; stir into meat mixture.

3. In a 13-in. x 9-in. baking dish coated with cooking spray, layer half of the meat mixture and all of the spinach mixture. Top with remaining meat mixture.

4. Cover and bake at 350° for 30 minutes. Uncover; sprinkle with cheese. Bake 5 minutes longer or until cheese is melted. Sprinkle with olives and onions. Let stand for 10 minutes before serving.

PER SERVING *1 serving equals 328 cal., 9 g fat (4 g sat. fat), 40 mg chol., 855 mg sodium, 36 g carb., 4 g fiber, 25 g pro.* **Diabetic Exchanges:** *3 lean meat, 2 vegetable, 1½ starch.*

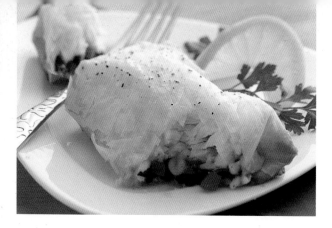

330 CALORIES Phyllo-Wrapped Halibut

I created these packets to convince my husband that seafood doesn't have to taste fishy. He really likes the flaky phyllo wrapping with mild fish and vegetables tucked inside.

—**CARRIE VAZZANO** ROLLING MEADOWS, IL

PREP: 20 MIN. • **BAKE:** 20 MIN. • **MAKES:** 2 SERVINGS

- 4 cups fresh baby spinach
- ¾ cup chopped sweet red pepper
- ¾ teaspoon salt-free lemon-pepper seasoning, divided
- ½ teaspoon lemon juice
- 6 sheets phyllo dough (14 inches x 9 inches)
- 2 tablespoons reduced-fat butter, melted
- 2 halibut fillets (4 ounces each)
- ¼ teaspoon salt
- ⅛ teaspoon pepper
- ¼ cup shredded part-skim mozzarella cheese

1. In a large nonstick skillet lightly coated with cooking spray, saute spinach and red pepper until tender. Add ½ teaspoon lemon-pepper and lemon juice. Remove from the heat; cool.

2. Line a baking sheet with foil and coat the foil with cooking spray; set aside. Place one sheet of phyllo dough on a work surface; brush with butter. (Until ready to use, keep phyllo dough covered with plastic wrap and a damp towel to prevent it from drying out.) Layer remaining phyllo over first sheet, brushing each with butter. Cut stack in half widthwise.

3. Place a halibut fillet in the center of each square; sprinkle with salt and pepper. Top with cheese and spinach mixture. Fold sides and bottom edge over fillet and roll up to enclose it; trim end of phyllo if necessary. Brush with remaining butter; sprinkle with remaining lemon-pepper.

4. Place seam side down on prepared baking sheet. Bake at 375° for 20-25 minutes or until golden brown. **NOTE** *This recipe was tested with Land O'Lakes light stick butter.*
PER SERVING *1 serving equals 330 cal., 12 g fat (6 g sat. fat), 64 mg chol., 676 mg sodium, 26 g carb., 4 g fiber, 33 g pro.* **Diabetic Exchanges:** *4 lean meat, 2 vegetable, 1 starch, 1 fat.*

272 CALORIES Cacciatore Chicken Breasts

This easy recipe is my version of traditional Chicken Cacciatore. The tasty sauce and chicken can be served over rice or noodles. If you want to lower the sodium, you can use garlic powder instead of garlic salt.

—**JOANN MCCAULEY** DUBUQUE, IA

START TO FINISH: 30 MIN. • **MAKES:** 2 SERVINGS

- ½ medium onion, sliced and separated into rings
- ½ medium green pepper, sliced
- 1 tablespoon olive oil
- 2 boneless skinless chicken breast halves (5 ounces each)
- ¾ cup canned stewed tomatoes
- 2 tablespoons white wine or chicken broth
- ¼ teaspoon garlic salt
- ¼ teaspoon dried rosemary, crushed
- ⅛ teaspoon pepper

1. In a large skillet, saute onion and green pepper in oil until crisp-tender. Remove and set aside. Cook chicken

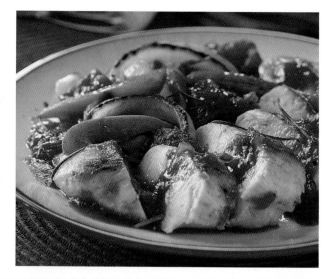

over medium-high heat for 4-5 minutes on each side or until juices run clear. Remove and keep warm.

2. Add the tomatoes, wine, garlic salt, rosemary and pepper to the skillet. Stir in onion mixture and heat through. Serve with chicken.

PER SERVING *1 chicken breast half with ¾ cup vegetables equals 272 cal., 10 g fat (2 g sat. fat), 78 mg chol., 462 mg sodium, 12 g carb., 2 g fiber, 30 g pro.* **Diabetic Exchanges:** *4 lean meat, 2 vegetable, 1½ fat.*

323 CALORIES

Pork Medallions with Dijon Sauce

I lightened up this recipe years ago, and I've been using it ever since. I brown lean pork medallions in a skillet before stirring up a succulent sauce.

—LOIS KINNEBERG PHOENIX, AZ

START TO FINISH: 25 MIN. • **MAKES:** 3 SERVINGS

- 1 **pork tenderloin (1 pound)**
- ⅓ **cup all-purpose flour**
- ¼ **teaspoon salt**
- ¼ **teaspoon pepper**
- 1 **tablespoon butter**
- 3 **green onions**
- ⅓ **cup white wine or chicken broth**
- ½ **cup fat-free evaporated milk**
- 4 **teaspoons Dijon mustard**

1. Cut pork widthwise into six pieces; flatten to ¼-in. thickness. In a large resealable plastic bag, combine flour, salt and pepper. Add pork, a few pieces at a time, and shake to coat. In a large nonstick skillet, brown pork in butter over medium-high heat. Remove and keep warm.

2. Slice green onions, separating the white and green portions; reserve green portion for garnish. In the same skillet, saute the white portion of green onions for 1 minute. Add wine.

3. Bring to a boil; cook until liquid is reduced to about 2 tablespoons. Add milk. Reduce heat; simmer, uncovered, for 1-2 minutes or until slightly thickened. Whisk in mustard. Serve pork with Dijon sauce. Garnish with reserved green onions.

PER SERVING *1 serving equals 323 cal., 10 g fat (4 g sat. fat), 96 mg chol., 516 mg sodium, 18 g carb., 1 g fiber, 35 g pro.* **Diabetic Exchanges:** *4 lean meat, 1 starch, ½ fat.*

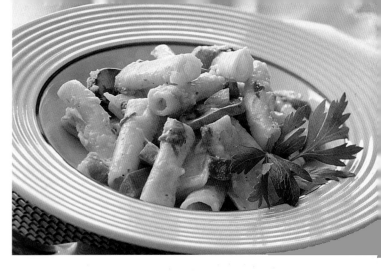

340 CALORIES Creamy Pepperoni Ziti

You can easily feed a crowd with this simple dish that's ready in about 40 minutes. The rich and cheesy sauce will make it a fast favorite at your next potluck or weeknight dinner.

—CHARLANE GATHY LEXINGTON, KY

PREP: 15 MIN. • **BAKE:** 25 MIN. • **MAKES:** 9 SERVINGS

- 1 **package (16 ounces) ziti or small tube pasta**
- 1 **can (10¾ ounces) condensed cream of mushroom soup, undiluted**
- ¾ **cup shredded part-skim mozzarella cheese**
- ¾ **cup chopped pepperoni**
- ½ **cup each chopped onion, mushrooms, green pepper and tomato**
- ½ **cup half-and-half cream**
- ¼ **cup chicken broth**
- ¼ **teaspoon salt**
- ¼ **teaspoon garlic powder**
- ¼ **teaspoon pepper**
- ½ **cup grated Parmesan cheese**

1. Cook pasta according to package directions; drain. In a large bowl, combine the pasta, soup, mozzarella cheese, pepperoni, onion, mushrooms, green pepper, tomato, cream, broth and seasonings.

2. Transfer to a greased 13-in. x 9-in. baking dish. Sprinkle with Parmesan cheese. Cover and bake at 350° for 20 minutes. Uncover; bake 5-10 minutes longer or until bubbly.

PER SERVING *1 cup equals 340 cal., 12 g fat (6 g sat. fat), 27 mg chol., 696 mg sodium, 43 g carb., 2 g fiber, 15 g pro.* **Diabetic Exchanges:** *3 starch, 1 high-fat meat, ½ fat.*

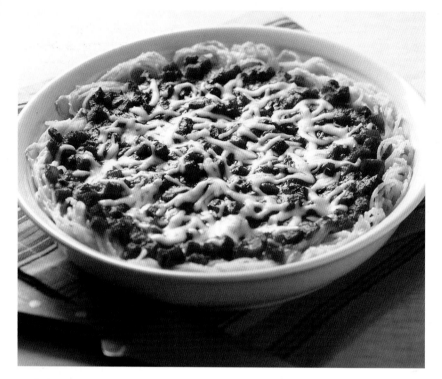

Turkey Mushroom Tetrazzini

Your family will flip over my turkey and mushroom casserole! The creamy Parmesan-topped tetrazzini is so satisfying, no one ever seems to suspect that it's low in fat.

—IRENE BANEGAS LAS CRUCES, NM

PREP: 25 MIN. • **BAKE:** 25 MIN.
MAKES: 6 SERVINGS

- ½ pound uncooked spaghetti
- ¼ cup finely chopped onion
- 1 tablespoon butter
- 1 garlic clove, minced
- 3 tablespoons cornstarch
- 1 can (14½ ounces) reduced-sodium chicken broth
- 1 can (12 ounces) fat-free evaporated milk
- 2½ cups cubed cooked turkey breast
- 1 can (4 ounces) mushroom stems and pieces, drained
- ½ teaspoon seasoned salt
  Dash pepper
- 2 tablespoons grated Parmesan cheese
- ¼ teaspoon paprika

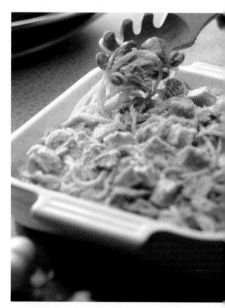

341 CALORIES

Sausage Spaghetti Pie

I adapted a classic family-favorite recipe to our healthy lifestyle, using ingredients that my family prefers. It is wonderful and has been a big hit with all who have sampled it.

—SUE ANN O'BUCK
SINKING SPRING, PA

PREP: 20 MIN. • **BAKE:** 25 MIN.
MAKES: 4 SERVINGS

- 4 ounces uncooked spaghetti
- ½ pound smoked turkey kielbasa, diced
- 1 cup garden-style spaghetti sauce
- 1 cup reduced-fat ricotta cheese
- 3 egg whites
- ⅓ cup grated Parmesan cheese
- ¼ cup shredded part-skim mozzarella cheese

1. Cook spaghetti according to package directions. Meanwhile, in a small nonstick skillet, saute sausage for 3-4 minutes or until browned; stir in spaghetti sauce.

2. In a small bowl, combine ricotta cheese and 1 egg white; set aside. Drain spaghetti; add Parmesan cheese and remaining egg whites. Press onto the bottom and up the sides of a 9-in. deep-dish pie plate coated with cooking spray. Spoon ricotta mixture into crust. Top with sausage mixture.

3. Bake, uncovered, at 350° for 20 minutes. Sprinkle with mozzarella cheese. Bake 5 minutes longer or until cheese is melted and filling is heated through. Let stand for 5 minutes before slicing.

PER SERVING *1 piece equals 341 cal., 9 g fat (4 g sat. fat), 47 mg chol., 980 mg sodium, 38 g carb., 2 g fiber, 24 g pro.*
Diabetic Exchanges: *3 lean meat, 2 starch, 1 vegetable.*

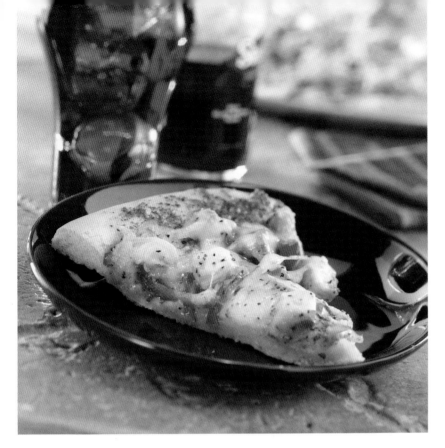

1. Cook spaghetti according to package directions; drain.
2. In a large saucepan, saute onion in butter until tender. Add garlic; cook 1 minute longer. Combine cornstarch and broth until smooth; stir into the onion mixture. Bring to a boil; cook and stir for 2 minutes or until thickened.
3. Reduce heat to low. Add milk; cook and stir for 2-3 minutes. Stir in the spaghetti, turkey, mushrooms, seasoned salt and pepper.
4. Transfer to an 8-in. square baking dish coated with cooking spray. Cover and bake at 350° for 20 minutes. Uncover; sprinkle with cheese and paprika. Bake 5-10 minutes longer or until heated through.
PER SERVING *1¼ cups equals 331 cal., 5 g fat (2 g sat. fat), 51 mg chol., 544 mg sodium,*

41 g carb., 1 g fiber, 28 g pro.
Diabetic Exchanges: 3 lean meat, 2 starch, 1 vegetable, ½ fat-free milk.

293 CALORIES

Chicken Pesto Pizza

This is the only pizza I make now. We love it! Keeping the spices simple helps the flavor of the chicken and vegetables come through. This pizza tastes great and is good for you, too.

—HEATHER THOMPSON
WOODLAND HILLS, CA

PREP: 35 MIN. + RISING • **BAKE:** 20 MIN.
MAKES: 8 SLICES

- 2 teaspoons active dry yeast
- 1 cup warm water (110° to 115°)
- 2¾ cups bread flour
- 1 tablespoon plus 2 teaspoons olive oil, divided
- 1 tablespoon sugar

- 1½ teaspoons salt, divided
- ½ pound boneless skinless chicken breasts, cut into ½-inch pieces
- 1 small onion, halved and thinly sliced
- ½ each small green, sweet red and yellow peppers, julienned
- ½ cup sliced fresh mushrooms
- 3 tablespoons prepared pesto
- 1½ cups (6 ounces) shredded part-skim mozzarella cheese
- ¼ teaspoon pepper

1. In a large bowl, dissolve yeast in warm water. Beat in 1 cup flour, 1 tablespoon oil, sugar and 1 teaspoon salt. Add remaining flour; beat until combined.
2. Turn onto a lightly floured surface; knead until smooth and elastic, about 6-8 minutes. Place in a bowl coated with cooking spray, turning once to coat top. Cover and let rise in a warm place until doubled, about 1 hour.
3. In a large nonstick skillet over medium heat, cook chicken, onion, peppers and mushrooms in remaining oil until chicken is no longer pink and vegetables are tender. Remove from heat; set aside.
4. Punch dough down; roll into a 15-in. circle. Transfer to a 14-in. pizza pan. Build up edges slightly. Spread with pesto. Top with chicken mixture and cheese. Sprinkle with pepper and remaining salt.
5. Bake at 400° for 18-20 minutes or until the crust and cheese are lightly browned.
PER SERVING *1 slice equals 293 cal., 10 g fat (3 g sat. fat), 30 mg chol., 601 mg sodium, 35 g carb., 2 g fiber, 18 g pro.*
Diabetic Exchanges: 2 starch, 1 lean meat, 1 fat.

274 CALORIES

Country Chicken with Gravy

This lightened-up dinner entree is so quick and simple! It's always a hit when I serve it to guests.

—RUTH HELMUTH ABBEVILLE, SC

START TO FINISH: 30 MIN. • **MAKES:** 4 SERVINGS

- ¾ cup crushed cornflakes
- ½ teaspoon poultry seasoning
- ½ teaspoon paprika
- ¼ teaspoon salt
- ¼ teaspoon dried thyme
- ¼ teaspoon pepper
- 2 tablespoons fat-free evaporated milk
- 4 boneless skinless chicken breast halves (4 ounces each)
- 2 teaspoons canola oil

GRAVY
- 1 tablespoon butter
- 1 tablespoon all-purpose flour
- ¼ teaspoon pepper
- ⅛ teaspoon salt
- ½ cup fat-free evaporated milk
- ¼ cup condensed chicken broth, undiluted
- 1 teaspoon sherry or additional condensed chicken broth
- 2 tablespoons minced chives

1. In a shallow bowl, combine the first six ingredients. Place milk in another shallow bowl. Dip chicken in milk, then roll in cornflake mixture.

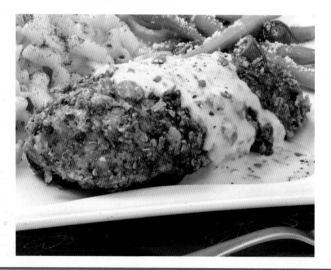

2. In a large nonstick skillet coated with cooking spray, cook chicken in oil over medium heat for 6-8 minutes on each side or until a thermometer reads 170°.

3. Meanwhile, in a small saucepan, melt butter. Stir in the flour, pepper and salt until smooth. Gradually stir in the milk, broth and sherry. Bring to a boil; cook and stir for 1-2 minutes or until thickened. Stir in chives. Serve with chicken.

PER SERVING *1 chicken breast half with 2 tablespoons gravy equals 274 cal., 8 g fat (3 g sat. fat), 72 mg chol., 569 mg sodium, 20 g carb., trace fiber, 28 g pro.* **Diabetic Exchanges:** *3 lean meat, 1 starch, ½ fat.*

263 CALORIES Glazed Pork Tenderloin

Here's a well-seasoned recipe originally for the grill. But we liked it so much that I changed it for the oven just so we could enjoy it all year long!

—VIRGINIA SMITH PEORIA, IL

PREP: 20 MIN. + CHILLING • **BAKE:** 40 MIN.
MAKES: 2 SERVINGS

- 2 teaspoons dried oregano
- 1 teaspoon dried parsley flakes
- ½ teaspoon dried rosemary, crushed
- ½ teaspoon dried thyme
- ½ teaspoon garlic powder
- ½ teaspoon seasoned salt
  Dash pepper
  Dash cayenne pepper
- 1 pork tenderloin (¾ pound)

GLAZE
- 4½ teaspoons brown sugar
- 4½ teaspoons Dijon mustard
- ¼ teaspoon honey

1. In a small bowl, combine the first eight ingredients. Rub over pork. Place in a large resealable plastic bag. Seal bag and refrigerate overnight.

2. Combine the glaze ingredients. Place tenderloin on a rack in a foil-lined shallow roasting pan. Bake, uncovered, at 350° for 40-45 minutes or until a thermometer reads 160°, basting occasionally with glaze. Let stand for 5 minutes before slicing.

PER SERVING *5 ounces cooked pork equals 263 cal., 7 g fat (2 g sat. fat), 95 mg chol., 737 mg sodium, 14 g carb., 1 g fiber, 35 g pro.* **Diabetic Exchanges:** *5 lean meat, 1 starch.*

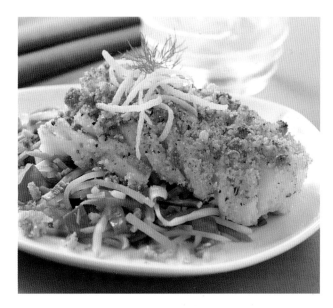

316 CALORIES Crispy Cod with Veggies

Take the chill off brisk evenings and warm the body and soul with our golden-brown baked cod. Round out the meal with a loaf of crusty bread.
—**TASTE OF HOME TEST KITCHEN**

PREP: 15 MIN. • **BAKE:** 25 MIN. • **MAKES:** 2 SERVINGS

- 2 **cups broccoli coleslaw mix**
- ½ **cup chopped fresh tomato**
- 4 **teaspoons chopped green onion**
- 2 **garlic cloves, minced**
- 2 **cod fillets (6 ounces each)**
  Pepper to taste
- ¼ **cup crushed potato sticks**
- 3 **tablespoons seasoned bread crumbs**
- 2 **tablespoons grated Parmesan cheese**
- 4 **teaspoons butter, melted**

1. In a large bowl, combine the coleslaw mix, tomato, onion and garlic; spread into an 11-in. x 7-in. baking pan coated with cooking spray. Top with cod fillets; sprinkle with pepper.

2. Combine the potato sticks, bread crumbs, cheese and butter; sprinkle over fillets. Bake, uncovered, at 450° for 25-30 minutes or until fish flakes easily with a fork.

PER SERVING *1 fillet with 1 cup vegetables equals 316 cal., 12 g fat (6 g sat. fat), 89 mg chol., 445 mg sodium, 18 g carb., 3 g fiber, 34 g pro.* **Diabetic Exchanges:** *5 lean meat, 2 fat, 1 vegetable, ½ starch.*

278 CALORIES Homemade Fish Sticks

I'm a nutritionist and needed a healthy fish fix. Moist inside and crunchy outside, these sticks are great with oven fries or roasted veggies and low-fat homemade tartar sauce.
—**JENNIFER ROWLAND** ELIZABETHTOWN, KY

START TO FINISH: 25 MIN. • **MAKES:** 2 SERVINGS

- ½ **cup all-purpose flour**
- 1 **egg, beaten**
- ½ **cup dry bread crumbs**
- ½ **teaspoon salt**
- ½ **teaspoon paprika**
- ½ **teaspoon lemon-pepper seasoning**
- ¾ **pound cod fillets, cut into 1-inch strips**
  Butter-flavored cooking spray

1. Place flour and egg in separate shallow bowls. In another shallow bowl, combine bread crumbs and seasonings. Dip fish in the flour, then egg, then roll in the crumb mixture.

2. Place on a baking sheet coated with cooking spray. Spritz fish sticks with butter-flavored spray. Bake at 400° for 10-12 minutes or until fish flakes easily with a fork, turning once.

PER SERVING *1 serving equals 278 cal., 4 g fat (1 g sat. fat), 129 mg chol., 718 mg sodium, 25 g carb., 1 g fiber, 33 g pro.* **Diabetic Exchanges:** *4 lean meat, 1½ starch.*

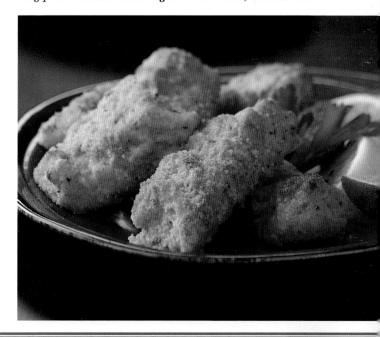

343 CALORIES Spicy Turkey Quesadillas

A bit of hot sauce and green chilies liven up mild cranberries and turkey, while fat-free cream cheese rounds out the bold flavors in this easy dish.

—TASTE OF HOME TEST KITCHEN

START TO FINISH: 25 MIN.
MAKES: 2 SERVINGS

- 3 ounces fat-free cream cheese
- ¼ cup chopped fresh or frozen cranberries, thawed
- 1 tablespoon chopped green chilies
- 1½ teaspoons honey
- 1 teaspoon Louisiana-style hot sauce
- 4 flour tortillas (6 inches)
- 1 cup diced cooked turkey breast

1. In a small bowl, beat cream cheese until smooth. Stir in the cranberries, chilies, honey and hot sauce until blended. Spread over one side of each tortilla. Place turkey on two tortillas; top with remaining tortillas.

2. Cook in a large nonstick skillet over medium heat for 2-3 minutes on each side or until lightly browned. Cut into wedges.

PER SERVING *1 quesadilla equals 343 cal., 7 g fat (1 g sat. fat), 64 mg chol., 751 mg sodium, 35 g carb., 1 g fiber, 33 g pro.* **Diabetic Exchanges:** *3 lean meat, 2 starch.*

272 CALORIES Spinach-Feta Chicken Rolls

I was inspired by my favorite Greek appetizer when I created these spirals. They're worth the bit of extra work.

—LINDA GREGG SPARTANBURG, SC

PREP: 25 MIN. • **BAKE:** 45 MIN.
MAKES: 6 SERVINGS

- ½ cup sun-dried tomatoes (not packed in oil)
- 1 cup boiling water
- 1 package (10 ounces) frozen chopped spinach, thawed and squeezed dry
- 1 cup (4 ounces) crumbled feta cheese

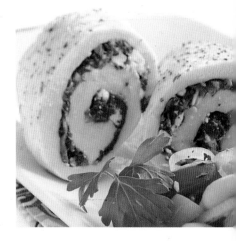

- 4 green onions, thinly sliced
- ¼ cup Greek olives, chopped
- 1 garlic clove, minced
- 6 boneless skinless chicken breast halves (6 ounces each)
- ¼ teaspoon salt
- ¼ teaspoon pepper

1. Place tomatoes in a small bowl; add boiling water. Let stand for 5 minutes. In another bowl, combine the spinach, feta, onions, olives and garlic. Drain and chop tomatoes; add to spinach mixture.

2. Flatten chicken to ¼-in. thickness; sprinkle with salt and pepper. Spread spinach mixture over chicken. Roll up and secure with toothpicks. Place in a 13-in. x 9-in. baking dish coated with cooking spray.

3. Cover and bake at 350° for 30 minutes. Uncover; bake 15-20 minutes longer or until a thermometer reads 170°. Discard toothpicks.

PER SERVING *1 stuffed chicken breast half equals 272 cal., 9 g fat (3 g sat. fat), 104 mg chol., 583 mg sodium, 7 g carb., 3 g fiber, 40 g pro.* **Diabetic Exchanges:** *5 lean meat, 1 vegetable.*

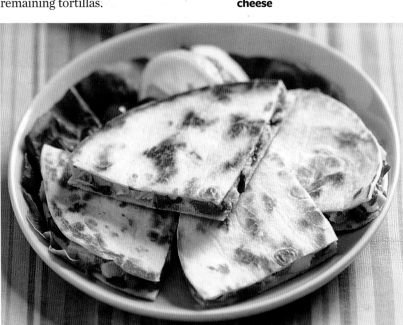

284 CALORIES Southwest Vegetarian Bake

This hearty casserole hits the spot whenever I have a taste for Mexican food with all the fixings!

—PATRICIA GALE MONTICELLO, IL

PREP: 40 MIN. • **BAKE:** 35 MIN. + STANDING
MAKES: 8 SERVINGS

- ¾ cup uncooked brown rice
- 1½ cups water
- 1 can (15 ounces) black beans, rinsed and drained
- 1 can (11 ounces) Mexicorn, drained
- 1 can (10 ounces) diced tomatoes and green chilies
- 1 cup salsa
- 1 cup (8 ounces) reduced-fat sour cream
- 1 cup (4 ounces) shredded reduced-fat cheddar cheese
- ¼ teaspoon pepper
- ½ cup chopped red onion
- 1 can (2¼ ounces) sliced ripe olives, drained
- 1 cup (4 ounces) shredded reduced-fat Mexican cheese blend

1. In a large saucepan, bring rice and water to a boil. Reduce heat; cover and simmer 35-40 minutes or until tender. Preheat oven to 350°. In a large bowl, combine beans, Mexicorn, tomatoes, salsa, sour cream, cheddar cheese, pepper and rice. Transfer to a shallow 2½-qt. baking dish coated with cooking spray. Sprinkle with onion and olives.

2. Bake, uncovered, 30 minutes. Sprinkle with Mexican cheese. Bake 5-10 minutes or until heated through and cheese is melted. Let stand 10 minutes before serving.

PER SERVING *1 cup equals 284 cal., 10 g fat (6 g sat. fat), 30 mg chol., 879 mg sodium, 35 g carb., 6 g fiber, 15 g pro.* ***Diabetic Exchanges:*** *2 starch, 1 lean meat, 1 fat.*

339 CALORIES
Stovetop Beef 'n' Shells

Here's an easy dish I make when I'm pressed for time. It's as tasty as it is fast. Team it with salad, bread and fruit for a comforting meal.

—DONNA ROBERTS MANHATTAN, KS

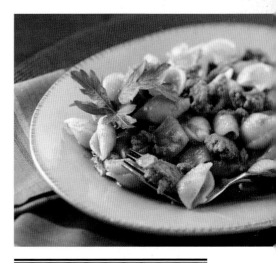

START TO FINISH: 30 MIN.
MAKES: 4 SERVINGS

- 1½ cups uncooked medium pasta shells
- 1 pound lean ground beef (90% lean)
- 1 medium onion, chopped
- 1 garlic clove, minced
- 1 can (15 ounces) crushed tomatoes
- 1 can (8 ounces) tomato sauce
- 1 teaspoon sugar
- ½ teaspoon salt
- ½ teaspoon pepper

1. Cook pasta according to package directions. Meanwhile, in a large saucepan, cook beef and onion over medium heat until meat is no longer pink. Add garlic; cook 1 minute longer. Drain.

2. Stir in the tomatoes, tomato sauce, sugar, salt and pepper. Bring to a boil. Reduce heat; simmer, uncovered, for 10-15 minutes. Drain pasta; stir into beef mixture and heat through.

PER SERVING *1¼ cups equals 339 cal., 9 g fat (4 g sat. fat), 56 mg chol., 772 mg sodium, 36 g carb., 4 g fiber, 29 g pro.* ***Diabetic Exchanges:*** *3 lean meat, 3 vegetable, 1½ starch.*

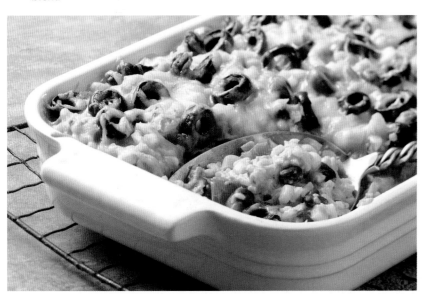

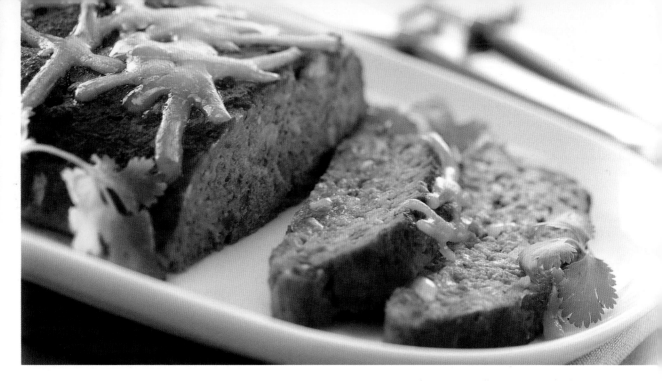

266 CALORIES Mexican Meat Loaf

This great-tasting meat loaf just may become the new family treasure! It's moist, tender and chock-full of green pepper, onion and zesty tomato flavor. What's not to love?
—**CONNIE STAAL** GREENBRIER, AR

PREP: 20 MIN. • **BAKE:** 45 MIN. • **MAKES:** 6 SERVINGS

- 1 large onion, chopped
- 1 medium green pepper, chopped
- 2 teaspoons olive oil
- 2 garlic cloves, minced
- ¾ cup dry bread crumbs
- ¾ cup shredded reduced-fat cheddar cheese
- ½ cup tomato sauce
- ¼ cup fat-free plain yogurt
- 2 tablespoons minced fresh parsley
- 2 teaspoons Worcestershire sauce
- 1 teaspoon chili powder
- ¾ pound lean ground turkey
- ¼ pound lean ground beef (90% lean)

TOPPING

- ¼ cup tomato sauce
- 1 teaspoon Worcestershire sauce
- ½ teaspoon chili powder
- ¼ cup shredded reduced-fat cheddar cheese

1. In a nonstick skillet, saute onion and green pepper in oil until tender. Add garlic; cook 1 minute longer.
2. Transfer to a large bowl. Stir in the bread crumbs, cheese, tomato sauce, yogurt, parsley, Worcestershire sauce and chili powder. Crumble turkey and beef over mixture and mix well.
3. Shape into a loaf. Place in an 11-in. x 7-in. baking dish coated with cooking spray. Bake, uncovered, at 350° for 25 minutes; drain.
4. Combine the tomato sauce, Worcestershire sauce and chili powder; spread over meat loaf. Bake for 15 minutes or until no pink remains and a thermometer reads 165°. Sprinkle with cheese; bake 2-3 minutes longer or until cheese is melted.
PER SERVING *1 slice equals 266 cal., 13 g fat (5 g sat. fat), 70 mg chol., 480 mg sodium, 17 g carb., 2 g fiber, 21 g pro.* **Diabetic Exchanges:** *3 lean meat, 1 starch, ½ fat.*

339 CALORIES Polynesian Stir-Fry

Here's a restaurant-quality meal that blends the sweet taste of pineapple with crunchy veggies and tender pork. The peanuts add a special touch.
—**SUSIE VAN ETTEN** CHAPMANSBORO, TN

START TO FINISH: 30 MIN. • **MAKES:** 4 SERVINGS

1 can (8 ounces) unsweetened pineapple chunks
1 tablespoon cornstarch
2 tablespoons cold water
1 tablespoon reduced-sodium soy sauce
2 tablespoons reduced-sugar apricot preserves
1 pork tenderloin (1 pound), thinly sliced
3 teaspoons canola oil, divided
1 medium onion, halved and sliced
1 small green pepper, cut into 1-inch pieces
1 small sweet red pepper, cut into 1-inch pieces
2 cups hot cooked rice
  Chopped unsalted peanuts, optional

1. Drain pineapple, reserving juice; set aside. For sauce, in a small bowl, combine cornstarch and water until smooth. Stir in the soy sauce, preserves and reserved pineapple juice; set aside.
2. In a large nonstick skillet or wok, stir-fry pork in 2 teaspoons oil until no longer pink. Remove; keep warm.
3. Stir-fry onion and peppers in remaining oil for 3 minutes. Add pineapple; stir-fry 2-3 minutes longer or until vegetables are crisp-tender.
4. Stir cornstarch mixture and add to the pan. Bring to a boil; cook and stir for 2 minutes or until thickened. Add pork; heat through. Serve with rice. Just before serving, sprinkle each serving with peanuts if desired.
PER SERVING *1 cup stir-fry with ½ cup rice (calculated without peanuts) equals 339 cal., 8 g fat (2 g sat. fat), 63 mg chol., 204 mg sodium, 40 g carb., 2 g fiber, 26 g pro.* **Diabetic Exchanges:** *3 lean meat, 1½ starch, 1 vegetable, ½ fruit, ½ fat.*

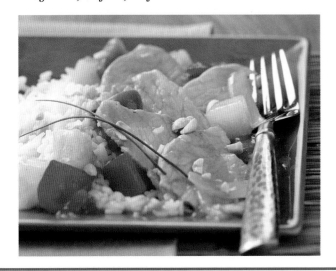

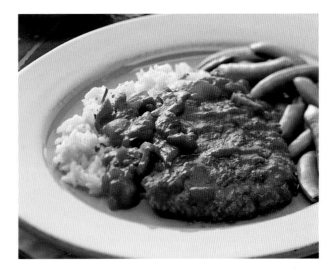

255 CALORIES Swiss Steak

Try a classic dinner that takes little time to get started, then simmers on its own. We like it with mashed potatoes or rice.
—**BETTY RICHARDSON** SPRINGFIELD, IL

PREP: 10 MIN. • **COOK:** 1½ HOURS • **MAKES:** 4 SERVINGS

4 beef cubed steaks (4 ounces each)
1 tablespoon canola oil
1 medium onion, chopped
1 celery rib with leaves, chopped
1 garlic clove, minced
1 can (14½ ounces) stewed tomatoes, cut up
1 can (8 ounces) tomato sauce
1 teaspoon beef bouillon granules
1 tablespoon cornstarch
2 tablespoons cold water

1. In a large nonstick skillet, brown cubed steaks on both sides in oil over medium-high heat; remove and set aside. In the same skillet, saute the onion, celery and garlic for 3-4 minutes or until tender. Add the tomatoes, tomato sauce and bouillon. Return steaks to the pan. Bring to a boil. Reduce heat; cover and simmer for 1¼ to 1¾ hours or until meat is tender.
2. Combine cornstarch and water until smooth; stir into tomato mixture. Bring to a boil; cook and stir for 2 minutes or until thickened.
PER SERVING *1 steak with ¾ cup sauce equals 255 cal., 8 g fat (2 g sat. fat), 65 mg chol., 746 mg sodium, 18 g carb., 3 g fiber, 28 g pro.* **Diabetic Exchanges:** *3 lean meat, 3 vegetable, ½ fat.*

340 CALORIES · Scallops with Angel Hair

Scallops taste extravagant, but they're actually low in fat. The seafood pairs well with delicate angel hair that's lightly coated with a sauce of white wine, garlic and lemon.

—**NANCY MUELLER** MENOMONEE FALLS, WI

START TO FINISH: 30 MIN. • **MAKES:** 4 SERVINGS

- **8 ounces uncooked angel hair pasta**
- **¾ pound bay scallops**
- **2 teaspoons olive oil, divided**
- **1 small onion, chopped**
- **2 garlic cloves, minced**
- **1 cup vegetable broth**
- **¼ cup dry white wine or additional vegetable broth**
- **2 tablespoons lemon juice**
- **¼ teaspoon salt**
- **⅛ teaspoon pepper**
- **2 teaspoons cornstarch**
- **2 teaspoons cold water**
- **¼ cup minced fresh parsley**
  Shredded Parmesan cheese and thinly sliced green onions, optional

1. Cook pasta according to package directions. Meanwhile, in a large nonstick skillet coated with cooking spray, cook scallops in 1 teaspoon oil over medium heat until firm and opaque; remove and keep warm.

2. In same skillet, saute onion in remaining oil until tender. Add garlic; cook 1 minute longer. Stir in broth, wine, lemon juice, salt and pepper. Bring to a boil.

3. Combine cornstarch and water until smooth. Gradually stir into the pan. Bring to a boil; cook and stir for 2 minutes or until thickened. Stir in parsley and reserved scallops; heat through.

4. Drain pasta; serve with scallops. Sprinkle with cheese and green onions if desired.

PER SERVING *⅓ cup scallop mixture with 1 cup pasta (calculated without cheese) equals 340 cal., 4 g fat (1 g sat. fat), 28 mg chol., 527 mg sodium, 50 g carb., 2 g fiber, 22 g pro.*

310 CALORIES
Makeover Swiss Chicken Supreme

Even though this recipe is slimmed down from its original version with reduced-fat ingredients, it still reigns supreme at our house!

—**STEPHANIE BELL** KAYSVILLE, UTAH

PREP: 15 MIN. • **BAKE:** 30 MIN. • **MAKES:** 4 SERVINGS

- **4 boneless skinless chicken breast halves (4 ounces each)**
- **1 tablespoon dried minced onion**
- **½ teaspoon garlic powder**
- **¼ teaspoon salt**
- **⅛ teaspoon pepper**
- **4 slices (¾ ounce each) reduced-fat Swiss cheese**
- **1 can (10¾ ounces) reduced-fat reduced-sodium condensed cream of chicken soup, undiluted**
- **⅓ cup reduced-fat sour cream**
- **½ cup fat-free milk**
- **⅓ cup crushed reduced-fat butter-flavored crackers (about 8 crackers)**
- **1 teaspoon butter, melted**

1. Place chicken in a 13-in. x 9-in. baking dish coated with cooking spray. Sprinkle with minced onion, garlic powder, salt and pepper. Top each with a slice of cheese.

2. In a small bowl, combine soup, sour cream and milk; pour over chicken. Toss the cracker crumbs and butter; sprinkle over chicken. Bake, uncovered, at 350° for 30-40 minutes or until a thermometer reads 170°.

PER SERVING *1 serving equals 310 cal., 11 g fat (5 g sat. fat), 89 mg chol., 567 mg sodium, 17 g carb., trace fiber, 34 g pro.* **Diabetic Exchanges:** *3 lean meat, 2 fat, 1 starch.*

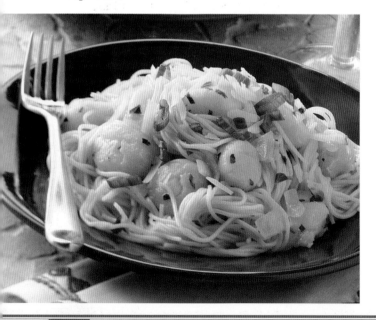

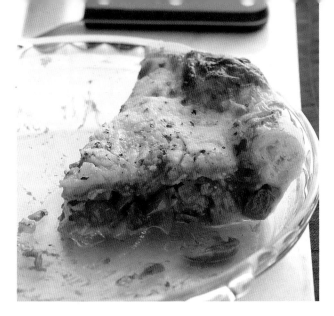

Pizza Lover's Pie

Love pizza? Then you'll really go for the tasty spin this recipe puts on it. Plus, it's easy to tailor to picky eaters' tastes.
—**CAROL GILLESPIE** CHAMBERSBURG, PA

PREP: 20 MIN. • BAKE: 20 MIN. • MAKES: 8 SERVINGS

- ¼ pound bulk pork sausage
- ½ cup chopped green pepper
- ¼ cup chopped onion
- 1 loaf (1 pound) frozen bread dough, thawed and halved
- 2 cups (8 ounces) shredded part-skim mozzarella cheese
- ½ cup grated Parmesan cheese
- 1 can (8 ounces) pizza sauce
- 8 slices pepperoni
- 1 can (4 ounces) mushroom stems and pieces, drained
- ¼ teaspoon dried oregano

1. In a large skillet, cook the sausage, pepper and onion over medium heat until meat is no longer pink; drain. Set aside.
2. Roll half of dough into a 12-in. circle. Transfer to a greased 9-in. deep-dish pie plate. Layer with half of the mozzarella cheese, Parmesan cheese and pizza sauce. Top with the sausage mixture, pepperoni, mushrooms and ⅛ teaspoon oregano.
3. Roll out remaining dough to fit top of pie. Place over filling; seal edges. Layer with remaining pizza sauce, cheeses and oregano.
4. Bake at 400° for 18-22 minutes or until golden brown.

PER SERVING *1 piece equals 305 cal., 12 g fat (5 g sat. fat), 27 mg chol., 743 mg sodium, 32 g carb., 3 g fiber, 17 g pro.* **Diabetic Exchanges:** *2 starch, 2 medium-fat meat.*

Crunchy Onion Barbecue Chicken

I threw this recipe together one night when I had some chicken breasts to use up. I was thrilled with how moist, crunchy and flavorful they turned out. My husband was, too!
—**JANE HOLEY** CLAYTON, MI

PREP: 10 MIN. • BAKE: 25 MIN. • MAKES: 4 SERVINGS

- ½ cup barbecue sauce
- 1⅓ cups French-fried onions, crushed
- ¼ cup grated Parmesan cheese
- ½ teaspoon pepper
- 4 boneless skinless chicken breast halves (6 ounces each)

1. Place barbecue sauce in a shallow bowl. In another shallow bowl, combine the onions, cheese and pepper. Dip both sides of chicken in barbecue sauce, then one side in onion mixture.
2. Place chicken, crumb side up, on a baking sheet coated with cooking spray. Bake at 400° for 22-27 minutes or until a thermometer reads 170°.
PER SERVING *1 chicken breast half equals 286 cal., 10 g fat (3 g sat. fat), 97 mg chol., 498 mg sodium, 9 g carb., trace fiber, 36 g pro.* **Diabetic Exchanges:** *5 lean meat, 1 fat, ½ starch.*

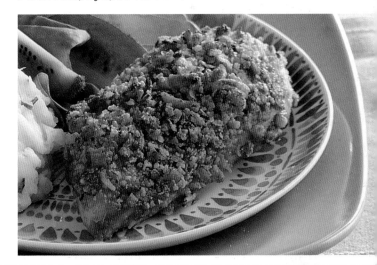

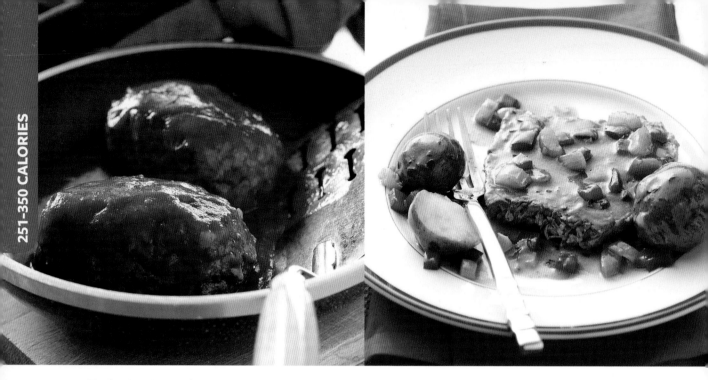

Stovetop Meat Loaves

Who says meat loaf has to bake in the oven for hours? With this convenient recipe, all you need is your stovetop and 30 minutes. It's a fast-and-easy recipe to make for one or two people.

—**EMILY SUND** GENESEO, IL

START TO FINISH: 30 MIN.
MAKES: 2 SERVINGS

- 3 tablespoons 2% milk
- 2 tablespoons quick-cooking oats
- 1 tablespoon chopped onion
- ¼ teaspoon salt
- ½ pound lean ground beef
- ½ teaspoon cornstarch
- ½ cup Italian tomato sauce
- ¼ cup cold water

1. In a small bowl, combine the milk, oats, onion and salt. Crumble beef over mixture and mix well. Shape into two loaves.
2. In a small nonstick skillet, brown loaves on all sides; drain. Combine the cornstarch, tomato sauce and water until smooth. Pour over meat loaves. Bring to a boil. Reduce heat to medium-low; cover and cook for 15-20 minutes or until meat is no longer pink.

PER SERVING *1 meat loaf equals 259 cal., 10 g fat (4 g sat. fat), 71 mg chol., 922 mg sodium, 16 g carb., 2 g fiber, 25 g pro.* **Diabetic Exchanges:** *3 lean meat, 1 starch.*

Round Steak with Potatoes

Have a delicious steak-and-potatoes dinner tonight! Baking the round steak for an extended amount of time guarantees tender results.

—**TARYN KUEBELBECK**
PLYMOUTH, MN

PREP: 20 MIN. • **BAKE:** 2½ HOURS
MAKES: 6 SERVINGS

- 2 pounds beef top round steak
- 1 teaspoon salt
- ½ teaspoon pepper
- 2 tablespoons canola oil
- 1 can (10¾ ounces) condensed golden mushroom soup, undiluted
- 1¼ cups water
- 1 cup chopped celery
- 1 cup chopped sweet red pepper
- ½ cup chopped onion
- ¼ teaspoon dried thyme
- 12 small red potatoes

1. Cut steak into six pieces; sprinkle with salt and pepper. In an ovenproof Dutch oven, brown meat in oil on both sides. Stir in the soup, water, celery, red pepper, onion and thyme. Cover and bake at 350° for 1 hour.
2. Add potatoes; cover and bake 1½ hours longer or until steak and vegetables are tender.

PER SERVING *1 serving equals 344 cal., 11 g fat (2 g sat. fat), 87 mg chol., 829 mg sodium, 22 g carb., 3 g fiber, 37 g pro.*

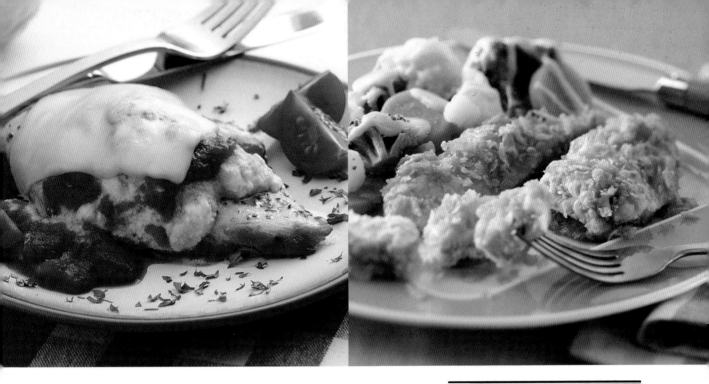

252 CALORIES Smothered Chicken Italiano

This is one of my husband's favorites and has become a reliable dish to serve our dinner guests. It's impressive and tasty, but so easy to prepare.

—MARY KRETSCHMER MIAMI, FL

PREP: 15 MIN. • **BAKE:** 20 MIN.
MAKES: 4 SERVINGS

- ½ teaspoon dried oregano
- ¼ teaspoon garlic powder
- ¼ teaspoon salt, divided
- ¼ teaspoon pepper, divided
- 4 boneless skinless chicken breast halves (4 ounces each)
- 2 teaspoons canola oil
- 1 cup part-skim ricotta cheese
- 1 cup crushed tomatoes
- 4 slices part-skim mozzarella cheese

1. In a small bowl, combine the oregano, garlic powder, ⅛ teaspoon salt and ⅛ teaspoon pepper; rub over chicken. In a large nonstick skillet coated with cooking spray, brown chicken in oil for 3-4 minutes on each side.

2. Transfer to an 11-in. x 7-in. baking dish coated with cooking spray. Combine ricotta cheese and remaining salt and pepper; spoon over chicken. Top with tomatoes.

3. Bake, uncovered, at 350° for 15 minutes. Top with cheese. Bake 5-10 minutes longer or until a thermometer reads 170°.

PER SERVING *1 serving equals 252 cal., 11 g fat (5 g sat. fat), 85 mg chol., 341 mg sodium, 6 g carb., 1 g fiber, 32 g pro.* **Diabetic Exchanges:** *4 lean meat, ½ fat.*

281 CALORIES
Easy Chicken Strips

I came up with these crispy strips one night when I was looking for a fast new way to serve chicken. I've been told they taste like those served in restaurants!

—CRYSTAL SHECKLES-GIBSON
BEESPRING, KY

START TO FINISH: 30 MIN.
MAKES: 6 SERVINGS

- ¼ cup all-purpose flour
- ¾ teaspoon seasoned salt
- 1¼ cups crushed cornflakes
- ⅓ cup butter, melted
- 1½ pounds boneless skinless chicken breasts, cut into 1-inch strips

1. In a shallow bowl, combine flour and seasoned salt. Place cornflakes and butter in separate shallow bowls. Coat chicken with flour mixture, then dip in butter and coat with cornflakes.

2. Transfer to an ungreased baking sheet. Bake at 400° for 15-20 minutes or until no longer pink.

PER SERVING *1 serving equals 281 cal., 12 g fat (7 g sat. fat), 87 mg chol., 430 mg sodium, 18 g carb., trace fiber, 24 g pro.* **Diabetic Exchanges:** *3 lean meat, 2 fat, 1 starch.*

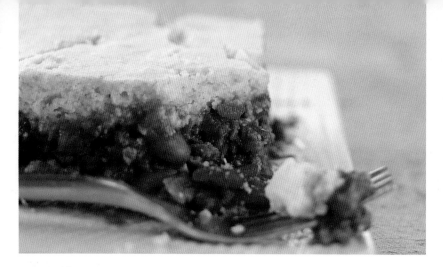

339 CALORIES Hamburger Corn Bread Casserole

Welcome friends in from the cold with a comforting dish that all ages will love. A layer of corn bread makes this meal in one both filling and delicious!

—**KATHY GARRISON** FORT WORTH, TX

PREP: 25 MIN. • **BAKE:** 15 MIN.
MAKES: 6 SERVINGS

- 1 **pound lean ground beef (90% lean)**
- 1 **small onion, chopped**
- 1 **can (15 ounces) Ranch Style beans (pinto beans in seasoned tomato sauce)**
- 1 **can (14½ ounces) diced tomatoes, undrained**
- 1 **teaspoon chili powder**
- 1 **teaspoon Worcestershire sauce**

TOPPING

- ½ **cup all-purpose flour**
- ½ **cup cornmeal**
- 2 **tablespoons sugar**
- 2 **teaspoons baking powder**
- ¼ **teaspoon salt**
- 1 **egg, beaten**
- ½ **cup fat-free milk**
- 1 **tablespoon canola oil**

1. In a large skillet, cook beef and onion over medium heat until meat is no longer pink; drain. Add the beans, tomatoes, chili powder and Worcestershire sauce; bring to a boil. Reduce heat; simmer, uncovered, for 5 minutes.

2. Transfer to an 11-in. x 7-in. baking dish coated with cooking spray. For topping, in a bowl, combine flour, cornmeal, sugar, baking powder and salt. Combine egg, milk and oil; stir into dry ingredients just until moistened. Spoon over filling; gently spread to cover top.

3. Bake, uncovered, at 425° for 14-18 minutes or until filling is bubbly and a toothpick inserted into topping comes out clean. Let stand for 5 minutes before cutting.

PER SERVING *1 serving equals 339 cal., 10 g fat (3 g sat. fat), 73 mg chol., 722 mg sodium, 38 g carb., 6 g fiber, 22 g pro.* **Diabetic Exchanges:** *3 lean meat, 2 starch, 1 vegetable, ½ fat.*

308 CALORIES Glazed Beef Tournedos

I found this quick recipe in a cookbook years ago. It's been a standby for special occasions ever since! I like to serve it with twice-baked potatoes and a crisp spinach salad.

—**JANET SINGLETON** BELLEVUE, OH

START TO FINISH: 20 MIN.
MAKES: 4 SERVINGS

- 3 **tablespoons steak sauce**
- 2 **tablespoons ketchup**
- 2 **tablespoons orange marmalade**
- 1 **tablespoon lemon juice**
- 1 **tablespoon finely chopped onion**
- 1 **garlic clove, minced**
- 4 **beef tenderloin steaks (6 ounces each)**

1. In a small bowl, combine the steak sauce, ketchup, marmalade, lemon juice, onion and garlic. Set aside ¼ cup for serving.

2. Moisten a paper towel with cooking oil; using long-handled tongs, lightly coat the grill rack. Grill steaks, uncovered, over medium heat or broil 4 in. from the heat for 5-7 minutes on each side or until meat reaches desired doneness (for medium-rare, a thermometer should read 145°; medium, 160°; well-done, 170°), basting frequently with remaining sauce.

3. Just before serving, brush steaks with reserved sauce.

PER SERVING *1 serving equals 308 cal., 12 g fat (5 g sat. fat), 106 mg chol., 385 mg sodium, 12 g carb., trace fiber, 36 g pro.* **Diabetic Exchanges:** *5 lean meat, 1 starch.*

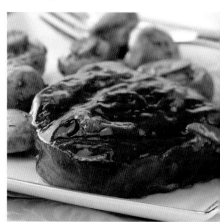

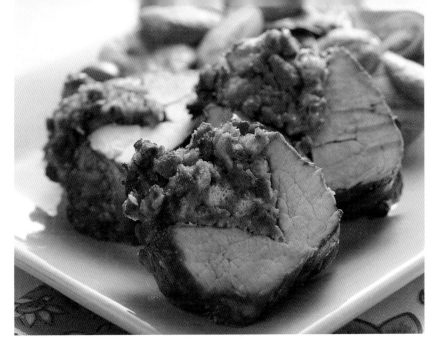

296 CALORIES Grilled Stuffed Pork Tenderloin

We serve this tenderloin with salad and wine. It's so easy you won't believe it!
—**BOBBIE CARR** LAKE OSWEGO, OR

PREP: 20 MIN. + MARINATING
GRILL: 25 MIN. • **MAKES:** 6 SERVINGS

- 2 **pork tenderloins (¾ pound each)**
- ¾ **cup dry red wine or reduced-sodium beef broth**
- ⅓ **cup packed brown sugar**
- ¼ **cup ketchup**
- 2 **tablespoons reduced-sodium soy sauce**
- 2 **garlic cloves, minced**
- 1 **teaspoon curry powder**
- ½ **teaspoon minced fresh gingerroot**
- ¼ **teaspoon pepper**
- 1¼ **cups water**
- 2 **tablespoons butter**
- 1 **package (6 ounces) stuffing mix**

1. Cut a lengthwise slit down the center of each tenderloin to within ½ in. of bottom. In a large resealable plastic bag, combine the wine, brown sugar, ketchup, soy sauce, garlic, curry, ginger and pepper; add pork. Seal bag and turn to coat; refrigerate for 2-3 hours.

2. In a small saucepan, bring water and butter to a boil. Stir in stuffing mix. Remove from the heat; cover and let stand for 5 minutes. Cool.

3. Drain and discard marinade. Open tenderloins so they lie flat; spread stuffing down the center of each. Close tenderloins; tie at 1½-in. intervals with kitchen string.

4. Prepare grill for indirect heat. Moisten a paper towel with cooking oil; using long-handled tongs, lightly coat the grill rack. Grill pork, covered, over indirect medium-hot heat for 25-40 minutes or until a thermometer reads 160°. Let stand for 5 minutes before slicing.

PER SERVING *1 serving equals 296 cal., 9 g fat (4 g sat. fat), 73 mg chol., 678 mg sodium, 24 g carb., 1 g fiber, 27 g pro.* **Diabetic Exchanges:** *3 lean meat, 1½ starch, 1 fat.*

202 CALORIES Southwest Lasagna Rolls

We love this south-of-the-border lasagna. The cheesy dish comes together fast with a can of vegetarian chili. Add a green salad and baked tortilla chips—and dinner is served!
—**TRISHA KRUSE** EAGLE, ID

PREP: 20 MIN. • **BAKE:** 35 MIN.
MAKES: 8 SERVINGS

- 1 **can (15 ounces) vegetarian chili with beans**
- 1 **carton (15 ounces) reduced-fat ricotta cheese**
- 1 **cup (4 ounces) shredded reduced-fat Mexican cheese blend**
- 1 **can (4 ounces) chopped green chilies**
- 1 **teaspoon taco seasoning**
- ¼ **teaspoon salt**
- 8 **lasagna noodles, cooked and drained**
- 1 **jar (16 ounces) salsa**

1. In a large bowl, combine the first six ingredients. Spread about ½ cup on each noodle; carefully roll up. Place seam side down in a 13-in. x 9-in. baking dish coated with cooking spray.

2. Cover and bake at 350° for 25 minutes. Uncover; top with salsa. Bake 10 minutes longer or until heated through.

PER SERVING *1 lasagna roll equals 259 cal., 6 g fat (3 g sat. fat), 23 mg chol., 648 mg sodium, 31 g carb., 6 g fiber, 15 g pro.* **Diabetic Exchanges:** *2 starch, 1 lean meat, 1 vegetable.*

263 CALORIES

Pork Chops with Blue Cheese Sauce

These wonderful chops have a unique kick. The recipe makes a decadent but quick-and-easy weeknight meal. Even if you aren't a blue cheese fan, you'll enjoy the mild-flavored sauce.

—KATHLEEN SPECHT CLINTON, MT

START TO FINISH: 25 MIN. • **MAKES:** 4 SERVINGS

- 4 bone-in pork loin chops (7 ounces each)
- 1 teaspoon coarsely ground pepper

SAUCE
- 1 green onion, finely chopped
- 1 garlic clove, minced
- 1 teaspoon butter
- 1 tablespoon all-purpose flour
- ⅔ cup fat-free milk
- 3 tablespoons crumbled blue cheese
- 1 tablespoon white wine or reduced-sodium chicken broth

1. Sprinkle pork chops on both sides with pepper. Broil 4-5 in. from the heat for 4-5 minutes on each side or until a thermometer reads 145°. Let stand 5 minutes before serving.
2. Meanwhile, in a small saucepan, saute onion and garlic in butter until tender. Sprinkle with flour; stir until blended. Gradually add milk. Bring to a boil; cook and stir for 2 minutes or until thickened. Add cheese and wine; heat through. Serve sauce with chops.
PER SERVING *1 pork chop with 3 tablespoons sauce equals 263 cal., 11 g fat (5 g sat. fat), 94 mg chol., 176 mg sodium, 5 g carb., trace fiber, 33 g pro.* **Diabetic Exchange:** *5 lean meat.*

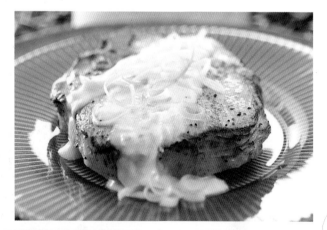

274 CALORIES Romano Chicken Supreme

Romano cheese and golden-brown bread crumbs add delicious crunch to my chicken recipe.

—ANNA MINEGAR ZOLFO SPRINGS, FL

PREP: 20 MIN. • **BAKE:** 20 MIN. • **MAKES:** 6 SERVINGS

- 6 boneless skinless chicken breast halves (5 ounces each)
- ¼ teaspoon salt
- 1 pound fresh mushrooms, chopped
- 3 tablespoons butter
- 1 tablespoon lemon juice
- 1 teaspoon dried basil
- 2 garlic cloves, minced
- ½ cup reduced-sodium chicken broth
- 2 tablespoons orange juice
- 1 cup soft bread crumbs
- ⅓ cup grated Romano cheese

1. In a large skillet coated with cooking spray, brown chicken on both sides over medium heat. Transfer to a 13-in. x 9-in. baking dish coated with cooking spray; sprinkle with salt.
2. In the same skillet, saute mushrooms in butter until tender. Stir in the lemon juice, basil and garlic; cook 1 minute longer. Add broth and orange juice; heat through. Spoon over chicken; sprinkle with bread crumbs and cheese.
3. Bake, uncovered, at 400° for 20-25 minutes or until a thermometer reads 170°.
PER SERVING *1 chicken breast half with about ¼ cup mushroom mixture equals 274 cal., 11 g fat (6 g sat. fat), 100 mg chol., 413 mg sodium, 8 g carb., 1 g fiber, 34 g pro.* **Diabetic Exchanges:** *4 lean meat, 1 fat, ½ starch.*

312 CALORIES Tender Turkey Meatballs

I tweaked one of my old recipes to come up with this healthier version. These tender marjoram-seasoned meatballs are always popular.

—JANE THOMA MONROE, MI

PREP: 25 MIN. • **COOK:** 20 MIN. • **MAKES:** 6 SERVINGS

- ½ cup chopped onion
- ¼ cup egg substitute
- ¼ cup toasted wheat germ
- ¼ cup chopped green pepper
- ¼ cup ketchup

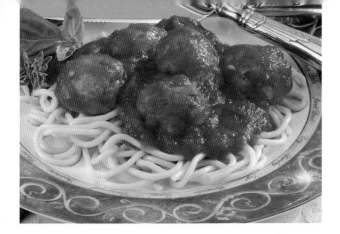

1 teaspoon chili powder
½ teaspoon dried marjoram
½ teaspoon pepper
1 pound lean ground turkey
1 package (12 ounces) spaghetti
5 cups meatless spaghetti sauce

1. In a bowl, combine the first eight ingredients. Crumble turkey over mixture and mix well. Shape into 30 balls, about 1 in. each. Place meatballs on a rack coated with cooking spray in a shallow baking pan. Bake at 400° for 13-16 minutes or until the juices run clear; drain.

2. Meanwhile, cook spaghetti according to package directions. Transfer meatballs to a large saucepan; add spaghetti sauce. Heat through. Drain spaghetti; top with meatballs and sauce.

PER SERVING *5 meatballs with sauce and 1 cup spaghetti equals 312 cal., 7 g fat (2 g sat. fat), 60 mg chol., 1,047 mg sodium, 40 g carb., 5 g fiber, 22 g pro.* **Diabetic Exchanges:** *2½ starch, 2 lean meat.*

346 CALORIES

Makeover Spinach Tuna Casserole

My family has savored this thick, gooey tuna casserole for years. Reduced-fat sour cream and fat-free mayo keep it on the light side, while spinach adds a boost of nutrition.
—**KARLA HAMRICK** WAPAKONETA, OH

PREP: 25 MIN. • **BAKE:** 40 MIN. • **MAKES:** 8 SERVINGS

5 cups uncooked egg noodles
1 cup (8 ounces) reduced-fat sour cream
½ cup fat-free mayonnaise
2 to 3 teaspoons lemon juice
2 tablespoons butter
¼ cup all-purpose flour
2 cups fat-free milk
⅓ cup plus 2 tablespoons shredded Parmesan cheese, divided
1 package (10 ounces) frozen chopped spinach, thawed and squeezed dry
1 package (6 ounces) reduced-sodium chicken stuffing mix
⅓ cup seasoned bread crumbs
2 cans (6 ounces each) light water-packed tuna, drained and flaked

1. Cook noodles according to package directions. Meanwhile, in a small bowl, combine the sour cream, mayonnaise and lemon juice; set aside.

2. In a large saucepan, melt butter. Stir in flour until blended. Gradually stir in milk. Bring to a boil; cook and stir for 2 minutes or until thickened. Reduce heat; stir in ⅓ cup cheese until melted. Remove from the heat; stir in the sour cream mixture. Add the spinach, stuffing mix, bread crumbs and tuna.

3. Drain noodles and place in a 13-in. x 9-in. baking dish coated with cooking spray. Top with tuna mixture; sprinkle with remaining cheese.

4. Cover and bake at 350° for 35 minutes. Uncover; bake 5-10 minutes longer or until lightly browned and heated through.

PER SERVING *1 serving equals 346 cal., 9 g fat (5 g sat. fat), 50 mg chol., 734 mg sodium, 41 g carb., 2 g fiber, 24 g pro.* **Diabetic Exchanges:** *2½ starch, 2 lean meat, 1½ fat.*

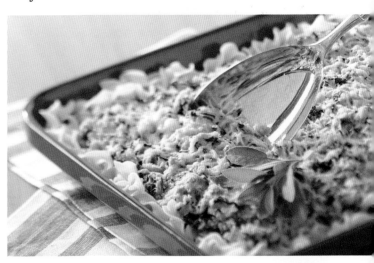

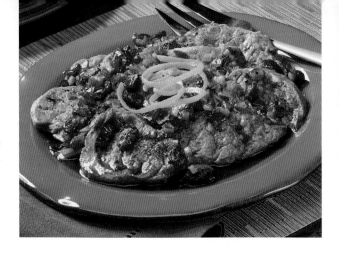

335 CALORIES **Easy Chicken Potpie**

Biscuit mix, canned soup and precut frozen veggies let me make this heartwarming favorite any time. I like to serve it with cranberry sauce.

—MARTHA EVANS OMAHA, NE

PREP: 20 MIN. • **BAKE:** 40 MIN. • **MAKES:** 6 SERVINGS

- 1 can (10¾ ounces) reduced-fat reduced-sodium condensed cream of chicken soup, undiluted
- 1 can (10¾ ounces) reduced-fat reduced-sodium condensed cream of mushroom soup, undiluted
- ½ cup plus ⅔ cup fat-free milk, divided
- ½ teaspoon dried thyme
- ¼ teaspoon pepper
- ⅛ teaspoon poultry seasoning
- 2 packages (16 ounces each) frozen mixed vegetables, thawed
- 1½ cups cubed cooked chicken breast
- 1½ cups reduced-fat biscuit/baking mix

1. In a large bowl, combine the soups, ½ cup milk, thyme, pepper and poultry seasoning. Stir in vegetables and chicken.

2. Transfer to a 13-in. x 9-in. baking dish coated with cooking spray. In a small bowl, stir biscuit mix and remaining milk just until blended. Drop by 12 rounded tablespoonfuls onto chicken mixture.

3. Bake, uncovered, at 350° for 40-50 minutes or until filling is bubbly and biscuits are golden brown.

PER SERVING *1⅓ cups chicken mixture with 2 biscuits equals 335 cal., 5 g fat (2 g sat. fat), 34 mg chol., 832 mg sodium, 53 g carb., 8 g fiber, 20 g pro.*

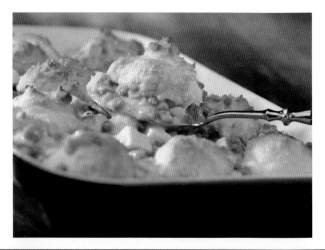

339 CALORIES
Cran-Orange Pork Medallions

Talk about versatile recipes! This is a longtime favorite just as it is, but occasionally, I jazz up the recipe with jalapeno peppers and fresh ginger. I've also made it with peach preserves and dried cherries for a change of pace.

—JULIE WESSON WILTON, WI

START TO FINISH: 30 MIN. • **MAKES:** 4 SERVINGS

- 1 pork tenderloin (1 pound), cut into 1-inch slices
- ½ teaspoon salt
- ½ teaspoon garlic powder
- ½ teaspoon ground coriander
- ¼ teaspoon pepper
- 2 tablespoons olive oil
- 1 medium red onion, chopped
- ½ cup orange marmalade
- ¼ cup orange juice
- ¼ cup dried cranberries
- 2 tablespoons balsamic vinegar

1. Flatten pork slices to ¼-in. thickness. Combine the salt, garlic powder, coriander and pepper; sprinkle over both sides of pork.

2. In a large skillet, cook pork in oil for 3 minutes on each side or until no longer pink. Remove and keep warm.

3. In the same skillet, saute onion in pan juices for 5 minutes or until tender. Stir in the marmalade, orange juice, cranberries and vinegar. Bring to a boil. Reduce heat; return pork to skillet. Simmer, uncovered, for 5 minutes or until sauce is thickened.

PER SERVING *1 serving equals 339 cal., 11 g fat (2 g sat. fat), 63 mg chol., 365 mg sodium, 38 g carb., 1 g fiber, 23 g pro.*

311 CALORIES Turkey 'n' Squash Lasagna

I came up with this lasagna recipe when spaghetti squash was on sale at the supermarket, and it was a hit with all my friends. I used ground turkey because I'm trying to cook healthier.
—**NANCY BEALL** COLORADO SPRINGS, CO

PREP: 70 MIN. • **BAKE:** 50 MIN. + STANDING • **MAKES:** 12 SERVINGS

- 1 **medium spaghetti squash (2 to 2½ pounds)**
- 1 **pound lean ground turkey**
- 1 **large onion, chopped**
- 1 **tablespoon olive oil, divided**
- 2 **garlic cloves, minced**
- 2 **cans (28 ounces each) crushed tomatoes**
- 1 **can (6 ounces) tomato paste**
- ⅓ **cup minced fresh parsley**
- 1 **teaspoon sugar**
- 1 **teaspoon dried basil**
- 1 **teaspoon dried oregano**
- ½ **teaspoon salt**
- ¼ **teaspoon pepper**
- 1 **egg, lightly beaten**
- 1 **carton (15 ounces) reduced-fat ricotta cheese**
- ¾ **cup plus 2 tablespoons grated Parmesan cheese, divided**
- 2 **medium zucchini, sliced**
- 6 **lasagna noodles, cooked and drained**
- 2 **cups (8 ounces) shredded part-skim mozzarella cheese, divided**

1. With a sharp knife, pierce spaghetti squash 10 times. Place on a microwave-safe plate; microwave on high for 5-6 minutes. Turn; cook 4-5 minutes longer or until fork-tender. Cover and let stand for 15 minutes. Cut squash in half lengthwise; discard seeds. Scoop out squash, separating strands with a fork; set aside.

2. In a large saucepan, cook turkey and onion in 1½ teaspoons oil over medium heat until meat is no longer pink. Add garlic; cook 1 minute longer. Drain. Stir in the tomatoes, tomato paste, parsley, sugar and seasonings. Bring to a boil. Reduce heat; cover and simmer for 30 minutes.

3. In a small bowl, combine the egg, ricotta and ¾ cup Parmesan until blended. In a small skillet, saute zucchini in remaining oil until crisp-tender.

4. Spread 1½ cups meat sauce into a 13-in. x 9-in. baking dish coated with cooking spray. Layer with three noodles and half of the zucchini, spaghetti squash and ricotta mixture. Sprinkle with 1½ cups mozzarella and half of remaining sauce. Top with the remaining noodles, zucchini, spaghetti squash, ricotta mixture and sauce (dish will be full).

5. Place dish on a baking sheet. Bake, uncovered, at 350° for 45-55 minutes or until edges are bubbly. Sprinkle with remaining mozzarella and Parmesan cheeses. Bake 5 minutes longer or until cheese is melted. Let stand for 10 minutes before cutting.

NOTE *This recipe was tested in a 1,100-watt microwave.*
PER SERVING *1 serving equals 311 cal., 12 g fat (5 g sat. fat), 72 mg chol., 548 mg sodium, 31 g carb., 5 g fiber, 22 g pro.* **Diabetic Exchanges:** *2 starch, 2 lean meat, 1 fat.*

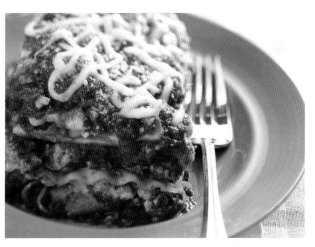

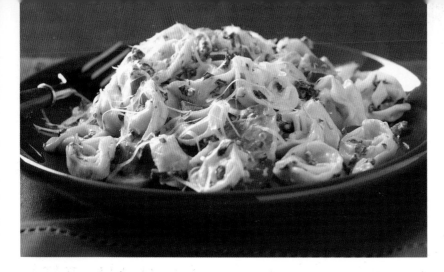

341 CALORIES
Tortellini Primavera

This decadent tortellini with spinach, mushrooms and tomatoes always brings compliments. Parmesan cheese makes it taste so rich that no one even notices it's a vegetarian dish!

—SUSIE PIETROWSKI BELTON, TX

START TO FINISH: 30 MIN.
MAKES: 5 SERVINGS

- 1 package (19 ounces) frozen cheese tortellini
- ½ pound sliced fresh mushrooms
- 1 small onion, chopped
- 2 teaspoons butter
- 2 garlic cloves, minced
- ⅔ cup fat-free milk
- 1 package (8 ounces) fat-free cream cheese, cubed
- 1 package (10 ounces) frozen chopped spinach, thawed and squeezed dry
- 1 teaspoon Italian seasoning
- 1 large tomato, chopped
- ¼ cup shredded Parmesan cheese

1. Cook tortellini according to package directions. Meanwhile, in a large nonstick skillet coated with cooking spray, saute mushrooms and onion in butter until tender. Add garlic; cook 1 minute longer. Stir in milk; heat through. Stir in cream cheese until blended. Add spinach and Italian seasoning; heat through.

2. Drain tortellini; toss with sauce and tomato. Sprinkle with the Parmesan cheese.

PER SERVING *1¼ cups equals 341 cal., 10 g fat (5 g sat. fat), 28 mg chol., 671 mg sodium, 41 g carb., 4 g fiber, 23 g pro.* **Diabetic Exchanges:** *2½ starch, 2 lean meat, 1 vegetable.*

258 CALORIES
Pork Tenderloin with Horseradish Sauce

My zesty pork recipe gets rave reviews every time. The sauce also doubles as an excellent dip for fresh veggies!

—ANN BERGER OSOWSKI
ORANGE CITY, FL

PREP: 15 MIN. • **BAKE:** 30 MIN. + STANDING
MAKES: 2 SERVINGS

- ½ teaspoon steak seasoning
- ½ teaspoon dried rosemary, crushed
- ½ teaspoon dried thyme
- 1 pork tenderloin (¾ pound)
- 2 garlic cloves, peeled and quartered
- 1 teaspoon balsamic vinegar
- 1 teaspoon olive oil

HORSERADISH SAUCE

- 2 tablespoons fat-free mayonnaise
- 2 tablespoons reduced-fat sour cream
- 1 teaspoon prepared horseradish
- ⅛ teaspoon grated lemon peel
  Dash salt and pepper

1. In a small bowl, combine the steak seasoning, rosemary and thyme; rub over meat. Using the point of a sharp knife, make eight slits in the tenderloin. Insert garlic into slits. Place meat on a rack in a foil-lined shallow roasting pan. Drizzle with vinegar and oil.

2. Bake, uncovered, at 350° for 30-40 minutes or until a thermometer reads 160°. Let stand for 10 minutes before slicing. Meanwhile, combine the sauce ingredients; chill until serving. Serve with pork.

PER SERVING *4 ounces cooked pork with 2 tablespoons sauce equals 258 cal., 10 g fat (3 g sat. fat), 101 mg chol., 450 mg sodium, 5 g carb., 1 g fiber, 35 g pro.* **Diabetic Exchanges:** *5 lean meat, 1 fat.*

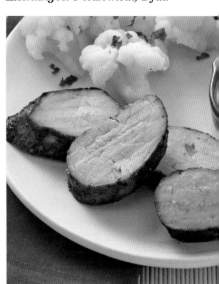

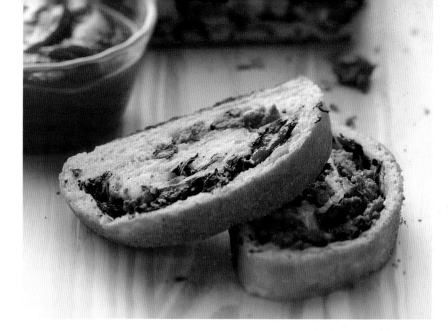

316 CALORIES Pizza Roll-Up

Here's a great dish for snacking or for dinner. It's also tasty made with ground turkey or Italian sausage instead of the ground beef.

—JANICE CHRISTOFFERSON
EAGLE RIVER, WI

PREP: 15 MIN. • **BAKE:** 25 MIN.
MAKES: 6 SERVINGS

- ½ **pound lean ground beef (90% lean)**
- 1 **tube (13.8 ounces) refrigerated pizza crust**
- 1 **package (10 ounces) frozen chopped spinach, thawed and squeezed dry**
- 1 **jar (7 ounces) roasted sweet red peppers, drained and sliced**
- 1 **cup (4 ounces) shredded part-skim mozzarella cheese**
- ½ **teaspoon onion powder**
- ½ **teaspoon pepper**
- ½ **cup loosely packed basil leaves Cooking spray**
- 1 **tablespoon grated Parmesan cheese**
- 1 **can (8 ounces) pizza sauce, warmed**

1. In a small nonstick skillet, cook beef over medium heat until no longer pink; drain.

2. Unroll dough into one long rectangle; top with spinach, beef, roasted peppers and mozzarella cheese. Sprinkle with onion powder and pepper. Top with basil.

3. Roll up jelly-roll style, starting with a short side; tuck ends under and pinch seam to seal. Place roll-up on a baking sheet coated with cooking spray; spritz top and sides with additional cooking spray. Sprinkle with Parmesan cheese.

4. Bake at 375° for 25-30 minutes or until golden brown. Let stand for 5 minutes. Cut into scant 1-in. slices. Serve with pizza sauce.

PER SERVING *2 slices with 2 tablespoons pizza sauce equals 316 cal., 8 g fat (3 g sat. fat), 30 mg chol., 824 mg sodium, 37 g carb., 3 g fiber, 20 g pro.*

262 CALORIES Berry Barbecued Pork Roast

Tender pork loin roast topped with ruby-red cranberry sauce is sure to please your dinner guests!

—DORIS HEATH FRANKLIN, NC

PREP: 15 MIN. • **BAKE:** 1 HOUR + STANDING
MAKES: 12 SERVINGS

- 1 **boneless rolled pork loin roast (3 pounds)**
- ¼ **teaspoon salt**
- ¼ **teaspoon pepper**
- 4 **cups fresh or frozen cranberries**
- 1 **cup sugar**
- ½ **cup orange juice**
- ½ **cup barbecue sauce**

1. Sprinkle roast with salt and pepper. Place with fat side up on a rack in a shallow roasting pan. Bake, uncovered, at 350° for 45 minutes.

2. Meanwhile, in a saucepan, combine the cranberries, sugar, orange juice and barbecue sauce. Bring to a boil. Reduce heat to medium-low; cook and stir for 10-12 minutes or until cranberries pop and sauce is thickened.

3. Brush some of the sauce over roast. Bake 15-20 minutes longer or until a thermometer reads 145°, brushing often with sauce. Let stand for 10 minutes before slicing. Serve with remaining sauce.

PER SERVING *3 ounces cooked pork with ¼ cup sauce equals 262 cal., 8 g fat (3 g sat. fat), 67 mg chol., 190 mg sodium, 23 g carb., 1 g fiber, 24 g pro.* ***Diabetic Exchanges:*** *3 lean meat, 1 starch, ½ fruit.*

277 CALORIES Meatball Sandwiches

My husband and I like classic meatball subs, but I wanted to come up with a version that's fast to make after a long day. My recipe comes together in a snap.
—**KAREN BARTHEL** NORTH CANTON, OH

PREP: 30 MIN. • **COOK:** 30 MIN. • **MAKES:** 8 SERVINGS

- ¼ cup egg substitute
- ½ cup soft bread crumbs
- ¼ cup finely chopped onion
- 2 garlic cloves, minced
- ½ teaspoon onion powder
- ½ teaspoon dried oregano
- ½ teaspoon dried basil
- ¼ teaspoon pepper
  Dash salt
- 1¼ pounds lean ground beef (90% lean)
- 2 cups garden-style pasta sauce
- 4 hoagie buns, split
- 2 tablespoons shredded part-skim mozzarella cheese
  Shredded Parmesan cheese, optional

1. In a large bowl, combine the first nine ingredients. Crumble beef over mixture and mix well. Shape into 40 meatballs. In a large skillet coated with cooking spray, brown meatballs in batches; drain.
2. Place meatballs in a large saucepan. Add pasta sauce; bring to a boil. Reduce heat; cover and simmer for 10-15 minutes or until meat is no longer pink. Spoon meatballs and sauce onto bun halves; sprinkle with mozzarella and Parmesan cheese if desired.
PER SERVING *1 sandwich (calculated without Parmesan cheese) equals 277 cal., 10 g fat (4 g sat. fat), 47 mg chol., 506 mg sodium, 28 g carb., 3 g fiber, 20 g pro.*

312 CALORIES
Mexican-Inspired Turkey Burgers

We adore burgers on the grill—but turkey burgers can be bland, and beef burgers can be fatty. To create flavorful turkey burgers, I used a spice combination from a taco recipe and then tinkered with different cheeses and toppings.
—**HEATHER BYERS** PITTSBURGH, PA

START TO FINISH: 25 MIN. • **MAKES:** 4 SERVINGS

- ½ cup salsa, divided
- ¼ cup shredded reduced-fat cheddar cheese
- 3 teaspoons paprika
- 1 teaspoon dried oregano
- 1 teaspoon ground cumin
- ¾ teaspoon sugar
- ¾ teaspoon garlic powder
- ½ teaspoon dried thyme
- ¼ teaspoon salt
- ¼ teaspoon cayenne pepper
- 1 pound extra-lean ground turkey
- ¼ cup reduced-fat sour cream
- 4 hamburger buns, split
- ½ cup torn curly endive
- 1 medium tomato, chopped

1. In a large bowl, combine ¼ cup salsa, cheese, paprika, oregano, cumin, sugar, garlic powder, thyme, salt and cayenne. Crumble turkey over mixture and mix well. Shape into four burgers.
2. Moisten a paper towel with cooking oil; using long-handled tongs, lightly coat the grill rack. Grill, covered, over medium heat or broil 4 in. from the heat for 5-7 minutes on each side or until a thermometer reads 165° and juices run clear.

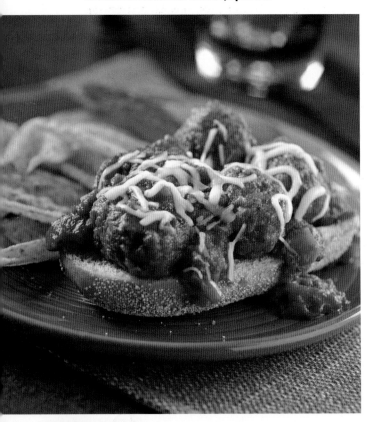

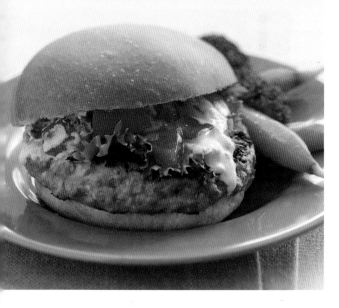

3. In a small bowl, combine sour cream and remaining salsa. Place burgers on buns; top with endive, tomato and sour cream mixture.

PER SERVING *1 burger equals 312 cal., 7 g fat (2 g sat. fat), 55 mg chol., 599 mg sodium, 29 g carb., 3 g fiber, 36 g pro.* **Diabetic Exchanges:** *4 lean meat, 2 starch.*

Marvelous Chicken Enchiladas

I love Mexican food, and this light recipe is one of my favorites. Try using Monterey Jack cheese in place of the cheddar for a slightly milder flavor.

—REBEKAH SABO ROCHESTER, NY

PREP: 30 MIN. • **BAKE:** 25 MIN. • **MAKES:** 6 ENCHILADAS

- 1 **pound boneless skinless chicken breasts, cut into thin strips**
- 4 **teaspoons chili powder**
- 2 **teaspoons olive oil**
- 2 **tablespoons all-purpose flour**
- 1½ **teaspoons ground coriander**
- 1 **teaspoon baking cocoa**
- 1 **cup fat-free milk**
- 1 **cup frozen corn, thawed**
- 4 **green onions, chopped**
- 1 **can (4 ounces) chopped green chilies, drained**
- ½ **teaspoon salt**
- ½ **cup minced fresh cilantro, divided**
- 6 **whole wheat tortillas (8 inches)**
- ½ **cup salsa**
- ½ **cup tomato sauce**
- ½ **cup shredded reduced-fat cheddar cheese**

1. Sprinkle chicken with chili powder. In a large nonstick skillet coated with cooking spray, cook chicken in oil over medium heat until no longer pink. Sprinkle with flour, coriander and cocoa; stir until blended.
2. Gradually stir in milk. Bring to a boil; cook and stir for 2 minutes or until thickened. Add the corn, onions, chilies and salt; cook and stir 2 minutes longer or until heated through. Remove from the heat. Stir in ¼ cup of cilantro.
3. Spread ⅔ cup filling down the center of each tortilla. Roll up and place seam side down in a 13-in. x 9-in. baking dish coated with cooking spray.
4. In a small bowl, combine the salsa, tomato sauce and remaining cilantro; pour over enchiladas. Sprinkle with cheese. Cover and bake at 375° for 25 minutes or until heated through.

PER SERVING *1 enchilada equals 336 cal., 9 g fat (2 g sat. fat), 49 mg chol., 749 mg sodium, 37 g carb., 4 g fiber, 25 g pro.* **Diabetic Exchanges:** *3 lean meat, 2½ starch, ½ fat.*

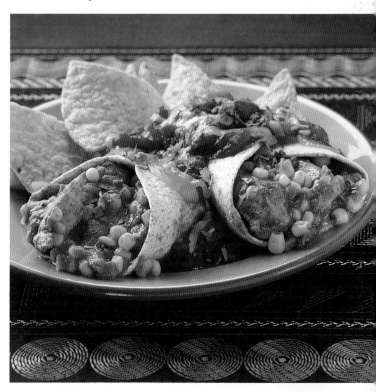

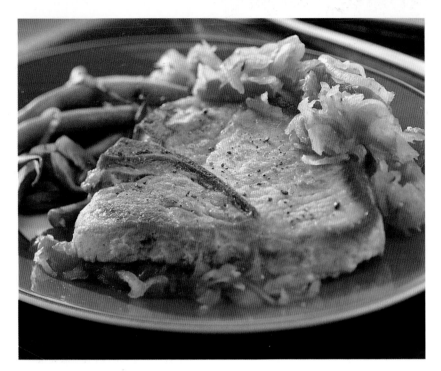

247 CALORIES
Chicken Rice Dish

Fresh early-spring asparagus and a touch of lemon dress up this tasty chicken main dish. I like to serve it with a fresh green salad.

—**REBECCA VANDIVER** BETHANY, OK

START TO FINISH: 25 MIN.
MAKES: 4 SERVINGS

- 2 **cups water**
- 2 **cups cut fresh asparagus (1-inch diagonal pieces)**
- 1 **package (6 ounces) long grain and wild rice mix**
- ¼ **cup reduced-fat butter, divided**
- ¾ **pound boneless skinless chicken breasts, cut into 1-inch strips**
- ¼ **teaspoon salt**
- 1 **medium carrot, shredded**
- 2 **tablespoons lemon juice**
- 1 **teaspoon minced garlic**
- ½ **teaspoon grated lemon peel, optional**

1. In a large saucepan, combine the water, asparagus, rice mix with contents of seasoning packet and 2 tablespoons butter. Bring to a boil; reduce heat. Cover and simmer for 10-15 minutes or until the water is absorbed.

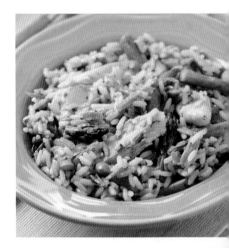

311 CALORIES
Chops 'n' Kraut

Diced tomatoes lend color to this hearty entree, and brown sugar adds a hint of sweetness to the sauerkraut.

—**RUTH TAMUL** MOREHEAD CITY, NC

PREP: 25 MIN. • **BAKE:** 20 MIN.
MAKES: 6 SERVINGS

- 6 **bone-in pork loin chops (7 ounces each)**
- ¼ **teaspoon salt**
- ¼ **teaspoon pepper**
- 3 **teaspoons canola oil, divided**
- 1 **medium onion, thinly sliced**
- 2 **garlic cloves, minced**
- 1 **can (14½ ounces) petite diced tomatoes, undrained**
- 1 **can (14 ounces) sauerkraut, rinsed and well drained**
- ⅓ **cup packed brown sugar**
- 1½ **teaspoons caraway seeds**

1. Sprinkle both sides of pork chops with salt and pepper. In a large nonstick skillet coated with cooking spray, cook three chops in 1 teaspoon oil for 2-3 minutes on each side or until browned; drain. Repeat with remaining chops and 1 teaspoon oil.

2. Place pork chops in a 13-in. x 9-in. baking dish coated with cooking spray; set aside. In the same skillet, cook onion in remaining oil until tender. Add garlic; cook 1 minute longer. Stir in the tomatoes, sauerkraut, brown sugar and caraway seeds. Cook and stir until mixture comes to a boil.

3. Carefully pour over chops. Cover and bake at 350° for 20-25 minutes or until a thermometer reads 160°.
PER SERVING *1 pork chop with ⅔ cup sauerkraut mixture equals 311 cal., 11 g fat (3 g sat. fat), 86 mg chol., 691 mg sodium, 21 g carb., 3 g fiber, 32 g pro.* **Diabetic Exchanges:** *4 lean meat, 1 vegetable, ½ starch, ½ fat.*

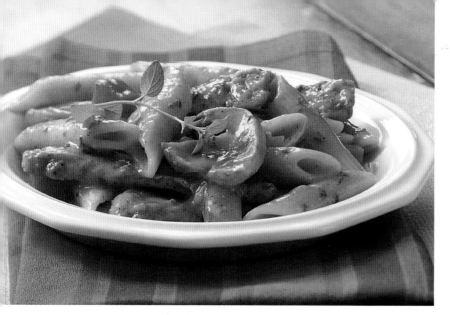

2. Meanwhile, in a large skillet, saute chicken and salt in remaining butter until chicken is no longer pink. Add the carrot, lemon juice, garlic and lemon peel if desired; cook and stir for 1-2 minutes or until carrot is crisp-tender. Stir into the rice mixture.

PER SERVING *1¼ cups equals 247 cal., 7 g fat (4 g sat. fat), 54 mg chol., 668 mg sodium, 29 g carb., 2 g fiber, 20 g pro.* **Diabetic Exchanges:** *2 lean meat, 1½ starch, 1 vegetable.*

264 CALORIES
Pork 'n' Penne Skillet

I enjoy this one-pan skillet supper because it's quick, and cleanup is so easy. Toss a salad while it's cooking and add hot rolls or biscuits for a complete and satisfying meal.

—DAWN GOODISON ROCHESTER, NY

START TO FINISH: 30 MIN.
MAKES: 8 SERVINGS

- 2 tablespoons all-purpose flour
- 1 teaspoon chili powder
- ¾ teaspoon salt
- ¾ teaspoon pepper
- 1 pound boneless pork loin chops, cut into strips
- 2 cups sliced fresh mushrooms
- 1 cup chopped onion
- 1 cup chopped sweet red pepper
- 1 teaspoon dried oregano
- 1 tablespoon canola oil
- 1 tablespoon butter
- 1 teaspoon minced garlic
- 3 cups 2% milk
- 1 can (15 ounces) tomato sauce
- 2 cups uncooked penne

1. In a large resealable plastic bag, combine flour, chili powder, salt and pepper. Add pork, a few pieces at a time, and shake to coat.
2. In a large skillet, cook the pork, mushrooms, onion, red pepper and oregano in oil and butter over medium heat for 4-6 minutes or until pork is browned. Add garlic; cook 1 minute longer.
3. Add milk, tomato sauce and pasta. Bring to a boil. Reduce heat; simmer, uncovered, 15-20 minutes or until meat is tender.
PER SERVING *1 cup equals 264 cal., 10 g fat (4 g sat. fat), 44 mg chol., 546 mg sodium, 26 g carb., 2 g fiber, 18 g pro.*

291 CALORIES
Southwestern Beef Strips

Taco seasoning gives this filling main dish some zip. Keep it on hand to season ground beef or turkey for all kinds of Southwest specialties.

—TASTE OF HOME TEST KITCHEN

START TO FINISH: 20 MIN.
MAKES: 6 SERVINGS

- 1½ pounds beef top sirloin steak, cut into thin strips
- 1 medium onion, sliced
- 1 medium sweet red pepper, cut into thin strips
- 2 tablespoons taco seasoning
- ¼ teaspoon salt
- ¼ teaspoon pepper
- 2 tablespoons canola oil
- 1 can (15 ounces) black beans, rinsed and drained
- 1½ cups frozen corn, thawed
- ½ cup picante sauce
- 2 teaspoons dried cilantro flakes
  Hot cooked fettuccine, optional

1. In a large skillet, stir-fry the beef, onion, red pepper, taco seasoning, salt and pepper in oil until meat is no longer pink.
2. Stir in the beans, corn, picante sauce and cilantro; heat through. Serve with fettuccine if desired.
PER SERVING *1⅓ cups beef mixture (calculated without fettuccine) equals 291 cal., 11 g fat (3 g sat. fat), 63 mg chol., 777 mg sodium, 22 g carb., 5 g fiber, 27 g pro.*

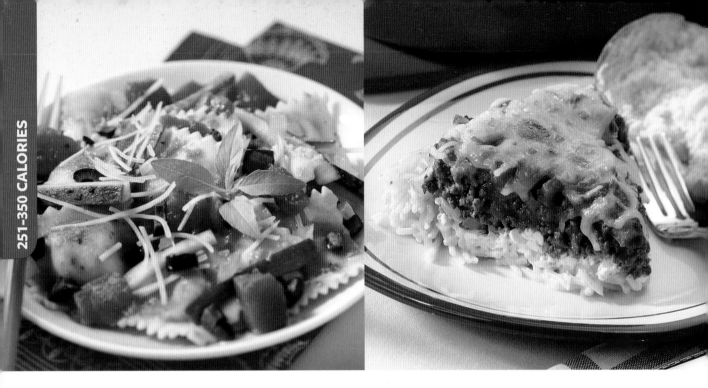

Veggie Cheese Ravioli

Have the best of both worlds with my 20-minute main dish. It tastes light and good for you, but the ravioli makes it hearty and satisfying.

—GERTRUDIS MILLER EVANSVILLE, IN

START TO FINISH: 20 MIN.
MAKES: 3 SERVINGS

- 1 package (9 ounces) refrigerated cheese ravioli
- 2 small zucchini, julienned
- 1 medium onion, chopped
- 1 can (14½ ounces) diced tomatoes, undrained
- 2 tablespoons chopped ripe olives
- ¾ teaspoon Italian seasoning
- 3 tablespoons shredded Parmesan cheese

1. Cook ravioli according to package directions. Meanwhile, in a large nonstick skillet coated with cooking spray, cook and stir zucchini and onion until tender. Stir in tomatoes, olives and Italian seasoning. Bring to a boil. Reduce heat; simmer, uncovered, for 5 minutes.

2. Drain ravioli and add to the pan; stir gently to combine. Sprinkle with cheese.

PER SERVING *1½ cups equals 322 cal., 8 g fat (4 g sat. fat), 37 mg chol., 649 mg sodium, 48 g carb., 6 g fiber, 17 g pro.* **Diabetic Exchanges:** *2 starch, 2 vegetable, 1 lean meat, 1 fat.*

Spaghetti Pie

A classic Italian combination is remade into a creamy, family-pleasing casserole in this quick and easy dish. The recipe was given to me several years ago. My family never grows tired of it.

—ELLEN THOMPSON SPRINGFIELD, OH

PREP: 25 MIN. • **BAKE:** 25 MIN.
MAKES: 6 SERVINGS

- 1 pound lean ground beef (90% lean)
- ½ cup finely chopped onion
- ¼ cup chopped green pepper
- 1 cup canned diced tomatoes, undrained
- 1 can (6 ounces) tomato paste
- 1 teaspoon dried oregano
- ¾ teaspoon salt
- ½ teaspoon garlic powder
- ¼ teaspoon sugar
- ¼ teaspoon pepper
- 6 ounces spaghetti, cooked and drained
- 1 tablespoon butter, melted
- 2 egg whites, lightly beaten
- ¼ cup grated Parmesan cheese
- 1 cup (8 ounces) fat-free cottage cheese
- ½ cup shredded part-skim mozzarella cheese

1. In a nonstick skillet, cook the beef, onion and green pepper over medium heat until meat is no longer pink; drain. Stir in the tomatoes, tomato paste, oregano, salt, garlic powder, sugar and pepper; set aside.

2. In a large bowl, combine the

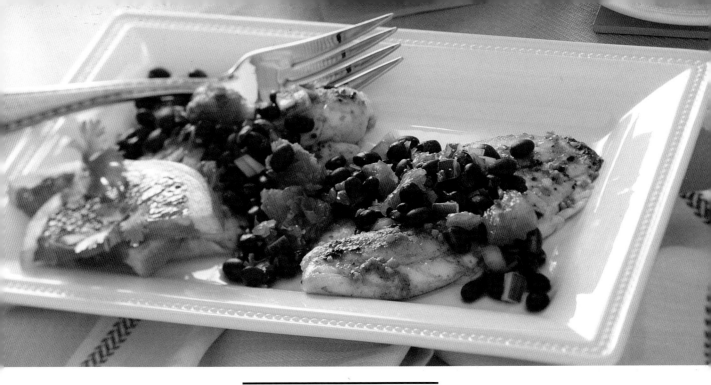

spaghetti, butter, egg whites and Parmesan cheese. Press onto the bottom and up the sides of a 9-in. deep-dish pie plate coated with cooking spray. Top with cottage cheese and beef mixture.

3. Bake, uncovered, at 350° for 20 minutes. Sprinkle with mozzarella cheese. Bake for 5-10 minutes longer or until cheese is melted and filling is heated through. Let stand for 5 minutes before cutting.

PER SERVING *1 serving equals 348 cal., 10 g fat (5 g sat. fat), 52 mg chol., 690 mg sodium, 33 g carb., 4 g fiber, 29 g pro.* ***Diabetic Exchanges:*** *3 lean meat, 2 vegetable, 1½ starch, 1 fat.*

264 CALORIES Tilapia with Grapefruit Salsa

Delicate, nutritious tilapia fillets are topped with an attractive black bean and grapefruit salsa in this easy recipe.
—EMILY SEEFELDT RED WING, MN

PREP: 25 MIN. + MARINATING
COOK: 10 MIN. • **MAKES:** 2 SERVINGS

- ⅓ cup unsweetened grapefruit juice
- ½ teaspoon ground cumin
- 1 garlic clove, minced
- ¼ teaspoon grated grapefruit peel
- ⅛ teaspoon salt
- ⅛ teaspoon pepper
  Dash to ⅛ teaspoon cayenne pepper
- 2 tilapia fillets (6 ounces each)
- ½ cup canned black beans, rinsed and drained
- ⅓ cup chopped pink grapefruit sections
- ¼ cup chopped red onion
- 1 tablespoon minced fresh cilantro
- 1 to 2 teaspoons chopped jalapeno pepper
- 2 teaspoons butter

1. For marinade, in a small bowl, combine the first seven ingredients. Set aside 1 tablespoon. Place tilapia in a large resealable plastic bag; add remaining marinade. Seal bag and turn to coat. Refrigerate for 1 hour.

2. For the salsa, in a small bowl, combine the beans, grapefruit sections, onion, cilantro, jalapeno and reserved marinade. Cover and refrigerate until serving.

3. Drain and discard marinade. In a small skillet over medium heat, cook tilapia in butter for 4-5 minutes on each side or until fish flakes easily with a fork. Serve with the salsa.

NOTE *Wear disposable gloves when cutting hot peppers; the oils can burn skin. Avoid touching your face.*
PER SERVING *1 fillet with ½ cup salsa equals 264 cal., 6 g fat (3 g sat. fat), 93 mg chol., 369 mg sodium, 18 g carb., 4 g fiber, 36 g pro.* ***Diabetic Exchanges:*** *5 lean meat, 1 starch, 1 fat.*

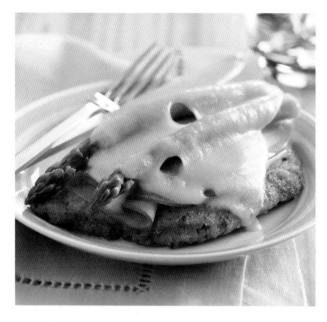

PER SERVING *1 serving equals 291 cal., 12 g fat (6 g sat. fat), 100 mg chol., 595 mg sodium, 16 g carb., 1 g fiber, 31 g pro.* **Diabetic Exchanges:** *3 lean meat, 2 fat, 1 starch.*

304 CALORIES Stir-Fried Steak & Veggies

Here's a complete and healthful meal that's table-ready in less than 30 minutes! You'll want to make it often.
—**VICKY PRIESTLEY** ALUM CREEK, WV

START TO FINISH: 25 MIN. • **MAKES:** 6 SERVINGS

- 1½ cups uncooked instant brown rice
- 1 tablespoon cornstarch
- 1 tablespoon brown sugar
- ¾ teaspoon ground ginger
- ½ teaspoon chili powder
- ¼ teaspoon garlic powder
- ¼ teaspoon pepper
- ½ cup cold water
- ¼ cup reduced-sodium soy sauce
- 1 pound beef top sirloin steak, cut into ½-inch cubes
- 2 tablespoons canola oil, divided
- 1 package (16 ounces) frozen stir-fry vegetable blend, thawed

291 CALORIES Turkey Asparagus Divan

It looks and tastes decadent, but at just 291 calories per serving, this classic entree isn't much of a splurge. Pair it with a side salad and slice of whole grain bread for a complete meal.
—**TASTE OF HOME TEST KITCHEN**

START TO FINISH: 30 MIN. • **MAKES:** 8 SERVINGS

- 1½ cups water
- 16 fresh asparagus spears, trimmed
- 2 egg whites
- 1 egg
- 2 tablespoons fat-free milk
- 1¼ cups seasoned bread crumbs
- 1 package (17.6 ounces) turkey breast cutlets
- ¼ cup butter
- 8 slices deli ham
- 8 slices reduced-fat Swiss cheese

1. In a large skillet, bring water to a boil. Add asparagus; cover and boil for 3 minutes. Drain and pat dry.
2. In a shallow bowl, beat the egg whites, egg and milk. Place bread crumbs in another shallow bowl. Dip turkey in egg mixture, then coat with crumbs.
3. In a large skillet, cook turkey in butter in batches for 2-3 minutes on each side or until no longer pink. Layer each cutlet with a ham slice, two asparagus spears and cheese. Cover and cook for 1 minute or until cheese is melted. Transfer to a platter; keep warm.

1. Cook rice according to package directions. Meanwhile, in a small bowl, combine the cornstarch, brown sugar and seasonings. Stir in water and soy sauce until smooth; set aside.

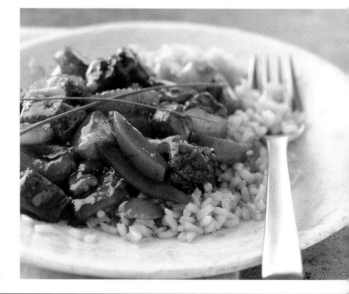

2. In a large nonstick skillet or wok coated with cooking spray, stir-fry beef in 1 tablespoon oil until no longer pink. Remove and keep warm. Stir-fry vegetables in remaining oil until crisp-tender.

3. Stir cornstarch mixture and add to the pan. Bring to a boil; cook and stir for 2 minutes or until thickened. Add beef; heat through. Serve with rice.

PER SERVING *¾ cup stir-fry with ½ cup rice equals 304 cal., 8 g fat (2 g sat. fat), 42 mg chol., 470 mg sodium, 37 g carb., 3 g fiber, 19 g pro. **Diabetic Exchanges:** 2 lean meat, 2 vegetable, 1½ starch, 1 fat.*

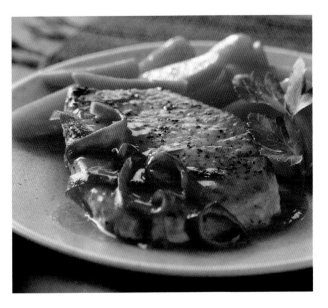

`326 CALORIES`
Veggie-Cheese Stuffed Shells

Need a great-tasting meatless dish you can count on? These pleasing pasta shells are packed with veggies, three kinds of cheese and wonderful flavor!

—SHARON DELANEY-CHRONIS SOUTH MILWAUKEE, WI

PREP: 20 MIN. • **BAKE:** 35 MIN. • **MAKES:** 2 SERVINGS

- 6 uncooked jumbo pasta shells
- ⅔ cup reduced-fat ricotta cheese
- ½ cup shredded part-skim mozzarella cheese, divided
- ¼ cup shredded carrot
- ¼ cup shredded zucchini
- 2 tablespoons grated Parmesan cheese
- ½ teaspoon dried parsley flakes
- ½ teaspoon dried oregano
- ⅛ teaspoon garlic powder
- ⅛ teaspoon pepper
- ¾ cup meatless spaghetti sauce, divided

1. Cook pasta according to package directions. Meanwhile, in a small bowl, combine the ricotta cheese, ¼ cup mozzarella cheese, carrot, zucchini, Parmesan cheese, parsley, oregano, garlic powder and pepper.

2. Spread ¼ cup spaghetti sauce in a 3-cup baking dish coated with cooking spray. Drain shells; stuff with cheese mixture. Place in prepared baking dish. Top with remaining spaghetti sauce.

3. Cover and bake at 350° for 25 minutes. Uncover; sprinkle with remaining mozzarella. Bake 10-15 minutes longer or until bubbly.

PER SERVING *3 stuffed shells equals 326 cal., 10 g fat (6 g sat. fat), 40 mg chol., 721 mg sodium, 37 g carb., 3 g fiber, 21 g pro. **Diabetic Exchanges:** 2 medium-fat meat, 2 vegetable, 1½ starch.*

`261 CALORIES` Onion-Dijon Pork Chops

Coated in a flavorful sauce, these chops are cooked to tender perfection. Serve with rice and carrots for a nutritious meal.

—TASTE OF HOME TEST KITCHEN

START TO FINISH: 25 MIN. • **MAKES:** 4 SERVINGS

- 4 boneless pork loin chops (5 ounces each)
- ¼ teaspoon salt
- ¼ teaspoon pepper
- ¾ cup thinly sliced red onion
- ¼ cup water
- ¼ cup cider vinegar
- 3 tablespoons brown sugar
- 2 tablespoons honey Dijon mustard

1. Sprinkle pork chops with salt and pepper. In a large nonstick skillet coated with cooking spray, cook pork over medium heat for 4-6 minutes on each side or until lightly browned. Remove and keep warm.

2. Add the remaining ingredients to the skillet, stirring to loosen browned bits from pan. Bring to a boil; cook and stir for 2 minutes or until thickened. Return chops to the pan. Reduce heat; cover and simmer for 3-4 minutes or until a thermometer reads 145°. Let stand for 5 minutes before serving.

PER SERVING *1 pork chop with 2 tablespoons onion mixture equals 261 cal., 9 g fat (3 g sat. fat), 69 mg chol., 257 mg sodium, 17 g carb., 1 g fiber, 28 g pro. **Diabetic Exchanges:** 4 lean meat, 1 starch.*

Weekday Lasagna

This lasagna is my husband's favorite dish. I love it because it's low in fat and a real time-saver since you don't have to cook the noodles before baking.
—**KAREN MCCABE** PROVO, UTAH

PREP: 35 MIN. • **BAKE:** 1 HOUR + STANDING
MAKES: 9 SERVINGS

- 1 **pound lean ground beef (90% lean)**
- 1 **small onion, chopped**
- 1 **can (28 ounces) crushed tomatoes**
- 1¾ **cups water**
- 1 **can (6 ounces) tomato paste**
- 1 **envelope spaghetti sauce mix**
- 1 **egg, lightly beaten**
- 2 **cups (16 ounces) fat-free cottage cheese**
- 2 **tablespoons grated Parmesan cheese**
- 6 **uncooked lasagna noodles**
- 1 **cup (4 ounces) shredded part-skim mozzarella cheese**

1. In a large saucepan, cook beef and onion over medium heat until meat is no longer pink; drain. Stir in the tomatoes, water, tomato paste and spaghetti sauce mix. Bring to a boil. Reduce heat; cover and simmer for 15-20 minutes, stirring occasionally.

2. In a small bowl, combine the egg, cottage cheese and the Parmesan cheese.

3. Spread 2 cups meat sauce in a 13-in. x 9-in. baking dish coated with cooking spray. Layer with three noodles, half of the cottage cheese mixture and half of the remaining meat sauce. Repeat the layers.

4. Cover and bake at 350° for 50 minutes or until a thermometer reads 160°. Uncover; sprinkle with mozzarella cheese. Bake for 10-15 minutes longer or until bubbly and cheese is melted. Let stand for 15 minutes before cutting.

PER SERVING *1 piece equals 280 cal., 7 g fat (3 g sat. fat), 65 mg chol., 804 mg sodium, 29 g carb., 4 g fiber, 25 g pro.* **Diabetic Exchanges:** *3 lean meat, 2 vegetable, 1 starch.*

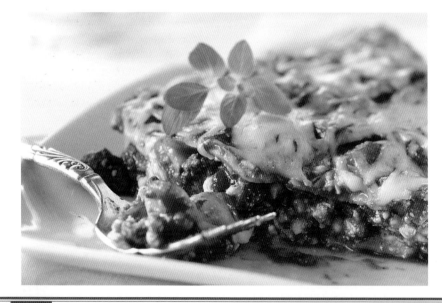

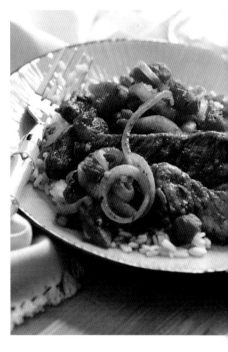

Sirloin Strips over Rice

I found this wonderful recipe in a magazine some 20 years ago. Its great flavor and the fact that leftovers just get better have made it a family winner!
—**KAREN DUNN** KANSAS CITY, MO

PREP: 15 MIN. • **COOK:** 30 MIN.
MAKES: 6 SERVINGS

- 1½ **pounds beef top sirloin steak, cut into thin strips**
- 1 **teaspoon salt**
- ¼ **teaspoon pepper**
- 2 **teaspoons olive oil, divided**
- 2 **medium onions, thinly sliced**
- 1 **garlic clove, minced**
- 1 **can (14½ ounces) diced tomatoes, undrained**
- ½ **cup reduced-sodium beef broth**
- ⅓ **cup dry red wine or additional reduced-sodium beef broth**
- 1 **bay leaf**
- ½ **teaspoon dried basil**
- ½ **teaspoon dried thyme**
- 3 **cups hot cooked rice**

1. Sprinkle beef strips with salt and pepper. In a large nonstick skillet coated with cooking spray, brown beef in 1 teaspoon oil. Remove and keep warm.

2. In the same skillet, saute onions in remaining oil until tender. Add garlic; cook 1 minute longer. Stir in the tomatoes, broth, wine, bay leaf, basil and thyme. Bring to a boil. Reduce heat; simmer, uncovered, for 10 minutes.

3. Return beef to the pan; cook for 2-4 minutes or until tender. Discard bay leaf. Serve with rice.

PER SERVING *⅔ cup beef mixture with ½ cup rice equals 299 cal.,* *7 g fat (2 g sat. fat), 63 mg chol., 567 mg sodium, 31 g carb., 3 g fiber, 25 g pro.* **Diabetic Exchanges:** *3 lean meat, 1½ starch, 1 vegetable, ½ fat.*

---

293 CALORIES

Pork Tenderloin Stew

My family often asks for this thick, creamy stew. It does an especially good job of warming us up on cold winter nights. Potatoes, carrots and mushrooms make it so satisfying.

—JANET ALLEN BELLEVILLE, IL

PREP: 20 MIN. • **COOK:** 40 MIN.
MAKES: 8 SERVINGS

- 2 **pork tenderloins (1 pound each),** cut into 1-inch cubes
- 1 **tablespoon olive oil**
- 1 **medium onion, chopped**
- 1 **garlic clove, minced**
- 1 **can (14½ ounces) reduced-sodium chicken broth**
- 2 **pounds red potatoes, peeled and cubed**
- 1 **cup sliced fresh carrots**
- 1 **cup sliced celery**
- ½ **pound sliced fresh mushrooms**
- 2 **tablespoons cider vinegar**
- 2 **teaspoons sugar**
- 1½ **teaspoons dried tarragon**
- 1 **teaspoon salt**
- 2 **tablespoons all-purpose flour**
- ½ **cup fat-free milk**
- ½ **cup reduced-fat sour cream**

1. In a large nonstick skillet over medium heat, cook pork in batches in oil until no longer pink; remove and keep warm.

2. In the same pan, saute onion until crisp-tender. Add garlic; cook 1 minute longer. Add the broth, vegetables, vinegar, sugar, tarragon and salt; bring to a boil. Reduce heat; cover and simmer for 25-30 minutes or until the vegetables are tender.

3. Combine flour and milk until smooth; gradually stir into vegetable mixture. Bring to a boil; cook and stir for 2 minutes or until thickened. Add pork and heat through. Stir in sour cream just before serving (do not boil).

PER SERVING *1¼ cups equals 293 cal., 7 g fat (3 g sat. fat), 68 mg chol., 521 mg sodium, 28 g carb., 3 g fiber, 28 g pro.*

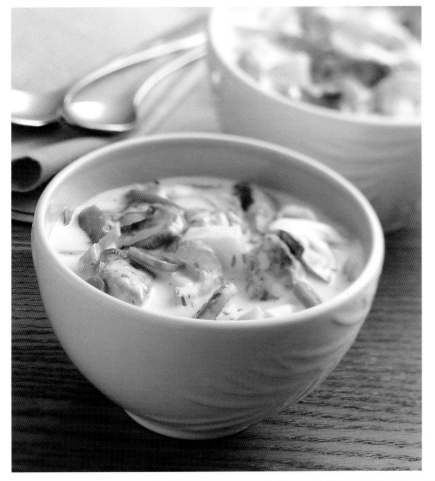

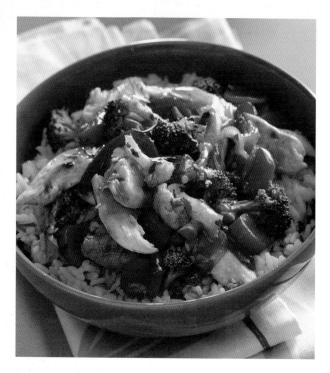

1. Combine the cornstarch, broth and soy sauce until smooth; set aside.
2. In a large nonstick skillet or wok, stir-fry the chicken in 1 tablespoon oil until no longer pink. Remove and keep warm.
3. Stir-fry the cauliflower, broccoli, carrots, red pepper and onion in remaining oil until crisp-tender. Add the garlic, salt, pepper and pepper flakes; cook 1 minute longer.
4. Stir cornstarch mixture and add to the pan. Bring to a boil; cook and stir for 2 minutes or until thickened. Add chicken; heat through. Serve with rice. Sprinkle each serving with cilantro.

PER SERVING *1 cup stir-fry with ½ cup rice equals 297 cal., 8 g fat (1 g sat. fat), 50 mg chol., 670 mg sodium, 32 g carb., 3 g fiber, 23 g pro.* **Diabetic Exchanges:** *2 lean meat, 1½ starch, 1 vegetable, 1 fat.*

---

297 CALORIES

Chicken & Vegetable Stir-Fry

You can't beat a stir-fry when you want a light entree that's quick, filling and loaded with flavor. Pepper flakes give the classic dish a bit of extra zip.

—SAMUEL ONIZUK ELKTON, MD

PREP: 20 MIN. • **COOK:** 15 MIN. • **MAKES:** 5 SERVINGS

- 4 teaspoons cornstarch
- 1 cup reduced-sodium chicken broth
- 2 tablespoons reduced-sodium soy sauce
- 1 pound boneless skinless chicken breasts, cut into ¼-inch strips
- 2 tablespoons olive oil, divided
- 1½ cups fresh cauliflowerets
- 1½ cups fresh broccoli florets
- 2 medium carrots, sliced
- 1 small sweet red pepper, julienned
- 1 small onion, halved and sliced
- 1 garlic clove, minced
- ½ teaspoon salt
- ½ teaspoon pepper
- ¼ to ½ teaspoon crushed red pepper flakes
- 2½ cups hot cooked rice
  Minced fresh cilantro

---

272 CALORIES

Grilled Snapper with Caper Sauce

This recipe uses snapper, but if you prefer a different fish, try mahi-mahi. It is a delicious firm, mild fish that won't fall apart on the grill.

—ALAINA SHOWALTER CLOVER, SC

PREP: 20 MIN. + MARINATING • **GRILL:** 10 MIN. • **MAKES:** 4 SERVINGS

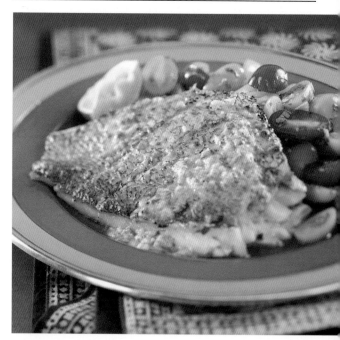

- ⅓ cup lime juice
- 1 jalapeno pepper, seeded
- 3 garlic cloves, peeled
- 1¼ teaspoons fresh thyme leaves or ¼ teaspoon dried thyme
- 1 teaspoon salt
- 1 teaspoon pepper
- 4 red snapper fillets (6 ounces each)

SAUCE
- 3 tablespoons lime juice
- 3 tablespoons olive oil
- 2 tablespoons water
- 2 teaspoons red wine vinegar
- ½ cup fresh cilantro leaves
- 1 shallot, peeled
- 1 tablespoon capers, drained
- 1½ teaspoons chopped seeded jalapeno pepper
- 1 garlic clove, peeled and halved
- ¼ teaspoon pepper

1. In a small food processor, combine the first six ingredients; cover and process until blended. Pour into a large resealable plastic bag. Add the fillets; seal bag and turn to coat. Refrigerate for 30 minutes.

2. Drain and discard marinade. Moisten a paper towel with cooking oil; using long-handled tongs, lightly coat the grill rack. Grill fillets, covered, over medium heat or broil 4 in. from the heat for 3-5 minutes on each side or until the fish flakes easily with a fork.

3. Meanwhile, combine sauce ingredients in a small food processor. Cover and process until blended. Serve with the fish.

NOTE *Wear disposable gloves when cutting hot peppers; the oils can burn skin. Avoid touching your face.*

PER SERVING *1 fillet with 3 tablespoons sauce equals 272 cal., 12 g fat (2 g sat. fat), 60 mg chol., 435 mg sodium, 5 g carb., 1 g fiber, 34 g pro.* **Diabetic Exchanges:** *5 lean meat, 2 fat.*

282 CALORIES Chicken Fajita Spaghetti

Save time and your sanity on busy nights with this dinner. I usually cut up the chicken, onion and peppers while our two young children are napping. Then, just before my husband gets home from work, I toss everything into the skillet while the pasta cooks on another burner.
—HEATHER BROWN FRISCO, TX

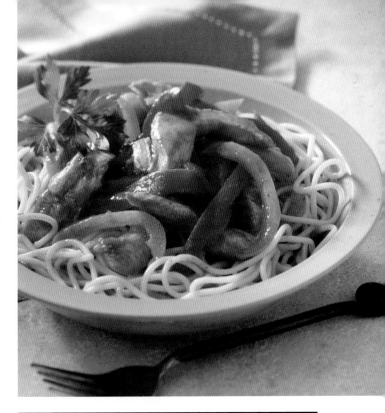

START TO FINISH: 20 MIN. • **MAKES:** 6 SERVINGS
- 8 ounces uncooked spaghetti
- 1 pound boneless skinless chicken breasts, cut into strips
- 1 tablespoon canola oil
- 1 small onion, sliced
- 1 small sweet red pepper, julienned
- 1 small sweet yellow pepper, julienned
- 1 can (4 ounces) chopped green chilies
- ½ cup water
- ½ cup taco sauce
- 1 envelope fajita seasoning mix

1. Cook the spaghetti according to package directions. Meanwhile, in a large skillet, cook chicken over medium heat in oil until no longer pink; remove and keep warm.

2. In the same skillet, saute onion and peppers until tender. Add the chicken, chilies, water, taco sauce and fajita seasoning; heat through. Drain spaghetti; toss with chicken mixture.

PER SERVING *1¼ cups equals 282 cal., 5 g fat (1 g sat. fat), 42 mg chol., 722 mg sodium, 37 g carb., 2 g fiber, 21 g pro.* **Diabetic Exchanges:** *2 starch, 2 lean meat, 1 vegetable.*

283 CALORIES Grilled Artichoke-Mushroom Pizza

We live on a lake and entertain lots of family and friends. This became one of our most-requested, go-to summer meals for quick cooking on the grill.

—BRENDA WATERS CLARKESVILLE, GA

PREP: 20 MIN. • **GRILL:** 15 MIN.
MAKES: 6 SERVINGS

- 1 prebaked 12-inch pizza crust
- ½ teaspoon olive oil
- ⅔ cup tomato and basil spaghetti sauce
- 2 plum tomatoes, sliced
- ¼ cup sliced fresh mushrooms
- ¼ cup water-packed artichoke hearts, rinsed, drained and chopped
- 2 tablespoons sliced ripe olives, optional
- 1 cup (4 ounces) shredded part-skim mozzarella cheese
- ½ cup crumbled tomato and basil feta cheese
- 1½ teaspoons minced fresh basil or ½ teaspoon dried basil
- 1½ teaspoons minced fresh rosemary or ½ teaspoon dried rosemary, crushed
- 1½ teaspoons minced chives

1. Brush crust with oil. Spread spaghetti sauce over crust to within 1 in. of edges. Top with tomatoes, mushrooms, artichokes and olives if desired. Sprinkle with cheeses.

2. Prepare grill for indirect heat. Grill, covered, over medium indirect heat for 12-15 minutes or until cheese is melted and crust is lightly browned. Sprinkle with herbs during the last 5 minutes of cooking. Let stand for 5 minutes before slicing.

PER SERVING *1 slice (calculated without olives) equals 283 cal., 10 g fat (3 g sat. fat), 17 mg chol., 712 mg sodium, 34 g carb., 1 g fiber, 14 g pro.* **Diabetic Exchanges:** *2 starch, 1½ fat, 1 lean meat.*

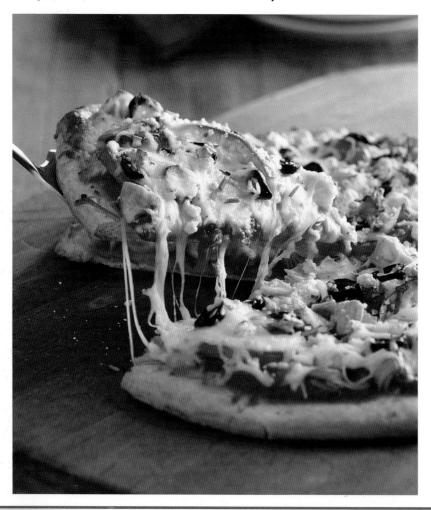

322 CALORIES Light-But-Hearty Tuna Casserole

My boyfriend grew up loving his mother's tuna casserole and says he can't tell at all that this one is light! We have it at least once a month. I usually serve it with a salad, but it has enough veggies to stand on its own.

—HEIDI CAROFANO BROOKLYN, NY

PREP: 20 MIN. • **BAKE:** 25 MIN.
MAKES: 4 SERVINGS

- 3 cups uncooked yolk-free noodles
- 1 can (10¾ ounces) reduced-fat reduced-sodium condensed cream of mushroom soup, undiluted
- ½ cup fat-free milk
- 2 tablespoons reduced-fat mayonnaise
- ½ teaspoon ground mustard
- 1 jar (6 ounces) sliced mushrooms, drained
- 1 can (5 ounces) albacore white tuna in water
- ¼ cup chopped roasted sweet red pepper

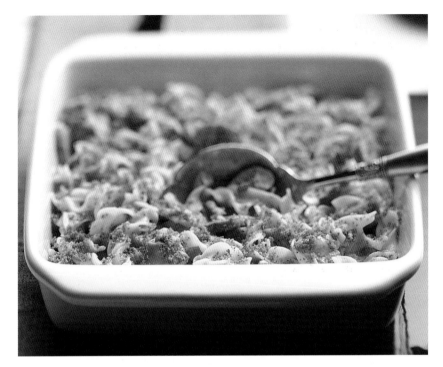

TOPPING

- ¼ cup dry bread crumbs
- 1 tablespoon butter, melted
- ½ teaspoon paprika
- ¼ teaspoon Italian seasoning
- ¼ teaspoon pepper

1. Cook noodles according to package directions.

2. In a large bowl, combine the soup, milk, mayonnaise and mustard. Stir in the mushrooms, tuna and red pepper. Drain the noodles; add to soup mixture and stir until blended. Transfer to an 8-in. square baking dish coated with cooking spray.

3. Combine topping ingredients; sprinkle over the casserole. Bake at 400° for 25-30 minutes or until bubbly.

PER SERVING *1½ cups equals 322 cal., 9 g fat (3 g sat. fat), 32 mg chol., 843 mg sodium, 39 g carb., 4 g fiber, 18 g pro.*

343 CALORIES Baked Vegetable Beef Stew

When my granddaughter was three, she had a toy bear that sang a song about root stew. She thought he was talking about tree roots, so I took her to the store to buy and learn about root veggies, and we made this stew.
—**ALICE MCCABE** CLIMAX, NY

PREP: 25 MIN. • **BAKE:** 1½ HOURS
MAKES: 6 SERVINGS

- 1½ pounds beef sirloin tip roast, cut into 1-inch cubes
- 3 cups cubed peeled potatoes
- 3 celery ribs, cut into 1-inch pieces
- 1½ cups cubed peeled sweet potatoes
- 3 large carrots, cut into 1-inch pieces
- 1 large onion, cut into 12 wedges
- 1 cup cubed peeled rutabaga
- 1 envelope reduced-sodium onion soup mix
- 2 teaspoons dried basil
- ½ teaspoon salt
- ¼ teaspoon pepper
- ½ cup water
- 1 can (14½ ounces) stewed tomatoes

1. In a large resealable plastic bag, combine the beef, vegetables, soup mix and seasonings. Seal bag and shake to coat.

2. Transfer to an oven-safe Dutch oven or a 13-in. x 9-in. baking dish coated with cooking spray (dish will be very full). Pour water over the beef mixture.

3. Cover and bake at 325° for 1 hour. Stir in tomatoes. Bake, uncovered, 30-50 minutes longer or until beef and vegetables are tender, stirring occasionally.

PER SERVING *1⅓cups equals 343 cal., 6 g fat (2 g sat. fat), 71 mg chol., 699 mg sodium, 42 g carb., 5 g fiber, 29 g pro.* **Diabetic Exchanges:** *3 lean meat, 3 vegetable, 1½ starch.*

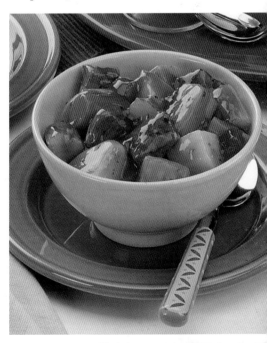

290 CALORIES Italian Chicken Wraps

After enjoying a chicken wrap at a restaurant, I experimented at home to create something similar. My version is as fast to make as it is yummy!

—CATHY HOFFLANDER ADRIAN, MI

START TO FINISH: 25 MIN. • **MAKES:** 6 SERVINGS

- 1 package (16 ounces) frozen stir-fry vegetable blend
- 2 packages (6 ounces each) ready-to-use grilled chicken breast strips
- ½ cup fat-free Italian salad dressing
- 3 tablespoons shredded Parmesan cheese
- 6 flour tortillas (8 inches), room temperature

1. In a large saucepan, cook vegetables according to package directions; drain. Stir in the chicken, salad dressing and cheese; heat through.

2. Spoon about ¾ cup down the center of each tortilla; roll up tightly.

PER SERVING *1 wrap equals 290 cal., 6 g fat (2 g sat. fat), 40 mg chol., 1,129 mg sodium, 38 g carb., 3 g fiber, 20 g pro.* **Diabetic Exchanges:** *2 lean meat, 2 vegetable, 1½ starch.*

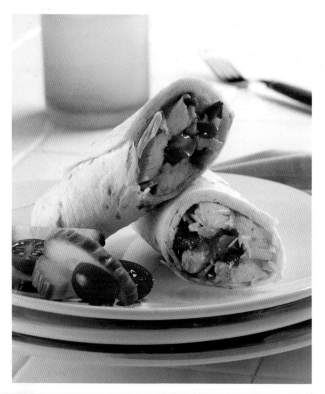

334 CALORIES Tilapia & Lemon Sauce

This delicious yet light pairing of fish and citrus will evoke thoughts of warm, summery days even when it's chilly outside.

—SUSAN TAUL BIRMINGHAM, AL

START TO FINISH: 30 MIN. • **MAKES:** 4 SERVINGS

- ¼ cup plus 1 tablespoon all-purpose flour, divided
- 1 teaspoon salt
- 4 tilapia fillets (4 ounces each)
- 2 tablespoons plus 2 teaspoons butter, divided
- ⅓ cup reduced-sodium chicken broth
- 2 tablespoons white wine or additional reduced-sodium chicken broth
- 1½ teaspoons lemon juice
- 1½ teaspoons minced fresh parsley
- 2 cups hot cooked rice
- ¼ cup sliced almonds, toasted

1. In a shallow bowl, combine ¼ cup flour and salt. Dip fillets in flour mixture.

2. In a large nonstick skillet coated with cooking spray, cook fillets in 2 tablespoons butter over medium-high heat for 4-5 minutes on each side or until fish flakes easily with a fork. Remove and keep warm.

3. In the same skillet, melt remaining butter. Stir in remaining flour until smooth; gradually add the broth, wine and lemon juice. Bring to a boil; cook and stir for 2 minutes or until thickened. Stir in parsley. Serve fish and sauce with rice; garnish with almonds.

PER SERVING *1 fillet with ½ cup rice, 1 tablespoon almonds and 4 teaspoons sauce equals 334 cal., 12 g fat (6 g sat. fat), 75 mg chol., 586 mg sodium, 30 g carb., 1 g fiber, 26 g pro.* **Diabetic Exchanges:** *3 lean meat, 2 starch, 2 fat.*

277 CALORIES
Orange-Glazed Pork Stir-Fry

To add extra color and tangy flavor, I like to stir drained mandarin orange segments in with the cooked pork. It makes such a fast, simple and delicious meal!

—EDIE DESPAIN LOGAN, UTAH

START TO FINISH: 20 MIN. • **MAKES:** 2 SERVINGS

- ½ pound pork tenderloin, cut into ¼-inch slices
- 2 teaspoons canola oil
- 1 cup fresh snow peas
- 1 small onion, sliced and separated into rings

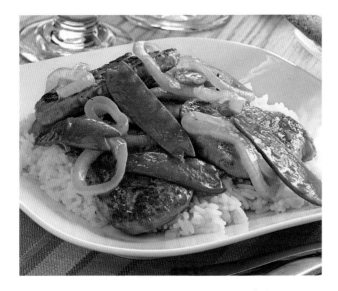

¼ cup reduced-sugar orange marmalade
1 tablespoon chili sauce
Hot cooked rice, optional

1. In a nonstick skillet or wok, stir-fry pork in oil until no longer pink. Remove and keep warm. Reduce heat to medium; add snow peas, onion, marmalade and chili sauce. Cook and stir until vegetables are crisp-tender.
2. Return pork to the pan and heat through. Serve with rice if desired.
PER SERVING *1½ cups pork mixture (calculated without rice) equals 277 cal., 9 g fat (2 g sat. fat), 63 mg chol., 164 mg sodium, 23 g carb., 3 g fiber, 26 g pro.* **Diabetic Exchanges:** *3 lean meat, 1 starch, 1 vegetable, 1 fat.*

272 CALORIES Meatless Zucchini Lasagna
Here's a meatless lasagna that's chock-full of healthful zucchini and delicious cheeses. You'll be surprised that such a generous portion still weighs in at under 300 calories!
—RUTH VAUGHT TEMPE, AZ

PREP: 45 MIN. • **BAKE:** 30 MIN. + STANDING • **MAKES:** 9 SERVINGS

6 lasagna noodles
1 medium onion, chopped
2 teaspoons olive oil
2 garlic cloves, minced
2 cups water
2 cans (6 ounces each) tomato paste
2½ teaspoons each dried thyme, basil and oregano
¾ teaspoon salt
3 medium zucchini, thinly sliced
1 egg, lightly beaten
1 carton (15 ounces) part-skim ricotta cheese
2 cups (8 ounces) shredded part-skim mozzarella cheese
¼ cup grated Parmesan cheese

1. Cook noodles according to package directions. Meanwhile, in a large nonstick skillet, saute onion in oil until tender. Add garlic; cook 1 minute longer. Stir in the water, tomato paste and seasonings. Bring to a boil. Reduce heat; cover and simmer for 10 minutes.
2. Place zucchini in a large saucepan; add ½ in. water. Bring to a boil. Reduce heat; cover and cook 5 minutes. Drain and set aside. In a small bowl, combine egg and ricotta cheese.
3. Drain noodles. Place ½ cup tomato sauce in a 13-in. x 9-in. baking dish coated with cooking spray; top with three noodles. Layer with half of the ricotta mixture and zucchini. Top with half of the remaining tomato sauce and 1 cup mozzarella cheese. Repeat layers.
4. Cover and bake at 375° for 25 minutes. Uncover; sprinkle with Parmesan cheese. Bake 5-10 minutes longer or until bubbly. Let lasagna stand for 10 minutes before cutting.
PER SERVING *1 piece equals 272 cal., 10 g fat (6 g sat. fat), 55 mg chol., 454 mg sodium, 28 g carb., 4 g fiber, 18 g pro.* **Diabetic Exchanges:** *2 medium-fat meat, 2 vegetable, 1 starch.*

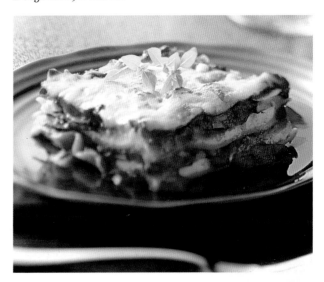

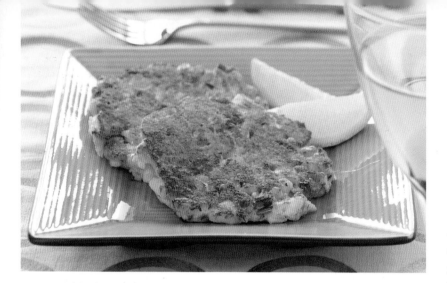

311 CALORIES Crab Cakes with Fresh Lemon

Fresh lemon brings out all the great flavors in these crispy crab cakes. Be careful not to overcook or they'll be dry, instead of moist and delicate.
—**EDIE DESPAIN** LOGAN, UTAH

PREP: 25 MIN. • **COOK:** 10 MIN./BATCH
MAKES: 4 SERVINGS

- ⅔ **cup yellow cornmeal**
- ⅓ **cup fat-free milk**
- 1 **small sweet red pepper, finely chopped**
- 4 **green onions, chopped**
- 1 **teaspoon canola oil**
- 3 **egg whites, lightly beaten**
- ⅓ **cup reduced-fat mayonnaise**
- ¼ **cup all-purpose flour**
- ¼ **cup minced fresh parsley**
- 2 **tablespoons lemon juice**
- ¼ **teaspoon seafood seasoning**
- ⅛ **teaspoon cayenne pepper**
- 2 **cups lump crabmeat, drained**
- 1 **cup frozen corn, thawed**
- 8 **lemon wedges**

1. In a large bowl, combine cornmeal and milk; set aside. In a large nonstick skillet, saute red pepper and onions in oil until tender. Remove from the heat.

2. Add the egg whites, mayonnaise, flour, parsley, lemon juice, seafood seasoning and cayenne to the reserved cornmeal mixture; mix well. Fold in the crab, corn and red pepper mixture.

3. Coat the same skillet with cooking spray; drop crab mixture by scant ½ cupfuls into the pan. Press into ¾-in.-thick patties. Cook in batches over medium heat for 4-6 minutes on each side or until golden brown. Serve with lemon wedges.
PER SERVING *2 crab cakes equals 311 cal., 9 g fat (1 g sat. fat), 67 mg chol., 764 mg sodium, 43 g carb., 5 g fiber, 17 g pro. **Diabetic Exchanges:** 3 starch, 2 lean meat, 1½ fat.*

276 CALORIES Open-Faced Chicken Sandwiches

Caramelized onions, mushrooms and two types of cheese make these my favorite sandwiches. I invented them for a last-minute party, using what I had on hand. They've been a hit with family and friends ever since.
—**LYNDA CLARK** SPOKANE, WA

START TO FINISH: 30 MIN.
MAKES: 8 SERVINGS

- 1 **pound sliced fresh mushrooms**
- 1 **large sweet onion, sliced**
- 1 **cup fat-free mayonnaise**
- ½ **cup crumbled blue cheese**
- ¼ **teaspoon pepper**
- 8 **slices French bread (1 inch thick)**
- 1 **pound boneless skinless chicken breasts, grilled and sliced**
- 1 **cup (4 ounces) shredded part-skim mozzarella cheese**

1. In a large nonstick skillet coated with cooking spray, saute the mushrooms and onion for 15-20 minutes or until onion is tender and golden brown; set aside.
2. In a small bowl, combine the mayonnaise, blue cheese and pepper. Spread blue cheese mixture over each bread slice. Top with chicken, mushroom mixture and mozzarella cheese.
3. Broil 4-6 in. from the heat for 3-4 minutes or until the cheese is melted.
PER SERVING *1 open-faced sandwich equals 276 cal., 8 g fat (4 g sat. fat), 66 mg chol., 618 mg sodium, 23 g carb., 3 g fiber, 27 g pro. **Diabetic Exchanges:** 3 lean meat, 1 starch, 1 vegetable.*

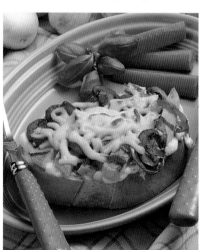

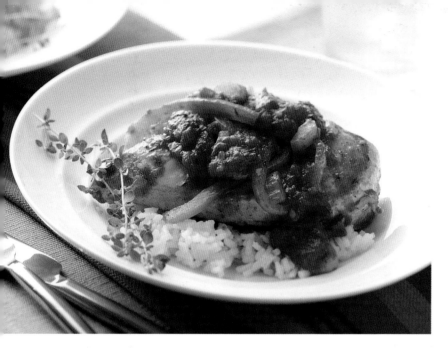

1 can (8 ounces) tomato sauce
½ cup uncooked elbow macaroni
½ cup water
¼ cup picante sauce
2 tablespoons shredded fat-free
  cheddar cheese
¼ cup crushed baked tortilla chip
  scoops
¼ cup chopped avocado
  Iceberg lettuce wedges and
  fat-free sour cream, optional

1. In a large nonstick skillet coated with cooking spray, cook the turkey, onion and green pepper over medium heat until turkey is no longer pink.
2. Stir in the tomato sauce, macaroni, water and picante sauce. Bring to a boil. Reduce heat; cover and simmer for 10-15 minutes or until macaroni is tender.
3. Divide between two plates; top with cheese, tortilla chips and avocado. Serve with lettuce and sour cream if desired.

PER SERVING *1 serving (calculated without sour cream) equals 267 cal., 9 g fat (2 g sat. fat), 46 mg chol., 795 mg sodium, 30 g carb., 3 g fiber, 18 g pro. **Diabetic Exchanges:** 2 lean meat, 1½ starch, 1 vegetable, ½ fat.*

320 CALORIES
Creole Chicken

Chili powder lends just a hint of heat to this full-flavored and oh-so-easy chicken entree. This recipe's a keeper!
—SUSAN SHIELDS ENGLEWOOD, FL

PREP: 15 MIN. • **COOK:** 25 MIN.
MAKES: 2 SERVINGS

  2 boneless skinless chicken breast
    halves (4 ounces each)
  1 teaspoon canola oil
  1 can (14½ ounces) stewed
    tomatoes, cut up
  ⅓ cup julienned green pepper
  ¼ cup chopped celery
  ¼ cup sliced onion
  ½ to 1 teaspoon chili powder
  ½ teaspoon dried thyme
  ⅛ teaspoon pepper
  1 cup hot cooked rice

1. In a small nonstick skillet coated with cooking spray, cook the chicken in oil over medium heat for 5-6 minutes on each side or until a thermometer reads 170°. Remove and keep warm.

2. In the same skillet, combine the tomatoes, green pepper, celery, onion, chili powder, thyme and pepper. Bring to a boil. Reduce heat; cover and simmer for 10 minutes or until vegetables are crisp-tender. Return chicken to pan; heat through. Serve with rice.

PER SERVING *1 chicken breast half with ⅔ cup sauce and ½ cup rice equals 320 cal., 5 g fat (1 g sat. fat), 63 mg chol., 447 mg sodium, 41 g carb., 3 g fiber, 27 g pro. **Diabetic Exchanges:** 3 lean meat, 3 starch, ½ fat.*

202 CALORIES Skillet Tacos

If you like Mexican food, you'll be whipping up these fast, healthy skillet tacos often.
—MARIA GOBEL GREENFIELD, WI

START TO FINISH: 30 MIN.
MAKES: 2 SERVINGS

  ¼ pound lean ground turkey
  2 tablespoons chopped onion
  2 tablespoons chopped green
    pepper

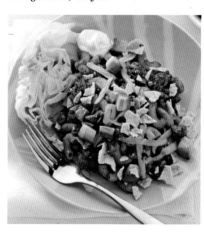

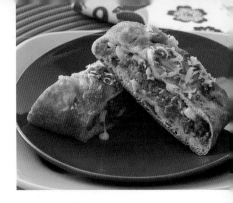

Italian Pasta Casserole

335 CALORIES

All the traditional Italian flavors abound in this dish reminiscent of lasagna. It's a zippy and hearty recipe that our family and guests really like.

—DENISE RASMUSSEN SALINA, KS

PREP: 30 MIN. • **BAKE:** 20 MIN.
MAKES: 6 SERVINGS

- 2 cups uncooked spiral pasta
- ½ pound lean ground beef (90% lean)
- ½ pound Italian turkey sausage links, casings removed
- 1 small onion, finely chopped
- 1 garlic clove, minced
- 2 cans (14½ ounces each) diced tomatoes, undrained
- ⅓ cup tomato paste
- ¾ teaspoon Italian seasoning
- ½ teaspoon chili powder
- ¼ teaspoon dried oregano
- ⅛ teaspoon salt
- ⅛ teaspoon garlic powder
- ⅛ teaspoon dried thyme
- ⅛ teaspoon pepper
- 2 ounces sliced turkey pepperoni
- 1 cup (4 ounces) shredded part-skim mozzarella cheese

1. Cook pasta according to package directions. Meanwhile, crumble beef and sausage into a large skillet; add onion. Cook and stir over medium heat until meat is no longer pink. Add garlic; cook 1 minute longer. Drain. Stir in the tomatoes, tomato paste and seasonings. Bring to a boil. Reduce the heat; simmer, uncovered, for 5 minutes.
2. Drain pasta; stir in meat mixture and pepperoni. Transfer half of the pasta mixture to a 2-qt. baking dish coated with cooking spray. Sprinkle with half of the cheese; repeat layers.
3. Cover and bake at 350° for 20-25 minutes or until bubbly.
PER SERVING *1 cup equals 335 cal., 11 g fat (4 g sat. fat), 64 mg chol., 752 mg sodium, 33 g carb., 4 g fiber, 26 g pro.* ***Diabetic Exchanges:*** *2 starch, 2 lean meat, 1½ fat.*

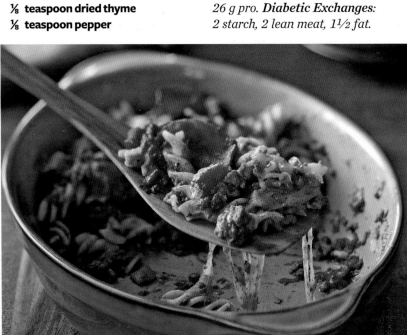

French Cheeseburger Loaf

277 CALORIES

Once you prepare this impressive-looking, yet simple-to-make sandwich, you'll probably never look at refrigerated bread dough the same. It's just so easy!

—NANCY DAUGHERTY CORTLAND, OH

PREP: 25 MIN. • **BAKE:** 25 MIN.
MAKES: 6 SERVINGS

- ¾ pound lean ground beef (90% lean)
- ½ cup chopped sweet onion
- 1 small green pepper, chopped
- 2 garlic cloves, minced
- 2 tablespoons all-purpose flour
- 2 tablespoons Dijon mustard
- 1 tablespoon ketchup
- 1 tube (11 ounces) refrigerated crusty French loaf
- 4 slices reduced-fat process American cheese product
- 1 egg white, lightly beaten
- 3 tablespoons shredded Parmesan cheese

1. In a large skillet, cook the beef, onion and pepper over medium heat until meat is no longer pink. Add garlic; cook 1 minute longer. Stir in the flour, mustard and ketchup; set aside.
2. Unroll dough starting at the seam. Pat into a 14-in. x 12-in. rectangle. Spoon meat mixture lengthwise down the center of the dough; top with cheese slices. Bring

long sides of dough to the center over filling; pinch seam to seal.

3. Place seam side down on a baking sheet coated with cooking spray. Brush with egg white. Sprinkle with Parmesan cheese.

4. With a sharp knife, cut diagonal slits in top of loaf. Bake at 350° for 25-30 minutes or until golden brown. Serve warm.

PER SERVING *1 slice equals 277 cal., 7 g fat (3 g sat. fat), 33 mg chol., 697 mg sodium, 30 g carb., 1 g fiber, 21 g pro.* **Diabetic Exchanges:** *2 starch, 2 lean meat.*

Colorful Beef Wraps

I stir-fry a combination of sirloin steak, onions and peppers for these hearty wraps. Spreading a little fat-free ranch salad dressing inside the tortillas really jazzes up the taste.
—**ROBYN CAVALLARO** EASTON, PA

START TO FINISH: 30 MIN.
MAKES: 6 SERVINGS

- 1 beef top sirloin steak (1 pound), cut into thin strips
- ¼ teaspoon pepper
- 3 tablespoons reduced-sodium soy sauce, divided
- 3 teaspoons olive oil, divided
- 1 medium red onion, cut into wedges
- 3 garlic cloves, minced
- 1 jar (7 ounces) roasted sweet red peppers, drained and cut into strips
- ¼ cup dry red wine or reduced-sodium beef broth
- 6 tablespoons fat-free ranch salad dressing
- 6 flour tortillas (8 inches)
- 1½ cups torn iceberg lettuce
- 1 medium tomato, chopped
- ¼ cup chopped green onions

1. In a large nonstick skillet coated with cooking spray, saute beef, pepper and 2 tablespoons soy sauce in 2 teaspoons oil until meat is no longer pink. Remove and keep warm.

2. Saute the onion and garlic in remaining oil for 1 minute. Stir in the red peppers, wine and remaining soy sauce; bring to a boil. Return beef to the pan; simmer for 5 minutes or until heated through.

3. Spread ranch dressing over one side of each tortilla; sprinkle with lettuce, tomato and green onions. Spoon about ¾ cup beef mixture down center of each tortilla; roll up.

PER SERVING *1 wrap equals 325 cal., 9 g fat (2 g sat. fat), 43 mg chol., 830 mg sodium, 39 g carb., 1 g fiber, 20 g pro.* **Diabetic Exchanges:** *2 starch, 2 lean meat, 1 vegetable, 1 fat.*

Easy Barbecued Pork Chops

Here's a good, thrifty skillet supper. I sometimes use a sweet red pepper instead of green for color and flavor. It makes an attractive main dish.
—**JORIE WELCH** ACWORTH, GA

PREP: 10 MIN. • **COOK:** 40 MIN.
MAKES: 4 SERVINGS

- 4 bone-in pork loin chops (6 ounces each)
- 2 teaspoons canola oil
- 1 medium green pepper, chopped
- ⅔ cup chopped celery
- ⅓ cup chopped onion
- 1 cup ketchup
- ¼ cup packed brown sugar
- ¼ cup reduced-sodium chicken broth
- 2 tablespoons chili powder

1. In a large nonstick skillet, brown pork chops in oil over medium-high heat. Remove chops and keep warm. Add green pepper, celery and onion to the skillet; cook and stir until vegetables begin to soften.

2. Return pork chops to the pan. In a bowl, combine the ketchup, brown sugar, broth and chili powder. Pour over chops and vegetables. Bring to a boil. Reduce heat; cover and simmer for 30 minutes or until meat is tender.

PER SERVING *1 pork chop with ⅓ cup sauce equals 312 cal., 9 g fat (2 g sat. fat), 66 mg chol., 867 mg sodium, 35 g carb., 3 g fiber, 24 g pro.* **Diabetic Exchanges:** *3 lean meat, 2 starch.*

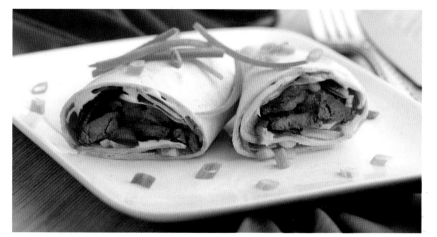

> My weight soared when a medical condition left me unable to exercise. Once I got my strength back, I started to cook to lose weight. I count calories and choose light options when I'm dining out. I'm so happy now that I can do all the things I love.

—REGINA LINDSEY

320 CALORIES Raspberry Chicken Salad

This pretty summer salad is a snap to make, but it looks as though you fussed. The simple raspberry dressing is also used to cook the chicken, which gives it a nice flavor.

—SUE ZIMONICK GREEN BAY, WI

START TO FINISH: 30 MIN. • **MAKES:** 4 SERVINGS

- 1 cup 100% raspberry spreadable fruit
- ⅓ cup raspberry vinegar
- 4 boneless skinless chicken breast halves (4 ounces each)
- 8 cups torn mixed salad greens
- 1 small red onion, thinly sliced
- 24 fresh raspberries

1. In a small bowl, combine spreadable fruit and vinegar; set aside ¾ cup for dressing. Broil chicken 4 in. from the heat for 5-7 minutes on each side or until a thermometer reads 170°, basting occasionally with remaining raspberry mixture. Cool for 10 minutes.

2. Meanwhile, arrange greens and onion on salad plates. Slice chicken; place over greens. Drizzle with reserved dressing. Garnish with raspberries.

PER SERVING *2 cups greens with 1 chicken breast half and 3 tablespoons dressing equals 320 cal., 3 g fat (1 g sat. fat), 63 mg chol., 97 mg sodium, 48 g carb., 3 g fiber, 25 g pro.* **Diabetic Exchanges:** *3 starch, 3 lean meat, 2 vegetable.*

275 CALORIES Veggie Tuna Burgers

You don't have to be a health nut to enjoy the flavor of these nutritious burgers. They're an easy way to get my children to eat their vegetables.

—LAURA DAVIS RUSTON, LA

START TO FINISH: 30 MIN. • **MAKES:** 6 SERVINGS

- ¼ cup finely chopped onion
- 1 garlic clove, minced
- 1 cup each shredded zucchini, yellow summer squash and carrots
- 1 egg, lightly beaten
- 2 cups soft whole wheat bread crumbs
- 1 can (6 ounces) light water-packed tuna, drained and flaked
- ¼ teaspoon salt
- ¼ teaspoon pepper
- 1 teaspoon butter
- 6 hamburger buns, split
- 6 slices reduced-fat cheddar cheese
- 6 lettuce leaves
- 6 slices tomato

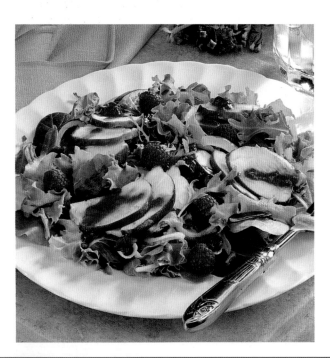

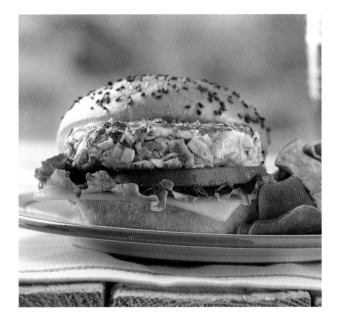

1. In a large nonstick skillet coated with cooking spray, saute onion and garlic for 1 minute. Add the zucchini, yellow squash and carrots; saute until tender. Drain and cool to room temperature.

2. In a large bowl, combine the egg, bread crumbs, tuna, salt and pepper. Add vegetable mixture. Shape into six 3¹/₂-in. patties.

3. Coat the same skillet again with cooking spray; cook patties in butter for 3-5 minutes on each side or until lightly browned. Serve on buns with cheese, lettuce and tomato.

PER SERVING *1 burger equals 275 cal., 8 g fat (4 g sat. fat), 58 mg chol., 643 mg sodium, 32 g carb., 3 g fiber, 20 g pro.* **Diabetic Exchanges:** *2 starch, 2 lean meat, 1 vegetable.*

274 CALORIES Spaghetti Pizza Casserole

I first tried this great-tasting dish at an office Christmas party, where it quickly became everyone's favorite. It's a wonderful alternative to ordinary spaghetti.
—**KIM NEER** KALAMAZOO, MI

PREP: 25 MIN. • **BAKE:** 25 MIN. • **MAKES:** 9 SERVINGS

- 1 package (7 ounces) spaghetti
- ½ cup egg substitute
- ¼ cup grated Parmesan cheese
- 1 pound lean ground beef (90% lean)
- 1 medium onion, chopped
- ½ cup chopped green pepper
- ½ cup chopped sweet yellow pepper
- 2 garlic cloves, minced
- 1 jar (24 ounces) spaghetti sauce
- 1 teaspoon Italian seasoning
- 1 teaspoon dried basil
- ½ teaspoon salt
- ¼ teaspoon pepper
- ½ pound sliced fresh mushrooms
- 1½ cups (6 ounces) shredded part-skim mozzarella cheese

1. Cook spaghetti according to package directions. Drain and rinse with cold water. In a large bowl, toss spaghetti with egg substitute and Parmesan cheese. Spread evenly into a 15-in. x 10-in. x 1-in. baking pan coated with cooking spray; set aside.

2. In a large nonstick skillet, cook the beef, onion and peppers over medium heat until meat is no longer pink; drain. Add garlic; cook 1 minute longer. Stir in spaghetti sauce and seasonings; heat through.

3. Spoon over spaghetti. Top with mushrooms and mozzarella cheese. Bake, uncovered, at 350° for 25-30 minutes or until lightly browned. Let stand for 5 minutes before serving.

PER SERVING *1 piece equals 274 cal., 8 g fat (4 g sat. fat), 37 mg chol., 685 mg sodium, 29 g carb., 3 g fiber, 22 g pro.* **Diabetic Exchanges:** *2 lean meat, 1¹/₂ starch, 1 vegetable.*

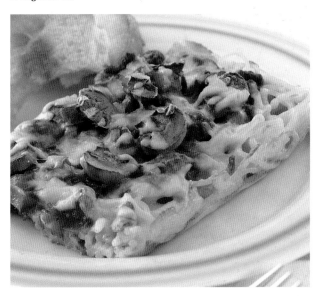

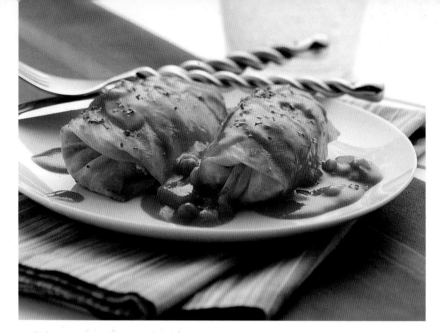

PER SERVING *2 cabbage rolls equals 293 cal., 10 g fat (3 g sat. fat), 74 mg chol., 582 mg sodium, 29 g carb., 4 g fiber, 22 g pro.* **Diabetic Exchanges:** *3 lean meat, 1½ starch, 1 vegetable.*

341 CALORIES

Home-Style Pot Roast

Tender meat, lots of vegetables and a tasty gravy make this meal so very satisfying and filling.

—OLGA MONTECORBOLI
MANCHESTER, CT

PREP: 15 MIN. • **COOK:** 3¼ HOURS
MAKES: 8 SERVINGS

- **1 beef eye round roast (2½ pounds)**
- **6 tablespoons all-purpose flour, divided**
- **1 tablespoon canola oil**
- **1½ cups plus ⅓ cup water, divided**
- **1½ cups dry red wine or reduced-sodium beef broth**
- **2 teaspoons beef bouillon granules**

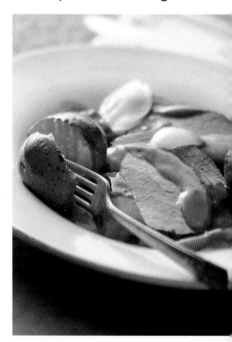

293 CALORIES Italian-Style Cabbage Rolls

Here's another great way to get your family to eat their veggies. Not only is this one of my gang's favorite dinners, but my son loves to help me roll the turkey filling into the cabbage leaves.

—ERIKA NIEHOFF EVELETH, MN

PREP: 45 MIN. • **BAKE:** 50 MIN.
MAKES: 5 SERVINGS

- **⅓ cup uncooked brown rice**
- **1 medium head cabbage**
- **½ cup shredded carrot**
- **¼ cup finely chopped onion**
- **¼ cup egg substitute**
- **1 can (10¾ ounces) reduced-sodium condensed tomato soup, undiluted, divided**
- **1 can (10¾ ounces) reduced-fat reduced-sodium condensed vegetable beef soup, undiluted, divided**
- **2 tablespoons Italian seasoning, divided**
- **¼ teaspoon cayenne pepper**
- **¼ teaspoon pepper**
- **1 pound lean ground turkey**

1. Cook rice according to package directions. Meanwhile, cook cabbage in boiling water just until leaves fall off head. Set aside 10 large leaves for rolls. (Refrigerate remaining cabbage for another use.) Cut out the thick vein from the bottom of each reserved leaf, making a V-shaped cut.

2. In a large bowl, combine carrot, onion, egg substitute, 2 tablespoons tomato soup, 2 tablespoons vegetable soup, 1 tablespoon Italian seasoning, cayenne, pepper and rice. Crumble turkey over mixture and mix well. Place about ⅓ cupful on each cabbage leaf. Overlap cut ends of leaf; fold in sides, beginning from the cut end. Roll up completely to enclose filling.

3. Place rolls seam side down in an 11-in. x 7-in. baking dish coated with cooking spray. Combine the remaining soups; pour over cabbage rolls. Sprinkle with the remaining Italian seasoning.

4. Cover and bake at 350° for 50-60 minutes or until cabbage is tender and a thermometer reads 165°.

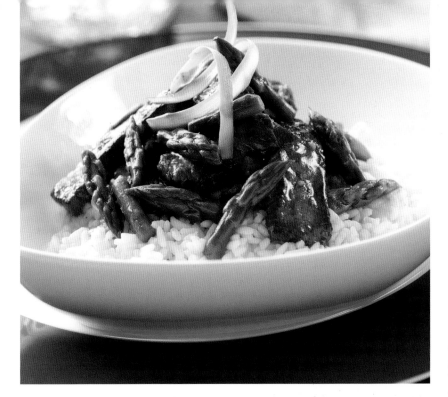

¼ teaspoon pepper
16 small red potatoes, halved
5 medium carrots, halved lengthwise and cut into 2-inch lengths
2 medium onions, quartered
½ teaspoon salt
½ teaspoon browning sauce, optional

1. Coat the roast with 2 tablespoons flour. In a nonstick Dutch oven, brown roast on all sides in oil over medium-high heat; drain. Add 1½ cups water, wine, bouillon and pepper. Bring to a boil. Reduce heat; cover and simmer for 2 hours.
2. Add the potatoes, carrots and onions; cover and simmer for 45 minutes or until meat and vegetables are tender. Remove meat and vegetables; keep warm.
3. Pour pan juices into a measuring cup; skim fat. Add enough water to measure 2 cups. In a small saucepan, combine remaining flour and water until smooth. Stir in salt and browning sauce if desired. Gradually stir in the 2 cups pan juices. Bring to a boil; cook and stir for 2 minutes or until thickened. Serve with roast and vegetables.

PER SERVING *1 serving equals 341 cal., 9 g fat (3 g sat. fat), 82 mg chol., 500 mg sodium, 32 g carb., 4 g fiber, 30 g pro.* **Diabetic Exchanges:** *4 lean meat, 1½ starch, 1 vegetable.*

347 CALORIES
Gingered Beef Stir-Fry
A friend who owns a bed and breakfast in Maryland shared this recipe with me. It's such a delicious and different way to serve fresh asparagus!
—**SONJA BLOW** NIXA, MO

PREP: 20 MIN. + MARINATING
COOK: 20 MIN. • **MAKES:** 4 SERVINGS

3 tablespoons reduced-sodium soy sauce, divided
1 tablespoon sherry
¼ teaspoon minced fresh gingerroot or dash ground ginger
½ pound beef flank steak, cut into thin strips
1 teaspoon cornstarch
½ cup beef broth
1½ teaspoons hoisin sauce
⅛ teaspoon sugar
2 tablespoons canola oil, divided
2 pounds fresh asparagus, cut into 1-inch lengths
1 garlic clove, minced
3 cups hot cooked rice

1. In a large resealable plastic bag, combine 2 tablespoons soy sauce, sherry and ginger; add beef. Seal bag and turn to coat; refrigerate for 30 minutes.
2. In a small bowl, combine cornstarch, broth, hoisin sauce, sugar and remaining soy sauce until smooth; set aside.
3. In a large skillet or wok, stir-fry beef in 1 tablespoon oil until no longer pink. Remove and set aside. Stir-fry asparagus in remaining oil until crisp-tender. Add garlic; cook 1 minute.
4. Stir cornstarch mixture and add to the pan. Bring to a boil; cook and stir 2 minutes or until thickened. Return beef to the pan; heat through. Serve with rice.

PER SERVING *1¼ cups stir-fry with ¾ cup rice equals 347 cal., 12 g fat (2 g sat. fat), 27 mg chol., 645 mg sodium, 41 g carb., 2 g fiber, 18 g pro.* **Diabetic Exchanges:** *2 starch, 2 fat, 1 lean meat, 1 vegetable.*

351-450 CALORIES

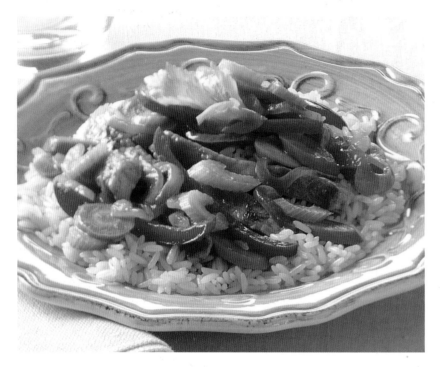

3. Stir cornstarch mixture and add to the pan. Bring to a boil; cook and stir for 1-2 minutes or until thickened. Serve with rice.

PER SERVING *1 cup pork mixture with ½ cup rice equals 370 cal., 8 g fat (2 g sat. fat), 36 mg chol., 494 mg sodium, 56 g carb., 3 g fiber, 18 g pro.*

362 CALORIES

Beefy Red Pepper Pasta

Chock-full of veggies and gooey with cheese, this hearty one-dish meal will warm the whole family to their toes! Pureed roasted red peppers add color and zing to the sauce.

—MARGE WERNER
BROKEN ARROW, OK

PREP: 20 MIN. • **COOK:** 25 MIN.
MAKES: 6 SERVINGS

- 1 jar (12 ounces) roasted sweet red peppers, drained
- 1 pound lean ground beef (90% lean)
- 1 small onion, chopped
- 1 can (14½ ounces) diced tomatoes, undrained
- 2 garlic cloves, minced

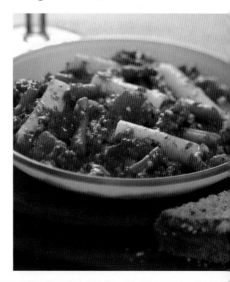

370 CALORIES

Apple Pork Stir-Fry

My super stir-fry offers a sweet twist with apple pie filling. Water chestnuts bring a slight crunch to the tender pork and crisp veggies.

—JO ANN ERPELDING CANTON, MI

START TO FINISH: 25 MIN.
MAKES: 3 SERVINGS

- ½ teaspoon cornstarch
- ½ cup apple cider or unsweetened apple juice
- 2 tablespoons reduced-sodium soy sauce
- ½ pound boneless pork loin chops, cut into strips
- 2 teaspoons canola oil
- ½ cup sliced celery
- ⅓ cup sliced fresh carrot
- ⅓ cup sliced onion
- ⅓ cup julienned sweet red pepper
- ⅓ cup sliced water chestnuts
- ¼ teaspoon ground ginger
- 1 cup apple pie filling
- 1½ cups hot cooked rice

1. In a small bowl, combine the cornstarch, cider and soy sauce until smooth; set aside. In a large skillet or wok, stir-fry pork in oil for 5-7 minutes or until no longer pink.
2. Add the celery, carrot, onion, red pepper, water chestnuts and ginger; stir-fry until vegetables are tender. Add pie filling.

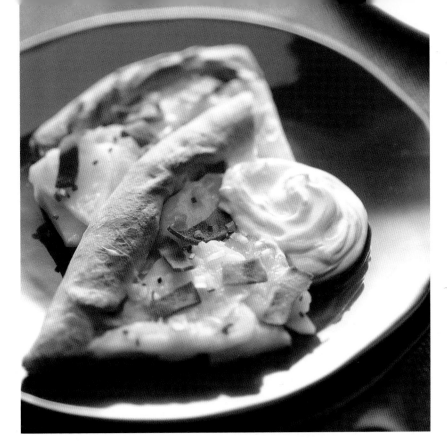

1 teaspoon dried oregano
1 teaspoon dried basil
¾ teaspoon salt
8 ounces uncooked ziti or small
  tube pasta
1½ cups cut fresh green beans
1½ cups (6 ounces) shredded
  part-skim mozzarella cheese

1. Place peppers in a food processor; cover and process until smooth. In a large skillet, cook beef and onion until meat is no longer pink; drain. Stir in the pepper puree, tomatoes, garlic, oregano, basil and salt. Bring to a boil. Reduce heat; simmer, uncovered, for 15 minutes.

2. Meanwhile, in a Dutch oven, cook pasta according to package directions, adding green beans during the last 5 minutes of cooking. Cook until pasta and green beans are tender; drain. Stir in meat sauce. Sprinkle with cheese; stir until melted.

PER SERVING *1⅔ cups equals 362 cal., 11 g fat (5 g sat. fat), 53 mg chol., 739 mg sodium, 38 g carb., 4 g fiber, 28 g pro.* **Diabetic Exchanges:** *3 lean meat, 2 starch, 1 vegetable.*

359 CALORIES
Baked Potato Pizza

I wanted to re-create a light version of a restaurant pizza my friends and I used to get all the time in college. Here's what I came up with!
—**CHARLOTTE GEHLE**
BROWNSTOWN, MI

PREP: 25 MIN. • **BAKE:** 25 MIN.
MAKES: 12 PIECES

3 medium potatoes, peeled and cut
  into ⅛-inch slices
1 loaf (1 pound) frozen pizza
  dough, thawed
3 tablespoons reduced-fat butter
4 garlic cloves, minced
¼ teaspoon salt
¼ teaspoon pepper
1 cup (4 ounces) shredded
  part-skim mozzarella cheese
¼ cup shredded Parmigiano-
  Reggiano cheese
6 turkey bacon strips, cooked and
  crumbled
2 green onions, chopped
2 tablespoons minced chives
  Reduced-fat sour cream, optional

1. Place potatoes in a small saucepan and cover with water. Bring to a boil. Reduce heat; cover and simmer for 15 minutes or until tender. Drain and pat dry.

2. Unroll dough onto a 14-in. pizza pan coated with cooking spray; flatten dough and build up edges slightly. In a microwave-safe bowl, melt butter with garlic; brush over the dough.

3. Arrange potato slices in a single layer over dough; sprinkle with salt and pepper. Top with cheeses. Bake at 400° for 22-28 minutes or until crust is golden and cheese is melted.

4. Sprinkle with bacon, onions and chives. Serve with sour cream if desired.

NOTE *This recipe was tested with Land O'Lakes light stick butter.*
PER SERVING *2 pieces (calculated without sour cream) equals 359 cal., 11 g fat (5 g sat. fat), 36 mg chol., 799 mg sodium, 48 g carb., 1 g fiber, 14 g pro.*

389 CALORIES Weeknight Beef Skillet

This mild but hearty family fare is chock-full of veggies, Italian seasoning and nutrition. It's a quick, easy meal that just might become one of your family's favorites!

—CLARA COULSON MINNEY
WASHINGTON COURT HOUSE, OH

START TO FINISH: 30 MIN. • **MAKES:** 4 SERVINGS

- 3 cups uncooked yolk-free whole wheat noodles
- 1 pound lean ground beef (90% lean)
- 1 medium green pepper, finely chopped
- 1 package (16 ounces) frozen mixed vegetables, thawed and drained
- 1 can (15 ounces) tomato sauce
- 1 tablespoon Worcestershire sauce
- 1½ teaspoons Italian seasoning
- 2 teaspoons sugar
- ¼ teaspoon salt
- ¼ cup minced fresh parsley

1. Cook noodles according to package directions. Meanwhile, in a large nonstick skillet over medium heat, cook beef and pepper until meat is no longer pink; drain.

2. Stir in the vegetables, tomato sauce, Worcestershire sauce, Italian seasoning, sugar and salt; heat through. Drain noodles and serve with meat mixture. Sprinkle with parsley.

PER SERVING *1¼ cups beef mixture with ¾ cup noodles equals 389 cal., 9 g fat (3 g sat. fat), 56 mg chol., 800 mg sodium, 49 g carb., 10 g fiber, 31 g pro.*
Diabetic Exchanges: *3 starch, 3 lean meat, 1 vegetable.*

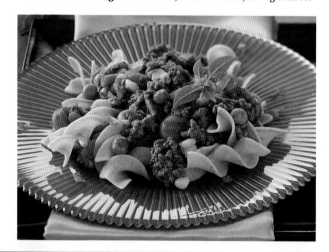

351 CALORIES Easy Arroz con Pollo

My children really look forward to dinner when they know I'm serving this. Best of all, it's a breeze to make.
—DEBBIE HARRIS TUCSON, AZ

PREP: 10 MIN. • **BAKE:** 1 HOUR • **MAKES:** 6 SERVINGS

- 1¾ cups uncooked instant rice
- 6 boneless skinless chicken breast halves (4 ounces each)
  Garlic salt and pepper to taste
- 1 can (14½ ounces) chicken broth
- 1 cup picante sauce
- 1 can (8 ounces) tomato sauce
- ½ cup chopped onion
- ½ cup chopped green pepper
- ½ cup shredded Monterey Jack cheese
- ½ cup shredded cheddar cheese

1. Spread the rice in a greased 13-in. x 9-in. baking dish. Sprinkle both sides of chicken with garlic salt and pepper; place over rice. In a large bowl, combine the broth, picante sauce, tomato sauce, onion and green pepper; pour over the chicken.

2. Cover and bake at 350° for 55 minutes or until a thermometer reads 170°. Sprinkle with cheeses. Bake, uncovered, 5 minutes longer or until cheese is melted.

PER SERVING *1 serving equals 351 cal., 9 g fat (5 g sat. fat), 91 mg chol., 791 mg sodium, 30 g carb., 1 g fiber, 35 g pro.*

412 CALORIES Pineapple Beef Kabobs

I first tried this recipe after reading a similar one in a health magazine in my doctor's office. It's easy, colorful, and the basting helps keep the kabobs juicy and tender.
—MARGUERITE SHAEFFER SEWELL, NJ

PREP: 20 MIN. + MARINATING • **GRILL:** 10 MIN.
MAKES: 6 SERVINGS

- 1 can (6 ounces) unsweetened pineapple juice
- ⅓ cup honey
- ⅓ cup soy sauce
- 3 tablespoons cider vinegar
- 1½ teaspoons minced garlic
- 1½ teaspoons ground ginger
- 1½ pounds beef top sirloin steak, cut into 1-inch pieces
- 1 fresh pineapple, peeled and cut into 1-inch chunks
- 12 large fresh mushrooms

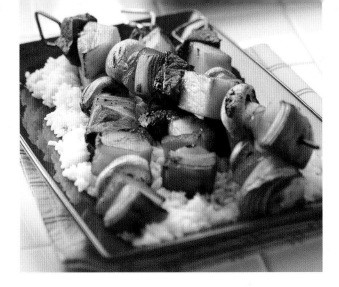

1 medium sweet red pepper, cut into 1-inch pieces
1 medium sweet yellow pepper, cut into 1-inch pieces
1 medium red onion, cut into 1-inch pieces
2½ cups uncooked instant rice

1. In a small bowl, combine the first six ingredients. Pour ¾ cup into a large resealable plastic bag; add beef. Seal bag and turn to coat; refrigerate for 1-4 hours. Cover and refrigerate remaining marinade for basting.

2. Drain and discard marinade. On 12 metal or soaked wooden skewers, alternately thread the beef, pineapple, mushrooms, peppers and onion. Moisten a paper towel with cooking oil; using long-handled tongs, lightly coat the grill rack.

3. Grill kabobs, covered, over medium-hot heat for 8-10 minutes or until meat reaches desired doneness, turning occasionally and basting frequently with reserved marinade. Cook rice according to package directions; serve with the kabobs.

PER SERVING *2 kabobs with ¾ cup rice equals 412 cal., 5 g fat (2 g sat. fat), 46 mg chol., 534 mg sodium, 60 g carb., 3 g fiber, 31 g pro.*

417 CALORIES Pot Roast with Vegetables

My mother made this pot roast at least once a week when I was a child—and I still love it! She always cooked Yorkshire pudding to go along with it, and that was one of my favorite meals.
—**CHERYL RIHN** BLOOMER, WI

PREP: 20 MIN. • **COOK:** 40 MIN. + COOLING • **MAKES:** 8 SERVINGS

1 beef sirloin tip roast (3 pounds)
2 tablespoons canola oil

4 large potatoes, peeled and quartered
4 large carrots, cut into 2-inch pieces
1 large onion, cut into wedges
2 cups water
1 teaspoon beef bouillon granules
½ teaspoon salt
¼ teaspoon pepper
3 tablespoons cornstarch
3 tablespoons cold water

1. In a pressure cooker, brown roast in oil on all sides. Add the potatoes, carrots, onion and water. Close cover securely; place pressure regulator on vent pipe. Bring cooker to full pressure over high heat. Reduce heat to medium-high; cook for 40 minutes. (Pressure regulator should maintain a slow steady rocking motion; adjust heat if needed.)

2. Remove from the heat; allow pressure to drop on its own. Remove meat and vegetables; keep warm. Bring cooking juices in pressure cooker to a boil. Add the bouillon, salt and pepper.

3. Combine cornstarch and cold water until smooth; stir into juices. Bring to a boil; cook and stir for 2 minutes or until thickened. Serve gravy with the roast and vegetables.

NOTE *This recipe was tested at 13 pounds of pressure (psi).*

PER SERVING *1 serving equals 417 cal., 11 g fat (3 g sat. fat), 90 mg chol., 343 mg sodium, 41 g carb., 4 g fiber, 36 g pro.*

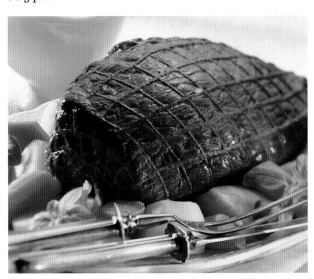

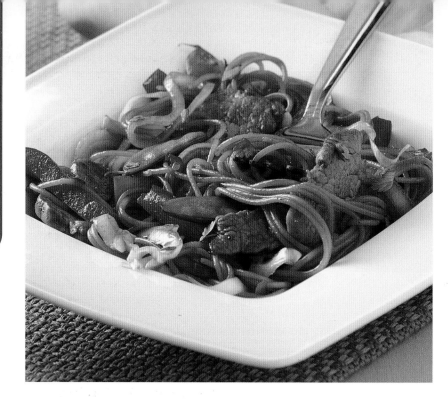

Chili Mac Casserole

With wagon wheel pasta and popular Tex-Mex ingredients, this fun main dish is sure to be a hit with both adults and kids. Simply add a green salad with your favorite low-calorie dressing for a complete dinner.

—JANET KANZLER YAKIMA, WA

PREP: 20 MIN. • **BAKE:** 25 MIN.
MAKES: 6 SERVINGS

- 1 **cup uncooked wagon wheel pasta**
- 1 **pound lean ground beef (90% lean)**
- ½ **cup chopped onion**
- ½ **cup chopped green pepper**
- 1 **can (15 ounces) turkey chili with beans**
- 1 **can (14½ ounces) stewed tomatoes, undrained**
- 1 **cup crushed baked tortilla chip scoops**
- 1 **cup (4 ounces) shredded reduced-fat cheddar cheese, divided**
- ¼ **cup uncooked instant rice**
- 1 **teaspoon chili powder**
- ¼ **teaspoon salt**
- ⅛ **teaspoon pepper**

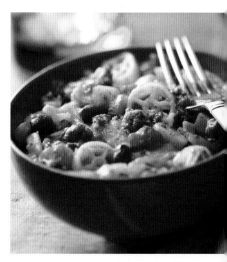

Chinese Pork 'n' Noodles

I based the recipe for these noodles on a similar dish I found in a magazine. I tweaked a few items, and my husband and I love it. It's just as good when you replace the pork with seafood.

—JENNIFER ENZER MANCHESTER, MI

PREP: 20 MIN. • **COOK:** 15 MIN.
MAKES: 4 SERVINGS

- 6 **ounces uncooked angel hair pasta**
- 3 **tablespoons hoisin sauce**
- 2 **tablespoons reduced-sodium soy sauce**
- 2 **teaspoons sesame oil**
- 1 **pork tenderloin (1 pound), halved and thinly sliced**
- 3 **teaspoons canola oil, divided**
- ¾ **cup julienned sweet red pepper**
- ¾ **cup halved fresh snow peas**
- ½ **cup sliced onion**
- 1 **cup sliced cabbage**
- ¼ **cup minced fresh cilantro**

1. Cook pasta according to package directions. Meanwhile, in a small bowl, combine the hoisin sauce, soy sauce and sesame oil; set aside.
2. In a large nonstick skillet or wok, stir-fry pork in 2 teaspoons canola oil for 3 minutes or until no longer pink. Remove and keep warm. In the same skillet, stir-fry the red pepper, peas and onion in remaining oil for 3 minutes. Add cabbage; stir-fry 2 minutes longer or until vegetables are crisp-tender.
3. Stir reserved hoisin sauce mixture and stir into skillet. Return pork to the pan; heat through. Drain pasta and add to skillet; toss to coat. Sprinkle each serving with 1 tablespoon cilantro.
PER SERVING *1½ cups equals 398 cal., 11 g fat (2 g sat. fat), 64 mg chol., 550 mg sodium, 43 g carb., 3 g fiber, 30 g pro.*
***Diabetic Exchanges:** 3 lean meat, 2½ starch, 1 vegetable, 1 fat.*

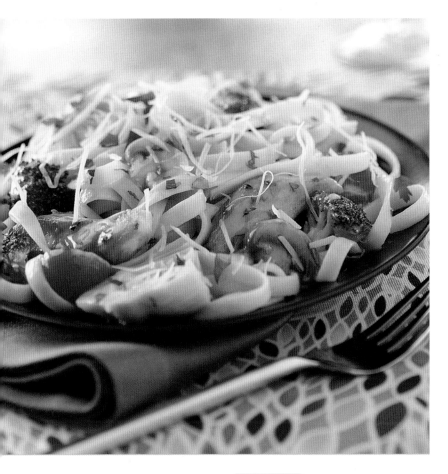

1 can (14 ounces) water-packed artichoke hearts, rinsed, drained and halved
½ teaspoon salt
½ teaspoon dried oregano
2 teaspoons all-purpose flour
¼ cup reduced-sodium chicken broth
⅓ cup white wine or additional reduced-sodium chicken broth
1 tablespoon minced fresh parsley
1 tablespoon shredded Parmesan cheese

1. Cook fettuccine according to the package directions. Meanwhile, in a large nonstick skillet coated with cooking spray, cook chicken in 2 teaspoons oil over medium heat until no longer pink. Remove and keep warm.

2. In the same skillet, cook and stir broccoli in remaining oil for 2 minutes. Stir in the mushrooms, tomatoes and garlic; cook 2 minutes longer. Add the artichokes, salt and oregano; heat through.

3. Combine the flour with broth and wine or additional broth until smooth; stir into the pan. Bring to a boil; cook and stir for 1-2 minutes or until thickened. Add parsley and reserved chicken.

4. Drain fettuccine; add to chicken mixture and toss to coat. Sprinkle with cheese.

PER SERVING *2 cups equals 378 cal., 8 g fat (2 g sat. fat), 64 mg chol., 668 mg sodium, 41 g carb., 2 g fiber, 33 g pro.* **Diabetic Exchanges:** *3 lean meat, 2 starch, 2 vegetable, 1 fat.*

1. Cook pasta according to package directions. Meanwhile, in a large nonstick skillet, cook the beef, onion and green pepper over medium heat until meat is no longer pink; drain. Stir in the chili, tomatoes, chips, ½ cup cheese, rice, chili powder, salt and pepper. Drain pasta; add to beef mixture.

2. Transfer to a 2-qt. baking dish coated with cooking spray. Sprinkle with the remaining cheese. Bake, uncovered, at 350° for 25-30 minutes or until cheese is melted.

PER SERVING *1 cup equals 358 cal., 11 g fat (5 g sat. fat), 60 mg chol., 847 mg sodium, 36 g carb., 4 g fiber, 28 g pro.* **Diabetic Exchanges:** *3 lean meat, 2 starch, 1 vegetable.*

378 CALORIES

Chicken Artichoke Pasta

Here's a delicious chicken dish that's easy enough for weeknights but special enough for guests. Oregano, garlic and a light wine sauce add lovely flavor to a medley of fresh vegetables.

—CATHY DICK ROANOKE, VA

START TO FINISH: 30 MIN.
MAKES: 4 SERVINGS

6 ounces uncooked fettuccine
1 pound boneless skinless chicken breasts, cut into thin strips
3 teaspoons olive oil, divided
½ cup fresh broccoli florets
½ cup sliced fresh mushrooms
½ cup cherry tomatoes, halved
2 garlic cloves, minced

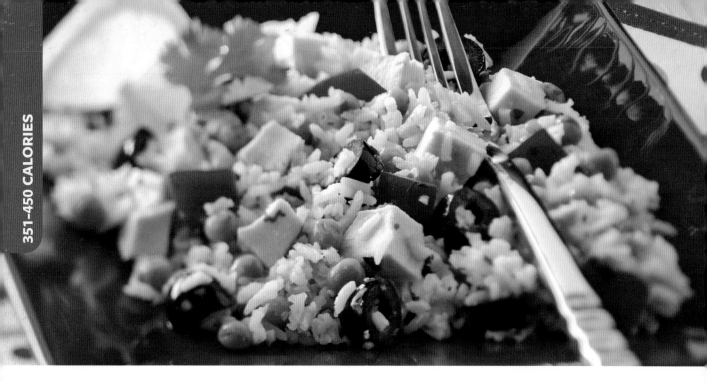

373 CALORIES

Skillet Arroz con Pollo

This chicken-and-rice dish is great for both family and special-occasion meals. It's a tasty main dish made all in one skillet...and the aroma while it cooks is simply amazing!

—CHERYL BATTAGLIA DALTON, PA

PREP: 15 MIN. • **COOK:** 25 MIN.
MAKES: 4 SERVINGS

- 1 medium onion, chopped
- 1 medium sweet red pepper, cut into ½-inch pieces
- 1 garlic clove, minced
- 2 teaspoons olive oil
- 1 cup uncooked long grain rice
- 1 can (14½ ounces) reduced-sodium chicken broth
- ¼ cup sherry or water
- ½ teaspoon grated lemon peel
- ¼ teaspoon salt
- ¼ teaspoon cayenne pepper
- 2 cups cubed cooked chicken breast
- 1 cup frozen peas, thawed
- ¼ cup sliced ripe olives, drained
- 2 tablespoons minced fresh cilantro

1. In a large nonstick skillet coated with cooking spray, saute the onion, red pepper and garlic in oil for 1 minute. Add rice; cook and stir for 4-5 minutes or until the rice is lightly browned.
2. Stir in the broth, sherry, lemon peel, salt and cayenne. Bring to a boil. Reduce heat; cover and simmer for 15 minutes.
3. Stir in the chicken, peas and olives. Cover and cook 3-6 minutes longer or until rice is tender and chicken is heated through. Sprinkle with cilantro.
PER SERVING *1½ cups equals 373 cal., 6 g fat (1 g sat. fat), 54 mg chol., 582 mg sodium, 49 g carb., 4 g fiber, 28 g pro. Diabetic Exchanges: 3 starch, 3 lean meat, 1 vegetable, ½ fat.*

390 CALORIES

Mexican Manicotti

Here's a creative spin on traditional manicotti. The Mexican flavors will leave you craving seconds.

—LARRY PHILLIPS SHREVEPORT, LA

PREP: 25 MIN. • **BAKE:** 25 MIN.
MAKES: 2 SERVINGS

- 4 uncooked manicotti shells
- 1 cup cubed cooked chicken breast
- 1 cup salsa, divided
- ½ cup reduced-fat ricotta cheese
- 2 tablespoons sliced ripe olives
- 4 teaspoons minced fresh parsley
- 1 tablespoon diced pimientos
- 1 green onion, thinly sliced
- 1 small garlic clove, minced
- ¼ to ½ teaspoon hot pepper sauce
- ⅓ cup shredded reduced-fat Monterey Jack cheese or reduced-fat Mexican cheese blend

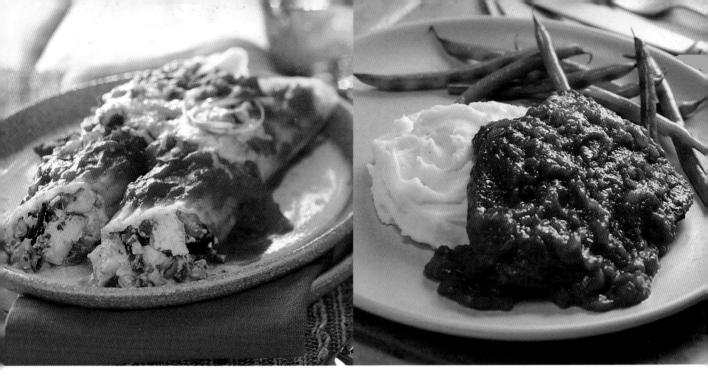

1. Cook manicotti according to package directions. In a small bowl, combine the chicken, ¼ cup salsa, ricotta cheese, olives, parsley, pimientos, green onion, garlic and pepper sauce. Drain manicotti; fill with chicken mixture.

2. Spread ¼ cup salsa in an 8-in. square baking dish coated with cooking spray. Top with manicotti shells and remaining salsa.

3. Cover and bake at 400° for 20 minutes. Uncover; sprinkle with Monterey Jack cheese and bake 5-10 minutes longer or until the cheese is melted and the filling is heated through.

PER SERVING *2 stuffed manicotti equals 390 cal., 10 g fat (4 g sat. fat), 81 mg chol., 783 mg sodium, 38 g carb., 2 g fiber, 35 g pro.*
***Diabetic Exchanges:** 4 lean meat, 2 starch, 1 vegetable.*

359 CALORIES

Steak with Sauce

My husband and I have enjoyed this recipe for years. The tomato sauce is wonderful, and the dish always brings back memories.
—VERA KLEIBER RALEIGH, NC

PREP: 20 MIN. • **BAKE:** 1½ HOURS
MAKES: 4 SERVINGS

- 2 **tablespoons all-purpose flour**
- ½ **to 1 teaspoon salt**
- ¼ **teaspoon pepper**
- 1½ **pounds beef top round steak**
- 2 **tablespoons canola oil**
- 2 **medium onions, chopped**
- 2 **cans (5½ ounces each) tomato juice**
- 1 **cup diced tomatoes**
- 4 **teaspoons lemon juice**
- 4 **teaspoons Worcestershire sauce**
- 2 **to 3 teaspoons packed brown sugar**
- 1 **teaspoon prepared mustard**

1. In a large resealable plastic bag, combine the flour, salt and pepper. Cut steak into four pieces. Add beef to bag, a few pieces at a time, and shake to coat. Remove the meat from bag and pound with a mallet to tenderize.

2. In a large skillet, brown meat in oil on both sides. Transfer to a shallow 2-qt. baking dish coated with cooking spray.

3. In the same skillet, saute onions in drippings until tender. Stir in the remaining ingredients. Pour over meat. Cover and bake at 350° for 1½ hours or until tender.

PER SERVING *1 serving equals 359 cal., 12 g fat (2 g sat. fat), 96 mg chol., 721 mg sodium, 20 g carb., 3 g fiber, 41 g pro.*
***Diabetic Exchanges:** 5 lean meat, 2 vegetable, 1½ fat, ½ starch.*

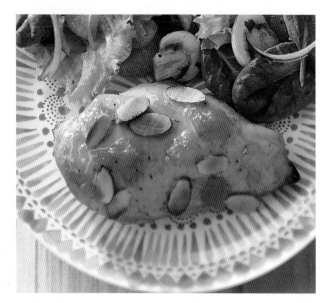

Poaching the cod before baking prevents it from watering out this wonderful casserole. With pasta and veggies, the satisfying dish is guaranteed to warm you up on chilly nights.
—**TASTE OF HOME TEST KITCHEN**

PREP: 25 MIN. • **BAKE:** 25 MIN. • **MAKES:** 6 SERVINGS

- 6 **cups water**
- 1 **teaspoon lemon-pepper seasoning**
- 1 **bay leaf**
- 2 **pounds cod fillets, cut into 1-inch pieces**
- 1 **cup uncooked small pasta shells**
- 1 **medium sweet red pepper, chopped**
- 1 **medium green pepper, chopped**
- 1 **medium onion, chopped**
- 1 **tablespoon butter**
- 3 **tablespoons all-purpose flour**
- 2½ **cups fat-free evaporated milk**
- ¾ **teaspoon salt**
- ½ **teaspoon dried thyme**
- ¼ **teaspoon pepper**
- 1 **cup (4 ounces) shredded Mexican cheese blend**

1. In a large skillet, bring the water, lemon-pepper and bay leaf to a boil. Reduce heat; carefully add cod. Cover and simmer for 5-8 minutes or until fish flakes easily with a fork; drain and set aside. Discard bay leaf.

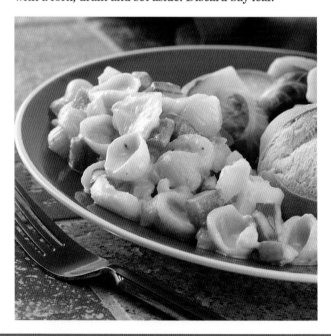

372 CALORIES

Apricot-Almond Chicken Breasts

This chicken dish is so delicious, even my picky eaters clamor for it! It takes only minutes to prepare, so on busy weeknights I can still put a healthy supper on the table. I'm frequently asked to share the recipe.
—**TRISHA KRUSE** EAGLE, ID

PREP: 10 MIN. • **BAKE:** 30 MIN. • **MAKES:** 4 SERVINGS

- 4 **boneless skinless chicken breast halves (6 ounces each)**
- ½ **teaspoon salt**
- ¼ **teaspoon pepper**
- ¾ **cup apricot preserves**
- ¼ **cup reduced-sodium chicken broth**
- 1 **tablespoon honey mustard**
- ¼ **cup sliced almonds**

1. Sprinkle chicken with salt and pepper. Place in a 13-in. x 9-in. baking dish coated with cooking spray. Bake, uncovered, at 350° for 15 minutes.
2. In a small bowl, combine the preserves, broth and mustard. Pour over chicken; sprinkle with almonds. Bake 15-20 minutes longer or until the chicken juices run clear.
PER SERVING *1 chicken breast half equals 372 cal., 7 g fat (1 g sat. fat), 94 mg chol., 468 mg sodium, 42 g carb., 1 g fiber, 36 g pro.* **Diabetic Exchanges:** *5 lean meat, 3 starch, ½ fat.*

2. Cook pasta according to package directions. Meanwhile, in a large saucepan, saute peppers and onion in butter over medium heat until tender. Stir in flour until blended. Gradually stir in milk. Bring to a boil; cook and stir for 2 minutes or until thickened. Stir in the salt, thyme and pepper. Remove from the heat; stir in cheese until melted.

3. Drain pasta. Stir fish and pasta into sauce. Transfer to a 2-qt. baking dish coated with cooking spray. Cover casserole and bake at 350° for 25-30 minutes or until heated through.

PER SERVING *1 cup equals 389 cal., 9 g fat (6 g sat. fat), 83 mg chol., 732 mg sodium, 35 g carb., 2 g fiber, 39 g pro.* **Diabetic Exchanges:** *4 lean meat, 1½ fat, 1 starch, 1 vegetable, 1 fat-free milk.*

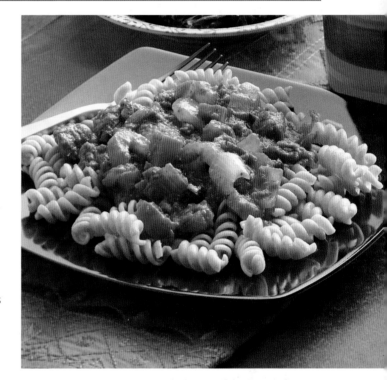

413 CALORIES Ragu Bolognese

I cook my hearty entree slowly, which creates a rich sauce that's absolutely fabulous. The veggies add fiber, and I use skim milk and turkey sausage to keep it lighter. This flavorful dish is great for family, but special enough for company.
—MARY BILYEU ANN ARBOR, MI

PREP: 30 MIN. • **COOK:** 1¼ HOURS • **MAKES:** 4 SERVINGS

- ½ pound Italian turkey sausage links, casings removed
- 1 large carrot, finely chopped
- 1 celery rib, finely chopped
- 1 small onion, finely chopped
- 1 can (15 ounces) crushed tomatoes
- ½ cup reduced-sodium chicken broth
- 2 tablespoons balsamic vinegar
- ¼ teaspoon crushed red pepper flakes
- ¾ cup fat-free milk
- 4 cups uncooked whole wheat spiral pasta
- 2 tablespoons prepared pesto
- 1 tablespoon chopped ripe olives

1. Crumble sausage into a nonstick Dutch oven. Add the carrot, celery and onion; cook and stir over medium heat until meat is no longer pink. Drain.

2. Stir in the tomatoes, broth, vinegar and pepper flakes. Bring to a boil. Stir in milk. Reduce heat; simmer, uncovered, for 1 to 1¼ hours or until thickened, stirring occasionally.

3. Cook pasta according to package directions. Stir pesto and olives into meat sauce. Drain pasta; serve with meat sauce.

PER SERVING *1 cup pasta with ⅔ cup meat sauce equals 413 cal., 11 g fat (2 g sat. fat), 38 mg chol., 674 mg sodium, 58 g carb., 6 g fiber, 21 g pro.*

Macaroni Scramble

This quick-and-easy dinner has all the pasta, cheese, meat and sweet tomato sauce that make for a family-pleasing classic. Serve with a green salad and crusty French bread for a surefire hit.

—**PATRICIA KILE** ELIZABETHTOWN, PA

START TO FINISH: 25 MIN.
MAKES: 3 SERVINGS

- 1 cup uncooked cellentani (spiral pasta) or elbow macaroni
- ½ pound lean ground beef (90% lean)
- 1 small onion, chopped
- 1 celery rib, chopped
- 1 small green pepper, chopped
- 1 garlic clove, minced
- 1 can (10¾ ounces) reduced-sodium condensed tomato soup, undiluted
- 1 tablespoon minced fresh parsley or 1 teaspoon dried parsley flakes
- 1 teaspoon dried oregano
- ¼ teaspoon salt
- ¼ teaspoon pepper
- ½ cup shredded reduced-fat cheddar cheese

1. Cook pasta according to package directions. Meanwhile, in a large skillet, cook the beef, onion, celery and green pepper over medium heat until meat is no longer pink. Add garlic; cook 1 minute longer. Drain.
2. Drain pasta; add to beef mixture. Stir in the soup, parsley, oregano, salt and pepper. Bring to a boil. Reduce heat; simmer, uncovered, for 4-5 minutes or until heated through. Sprinkle with cheese.

PER SERVING *1⅓ cups equals 351 cal., 11 g fat (5 g sat. fat), 50 mg chol., 758 mg sodium, 38 g carb., 3 g fiber, 24 g pro. Diabetic Exchanges: 3 lean meat, 2 starch, 1 vegetable, 1 fat.*

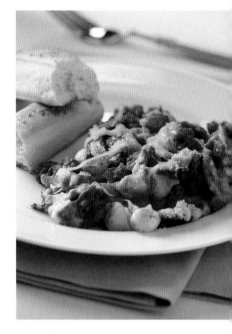

Italian Hot Dish

My husband had a poor perception of healthy food until he tried this satisfying casserole. The combination of pasta, oregano, mushrooms and green peppers makes it a favorite in our house.

—**THERESA SMITH** SHEBOYGAN, WI

PREP: 30 MIN. • **BAKE:** 40 MIN.
MAKES: 4 SERVINGS

- 1½ cups uncooked small pasta shells
- 1 pound lean ground beef (90% lean)
- 1 cup sliced fresh mushrooms, divided
- ½ cup chopped onion
- ½ cup chopped green pepper
- 1 can (15 ounces) tomato sauce
- 1 teaspoon dried oregano
- ½ teaspoon garlic powder
- ¼ teaspoon onion powder
- ⅛ teaspoon pepper
- ½ cup shredded part-skim mozzarella cheese, divided
- 4 teaspoons grated Parmesan cheese, divided

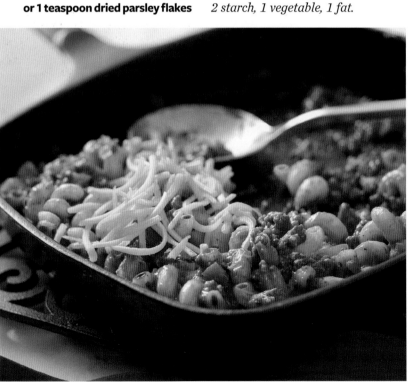

1. Cook pasta according to package directions. Meanwhile, in a large nonstick skillet coated with cooking spray, cook the beef, ½ cup of the mushrooms, onion and green pepper until meat is no longer pink; drain. Stir in the tomato sauce and seasonings. Bring mixture to a boil. Reduce heat; cover and simmer for 15 minutes.

2. Drain pasta; place in an 8-in. square baking dish coated with cooking spray. Top with meat sauce and remaining mushrooms. Sprinkle with ¼ cup mozzarella cheese and 2 teaspoons Parmesan cheese.

3. Cover and bake at 350° for 35 minutes. Uncover; sprinkle with remaining cheeses. Bake 5-10 minutes longer or until heated through and cheese is melted.

PER SERVING *1 serving equals 391 cal., 12 g fat (5 g sat. fat), 65 mg chol., 663 mg sodium, 36 g carb., 3 g fiber, 33 g pro.* **Diabetic Exchanges:** *3 lean meat, 2 starch, 2 vegetable, ½ fat.*

378 CALORIES

Jalapeno-Apricot Pork Tenderloin

A perfect blend of spices is what sets my dish apart. I often double the recipe and freeze the second tenderloin for later. The sweet-spicy glaze would also taste delicious over chicken.

—AMBER SHEA FORD
OVERLAND PARK, KS

PREP: 15 MIN. + CHILLING
BAKE: 20 MIN. • **MAKES:** 2 SERVINGS

2 teaspoons olive oil
1 garlic clove, minced
1 teaspoon dried oregano
½ teaspoon salt
½ teaspoon ground cumin
¼ teaspoon ground coriander
1 pork tenderloin (¾ pound)

GLAZE
⅓ cup apricot preserves
1 tablespoon lime juice
1 tablespoon diced seeded jalapeno pepper
¼ teaspoon ground cumin
⅛ teaspoon garlic salt

1. Combine the first six ingredients; rub over pork. Cover and refrigerate for up to 2 hours.

2. Place pork in an 11-in. x 7-in. baking dish coated with cooking spray. Bake, uncovered, at 400° for 15 minutes.

3. In a small bowl, combine the glaze ingredients; spoon ¼ cup over pork. Bake 5-10 minutes longer or until a thermometer reads 160°. Let pork stand for 5 minutes before slicing. Serve with the remaining glaze.

NOTE *Wear disposable gloves when cutting hot peppers; the oils can burn skin. Avoid touching your face.*
PER SERVING *5 ounces cooked pork with ¼ cup glaze equals 378 cal., 11 g fat (3 g sat. fat), 95 mg chol., 818 mg sodium, 37 g carb., 1 g fiber, 35 g pro.*

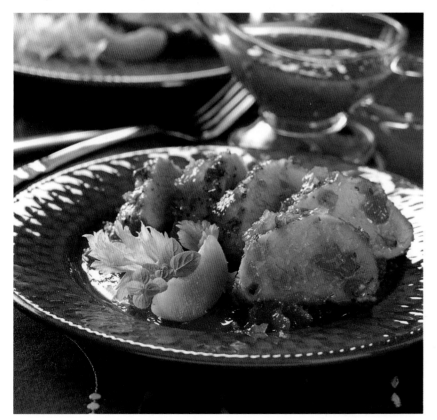

362 CALORIES Hearty Lentil Spaghetti

Packed full of lentils and Italian flavors, here's a vegetarian meal option that's thick, hearty and zesty.

—MARIE BENDER HENDERSON, NV

PREP: 15 MIN. • **COOK:** 70 MIN. • **MAKES:** 8 SERVINGS

- ¾ cup chopped onion
- 1 tablespoon olive oil
- 2 garlic cloves, minced
- 1½ cups dried lentils, rinsed
- 4 cups vegetable broth
- ½ teaspoon pepper
- ¼ teaspoon cayenne pepper
- 1 can (14½ ounces) Italian diced tomatoes
- 1 can (6 ounces) tomato paste
- 1 teaspoon white vinegar
- 1½ teaspoons dried basil
- 1½ teaspoons dried oregano
- 12 ounces uncooked spaghetti
- ¼ cup shredded Parmesan cheese

1. In a large saucepan coated with cooking spray, saute onion in oil until tender. Add garlic; cook 1 minute longer. Stir in the lentils, broth, pepper and cayenne. Bring to a boil. Reduce heat; cover and simmer for 20-30 minutes or until lentils are tender.

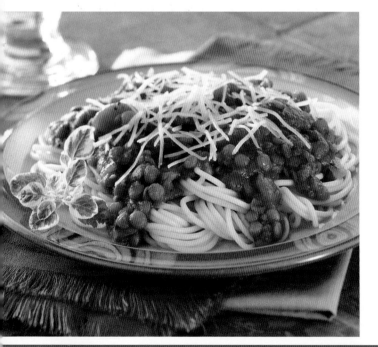

2. Stir in the tomatoes, tomato paste, vinegar, basil and oregano. Return to a boil. Reduce heat; cover and simmer for 40-45 minutes.

3. Cook spaghetti according to package directions; drain. Serve with lentil sauce. Sprinkle each serving with cheese.

PER SERVING *¾ cup sauce with ¾ cup spaghetti equals 362 cal., 4 g fat (1 g sat. fat), 2 mg chol., 764 mg sodium, 65 g carb., 14 g fiber, 19 g pro.*

360 CALORIES Dijon-Peach Pork Chops

I invented this dish one night when I was missing half the ingredients for the pork chop recipe I had planned to make. Tender chops are simmered with peaches, mustard and cloves.

—DEBBIE LIBERTON BOERNE, TX

START TO FINISH: 25 MIN. • **MAKES:** 4 SERVINGS

- 4 bone-in pork loin chops (7 ounces each)
- 1 can (15¼ ounces) sliced peaches, undrained
- ¼ cup packed brown sugar
- ¼ cup Dijon mustard
- ¼ teaspoon ground cloves

In a large skillet coated with cooking spray, brown pork chops over medium-high heat for 4-5 minutes on each side. Stir in the remaining ingredients. Bring to a boil. Reduce heat; cover and simmer for 10 minutes or until meat is tender.

PER SERVING *1 pork chop equals 360 cal., 10 g fat (3 g sat. fat), 86 mg chol., 456 mg sodium, 36 g carb., 1 g fiber, 31 g pro.* **Diabetic Exchanges:** *4 lean meat, 2½ starch.*

399 CALORIES

Bow Ties with Chicken & Shrimp

What a nourishing stovetop supper to keep your family warm and satisfied in cold weather! It's also simple, savory and special enough to serve company.

—JAN ARCHER KANSAS CITY, MO

PREP: 20 MIN. • **COOK:** 15 MIN. • **MAKES:** 7 SERVINGS

- 5¼ cups uncooked bow tie pasta
- ¾ pound boneless skinless chicken breasts, cubed
- 1 tablespoon butter
- 1 tablespoon olive oil
- 2 green onions, chopped
- 2 garlic cloves, minced

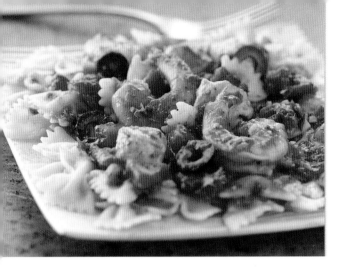

2 cans (14½ ounces each) Italian diced tomatoes, undrained
2 tablespoons minced fresh parsley, divided
1 tablespoon each dried basil, thyme and oregano
¼ teaspoon pepper
2 teaspoons cornstarch
½ cup reduced-sodium chicken broth
¾ pound cooked large shrimp, peeled and deveined
3 plum tomatoes, diced
10 large pitted ripe olives, sliced
   Minced fresh parsley, optional

1. Cook pasta according to package directions. Meanwhile, in a large nonstick skillet, saute chicken in butter and oil until no longer pink. Add onions and garlic; cook 1 minute longer. Stir in the canned tomatoes, parsley, basil, thyme, oregano and pepper.
2. Combine cornstarch and broth until smooth; stir into the pan. Bring to a boil; cook and stir for 2 minutes or until thickened. Add the shrimp, plum tomatoes and olives; heat through. Drain pasta; serve with chicken mixture. Sprinkle with parsley if desired.
PER SERVING *1 cup pasta with 1 cup sauce equals 399 cal., 8 g fat (2 g sat. fat), 105 mg chol., 661 mg sodium, 54 g carb., 3 g fiber, 29 g pro.*

411 CALORIES Citrus Fish Tacos
My fun fish tacos bring a deliciously different twist to this Southwest standby. I combine halibut or cod with a fruity salsa and a zesty seasoning.
—MARIA BALDWIN MESA, AZ

PREP: 15 MIN. + CHILLING • **BAKE:** 15 MIN. • **MAKES:** 4 SERVINGS

1½ cups finely chopped fresh pineapple
1 can (11 ounces) mandarin oranges, drained and cut in half
1 envelope reduced-sodium taco seasoning, divided
3 tablespoons thawed orange juice concentrate, divided
3 tablespoons lime juice, divided
1 jalapeno pepper, seeded and finely chopped
1½ pounds halibut or cod, cut into ¾-inch cubes
8 corn tortillas (6 inches), warmed
3 cups shredded lettuce

1. In a large bowl, combine the pineapple, oranges, 1 tablespoon taco seasoning, 1 tablespoon orange juice concentrate, 1 tablespoon lime juice and jalapeno pepper. Cover and refrigerate.
2. Place fish in an ungreased shallow 2-qt. baking dish. In a small bowl, combine the remaining taco seasoning, orange juice concentrate and lime juice. Pour over fish; toss gently to coat. Cover and bake at 375° for 12-16 minutes or until fish flakes easily with a fork.
3. Place a spoonful of the fish mixture down center of each tortilla. Top with lettuce and pineapple salsa; roll up.
NOTE *Wear disposable gloves when cutting hot peppers; the oils can burn skin. Avoid touching your face.*
PER SERVING *2 tacos equals 411 cal., 6 g fat (1 g sat. fat), 54 mg chol., 670 mg sodium, 52 g carb., 5 g fiber, 40 g pro.*

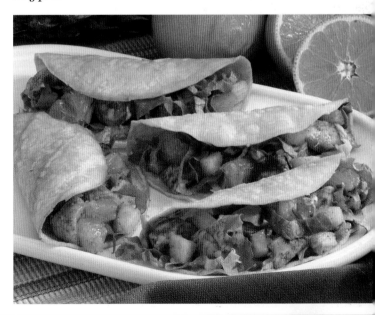

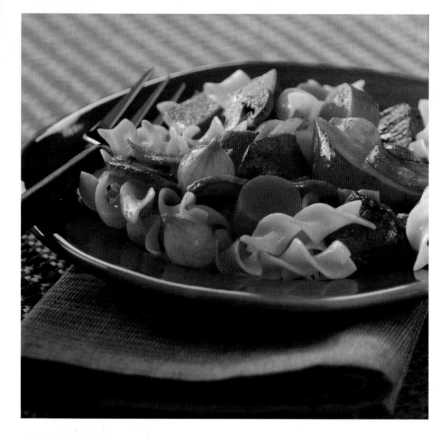

cooking juices if desired. Serve with egg noodles.

PER SERVING *1 cup stew with 1 cup noodles equals 388 cal., 7 g fat (2 g sat. fat), 70 mg chol., 434 mg sodium, 49 g carb., 4 g fiber, 26 g pro.* **Diabetic Exchanges:** *3 starch, 3 lean meat.*

---

358 CALORIES

Baked Fish 'n' Chips

Crunchy fillets with crispy potatoes add up to a quick and tasty light meal for the two of you.

—**JANICE MITCHELL** AURORA, CO

PREP: 20 MIN. • **BAKE:** 10 MIN.
MAKES: 2 SERVINGS

- 1 **tablespoon olive oil**
- ¼ **teaspoon pepper, divided**
- 2 **medium potatoes, peeled**
- 3 **tablespoons all-purpose flour**
- 1 **egg**
- 1 **tablespoon water**
- ⅓ **cup crushed cornflakes**
- 1½ **teaspoons grated Parmesan cheese**
  Dash cayenne pepper
- ½ **pound haddock fillets**
  Tartar sauce, optional

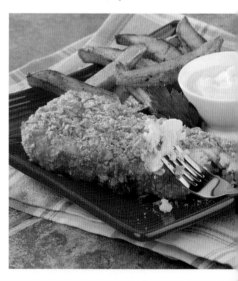

---

388 CALORIES

Burgundy Beef Stew

This stew is brimming with veggies and meat for plenty of hearty, home-cooked comfort. Special enough for company.

—**MINDY ILAR** ST ALBANS, WV

PREP: 25 MIN. • **COOK:** 1½ HOURS
MAKES: 6 SERVINGS

- ½ **cup all-purpose flour**
- 1 **pound beef top sirloin steak, cut into ½-inch pieces**
- 3 **turkey bacon strips, diced**
- 3 **garlic cloves, minced**
- 1 **bay leaf**
- 1 **teaspoon dried marjoram**
- ½ **teaspoon salt**
- ½ **teaspoon dried thyme**
- ¼ **teaspoon pepper**
- 1 **cup Burgundy wine**
- ½ **cup reduced-sodium beef broth**
- 8 **small red potatoes, halved**
- 2 **medium carrots, cut into 1-inch pieces**
- 1 **cup sliced fresh mushrooms**
- ¾ **cup frozen pearl onions, thawed**
- 6 **cups hot cooked egg noodles**

1. Place flour in a large resealable plastic bag. Add beef, a few pieces at a time, and shake to coat. In a Dutch oven coated with cooking spray, brown beef and turkey bacon on all sides.

2. Add the garlic, seasonings, wine and broth. Bring to a boil. Reduce heat; cover and simmer 40 minutes.

3. Stir in the vegetables. Cover and cook for 25-30 minutes or until meat and vegetables are tender. Discard the bay leaf. Thicken the

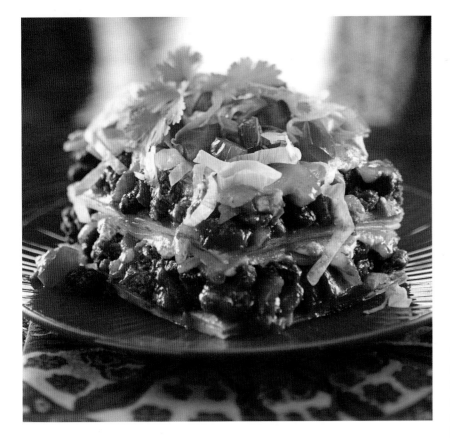

1. In a large bowl, combine oil and ⅛ teaspoon pepper. Cut potatoes lengthwise into ½-in. strips. Add to oil mixture and toss to coat. Place on a baking sheet coated with cooking spray. Bake at 425° for 25-30 minutes or until golden brown and crisp.

2. Meanwhile, in a shallow bowl, combine flour and remaining pepper. In another shallow bowl, beat egg and water. In a third bowl, combine the cornflakes, cheese and cayenne. Dredge fillets in flour, then dip in egg mixture and coat with crumbs.

3. Place on a baking sheet coated with cooking spray. Bake at 425° for 10-15 minutes or until fish flakes easily with a fork. Serve with chips and tartar sauce if desired.

PER SERVING *1 serving (calculated without tartar sauce) equals 358 cal., 10 g fat (2 g sat. fat), 131 mg chol., 204 mg sodium, 39 g carb., 2 g fiber, 28 g pro.* **Diabetic Exchanges:** *3 lean meat, 2½ starch, 2 fat.*

357 CALORIES

Enchilada Casser-Ole!

My husband loves this casserole, and it never lasts long at our house. Packed with black beans, cheese, tomatoes and Southwest flavor, it makes an impressive-looking entree that's as simple to make as it is simply delicious!
—**MARSHA WILLS** HOMOSASSA, FL

PREP: 25 MIN. • **BAKE:** 30 MIN
MAKES: 8 SERVINGS

1 pound lean ground beef (90% lean)
1 large onion, chopped
2 cups salsa
1 can (15 ounces) black beans, rinsed and drained
¼ cup reduced-fat Italian salad dressing
2 tablespoons reduced-sodium taco seasoning
¼ teaspoon ground cumin
6 flour tortillas (8 inches)
¾ cup reduced-fat sour cream
1 cup (4 ounces) shredded reduced-fat Mexican cheese blend
1 cup shredded lettuce
1 medium tomato, chopped
¼ cup minced fresh cilantro

1. In a large skillet, cook beef and onion over medium heat until meat is no longer pink; drain. Stir in the salsa, beans, salad dressing, taco seasoning and cumin.

2. Place three tortillas in an 11x7-in. baking dish coated with cooking spray. Layer with half of the meat mixture, half the sour cream and half the cheese. Repeat layers.

3. Cover and bake at 400° for 25 minutes. Uncover; bake 5-10 minutes longer or until heated through. Let stand for 5 minutes; top with lettuce, tomato and cilantro.

PER SERVING *1 piece equals 357 cal., 12 g fat (5 g sat. fat), 45 mg chol., 864 mg sodium, 37 g carb., 3 g fiber, 23 g pro.* **Diabetic Exchanges:** *3 lean meat, 2 starch, 1 vegetable, 1 fat.*

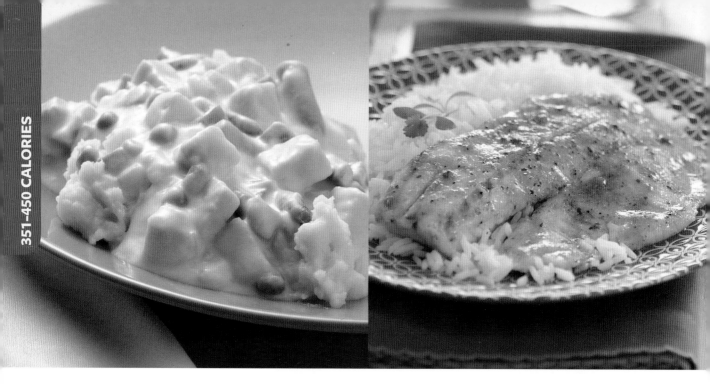

358 CALORIES

Creamed Turkey on Mashed Potatoes

Here's a true comfort-food classic. The creamy turkey mixture blends perfectly with tasty mashed potatoes.

—TASTE OF HOME TEST KITCHEN

START TO FINISH: 20 MIN.
MAKES: 4 SERVINGS

- ½ **cup chopped onion**
- 2 **tablespoons butter**
- 2 **tablespoons all-purpose flour**
- ¼ **teaspoon salt**
- ⅛ **teaspoon white pepper**
- 2 **cups fat-free milk**
- 2 **cups cubed cooked turkey breast**
- 1 **cup frozen mixed vegetables**
- 2 **cups mashed potatoes (with added milk and butter)**

1. In a large saucepan, saute the onion in butter until tender. Sprinkle with the flour, salt and pepper. Stir in the milk until blended.

2. Bring mixture to a boil; cook and stir for 2 minutes or until thickened and bubbly. Add the turkey and vegetables; cover and simmer until heated through. Serve turkey mixture over mashed potatoes.
PER SERVING *1 cup turkey mixture with ½ cup mashed potatoes equals equals 358 cal., 11 g fat (6 g sat. fat), 89 mg chol., 628 mg sodium, 35 g carb., 4 g fiber, 29 g pro. Diabetic Exchanges: 3 lean meat, 2 starch, 1½ fat, ½ fat-free milk.*

356 CALORIES Tilapia with Jasmine Rice

This zesty tilapia is to die for! Fragrant jasmine rice brings a special touch to the meal. But it gets even better: Each serving has only 5 grams of fat!

—SHIRL PARSONS CAPE CARTERET, NC

START TO FINISH: 30 MIN.
MAKES: 2 SERVINGS

- ¾ **cup water**
- ½ **cup uncooked jasmine rice**
- 1½ **teaspoons butter**
- ¼ **teaspoon ground cumin**
- ¼ **teaspoon seafood seasoning**
- ¼ **teaspoon pepper**
- ⅛ **teaspoon salt**
- 2 **tilapia fillets (6 ounces each)**
- ¼ **cup fat-free Italian salad dressing**

1. In a large saucepan, bring the water, rice and butter to a boil. Reduce heat; cover and simmer for 15-20 minutes or until liquid is absorbed and rice is tender.
2. Combine the seasonings; sprinkle over fillets. Place salad dressing in a large skillet; cook over medium heat until heated through. Add fish; cook for 3-4 minutes on each side or until fish flakes easily with a fork. Serve with rice.
PER SERVING *1 fillet with ¾ cup rice equals 356 cal., 5 g fat (3 g sat. fat), 91 mg chol., 743 mg sodium, 41 g carb., 1 g fiber, 35 g pro. Diabetic Exchanges: 4 lean meat, 3 starch, ½ fat.*

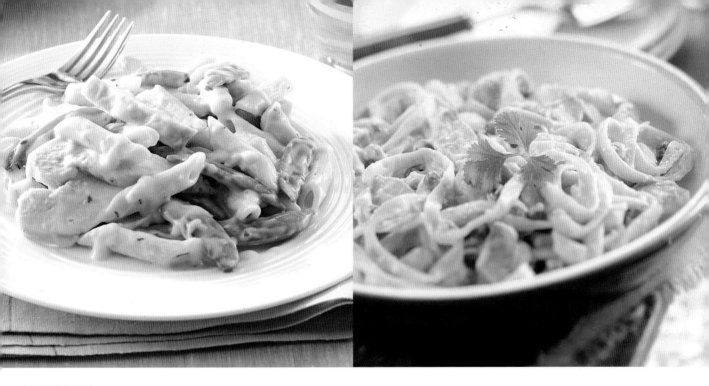

Garlic Chicken Penne

It takes just four ingredients to prepare my satisfying pasta dish. Chicken, snap peas and pasta star, and the garlicky sauce ties it all together nicely.
—**ANNE NOCK** AVON LAKE, OH

START TO FINISH: 20 MIN.
MAKES: 4 SERVINGS

- 8 **ounces uncooked penne pasta**
- 1½ **cups frozen sugar snap peas**
- 1 **package (1.6 ounces) garlic-herb pasta sauce mix**
- 1 **package (6 ounces) sliced cooked chicken**

1. In a large saucepan, cook pasta in boiling water for 6 minutes. Add the peas; return to a boil. Cook for 4-5 minutes or until pasta is tender. Meanwhile, prepare sauce mix according to the package directions.
2. Drain pasta mixture; add chicken. Drizzle with sauce and toss to coat.

PER SERVING *1⅓ cups equals 429 cal., 12 g fat (6 g sat. fat), 62 mg chol., 665 mg sodium, 54 g carb., 3 g fiber, 26 g pro.*

Chicken Fettuccine Alfredo

This fettuccine is very creamy and tasty. You'll be surprised that it's so low in fat! A filling dish that's also good for you, my recipe mixes tender chunks of chicken with peas, noodles and a rich homemade Alfredo sauce.
—**LADONNA REED** PONCA CITY, OK

START TO FINISH: 25 MIN.
MAKES: 4 SERVINGS

- 6 **ounces uncooked fettuccine**
- 1 **pound boneless skinless chicken breasts, cubed**
- 1 **small onion, chopped**
- 1 **tablespoon butter**
- 4 **garlic cloves, minced**
- ½ **teaspoon salt**
- ⅛ **teaspoon cayenne pepper**
- 4½ **teaspoons all-purpose flour**
- 1½ **cups fat-free half-and-half**
- 1 **cup frozen peas, thawed**
- ¼ **cup grated Parmesan cheese**

1. Cook fettuccine according to package directions. Meanwhile, in a large skillet, saute chicken and onion in butter until chicken is no longer pink. Add the garlic, salt and cayenne; cook 1 minute longer. Stir in flour until blended.
2. Gradually add the half-and-half, peas and cheese. Bring to a boil; cook and stir for 1-2 minutes or until thickened. Drain fettuccine; toss with chicken mixture.

PER SERVING *1 cup equals 425 cal., 8 g fat (4 g sat. fat), 75 mg chol., 577 mg sodium, 49 g carb., 4 g fiber, 36 g pro.*

❝ I took Zumba and spinning classes, kept track of my caloric intake and output, ate more produce and stayed away from fast food. In seven months, I went from 190 pounds to 125. It was liberating to reach my goal without crash dieting but with sheer determination! ❞

—ALLISON JOHNSON

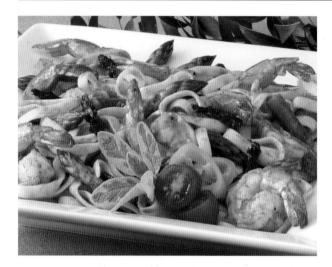

368 CALORIES

Mediterranean Shrimp 'n' Pasta

Sun-dried tomatoes and fresh asparagus take center stage in this dish that's loaded with tender shrimp and pasta.
—**SHIRLEY KUNDE** RHINELANDER, WI

PREP: 15 MIN. • **COOK:** 20 MIN. • **MAKES:** 4 SERVINGS

- 1 **cup boiling water**
- ½ **cup dry-pack sun-dried tomatoes, chopped**
- 6 **ounces uncooked fettuccine**
- 1 **can (8 ounces) tomato sauce**
- 2 **tablespoons clam juice**
- 2 **tablespoons unsweetened apple juice**
- 1 **teaspoon curry powder**
- ¼ **teaspoon pepper**
- 1 **pound fresh asparagus, trimmed and cut into 1-inch pieces**
- 1 **tablespoon olive oil**
- ½ **cup thinly sliced green onions**
- 2 **garlic cloves, minced**
- 1 **pound uncooked medium shrimp, peeled and deveined**

1. In a small bowl, pour boiling water over sun-dried tomatoes; let stand for 2 minutes. Drain and set aside. Cook fettuccine according to package directions.
2. Meanwhile, in a small bowl, combine the tomato sauce, clam juice, apple juice, curry powder and pepper; set aside. In a large nonstick skillet coated with cooking spray, cook asparagus in oil for 2 minutes. Add green onions and garlic; cook and stir 1 minute longer.
3. Stir in shrimp. Cook and stir 3 minutes longer or until shrimp turn pink. Stir in tomato sauce mixture and sun-dried tomatoes; heat through. Drain fettuccine and add to skillet; toss to coat.
PER SERVING 1½ cups equals 368 cal., 6 g fat (1 g sat. fat), 173 mg chol., 702 mg sodium, 46 g carb., 5 g fiber, 32 g pro. **Diabetic Exchanges:** 3 starch, 3 lean meat, ½ fat.

383 CALORIES Skillet Pasta Florentine

Here's an outstanding weeknight supper that's budget-friendly, healthy and liked by children. With such a thick, cheesy topping and so much flavor, who'd ever guess that it's lighter?
—**KELLY TURNBULL** JUPITER, FL

PREP: 20 MIN. • **COOK:** 35 MIN. • **MAKES:** 6 SERVINGS

- 3 **cups uncooked spiral pasta**
- 1 **egg, lightly beaten**
- 2 **cups (16 ounces) 2% cottage cheese**
- 1½ **cups reduced-fat ricotta cheese**
- 1 **package (10 ounces) frozen chopped spinach, thawed and squeezed dry**

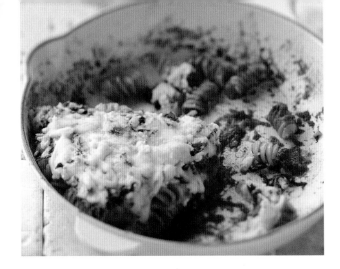

1 cup (4 ounces) shredded part-skim mozzarella cheese, divided
1 teaspoon each dried parsley flakes, oregano and basil
1 jar (14 ounces) meatless spaghetti sauce
2 tablespoons grated Parmesan cheese

1. Cook pasta according to package directions. Meanwhile, in a large bowl, combine the egg, cottage cheese, ricotta, spinach, ½ cup mozzarella and herbs.
2. Drain pasta. Place half of sauce in a large skillet; layer with pasta and remaining sauce. Top with the cheese mixture.
3. Bring to a boil. Reduce heat; cover and cook for 25-30 minutes or until a thermometer reads 160°.
4. Sprinkle with Parmesan cheese and remaining mozzarella cheese; cover and cook 5 minutes longer or until cheese is melted. Let the pasta stand for 5 minutes before serving.
PER SERVING *1 serving equals 383 cal., 9 g fat (5 g sat. fat), 73 mg chol., 775 mg sodium, 47 g carb., 4 g fiber, 27 g pro.*

400 CALORIES Malibu Chicken Bundles

The first time I made this, it was an instant hit, and the family agreed I wouldn't change a thing about the recipe. Mustard may seem like an odd ingredient, but it adds a really nice touch to this rich-tasting dish that's surprisingly light.
—BEVERLY NORRIS EVANSTON, WY

PREP: 25 MIN. • **BAKE:** 45 MIN. • **MAKES:** 4 SERVINGS

4 boneless skinless chicken breast halves (4 ounces each)
½ cup honey Dijon mustard, divided
4 thin slices deli ham
4 slices reduced-fat Swiss cheese
1 can (8 ounces) unsweetened crushed pineapple, well drained
1½ cups panko (Japanese) bread crumbs
¼ teaspoon salt
¼ teaspoon pepper
SAUCE
1 can (10¾ ounces) reduced-fat reduced-sodium condensed cream of chicken soup, undiluted
¼ cup reduced-fat sour cream
⅛ teaspoon dried tarragon

1. Flatten chicken breasts to ¼-in. thickness. Spread 1 tablespoon mustard over each; layer with ham, cheese and pineapple. Fold chicken over pineapple; secure with toothpicks. Brush bundles with remaining mustard.
2. In a shallow bowl, combine the bread crumbs, salt and pepper. Roll bundles in bread crumb mixture; place in an 11-in. x 7-in. baking dish coated with cooking spray. Bake, uncovered, at 350° for 45-50 minutes or until a thermometer reads 170°. Discard toothpicks.
3. Meanwhile, in a small saucepan, combine the sauce ingredients. Cook, stirring occasionally, until heated through. Serve with chicken.
PER SERVING *1 chicken bundle with ⅓ cup sauce equals 400 cal., 12 g fat (4 g sat. fat), 86 mg chol., 784 mg sodium, 41 g carb., 2 g fiber, 36 g pro.* **Diabetic Exchanges:** *4 lean meat, 2 starch, ½ fruit.*

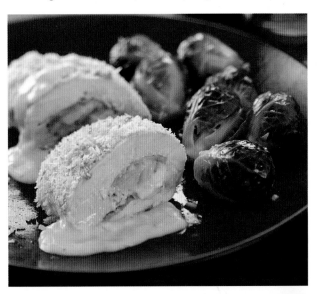

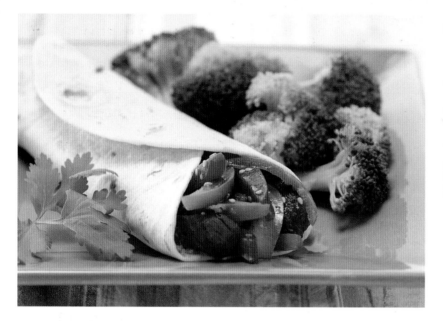

361 CALORIES

Turkey Fettuccine Skillet

I came up with this simple pasta dish as a way to use up leftover turkey from holiday dinners. Now, it's become a family tradition to enjoy it the day after Thanksgiving and Christmas.

—**KARI JOHNSTON** MARWAYNE, AB

PREP: 10 MIN. • **COOK:** 30 MIN.
MAKES: 6 SERVINGS

- 8 **ounces uncooked fettuccine**
- ½ **cup chopped onion**
- ½ **cup chopped celery**
- 4 **garlic cloves, minced**
- 1 **teaspoon canola oil**
- 1 **cup sliced fresh mushrooms**
- 2 **cups fat-free milk**
- 1 **teaspoon salt-free seasoning blend**
- ¼ **teaspoon salt**
- 2 **tablespoons cornstarch**
- ½ **cup fat-free half-and-half**
- ⅓ **cup grated Parmesan cheese**
- 3 **cups cubed cooked turkey breast**
- ¾ **cup shredded part-skim mozzarella cheese**

402 CALORIES

Asian Steak Wraps

Zesty marinade with a splash of fresh lime juice makes these sesame-flavored wraps a treat. To speed prep time, use a 1-pound package of frozen onion and pepper mix.

—**TRISHA KRUSE** EAGLE, ID

PREP: 20 MIN. + MARINATING
COOK: 10 MIN. • **MAKES:** 4 SERVINGS

- ¼ **cup lime juice**
- 3 **tablespoons honey**
- 1 **tablespoon reduced-sodium soy sauce**
- 2 **teaspoons sesame oil**
- 2 **teaspoons minced fresh gingerroot**
- 1½ **teaspoons minced fresh cilantro**
- 1 **pound beef top sirloin steak, cut into thin strips**
- ¼ **teaspoon salt**
- ¼ **teaspoon pepper**
- 1 **medium onion, halved and thinly sliced**
- 1 **large green pepper, julienned**
- 1 **large sweet red pepper, julienned**
- 4 **flour tortillas (8 inches), warmed**
- 2 **ounces reduced-fat cream cheese**
- 2 **teaspoons sesame seeds, toasted**

1. In a small bowl, combine first six ingredients. Pour ⅓ cup marinade into a large resealable plastic bag; add the beef. Seal bag and turn to coat; refrigerate for 1 hour. Add salt and pepper to remaining marinade; cover and refrigerate.

2. Drain beef and discard marinade. In a large nonstick skillet or wok coated with cooking spray, stir-fry beef until no longer pink; remove and keep warm. In the same pan, stir-fry onion and peppers until crisp-tender. Stir in reserved marinade. Return beef to the pan; heat through.

3. Spread tortillas with cream cheese; top with beef mixture and sprinkle with sesame seeds. Roll up.

PER SERVING *1 wrap equals 402 cal., 14 g fat (5 g sat. fat), 4 mg chol., 575 mg sodium, 41 g carb., 3 g fiber, 29 g pro.*
***Diabetic Exchanges:** 3 lean meat, 2 starch, 1 vegetable, 1 fat.*

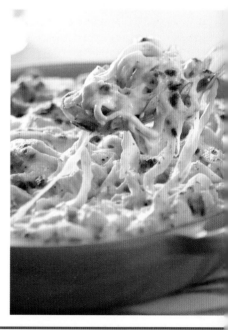

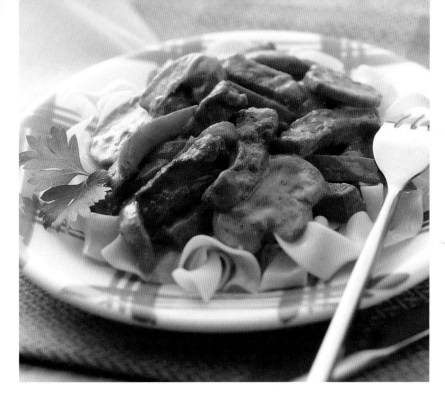

1. Cook fettuccine according to package directions. Meanwhile, in a large ovenproof skillet coated with cooking spray, saute the onion, celery and garlic in oil for 3 minutes. Add mushrooms; cook and stir until vegetables are tender. Stir in the milk, seasoning blend and salt. Bring to a boil.

2. Combine cornstarch and half-and-half until smooth; stir into skillet. Cook and stir for 2 minutes or until thickened and bubbly. Stir in the Parmesan cheese just until melted.

3. Stir in turkey. Drain fettuccine; add to turkey mixture. Heat through. Sprinkle with mozzarella cheese. Broil 4-6 in. from the heat for 2-3 minutes or until cheese is melted.

PER SERVING *1 cup equals 361 cal., 7 g fat (3 g sat. fat), 76 mg chol., 343 mg sodium, 38 g carb., 2 g fiber, 34 g pro.* **Diabetic Exchanges:** *4 lean meat, 2½ starch, ½ fat.*

414 CALORIES Paprika Beef Stroganoff

I am a busy home-schooling mother of two, and I love to make this wonderful meal! It simmers and fills my home with a delightful aroma, leaving me free to do other things. Definitely a family favorite.
—**LARA TAYLOR** VIRGINIA BEACH, VA

PREP: 15 MIN. • **COOK:** 55 MIN.
MAKES: 8 SERVINGS

- 2 **pounds beef top round steak, cut into thin strips**
- 1 **tablespoon plus 2 teaspoons canola oil, divided**
- 1 **large onion, sliced**
- 1 **large green pepper, cut into strips**
- ½ **pound sliced fresh mushrooms**
- 1¼ **cups reduced-sodium beef broth, divided**
- 1 **can (8 ounces) tomato sauce**
- ¾ **cup sherry or additional reduced-sodium beef broth**
- 2 **tablespoons Worcestershire sauce**
- 2 **tablespoons prepared mustard**
- 2 **teaspoons paprika**
- 1 **bay leaf**
- ½ **teaspoon dried thyme**
- ¼ **teaspoon pepper**
- 1 **package (12 ounces) yolk-free noodles**
- 3 **tablespoons all-purpose flour**
- 1 **cup (8 ounces) reduced-fat sour cream**

1. In a large nonstick skillet coated with cooking spray, cook beef in 1 tablespoon oil until no longer pink; drain and set aside.

2. In the same skillet, saute onion and green pepper in remaining oil for 1 minute. Stir in mushrooms; cook for 3-4 minutes or until tender. Stir in 1 cup broth, tomato sauce, sherry, Worcestershire sauce, mustard, paprika, bay leaf, thyme and pepper.

3. Return beef to the pan and bring to a boil. Reduce heat; cover and simmer for 40-50 minutes or until meat is tender.

4. Cook noodles according to package directions. Meanwhile, combine flour and remaining broth until smooth; gradually stir into beef mixture. Bring to a boil; cook and stir for 2 minutes or until thickened. Discard bay leaf. Remove from the heat; stir in sour cream until blended. Drain noodles; serve with Stroganoff.

PER SERVING *¾ cup stroganoff with 1 cup noodles equals 414 cal., 10 g fat (3 g sat. fat), 74 mg chol., 360 mg sodium, 42 g carb., 4 g fiber, 36 g pro.*

380 CALORIES

Santa Fe Chicken Pita Pizzas

With very little fuss, personal pizzas can be altered to please anyone, and that's why I call this dish easy. It's ideal for using up leftover chicken.

—**ATHENA RUSSELL** FLORENCE, SC

START TO FINISH: 30 MIN. • **MAKES:** 4 SERVINGS

- 4 whole pita breads
- ½ cup refried black beans
- ½ cup salsa
- 1 cup cubed cooked chicken breast
- 2 tablespoons chopped green chilies
- 2 tablespoons sliced ripe olives
- ¾ cup shredded Colby-Monterey Jack cheese
- 1 green onion, chopped
- ½ cup reduced-fat sour cream

1. Preheat oven to 350°. Place pita breads on an ungreased baking sheet; spread with beans. Top with salsa, chicken, chilies and olives; sprinkle with cheese.
2. Bake 8-10 minutes or until cheese is melted. Top with green onion; serve with sour cream.
PER SERVING *1 pizza equals 380 cal., 11 g fat (6 g sat. fat), 56 mg chol., 776 mg sodium, 44 g carb., 3 g fiber, 24 g pro.* **Diabetic Exchanges:** *3 starch, 2 lean meat, 1 fat.*

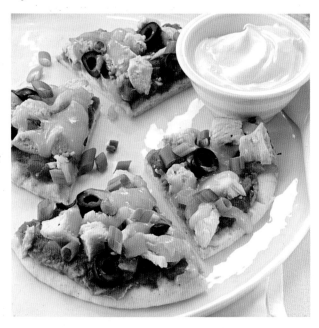

374 CALORIES # Chicken Hot Dish

You won't believe how simple this chicken recipe is to make! By layering a variety of delicious ingredients, you're sure to create a meal everyone will enjoy.

—**AMBER DUDLEY** NEW PRAGUE, MN

PREP: 5 MIN. • **BAKE:** 70 MIN. • **MAKES:** 6 SERVINGS

- 1 package (26 ounces) frozen shredded hash brown potatoes, thawed
- 1 package (24 ounces) frozen California-blend vegetables
- 3 cups cubed cooked chicken
- 1 can (10¾ ounces) reduced-fat reduced-sodium condensed cream of chicken soup, undiluted
- 1 can (10¾ ounces) reduced-fat reduced-sodium condensed cream of mushroom soup, undiluted
- 1 cup reduced-sodium chicken broth
- ¾ cup French-fried onions

1. In a greased 13-in. x 9-in. baking dish, layer the potatoes, vegetables and chicken. In a large bowl, combine soups and broth; pour over chicken (dish will be full).
2. Cover and bake at 375° for 1 hour. Uncover; sprinkle with French-fried onions. Bake 10 minutes longer or until heated through.
PER SERVING *1 serving equals 374 cal., 11 g fat (3 g sat. fat), 68 mg chol., 660 mg sodium, 39 g carb., 5 g fiber, 28 g pro.* **Diabetic Exchanges:** *3 lean meat, 2 starch, 1 vegetable.*

358 CALORIES # Herbed Pork and Potatoes

This recipe is wonderful because it's not only tasty, but the potatoes are a built-in side dish! We made it for our anniversary party, and our guests were more than impressed.

—**KATE COLLINS** AUBURN, WA

PREP: 25 MIN. • **BAKE:** 1 HOUR + STANDING • **MAKES:** 9 SERVINGS

- 3 tablespoons minced fresh rosemary
- 2 tablespoons minced fresh marjoram
- 8 garlic cloves, minced
- 4 teaspoons minced fresh sage
- 4 teaspoons olive oil, divided
- 2 teaspoons salt
- 2 teaspoons pepper
- 1 boneless pork loin roast (3 pounds)
- 4 pounds medium red potatoes, quartered

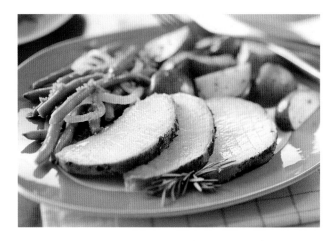

1. In a small bowl, combine the rosemary, marjoram, garlic, sage, 3 teaspoons oil, salt and pepper. Rub roast with 2 tablespoons herb mixture.

2. In a Dutch oven over medium-high heat, brown roast in remaining oil on all sides. Place in a roasting pan coated with cooking spray. Toss potatoes with remaining herb mixture; arrange around roast.

3. Cover and bake at 350° for 1 to 1¼ hours or until a thermometer reads 160°. Let stand for 10 minutes before slicing.

PER SERVING *4 ounces cooked pork with ¾ cup potatoes equals 358 cal., 9 g fat (3 g sat. fat), 75 mg chol., 581 mg sodium, 34 g carb., 4 g fiber, 33 g pro.*

371 CALORIES Turkey Burritos with Fresh Fruit Salsa

Packed with fruit, veggies, nutrition and flavor, this lighter, whole-grain twist on traditional burritos will definitely be a hit with your family. Even our pickiest eater goes for these with their sweet-spicy fruit salsa. Yum!
—**LISA EATON** KENNEBUNK, ME

PREP: 30 MIN. • **COOK:** 20 MIN. • **MAKES:** 10 SERVINGS

- 1 pint grape tomatoes, quartered
- 1 medium mango, peeled and chopped
- 2 medium kiwifruit, peeled and chopped
- 3 green onions, thinly sliced
- 3 tablespoons finely chopped red onion
- 1 jalapeno pepper, seeded and chopped
- 1 tablespoon lime juice

BURRITOS

- 1 pound lean ground turkey
- ½ teaspoon ground turmeric
- ¼ teaspoon ground cumin
- 1 tablespoon olive oil
- 2 garlic cloves, minced
- ½ cup Burgundy wine or reduced-sodium beef broth
- 1 jar (16 ounces) salsa
- 2 cups frozen corn, thawed
- 1 can (15 ounces) black beans, rinsed and drained
- 10 whole wheat tortilla (8 inches), warmed
- 1 cup (4 ounces) shredded reduced-fat cheddar cheese

1. For salsa, combine the first seven ingredients. Chill until serving.

2. In a large nonstick skillet, cook the turkey, turmeric and cumin in oil over medium heat until turkey is no longer pink. Add garlic; cook 1 minute longer. Drain. Stir in wine. Bring to a boil. Reduce heat; simmer, uncovered, for 3-5 minutes or until thickened.

3. Stir in the salsa, corn and black beans. Bring to a boil. Reduce heat; simmer, uncovered, for 10-15 minutes or until thickened. Remove from the heat.

4. Spoon about ½ cup turkey mixture off center on each tortilla. Sprinkle with cheese. Fold sides and ends over filling and roll up. Serve with salsa.

NOTE *Wear disposable gloves when cutting hot peppers; the oils can burn skin. Avoid touching your face.*

PER SERVING *1 burrito equals 371 cal., 11 g fat (3 g sat. fat), 44 mg chol., 553 mg sodium, 47 g carb., 6 g fiber, 18 g pro.* **Diabetic Exchanges:** *3 starch, 2 lean meat.*

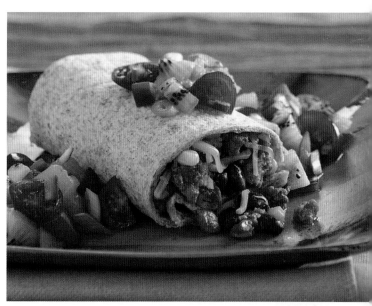

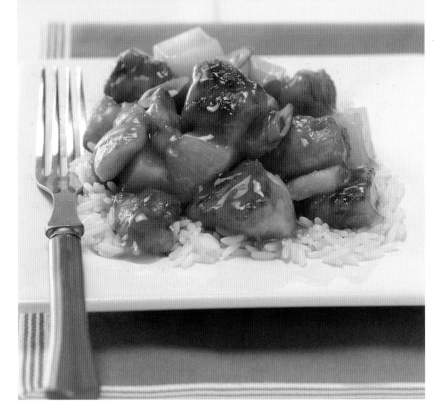

428 CALORIES Sweet and Sour Chicken

I first tasted this scrumptious dish at our friends' house. I immediately asked for the recipe, and we've enjoyed it ever since. In fact, it's called "favorite chicken" at our house!

—LORI BURTENSHAW TERRETON, ID

PREP: 20 MIN. + MARINATING
COOK: 15 MIN. • **MAKES:** 4 SERVINGS

- 1 tablespoon plus 2 teaspoons reduced-sodium soy sauce, divided
- 1 tablespoon sherry or reduced-sodium chicken broth
- ½ teaspoon salt
- ½ teaspoon garlic powder
- ½ teaspoon ground ginger
- 1 pound boneless skinless chicken breasts, cut into 1-inch cubes
- 1 can (20 ounces) unsweetened pineapple chunks
- 2 tablespoons plus ⅓ cup cornstarch, divided
- 2 tablespoons sugar
- ¼ cup cider vinegar
- ¼ cup ketchup
- 1 tablespoon canola oil
- 2 cups hot cooked rice

1. In a large resealable plastic bag, combine 1 tablespoon soy sauce, sherry, salt, garlic powder and ginger; add chicken. Seal bag and turn to coat; refrigerate 30 minutes.
2. Drain pineapple, reserving juice; set pineapple aside. Add enough water to juice to measure 1 cup. In a small bowl, combine 2 tablespoons cornstarch, sugar and pineapple juice mixture until smooth; stir in vinegar, ketchup and remaining soy sauce. Set aside.
3. Drain chicken and discard marinade. Place remaining cornstarch in a large resealable plastic bag. Add chicken, a few pieces at a time, and shake to coat. In a large nonstick skillet or wok coated with cooking spray, stir-fry chicken in oil until no longer pink. Remove and keep warm.
4. Stir pineapple juice mixture and add to pan. Bring to a boil; cook and stir for 2 minutes or until thickened. Add chicken and reserved pineapple; heat through. Serve with rice.

PER SERVING *1 cup chicken mixture with ½ cup rice equals 428 cal., 6 g fat (1 g sat. fat), 63 mg chol., 571 mg sodium, 65 g carb., 2 g fiber, 26 g pro.*

353 CALORIES Macaroni and Cheese

When my husband had heart problems, I searched for recipes to replace our full-fat standbys. Over the years, I've updated this dinner to accommodate new reduced-fat products, and my family continues to enjoy it.

—CORA JOHNSON SCHLOETZER
TOPEKA, KS

PREP: 20 MIN. • **BAKE:** 35 MIN. + STANDING
MAKES: 8 SERVINGS

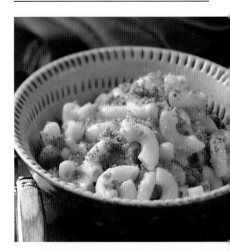

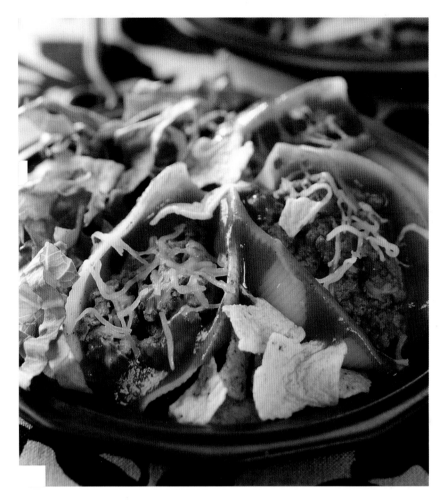

Taco Pasta Shells

Here's a kid-friendly dish so flavorful and fun, nobody is likely to guess that it's also lower in fat. It's a great family supper for busy weeknights. Crushed tortilla chips give it a nice crunch.

—ANNE THOMSEN WESTCHESTER, OH

PREP: 25 MIN. • **BAKE:** 25 MIN.
MAKES: 6 SERVINGS

- 18 uncooked jumbo pasta shells
- 1½ pounds lean ground beef (90% lean)
- 1 bottle (16 ounces) taco sauce, divided
- 3 ounces fat-free cream cheese, cubed
- 2 teaspoons chili powder
- ¾ cup shredded reduced-fat Mexican cheese blend, divided
- 20 baked tortilla chip scoops, coarsely crushed

1. Cook pasta according to package directions. Meanwhile, in a large nonstick skillet over medium heat, cook beef until no longer pink; drain. Add ½ cup taco sauce, cream cheese and chili powder; cook and stir until blended. Stir in ¼ cup cheese blend.
2. Drain pasta and rinse in cold water; stuff each shell with about 2 tablespoons beef mixture. Arrange in an 11-in. x 7-in. baking dish coated with cooking spray. Spoon remaining taco sauce over the top.
3. Cover and bake at 350° for 20 minutes. Uncover; sprinkle with remaining cheese blend. Bake 5-10 minutes longer or until heated through and cheese is melted. Sprinkle with chips.
PER SERVING *3 stuffed shells equals 384 cal., 13 g fat (5 g sat. fat), 67 mg chol., 665 mg sodium, 33 g carb., 3 g fiber, 33 g pro.*

- 3 cups uncooked elbow macaroni
- 12 ounces reduced-fat process cheese (Velveeta), sliced
- ½ cup finely chopped onion
- ⅓ cup all-purpose flour
- 2 teaspoons ground mustard
- ⅛ teaspoon pepper
- 1 can (12 ounces) fat-free evaporated milk
- 1¼ cups fat-free milk
- ½ cup dry bread crumbs
- 2 tablespoons butter, melted

1. Cook macaroni according to package directions; drain. In a 13-in. x 9-in. baking dish coated with cooking spray, layer a third of the macaroni, half of the cheese and half of the onion. Repeat layers. Top with remaining macaroni.
2. In a bowl, combine the flour, mustard, pepper, evaporated milk and milk; pour over layers. Combine bread crumbs and butter; sprinkle over top.
3. Cover and bake at 375° for 20 minutes. Uncover; bake 15 minutes longer or until bubbly. Let stand 10 minutes before serving.
PER SERVING *1 serving equals 353 cal., 7 g fat (4 g sat. fat), 25 mg chol., 161 mg sodium, 48 g carb., 2 g fiber, 22 g pro.*

362 CALORIES
Mushroom Turkey Tetrazzini

My creamy casserole is a fantastic way to use up that leftover Thanksgiving turkey. And it's a real family-pleaser!
—**LINDA HOWE** LISLE, IL

PREP: 35 MIN. • **BAKE:** 25 MIN. • **MAKES:** 8 SERVINGS

- 12 ounces uncooked spaghetti, broken into 2-inch pieces
- 2 teaspoons chicken bouillon granules
- ½ pound sliced fresh mushrooms
- 2 tablespoons butter
- 2 tablespoons all-purpose flour
- ¼ cup sherry or reduced-sodium chicken broth
- ¾ teaspoon salt-free lemon-pepper seasoning
- ½ teaspoon salt
- ⅛ teaspoon ground nutmeg
- 1 cup fat-free evaporated milk
- ⅔ cup grated Parmesan cheese, divided
- 4 cups cubed cooked turkey breast
- ¼ teaspoon paprika

1. Cook spaghetti according to package directions. Drain, reserving 2½ cups cooking liquid. Stir bouillon into cooking liquid and set aside. Place spaghetti in a 13-in. x 9-in. baking dish coated with cooking spray; set aside.
2. In a large nonstick skillet, saute mushrooms in butter until tender. Stir in flour until blended.

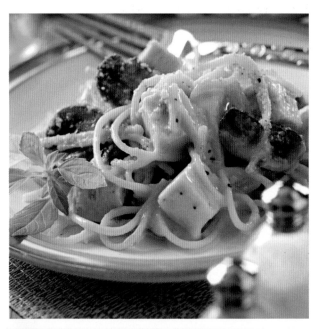

Gradually stir in sherry and reserved cooking liquid. Add the lemon-pepper, salt and nutmeg. Bring to a boil; cook and stir for 2 minutes or until thickened.
3. Reduce heat to low; stir in milk and ⅓ cup Parmesan cheese until blended. Add turkey; cook and stir until heated through.
4. Pour turkey mixture over spaghetti and toss to combine. Sprinkle with paprika and remaining Parmesan cheese. Cover and bake at 375° for 25-30 minutes or until bubbly.
PER SERVING *1 cup equals 362 cal., 7 g fat (3 g sat. fat), 75 mg chol., 592 mg sodium, 40 g carb., 2 g fiber, 33 g pro.* **Diabetic Exchanges:** *3 starch, 3 lean meat, ½ fat.*

353 CALORIES Makeover
Sloppy Joe Mac and Cheese

Decreasing the butter and replacing the half-and-half with milk helped cut a whopping 658 calories from this recipe. Now it offers all the heartwarming comfort of the original, without all the unnecessary fat!
—**TASTE OF HOME TEST KITCHEN**

PREP: 1 HOUR • **BAKE:** 30 MIN. • **MAKES:** 10 SERVINGS

- 1 package (16 ounces) elbow macaroni
- ¾ pound lean ground turkey
- ½ cup finely chopped celery
- ½ cup shredded carrot
- 1 can (14½ ounces) diced tomatoes, undrained
- 1 can (6 ounces) tomato paste
- ½ cup water
- 1 envelope sloppy joe mix
- 1 small onion, finely chopped
- 1 tablespoon butter
- ⅓ cup all-purpose flour
- 1 teaspoon ground mustard
- ¾ teaspoon salt
- ¼ teaspoon pepper
- 4 cups 2% milk
- 1 tablespoon Worcestershire sauce
- 8 ounces reduced-fat process cheese (Velveeta), cubed
- 2 cups (8 ounces) shredded cheddar cheese, divided

1. Cook macaroni according to package directions. Meanwhile, in a large nonstick skillet, cook the turkey, celery and carrot over medium heat until meat is no longer pink and vegetables are tender; drain. Add the tomatoes, tomato paste, water and sloppy joe mix. Bring

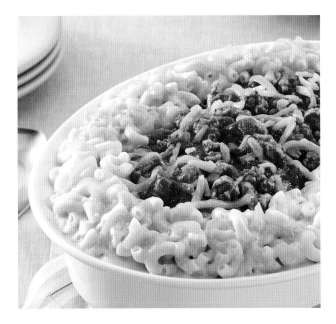

to a boil. Reduce heat; cover and simmer for 10 minutes, stirring occasionally.

2. Drain macaroni; set aside. In a large saucepan, saute onion in butter until tender. Stir in the flour, mustard, salt and pepper until smooth. Gradually add milk and Worcestershire sauce. Bring to a boil; cook and stir for 1-2 minutes or until thickened. Remove from the heat. Stir in the process cheese until melted. Add macaroni and 1 cup cheddar cheese; mix well.

3. Spread two-thirds of the macaroni mixture in a 13-in. x 9-in. baking dish coated with cooking spray. Spread turkey mixture to within 2 in. of edges. Spoon remaining macaroni mixture around edges of pan. Cover and bake at 375° for 30-35 minutes or until bubbly. Sprinkle with remaining cheddar cheese; cover and let stand until cheese is melted.

PER SERVING *1 cup equals 353 cal., 12 g fat (7 g sat. fat), 54 mg chol., 877 mg sodium, 42 g carb., 3 g fiber, 20 g pro.*

364 CALORIES Catfish Po'boys

When my neighbor prepared these large full-flavored sandwiches, I had to have the recipe. Strips of catfish are treated to a zesty Cajun cornmeal breading, then served on a bun with broccoli coleslaw.
—**MILDRED SHERRER** FORT WORTH, TX

START TO FINISH: 30 MIN. • **MAKES:** 4 SERVINGS

2 tablespoons fat-free mayonnaise
1 tablespoon fat-free sour cream
1 tablespoon white wine vinegar
1 teaspoon sugar
2 cups broccoli coleslaw mix
¼ cup cornmeal
2 teaspoons Cajun seasoning
½ teaspoon salt
⅛ teaspoon cayenne pepper
1 pound catfish fillets, cut into 2½-inch strips
2 tablespoons fat-free milk
2 teaspoons olive oil
4 kaiser rolls, split

1. In a small bowl, whisk the mayonnaise, sour cream, vinegar and sugar until smooth. Add coleslaw mix; toss to coat. Set aside.

2. In a large resealable plastic bag, combine the cornmeal, Cajun seasoning, salt and cayenne. In a shallow bowl, toss the catfish with milk. Place in bag, a few pieces at a time; seal bag and shake to coat.

3. In a large nonstick skillet, cook catfish over medium heat in oil for 4-5 minutes on each side or until fish flakes easily with a fork and coating is golden brown. Spoon coleslaw onto rolls; top with catfish.

PER SERVING *364 cal., 8 g fat (1 g sat. fat), 53 mg chol., 1,001 mg sodium, 44 g carb., 4 g fiber, 28 g pro.* ***Diabetic Exchanges:** 3 starch, 2½ lean meat.*

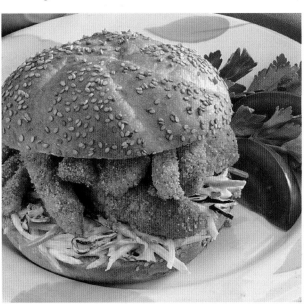

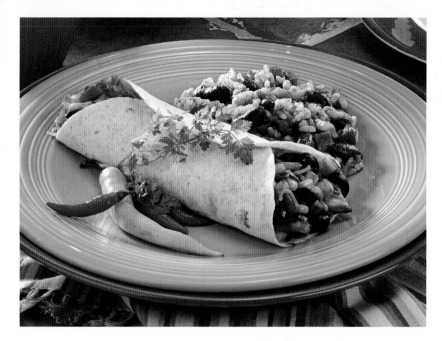

363 CALORIES
Corny Chicken Wraps

I'm a clinical dietitian, so I like to prepare foods that are both healthy and low-fat. This zippy Tex-Mex wrap is a quick alternative to a taco or sandwich for our on-the-go family. To increase the spicy flavor, use medium or hot salsa.

—SUSAN ALVERSON CHESTER, SD

START TO FINISH: 20 MIN.
MAKES: 6 SERVINGS

- 1 **pound boneless skinless chicken breasts, cut into strips**
- ½ **cup chopped green pepper**
- ¼ **cup chopped green onions**
- 2 **teaspoons canola oil**
- 1½ **cups frozen whole kernel corn, thawed**
- 1½ **cups salsa**
- ¼ **cup sliced ripe olives**
- ½ **teaspoon chili powder**
- 6 **flour tortillas (8 inches), warmed**
- 1 **cup (4 ounces) shredded reduced-fat cheddar cheese**

1. In a nonstick skillet, saute the chicken, green pepper and onions in oil for 3-4 minutes or until chicken juices run clear; drain. Stir in the corn, salsa, olives and chili powder. Cook and stir over medium heat for 3-4 minutes or until heated through.

2. Spoon about ½ cup chicken mixture over one side of each tortilla. Sprinkle with cheese; roll up and secure with toothpicks.

PER SERVING *1 wrap equals 363 cal., 11 g fat (4 g sat. fat), 55 mg chol., 740 mg sodium, 38 g carb., 4 g fiber, 26 g pro.* **Diabetic Exchanges:** *3 lean meat, 2½ starch.*

373 CALORIES Tomato-Basil
Chicken Spirals

After tasting a wonderful pasta dish at an Italian restaurant, I experimented until I came up with my tasty version. It's become one of our favorites. The riper the tomatoes, the better it is!

—SANDRA GIGUERE BREMEN, ME

- 2 **cups finely chopped sweet onion**
- 1 **cup chopped fresh basil**
- 4 **garlic cloves, minced**
- 1 **tablespoon olive oil**
- 5 **cups chopped seeded tomatoes**
- 1 **can (6 ounces) tomato paste**
- ½ **teaspoon crushed red pepper flakes**
- ½ **teaspoon salt**
- ¼ **teaspoon pepper**
- 1 **package (16 ounces) spiral pasta**
- 3 **cups cubed cooked chicken**
- ½ **cup shredded Parmesan cheese**

1. In a large saucepan or Dutch oven, saute the onion, basil and garlic in oil until onion is tender. Stir in the tomatoes, tomato paste, red pepper flakes, salt and pepper. Bring to a boil. Reduce heat; cover and simmer for 30-45 minutes.

2. Meanwhile, cook pasta according to package directions. Add chicken to the tomato mixture; heat through. Drain pasta. Top with chicken mixture; sprinkle with Parmesan cheese.

PER SERVING *373 cal., 6 g fat (2 g sat. fat), 44 mg chol., 291 mg sodium, 53 g carb., 5 g fiber, 27 g pro.* **Diabetic Exchanges:** *3 vegetable, 2½ starch, 2 lean meat.*

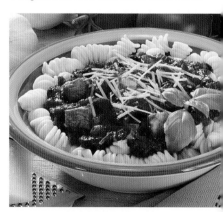

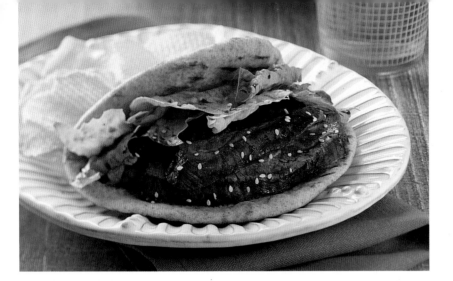

Flank Steak Pitas

The marinade in this yummy steak sandwich packs so much flavor, you won't even miss fatty ingredients like cheese or mayo.

—TAMMY KAMINSKI STANWOOD, WA

PREP: 15 MIN. + MARINATING
GRILL: 15 MIN. + STANDING
MAKES: 4 SERVINGS

- ¼ cup balsamic vinegar
- 2 tablespoons water
- 2 tablespoons reduced-sodium soy sauce
- 1 tablespoon hoisin sauce
- 2 garlic cloves, minced
- 1 teaspoon Thai chili sauce
- ¾ teaspoon pepper
- ½ teaspoon sesame oil
- 1 beef flank steak (1 pound)
- 4 whole pita breads
- 4 pieces leaf lettuce, torn
- ¼ teaspoon sesame seeds

1. In a small bowl, combine first eight ingredients. Pour ¼ cup marinade into a large resealable plastic bag; add the beef. Seal bag and turn to coat. Refrigerate for at least 8 hours or overnight. Cover and refrigerate remaining marinade.

2. Drain and discard marinade. Grill beef, covered, over medium heat for 6-8 minutes on each side or until meat reaches desired doneness (for medium-rare, a thermometer should read 145°; medium, 160°; well-done, 170°). Let stand for 10 minutes.

3. Meanwhile, grill pitas, uncovered, over medium heat for 1-2 minutes on each side or until warm. Thinly slice beef across the grain. In a large bowl, toss the beef, lettuce and reserved marinade. Serve in the pitas; sprinkle with sesame seeds.

PER SERVING *1 filled pita equals 362 cal., 10 g fat (4 g sat. fat), 54 mg chol., 703 mg sodium, 39 g carb., 2 g fiber, 28 g pro. Diabetic Exchanges: 3 lean meat, 2½ starch.*

Portobello Burgundy Beef

Nothing feels light about this rustic dish! Each bite is filled with mushrooms, beef and carrots draped in a Burgundy sauce. This is comfort food at its finest.

—MELANIE COLEMAN PITTSBURG, CA

PREP: 20 MIN. • **COOK:** 40 MIN.
MAKES: 4 SERVINGS

- ¼ cup plus 1 tablespoon all-purpose flour, divided
- 1 teaspoon dried marjoram, divided
- ½ teaspoon salt, divided
- 1 beef top round steak (1 pound), cut into ½-inch cubes
- 1 tablespoon olive oil
- 2 cups sliced baby portobello mushrooms
- 3 garlic cloves, minced
- 3 medium carrots, cut into ½-inch slices
- 1 can (14½ ounces) reduced-sodium beef broth, divided
- ½ cup Burgundy wine or additional reduced-sodium beef broth
- 1 bay leaf
- 4 cups cooked egg noodles

1. Place ¼ cup flour, ½ teaspoon marjoram and ¼ teaspoon salt in a large resealable plastic bag. Add beef, a few pieces at a time, and shake to coat. In a large nonstick skillet coated with cooking spray, brown beef in oil.

2. Add mushrooms and garlic; saute until mushrooms are tender. Stir in the carrots, 1½ cups broth, wine, bay leaf, remaining marjoram and salt. Bring to a boil. Reduce heat; cover and simmer 20-30 minutes or until beef and carrots are tender.

3. Combine remaining flour and broth; stir into pan. Bring to a boil; cook and stir for 2 minutes or until thickened. Discard bay leaf. Serve with noodles.

PER SERVING *1 cup beef mixture with 1 cup noodles equals 384 cal., 9 g fat (2 g sat. fat), 98 mg chol., 484 mg sodium, 39 g carb., 3 g fiber, 34 g pro. Diabetic Exchanges: 3 lean meat, 2 starch, 1 vegetable, ½ fat.*

Side Dishes

Counting calories doesn't mean settling for carrot sticks when it comes to rounding out meals. Dig into classics such as **coleslaw, potato salad** and even **mac 'n' cheese!** Make it a **500-calorie meal** by **pairing these side dishes** with your favorite dinner. Or use them to create a **satisfying** lunch.

CONTENTS

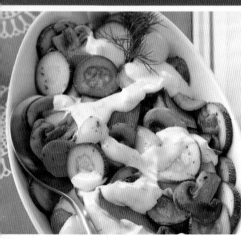

VEGETABLES IN DILL SAUCE
PAGE 365

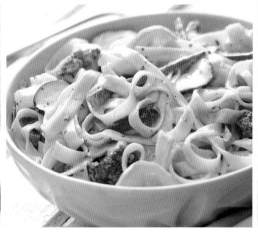

GARDEN PRIMAVERA FETTUCCINE
PAGE 382

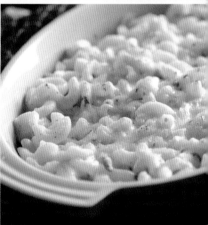

CREAMY MACARONI 'N' CHEESE
PAGE 387

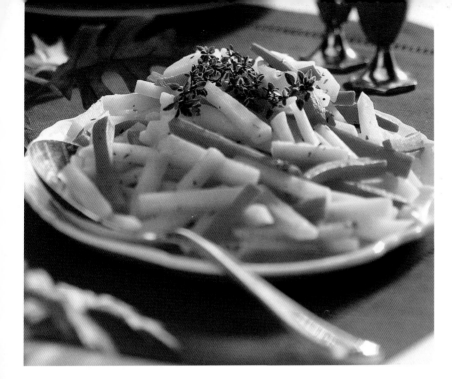

Winter Vegetables

The flavor of thyme shines through in this recipe, and the colorful array of vegetables is so appealing on the table! It's a great use for broccoli stalks, which too frequently go unused.

—CHARLENE AUGUSTYN
GRAND RAPIDS, MI

PREP: 25 MIN. • **COOK:** 20 MIN.
MAKES: 12 SERVINGS

- 3 medium turnips, peeled and cut into strips
- 1 large rutabaga, peeled and cut into strips
- 4 medium carrots, cut into strips
- 3 fresh broccoli spears
- 1 tablespoon butter
- 1 tablespoon minced fresh parsley
- ½ teaspoon salt
- ½ teaspoon dried thyme
  Pepper to taste

1. Place the turnips, rutabaga and carrots in a large saucepan and cover with water. Bring to a boil. Reduce heat; cover and cook for 10 minutes.

2. Meanwhile, cut florets from broccoli and save for another use. Cut broccoli stalks into strips; add to saucepan. Cover and cook for 5 minutes longer or until vegetables are crisp-tender; drain well.

3. In a large skillet, saute vegetables in butter. Stir in the parsley, salt, thyme and pepper.

PER SERVING *¾ cup equals 51 cal., 1 g fat (1 g sat. fat), 3 mg chol., 151 mg sodium, 10 g carb., 3 g fiber, 2 g pro. Diabetic Exchange: 2 vegetable.*

Warm Garlicky Grape Tomatoes

This is one of our favorite quick ways to use up a large crop of grape tomatoes.

—ROSE GULLEDGE CROFTON, MD

START TO FINISH: 30 MIN.
MAKES: 4 SERVINGS

- 2 cups grape tomatoes
- 3 garlic cloves, minced
- 1½ teaspoons minced fresh basil
- ½ teaspoon salt-free garlic seasoning blend
- ¼ teaspoon salt
- ⅛ teaspoon pepper
- 1 teaspoon olive oil, divided
- ¼ cup soft whole wheat bread crumbs
- ¼ cup crumbled feta cheese

1. In a small bowl, combine the tomatoes, garlic, basil, seasoning blend, salt and pepper. Add ½ teaspoon oil; toss to coat. Transfer to a 3-cup baking dish coated with cooking spray.

2. Bake at 425° for 15 minutes. Combine bread crumbs and remaining oil; sprinkle over the top. Sprinkle with cheese. Bake 5-10 minutes longer or until cheese is softened and tomatoes are tender.

PER SERVING *½ cup equals 64 cal., 3 g fat (1 g sat. fat), 4 mg chol., 259 mg sodium, 8 g carb., 2 g fiber, 3 g pro. Diabetic Exchanges: 1 vegetable, ½ fat.*

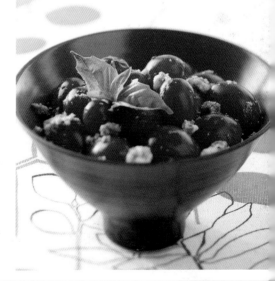

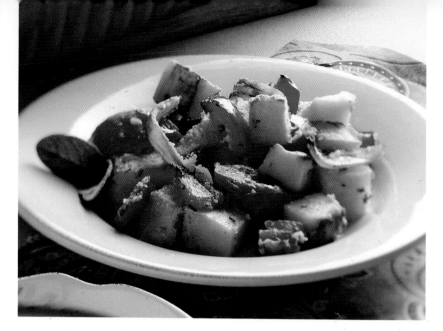

Parmesan Tomato

What a great way to use up all those fresh garden tomatoes—and what a simple but scrumptious side dish for entrees of all kinds! This quick and easy recipe is sure to become a summer standard at your house, too.

—MARCIA ORLANDO BOYERTOWN, PA

START TO FINISH: 30 MIN.
MAKES: 6 SERVINGS

- 3 **large tomatoes**
- 1 **tablespoon chicken bouillon granules**
- ¼ **cup grated Parmesan cheese**
- 1 **tablespoon butter**

1. Remove stems from tomatoes; cut in half widthwise. Place cut side up in an 11-in. x 7-in. baking dish coated with cooking spray.
2. Sprinkle with bouillon and cheese; dot with butter. Bake, uncovered, at 400° for 20-25 minutes or until heated through.
PER SERVING *1 tomato half equals 54 cal., 3 g fat (2 g sat. fat), 8 mg chol., 510 mg sodium, 5 g carb., 1 g fiber, 2 g pro.* **Diabetic Exchanges:** *1 vegetable, ½ fat.*

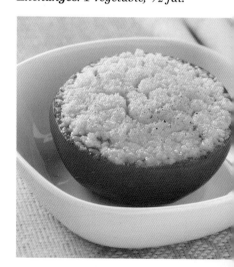

---

99 CALORIES ## Italian Squash Casserole

You can assemble this garlic-kissed veggie dish in advance, but wait to bake it until just before serving. The aroma from the oven will lure everyone in the house to the kitchen!

—PAUL VANSAVAGE BINGHAMTON, NY

PREP: 45 MIN. • **BAKE:** 30 MIN.
MAKES: 14 SERVINGS (¾ CUP EACH)

- 1 **whole garlic bulb**
- 2 **tablespoons olive oil, divided**
- 1 **medium butternut squash (about 3½ pounds), cut into 1-inch cubes**
- 2 **large sweet red peppers, cut into 1-inch pieces**
- 1 **large red onion, cut into wedges**
- 2 **medium tomatoes, cut into wedges**
- ¼ **cup dry bread crumbs**
- 3 **tablespoons minced fresh parsley**
- 1½ **teaspoons minced fresh rosemary or ½ teaspoon dried rosemary, crushed**
- 1 **teaspoon salt**
- ½ **teaspoon pepper**
- ½ **cup grated Parmesan cheese**

1. Remove papery outer skin from garlic (do not peel or separate cloves). Cut top off of garlic bulb. Brush with ½ teaspoon oil. Wrap bulb in heavy-duty foil. Bake at 425° for 30-35 minutes or until softened. Reduce heat to 400°. Cool the garlic for 10 minutes. Squeeze softened garlic into a bowl and mash.
2. Meanwhile, in a large skillet, saute squash in 1 tablespoon oil until golden brown; transfer to a large bowl. In the same skillet, saute peppers and onion in remaining oil until crisp-tender. Add to squash.
3. Stir in the tomatoes, garlic, bread crumbs, parsley, rosemary, salt and pepper. Transfer to a greased 13-in. x 9-in. baking dish; sprinkle with cheese. Bake, uncovered, for 30-40 minutes or until squash is tender.
PER SERVING *¾ cup equals 99 cal., 3 g fat (1 g sat. fat), 3 mg chol., 234 mg sodium, 17 g carb., 4 g fiber, 3 g pro.* **Diabetic Exchanges:** *1 starch, 1 vegetable.*

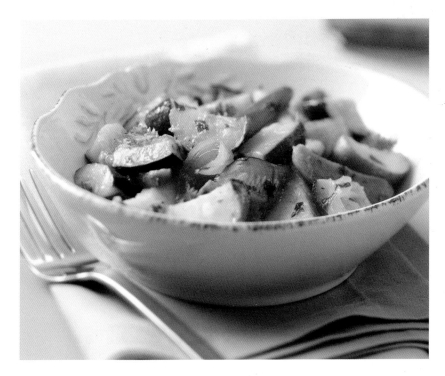

59 CALORIES Potato Vegetable Medley

Mom made this easy side with fresh vegetables from our garden. The fact that we kids had helped to plant, nurture and pick those veggies made it even more appealing to us!

—JOANN JENSEN LOWELL, IN

PREP: 10 MIN. • **BAKE:** 40 MIN.
MAKES: 6 SERVINGS

- 6 small red potatoes, quartered
- 16 baby carrots, halved lengthwise
- 1 small onion, cut into wedges
- ½ cup chicken broth
- 1¼ teaspoons seasoned salt, divided
- 2 medium zucchini, chopped
- 2 tablespoons minced fresh parsley

1. In a greased 2-qt. baking dish, combine the potatoes, carrots, onion, broth and 1 teaspoon seasoned salt.
2. Cover and bake at 400° for 30 minutes. Stir in zucchini and remaining seasoned salt. Bake 10-15 minutes longer or until vegetables are tender. Sprinkle with parsley.
PER SERVING *¾ cup equals 59 cal., trace fat (trace sat. fat), trace chol., 424 mg sodium, 13 g carb., 2 g fiber, 2 g pro.* **Diabetic Exchanges:** *1 vegetable, ½ starch.*

88 CALORIES Colorful Roasted Veggies

These delicious roasted vegetables are one of my mom's specialties. It's my favorite of all her side dishes.

—DIANE HARRISON
MECHANICSBURG, PA

PREP: 25 MIN. • **BAKE:** 20 MIN.
MAKES: 12 SERVINGS

- 4 medium carrots, julienned
- 1½ pounds fresh asparagus, trimmed and halved
- 1 large green pepper, julienned
- 1 medium sweet red pepper, julienned
- 1 medium red onion, sliced and separated into rings
- 5 cups fresh cauliflowerets
- 5 cups fresh broccoli florets
- ¼ to ½ cup olive oil
- 3 tablespoons lemon juice
- 3 garlic cloves, minced
- 1 tablespoon dried rosemary, crushed
- 1 teaspoon salt
- 1 teaspoon pepper

1. Preheat oven to 400°. In a large bowl, combine vegetables. In a small bowl, whisk oil, lemon juice, garlic, rosemary, salt and pepper until blended. Drizzle over the vegetables and toss to coat.
2. Transfer to two greased 15x10x1-in. baking pans. Bake, uncovered, 20-25 minutes or until tender, stirring occasionally.
PER SERVING *¾ cup (calculated with ¼ cup olive oil) equals 88 cal., 5 g fat (1 g sat. fat), 0 chol., 228 mg sodium, 10 g carb., 4 g fiber, 3 g pro.* **Diabetic Exchanges:** *2 vegetable, 1 fat.*

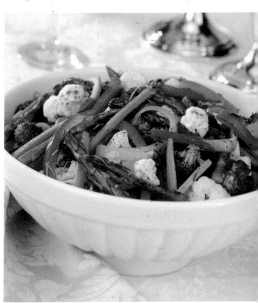

❝My family and I have tried at least 40 Comfort Food Diet recipes, and they are mostly winners! I'm starting to lose pounds and inches by combining the new recipes with daily workouts. We haven't forfeited taste for weight loss, which is the best part of this diet! ❞

—LISA MILLER

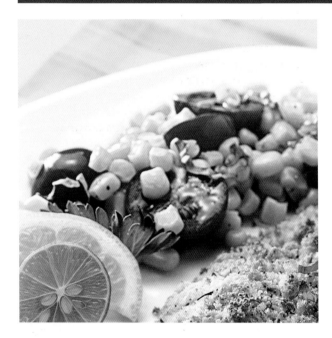

In a large skillet, saute corn in oil until crisp-tender. Stir in the tomatoes, salt and pepper; cook 1 minute longer. Remove from the heat; sprinkle with basil.

PER SERVING *¾ cup equals 85 cal., 4 g fat (1 g sat. fat), 0 chol., 161 mg sodium, 12 g carb., 2 g fiber, 2 g pro.*

64 CALORIES Ribboned Vegetables

Add a splash of color to your supper table with these vivid veggie strips. Cooked in lemon and horseradish, this simple side is a light and zippy complement to many a substantial cold-weather entree.

—**JULIE GWINN** HERSHEY, PA

START TO FINISH: 25 MIN. • **MAKES:** 4 SERVINGS

- 2 **medium carrots**
- 2 **small zucchini**
- 2 **small yellow summer squash**
- 1 **tablespoon butter**
- 2 **teaspoons lemon juice**
- 1 **teaspoon prepared horseradish**
- ½ **teaspoon salt**
- ⅛ **teaspoon pepper**

1. With a vegetable peeler or metal cheese slicer, cut very thin slices down the length of each carrot, zucchini and yellow squash, making long ribbons.

2. In a large skillet, saute vegetables in butter for 2 minutes. Stir in the remaining ingredients. Cook 2-4 minutes longer or until vegetables are crisp-tender, stirring occasionally.

PER SERVING *¾ cup equals 64 cal., 3 g fat (2 g sat. fat), 8 mg chol., 348 mg sodium, 9 g carb., 3 g fiber, 2 g pro.* **Diabetic Exchanges:** *2 vegetable, ½ fat.*

85 CALORIES
Sauteed Corn with Tomatoes & Basil

We harvest the veggies and basil from our backyard garden just minutes before fixing this recipe! It's so fresh and easy—and always delicious with grilled fish or meat.

—**PATRICIA NIEH** PORTOLA VALLEY, CA

START TO FINISH: 15 MIN. • **MAKES:** 4 SERVINGS

- 1 **cup fresh or frozen corn**
- 1 **tablespoon olive oil**
- 2 **cups cherry tomatoes, halved**
- ¼ **teaspoon salt**
- ¼ **teaspoon pepper**
- 3 **fresh basil leaves, thinly sliced**

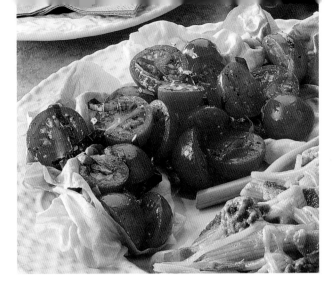

42 CALORIES Basil Cherry Tomatoes

These tomatoes are a quick and delicious side dish and will lend Italian flair to any dinner. Basil and olive oil are simple additions to sweet cherry tomatoes, and the flavors are wonderful together.
—**MELISSA STEVENS** ELK RIVER, MN

START TO FINISH: 10 MIN. • **MAKES:** 6 SERVINGS

- 3 pints cherry tomatoes, halved
- ½ cup chopped fresh basil
- 1½ teaspoons olive oil
  Salt and pepper to taste
  Lettuce leaves, optional

In a large bowl, combine the tomatoes, basil, oil, salt and pepper. Cover and refrigerate until serving. Serve on lettuce if desired.
PER SERVING *1 serving (calculated without salt) equals 42 cal., 2 g fat (trace sat. fat), 0 chol., 14 mg sodium, 7 g carb., 2 g fiber, 1 g pro.* **Diabetic Exchange:** *1 vegetable.*

70 CALORIES Mexican Veggies

I came up with this oh-so-easy combination while looking for a veggie side dish to complement my Mexican-style dinners. Corn, zucchini, salsa and fresh, crunchy flavor make this recipe a keeper!
—**PATRICIA MICKELSON** SAN JOSE, CA

START TO FINISH: 15 MIN. • **MAKES:** 2 SERVINGS

- 1 medium zucchini, diced
- ½ cup fresh or frozen corn
- ½ cup salsa or picante sauce

Place 1 in. of water in a small saucepan; add zucchini and corn. Bring to a boil. Reduce heat; cover and simmer for 3-4 minutes or until zucchini is almost tender. Drain. Stir in salsa; heat through.
PER SERVING *¾ cup equals 70 cal., trace fat (trace sat. fat), 0 chol., 284 mg sodium, 13 g carb., 4 g fiber, 2 g pro.* **Diabetic Exchanges:** *1 vegetable, ½ starch.*

66 CALORIES Baked Sweet Onion Rings

These are a real family favorite—especially when Vidalias are in season. You can boost the flavor even more with seasoned bread crumbs and a shake or two of different spices.
—**TONYA VOWELS** VINE GROVE, KY

START TO FINISH: 30 MIN. • **MAKES:** 4 SERVINGS

- ½ cup egg substitute
- ⅔ cup dry bread crumbs
- ½ teaspoon salt
- ¼ teaspoon pepper
- 1 sweet onion, sliced and separated into rings

1. Place egg substitute in a shallow dish. In another shallow dish, combine the bread crumbs, salt and pepper. Dip onion rings into egg, then roll in the bread crumb mixture.
2. Place on a baking sheet coated with cooking spray. Bake at 425° for 15-18 minutes or until golden brown, turning once.
PER SERVING *1 serving equals 66 cal., 1 g fat (trace sat. fat), 0 chol., 312 mg sodium, 12 g carb., 1 g fiber, 3 g pro.* **Diabetic Exchange:** *1 starch.*

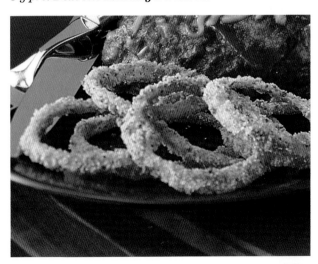

81 CALORIES

Zucchini Parmesan

You'll knock their socks off with this easy-to-prep side that's absolutely delicious. My favorite time to make it is when the zucchini is fresh out of my garden.

—**SANDI GUETTLER** BAY CITY, MI

START TO FINISH: 25 MIN.
MAKES: 6 SERVINGS

- 4 **medium zucchini, cut into ¼-inch slices**
- 1 **tablespoon olive oil**
- ½ **to 1 teaspoon minced garlic**
- 1 **can (14½ ounces) Italian diced tomatoes, undrained**
- 1 **teaspoon seasoned salt**
- ¼ **teaspoon pepper**
- ¼ **cup grated Parmesan cheese**

1. In a large skillet, saute zucchini in oil until crisp-tender. Add garlic; cook 1 minute longer.

2. Stir in the tomatoes, seasoned salt and pepper. Simmer, uncovered, for 9-10 minutes or until liquid is evaporated. Sprinkle with Parmesan cheese. Serve with a slotted spoon.
PER SERVING *½ cup equals 81 cal., 3 g fat (1 g sat. fat), 3 mg chol., 581 mg sodium, 10 g carb., 2 g fiber, 3 g pro.* **Diabetic Exchanges:** *2 vegetable, ½ fat.*

84 CALORIES

Tomato Corn Salad

The lightly dressed salad and colorful presentation in the tomato shell make this a great summer side dish. It goes well with all my barbecued entrees.

—**MARY RELYEA** CANASTOTA, NY

PREP: 20 MIN. + CHILLING
MAKES: 4 SERVINGS

- 4 **medium tomatoes**
- 1 **large ear sweet corn**
- ¼ **cup chopped red onion**

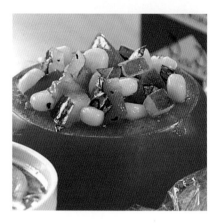

- ¼ **cup loosely packed fresh basil leaves, chopped**
- 2 **teaspoons olive oil**
- 1½ **teaspoons balsamic or white wine vinegar**
- ¼ **teaspoon garlic salt**
- ¼ **teaspoon pepper**

1. Cut a thin slice off the top of each tomato. Scoop out pulp, leaving ½-in. shells. Seed and chop enough of the pulp to equal 1 cup (discard any remaining pulp or save for another use). Place chopped tomato and tomato cups, inverted, on paper towels to drain.

2. In a large saucepan, cook corn in boiling water for 3-5 minutes or until tender. Drain and immediately place corn in ice water; drain. Cut corn off the cob.

3. In a small bowl, combine the corn, chopped tomato, onion and basil. In another bowl, whisk the oil, vinegar, garlic salt and pepper. Pour over corn mixture and toss to coat. Cover and refrigerate 30 minutes. Spoon into tomato cups.
PER SERVING *1 stuffed tomato equals 84 cal., 3 g fat (trace sat. fat), 0 chol., 127 mg sodium, 14 g carb., 3 g fiber, 3 g pro.* **Diabetic Exchanges:** *1 vegetable, ½ starch, ½ fat.*

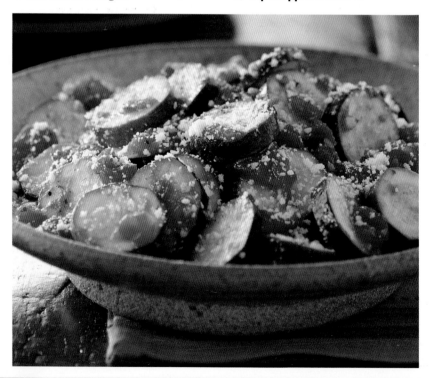

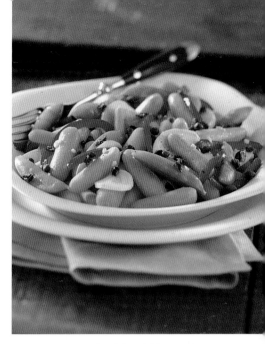

88 CALORIES
Special Cauliflower

I found this recipe in a local paper and it has become my favorite topping for cauliflower. I like it because the glaze adds color and also enhances the flavor with a little zip.

—RITA REINKE WAUWATOSA, WI

START TO FINISH: 20 MIN.
MAKES: 3 SERVINGS

- 2 cups fresh cauliflowerets
- 1 tablespoon plain yogurt
- 1 tablespoon mayonnaise
- ½ teaspoon Dijon mustard
- ⅛ teaspoon dill weed
- ⅛ teaspoon salt
- ⅛ teaspoon garlic powder
- ¼ cup shredded cheddar cheese

1. Place cauliflower in a steamer basket; place in a small saucepan over 1 in. of water. Bring to a boil; cover and steam for 6-8 minutes or until crisp-tender.

2. Meanwhile, in a small bowl, combine the yogurt, mayonnaise, mustard, dill, salt and garlic powder.

3. Transfer cauliflower to an ungreased 3-cup baking dish; top with yogurt mixture and cheese. Bake, uncovered, at 350° for 5 minutes or until heated through and cheese is melted.

PER SERVING ⅔ cup equals 88 cal., 7 g fat (3 g sat. fat), 12 mg chol., 222 mg sodium, 4 g carb., 2 g fiber, 4 g pro. **Diabetic Exchanges:** 1½ fat, 1 vegetable.

71 CALORIES
Sauteed Baby Carrot Medley

Convenient baby-cut carrots and crunchy sugar snap peas star in this quick-to-fix side dish. It's so nice on a holiday table.

—TASTE OF HOME TEST KITCHEN

START TO FINISH: 25 MIN.
MAKES: 8 SERVINGS

- 3 cups fresh baby carrots
- 2 tablespoons olive oil
- 1 small yellow summer squash, thinly sliced
- 1 small sweet red pepper, julienned
- 1½ cups fresh sugar snap peas
- 2 garlic cloves, minced
- ½ cup water
- 2 tablespoons sun-dried tomatoes (not packed in oil), finely chopped
- 1 tablespoon capers, drained
- ½ teaspoon salt
- ¼ teaspoon pepper

1. In a large skillet, saute carrots in oil for 1 minute. Add squash; saute 1 minute longer. Stir in the red pepper, peas and garlic; saute 1 minute more.

2. Add water. Reduce heat to medium. Cook and stir until liquid is evaporated and vegetables are crisp-tender. Stir in the tomatoes, capers, salt and pepper.

PER SERVING ⅔ cup equals 71 cal., 4 g fat (trace sat. fat), 0 chol., 240 mg sodium, 9 g carb., 2 g fiber, 2 g pro.

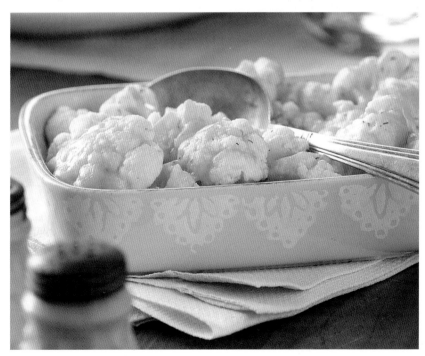

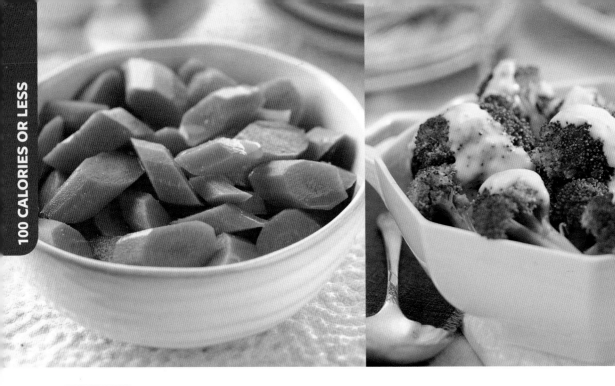

83 CALORIES
Spiced Glazed Carrots

Carrots sweetened with honey, apple juice and cinnamon are hard to pass up.

—NANCY ZIMMERMAN
CAPE MAY COURT HOUSE, NJ

START TO FINISH: 30 MIN.
MAKES: 4 SERVINGS

- 1 **pound fresh carrots, cut into ½-in. slices**
- ¾ **cup unsweetened apple juice**
- 1 **cinnamon stick (3 inches)**
- ¾ **teaspoon ground cumin**
- ½ **teaspoon ground ginger**
- ¼ **teaspoon ground coriander**
  Dash cayenne pepper
- 2 **teaspoons lemon juice**
- 2 **teaspoons honey**

1. In a large nonstick skillet coated with cooking spray, combine the first seven ingredients. Bring to a boil. Reduce heat; cover and simmer for 5-8 minutes or until carrots are crisp-tender.

2. Discard cinnamon stick. Add lemon juice and honey to carrots. Bring to a boil; cook, uncovered, for 2 minutes or until sauce is thickened.

PER SERVING *⅔ cup equals 83 cal., trace fat (trace sat. fat), 0 chol., 81 mg sodium, 20 g carb., 3 g fiber, 1 g pro.* **Diabetic Exchange:** *1 starch.*

76 CALORIES
Broccoli with Lemon Sauce

A tasty change from cheese, this lemon sauce is great with cauliflower, too!

—BARBARA FRASIER FYFFE, AL

START TO FINISH: 20 MIN.
MAKES: 10 SERVINGS (1¼ CUPS SAUCE)

- 3 **pounds fresh broccoli spears**
- 1 **cup chicken broth**
- 1 **tablespoon butter**
- 4½ **teaspoons cornstarch**
- ¼ **cup cold water**
- 2 **egg yolks, lightly beaten**
- 3 **tablespoons lemon juice**
- 2 **tablespoons grated lemon peel**

1. Place broccoli in a large saucepan; add 1 in. of water. Bring to a boil. Reduce heat; cover and cook for 5-8 minutes or until crisp-tender.

2. Meanwhile, in a small heavy saucepan, heat broth and butter until butter is melted. Combine the cornstarch and water until smooth; stir into broth mixture. Bring to a boil; cook and stir for 2 minutes or until thickened and bubbly.

3. Remove from the heat. Stir a small amount of hot mixture into egg yolks; return all to the pan, stirring constantly. Bring to a gentle boil; cook and stir 2 minutes longer. Remove from the heat. Gently stir in the lemon juice and peel. Drain broccoli; serve immediately with lemon sauce.

PER SERVING *¾ cup broccoli with 2 tablespoons sauce equals 76 cal., 3 g fat (1 g sat. fat), 44 mg chol., 164 mg sodium, 12 g carb., 5 g fiber, 4 g pro.* **Diabetic Exchanges:** *2 vegetable, ½ fat.*

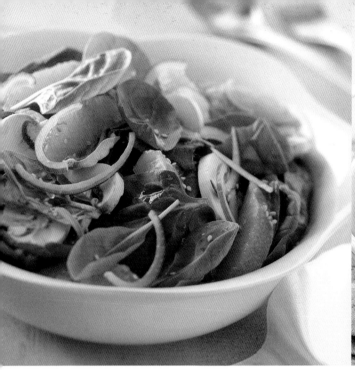
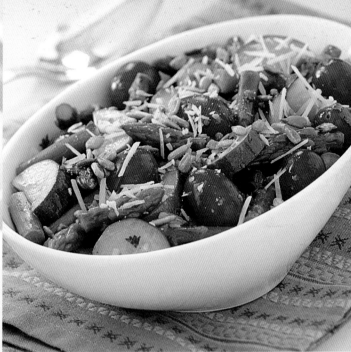

52 CALORIES

Spinach & Citrus Salad

Here's a simple way to get a healthy dose of vitamins A and C. Citrus lovers will appreciate the snappy dressing and bits of sweet orange in this crisp salad.

—**EDNA LEE** GREELEY, CO

START TO FINISH: 15 MIN.
MAKES: 9 SERVINGS

- 2 **tablespoons olive oil**
- 1 **tablespoon lime juice**
- 1 **teaspoon sesame seeds, toasted**
- ½ **teaspoon sugar**
- ½ **teaspoon grated lime peel**
- ¼ **teaspoon ground ginger**
- 4 **cups coarsely chopped fresh spinach**
- 2 **medium navel oranges, peeled and sectioned**
- 1 **cup sliced fresh mushrooms**
- ½ **small red onion, halved and thinly sliced**

1. In a small bowl, whisk the first six ingredients.

2. In a large salad bowl, combine the remaining ingredients. Just before serving, whisk dressing and pour over salad; toss to coat.

PER SERVING ¾ cup equals 52 cal., 3 g fat (trace sat. fat), 0 chol., 13 mg sodium, 6 g carb., 1 g fiber, 1 g pro. **Diabetic Exchanges:** 1 vegetable, ½ fat.

81 CALORIES ## Asparagus Tomato Salad

This crunchy, colorful salad was a hit with our church's cooking club.

—**DOROTHY BUHR** OGDEN, IL

START TO FINISH: 15 MIN.
MAKES: 6 SERVINGS

- 1 **pound fresh asparagus, cut into 1-inch lengths**
- 1 **small zucchini, halved and sliced**
- 1 **cup grape or cherry tomatoes**
- ¼ **cup sliced green onions**
- ¼ **cup minced fresh parsley**
- 3 **tablespoons olive oil**
- 2 **tablespoons red wine vinegar**
- 1 **garlic clove, minced**
- ¼ **teaspoon seasoned salt**
- ¼ **teaspoon Dijon mustard**
  Sunflower kernels and shredded Parmesan cheese, optional

1. Place the asparagus and zucchini in a steamer basket; place in a saucepan over 1 in. of water. Bring to a boil; cover and steam for 2 minutes. Rinse in cold water.

2. In a large bowl, combine the asparagus, zucchini, tomatoes, onions and parsley.

3. Whisk the oil, vinegar, garlic, seasoned salt and mustard; pour over asparagus mixture and toss to coat. Sprinkle with cheese and sunflower kernels if desired.

PER SERVING ¾ cup (calculated without optional ingredients) equals 81 cal., 7 g fat (1 g sat. fat), 0 chol., 78 mg sodium, 4 g carb., 1 g fiber, 2 g pro. **Diabetic Exchanges:** 1 vegetable, 1 fat.

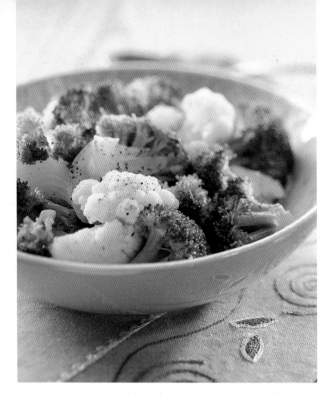

PER SERVING *1 cup equals 47 cal., 1 g fat (trace sat. fat), 0 chol., 262 mg sodium, 8 g carb., 3 g fiber, 2 g pro. Diabetic Exchange: 2 vegetable.*

96 CALORIES Lemon Garlic Mushrooms

I baste whole mushrooms with a lemony sauce to prepare this simple side dish. Using skewers or a grill basket makes it easy to turn the mushrooms.
—**DIANE HIXON** NICEVILLE, FL

START TO FINISH: 25 MIN. • **MAKES:** 4 SERVINGS

- ¼ cup lemon juice
- 3 tablespoons minced fresh parsley
- 2 tablespoons olive oil
- 3 garlic cloves, minced
  Pepper to taste
- 1 pound large fresh mushrooms

In a small bowl, combine the first five ingredients; set aside. Grill the mushrooms, covered, over medium-hot heat for 5 minutes. Brush generously with lemon mixture. Turn mushrooms; grill 5-8 minutes longer or until tender. Brush with remaining lemon mixture before serving.
PER SERVING *1 serving equals 96 cal., 7 mg sodium, 0 chol., 8 gm carb., 3 gm pro, 7 gm fat, 2 gm fiber. Diabetic Exchanges: 1½ fat, 1 vegetable.*

47 CALORIES Grilled Broccoli & Cauliflower

This is an ideal accompaniment for just about any meat. To change things up, add one chopped large baking potato, or mix in asparagus for a veggie extravaganza!
—**TARA DELGADO** WAUSEON, OH

START TO FINISH: 20 MIN. • **MAKES:** 2 SERVINGS

- 1 cup fresh broccoli florets
- 1 cup fresh cauliflowerets
- 1 small onion, cut into wedges
  Refrigerated butter-flavored spray
- ¼ teaspoon garlic salt
- ⅛ teaspoon paprika
- ⅛ teaspoon pepper

1. In a large bowl, combine the broccoli, cauliflower and onion; spritz with butter-flavored spray. Sprinkle with the garlic salt, paprika and pepper; toss to coat. Place vegetables on a double thickness of heavy-duty foil (about 18 in. x 12 in.); fold foil around vegetables and seal tightly.
2. Grill, covered, over medium heat for 10-15 minutes or until vegetables are tender. Open foil carefully to allow steam to escape.

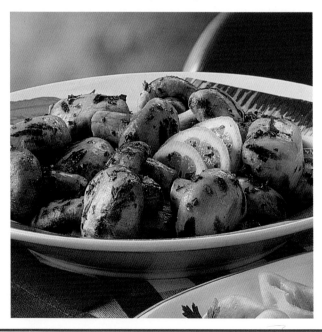

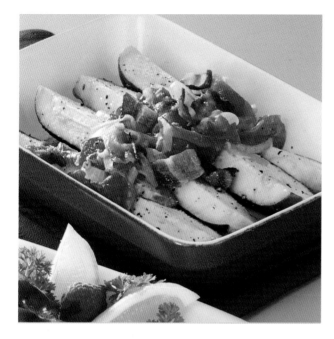

PER SERVING *1 cup equals 85 cal., 5 g fat (3 g sat. fat), 13 mg chol., 202 mg sodium, 6 g carb., 2 g fiber, 6 g pro.* **Diabetic Exchanges:** *1 medium-fat meat, 1 vegetable.*

87 CALORIES Holiday Peas

My mom used to dress up peas with buttered cracker crumbs when I was little, and it remains one of my favorite dishes. Just about any type of savory cracker can be used, including herb-flavored varieties.

—**SUE GRONHOLZ** BEAVER DAM, WI

START TO FINISH: 20 MIN. • **MAKES:** 12 SERVINGS

- 2 **packages (16 ounces each) frozen peas**
- 2 **teaspoons salt**
- 1 **cup finely crushed wheat crackers**
- 2 **tablespoons grated Parmesan cheese**
- 2 **tablespoons butter, melted**

1. Place peas in a large saucepan; add salt. Cover with water. Bring to a boil. Reduce heat; cover and simmer for 5-6 minutes or until tender.

2. Meanwhile, toss the cracker crumbs, cheese and butter. Drain peas and place in a serving bowl; top with crumb mixture.

PER SERVING *¾ cup equals 87 cal., 3 g fat (1 g sat. fat), 6 mg chol., 523 mg sodium, 12 g carb., 4 g fiber, 4 g pro.* **Diabetic Exchanges:** *1 starch, ½ fat.*

85 CALORIES Colorful Zucchini Spears

A bit of bacon lends hearty flavor to zucchini, while low-fat cheese helps keep the calories in check.

—**JAN CALDWELL** SHINGLE SPRINGS, CA

START TO FINISH: 30 MIN. • **MAKES:** 2 SERVINGS

- 1 **bacon strip, cut into 1-inch pieces**
- 1 **medium zucchini**
- ⅛ **teaspoon salt**
- ⅛ **teaspoon dried oregano**
- ⅛ **teaspoon garlic powder**
- ⅛ **teaspoon pepper**
- 1 **plum tomato, halved and sliced**
- ¼ **cup sliced onion**
- ¼ **cup shredded reduced-fat sharp cheddar cheese**

1. In a small nonstick skillet, cook bacon over medium heat until cooked but not crisp. Using a slotted spoon, remove bacon to paper towels to drain. Cut zucchini in half widthwise; cut halves lengthwise into quarters. Place in an ungreased shallow 1-qt. baking dish.

2. Combine the salt, oregano, garlic powder and pepper; sprinkle half over the zucchini. Top with tomato, onion, remaining seasonings and bacon. Bake, uncovered, at 350° for 15 minutes. Sprinkle with cheese; bake 5-10 minutes longer or until the zucchini is tender.

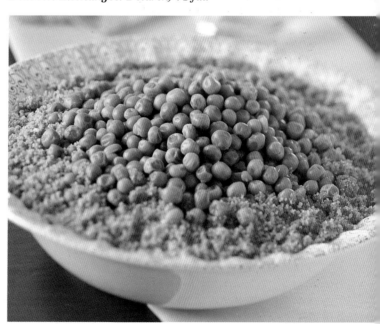

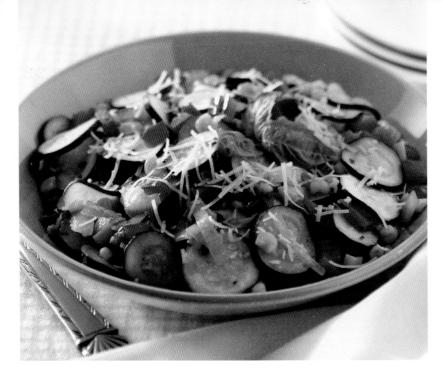

93 CALORIES Fast Italian Vegetable Skillet

This blend of sauteed vegetables is as pretty as it is tasty. The recipe was given to me by a dear friend, and it's become a family favorite. It's a quick summer side from our garden.
—**SUE SPENCER** COARSEGOLD, CA

START TO FINISH: 20 MIN.
MAKES: 6 SERVINGS

- 1 medium onion, halved and sliced
- 1 medium sweet red pepper, chopped
- 1 tablespoon olive oil
- 3 medium zucchini, thinly sliced
- 1 garlic clove, minced
- 1½ cups frozen corn, thawed
- 1 large tomato, chopped
- 2 teaspoons minced fresh basil
- ½ teaspoon salt
- ½ teaspoon Italian seasoning
- ¼ cup shredded Parmesan cheese

1. In a large nonstick skillet, saute onion and red pepper in oil for 2 minutes. Add zucchini; saute 4-5 minutes or until vegetables are crisp-tender. Add garlic; cook for 1 minute longer.

2. Stir in the corn, tomato, basil, salt and Italian seasoning; cook and stir until heated through. Sprinkle with cheese. Serve immediately.

PER SERVING *1 cup equals 93 cal., 4 g fat (1 g sat. fat), 3 mg chol., 266 mg sodium, 14 g carb., 3 g fiber, 4 g pro.* **Diabetic Exchanges:** *2 vegetable, ½ starch, ½ fat.*

74 CALORIES Melon 'n' Grape Medley

Our fruit salad has a zesty honey-orange dressing with a surprising twist—a hint of jalapeno!
—**TASTE OF HOME TEST KITCHEN**

PREP: 15 MIN. + CHILLING
MAKES: 6 SERVINGS

- 1½ cups cantaloupe balls
- 1½ cups watermelon balls
- 1½ cups green grapes

DRESSING

- ¼ cup orange juice
- 1 tablespoon honey
- 1 tablespoon lime juice
- 2 teaspoons chopped seeded jalapeno pepper
- ½ teaspoon grated lime peel

1. In a resealable plastic bag, combine the cantaloupe, watermelon and grapes.

2. Whisk the orange juice, honey and lime juice. Stir in the jalapeno and lime peel.

3. Pour over fruit. Seal the bag, removing as much air as possible, and turn to coat; refrigerate for at least 1 hour. Serve with a slotted spoon.

NOTE *Wear disposable gloves when cutting hot peppers; the oils can burn skin. Avoid touching your face.*

PER SERVING *¾ cup equals 74 cal., 1 g fat (trace sat. fat), 0 chol., 6 mg sodium, 18 g carb., 1 g fiber, 1 g pro.*

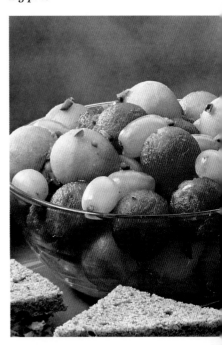

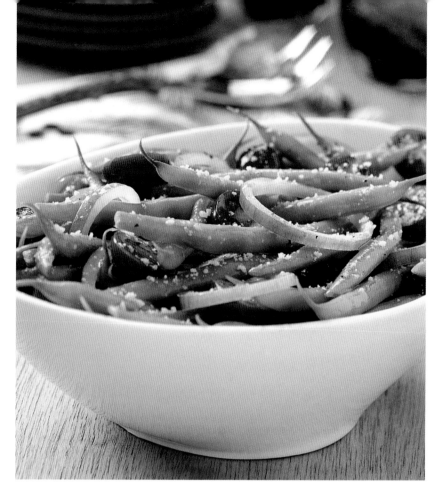

78 CALORIES Bravo Broccoli

Here's a fast, delicious way to dress up crisp-tender broccoli. Just toss it with a simple sweet-and-sour mixture that gets a bit of kick from red pepper flakes.

—TASTE OF HOME TEST KITCHEN

START TO FINISH: 20 MIN.
MAKES: 4 SERVINGS

- 1 **bunch broccoli, cut into florets**
- 1 **tablespoon butter, melted**
- 1 **tablespoon rice vinegar**
- 1½ **teaspoons brown sugar**
- ¼ **teaspoon salt**
- ¼ **teaspoon crushed red pepper flakes**
- ⅛ **teaspoon garlic powder**

1. Place broccoli in a steamer basket; place in a large saucepan over 1 in. of water. Bring to a boil; cover and steam for 3-4 minutes or until tender. Transfer to a large bowl.
2. Combine the remaining ingredients; drizzle over broccoli and gently toss to coat.
PER SERVING *¾ cup equals 78 cal., 3 g fat (2 g sat. fat), 8 mg chol., 210 mg sodium, 10 g carb., 5 g fiber, 5 g pro.* **Diabetic Exchanges:** *2 vegetable, ½ fat.*

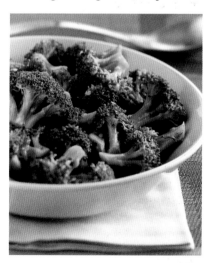

54 CALORIES
Dijon Green Beans

I love this recipe because it combines the freshness of crisp garden green beans and sweet tomatoes with a warm and tangy dressing. It's a wonderful, quick and nutritious side dish.

—JANNINE FISK MALDEN, MA

START TO FINISH: 20 MIN.
MAKES: 10 SERVINGS

- 1½ **pounds fresh green beans, trimmed**
- 2 **tablespoons red wine vinegar**
- 2 **tablespoons olive oil**
- 2 **teaspoons Dijon mustard**
- ½ **teaspoon salt**
- ¼ **teaspoon pepper**
- 1 **cup grape tomatoes, halved**
- ½ **small red onion, sliced**
- 2 **tablespoons grated Parmesan cheese**

1. Place beans in a large saucepan and cover with water. Bring to a boil. Cook, covered, for 10-15 minutes or until crisp-tender.
2. Meanwhile, whisk the vinegar, oil, mustard, salt and pepper in a small bowl. Drain beans; place in a large bowl. Add tomatoes and onion. Drizzle with dressing and toss to coat. Sprinkle with cheese.
PER SERVING *¾ cup equals 54 cal., 3 g fat (1 g sat. fat), 1 mg chol., 167 mg sodium, 6 g carb., 2 g fiber, 2 g pro.* **Diabetic Exchanges:** *1 vegetable, ½ fat.*

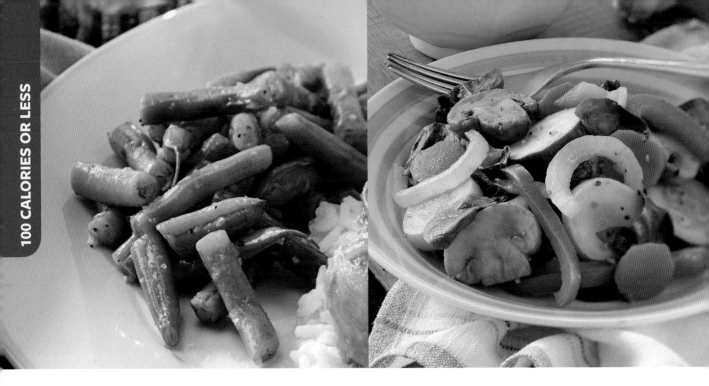

85 CALORIES Tangy Italian Green Beans

The sharpness of Parmesan cheese makes a nice accent for fresh green beans. This recipe has been a family tradition for many years.

—RUDY MARTINO LOMBARD, IL

START TO FINISH: 15 MIN.
MAKES: 2 SERVINGS

- ½ **pound fresh or frozen cut green beans**
- 2 **tablespoons water**
- 2¼ **teaspoons grated Parmesan cheese**
- 2¼ **teaspoons seasoned bread crumbs**
- ¼ **teaspoon garlic salt**
- ⅛ **teaspoon pepper**
- 1½ **teaspoons olive oil**

Place beans and water in a microwave-safe dish. Cover and microwave on high for 4-5 minutes or until crisp-tender. Meanwhile, in a small bowl, combine the cheese, bread crumbs, garlic salt and pepper. Drain beans; drizzle with olive oil. Sprinkle with cheese mixture and toss to coat.

NOTE *This recipe was tested in a 1,100-watt microwave.*
PER SERVING *¾ cup equals 85 cal., 4 g fat (1 g sat. fat), 1 mg chol., 309 mg sodium, 10 g carb., 4 g fiber, 3 g pro.* **Diabetic Exchanges:** *1 vegetable, ½ fat.*

51 CALORIES
Colorful Veggie Saute

A low-fat meal doesn't have to skimp on flavor with this tasty saute served on the side. The medley of garden-fresh ingredients is sparked up with garlic salt and hearty steak seasoning.

—PAMELA STEWART BELCHER, KY

START TO FINISH: 25 MIN.
MAKES: 5 SERVINGS

- 1 **small zucchini, sliced**
- 1 **yellow summer squash, sliced**
- 1 **small onion, halved and sliced**
- 1 **cup sliced fresh mushrooms**
- 1 **small green pepper, julienned**
- ½ **cup thinly sliced fresh carrots**
- 1 **tablespoon butter**
- 3 **cups coarsely chopped fresh spinach**
- ½ **teaspoon steak seasoning**
- ¼ **teaspoon garlic salt**

1. In a large skillet, saute the zucchini, yellow squash, onion, mushrooms, green pepper and carrots in butter until crisp-tender.
2. Add the spinach, steak seasoning and garlic salt; cook 3-4 minutes longer or just until the spinach is wilted.

NOTE *This recipe was tested with McCormick's Montreal Steak Seasoning. Look for it in the spice aisle at your grocery store.*
PER SERVING *¾ cup equals 51 cal., 3 g fat (2 g sat. fat), 6 mg chol., 202 mg sodium, 7 g carb., 2 g fiber, 2 g pro.* **Diabetic Exchanges:** *1 vegetable, ½ fat.*

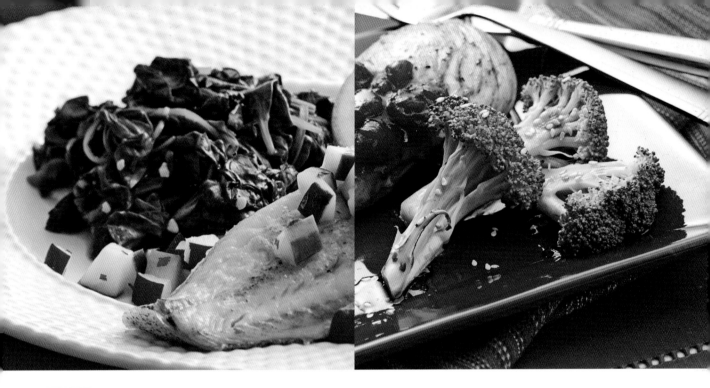

Wilted Garlic Spinach

You don't have to be a spinach fan to enjoy eating these healthful greens. Soy sauce gives my energy-packed dish an Asian twist. Also, try serving it over rice.

—DOTTY EGGE PELICAN RAPIDS, MN

START TO FINISH: 20 MIN.
MAKES: 4 SERVINGS

- 1 teaspoon cornstarch
- 1 teaspoon sugar
- 2 tablespoons chicken broth
- 1 tablespoon reduced-sodium soy sauce
- ½ teaspoon sesame oil
- 6 garlic cloves, minced
- 1 tablespoon canola oil
- ¾ pound fresh spinach, trimmed

1. In a small bowl, combine the cornstarch, sugar, broth, soy sauce and sesame oil until smooth; set aside. In a small skillet, saute garlic in oil for 1 minute. Stir broth mixture and add to skillet. Cook and stir over medium heat until slightly thickened.

2. Add spinach; cook and stir for 2 minutes or just until spinach is wilted and coated with sauce. Serve with a slotted spoon.

PER SERVING *½ cup equals 66 cal., 4 g fat (1 g sat. fat), 0 chol., 248 mg sodium, 6 g carb., 2 g fiber, 3 g pro.* **Diabetic Exchanges:** *1 vegetable, 1 fat.*

Sesame Broccoli

This delicious broccoli is often requested at our house. It's quick, easy and makes a colorful partner for any main dish.

—JANICE CAWMAN YAKIMA, WA

START TO FINISH: 25 MIN.
MAKES: 6 SERVINGS

- 1 pound fresh broccoli, cut into spears
- 1 tablespoon reduced-sodium soy sauce
- 2 teaspoons olive oil
- 2 teaspoons balsamic vinegar
- 1½ teaspoons honey
- 2 teaspoons sesame seeds, toasted

1. Place broccoli in a steamer basket; place in a saucepan over 1 in. of water. Bring to a boil; cover and steam for 10-15 minutes or until crisp-tender.

2. Meanwhile, in a small saucepan, combine the soy sauce, oil, vinegar and honey; cook and stir over medium-low heat until heated through.

3. Transfer broccoli to a serving bowl; drizzle with soy sauce mixture. Sprinkle with sesame seeds.

PER SERVING *¾ cup equals 48 cal., 2 g fat (trace sat. fat), 0 chol., 127 mg sodium, 6 g carb., 2 g fiber, 3 g pro.* **Diabetic Exchanges:** *1 vegetable, ½ fat.*

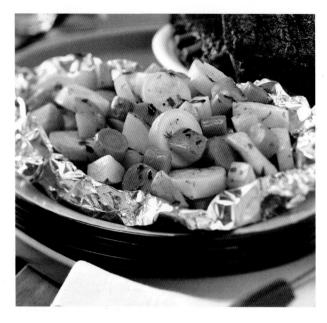

91 CALORIES Dilly Vegetable Medley

I love to eat what I grow, and I've tried many combinations of the fresh veggies from my garden. This one is really special! I never have leftovers when I serve it.

—REBECCA BARJONAH CORALVILLE, IA

PREP: 25 MIN. • **GRILL:** 20 MIN. • **MAKES:** 13 SERVINGS

- ¼ cup olive oil
- 2 tablespoons minced fresh basil
- 2 teaspoons dill weed
- ½ teaspoon salt
- ½ teaspoon pepper
- 7 small yellow summer squash, cut into ½-inch slices
- 1 pound Yukon Gold potatoes, cut into ½-inch cubes
- 5 small carrots, cut into ½-inch slices

1. In a large bowl, combine the first five ingredients. Add vegetables and toss to coat.

2. Place half of the vegetables on a double thickness of heavy-duty foil (about 18 in. square). Fold foil around the veggies and seal tightly. Repeat with the remaining vegetables.

3. Grill, covered, over medium heat for 20-25 minutes or until potatoes are tender, turning once. Open foil carefully to allow steam to escape.

PER SERVING *¾ cup equals 91 cal., 4 g fat (1 g sat. fat), 0 chol., 109 mg sodium, 12 g carb., 2 g fiber, 2 g pro. Diabetic Exchanges: 1 vegetable, 1 fat, ½ starch.*

85 CALORIES Grape Tomato Mozzarella Salad

After tasting something similar on a cruise, I created my own fuss-free salad. It makes such a speedy and summery light bite!

—LINDA HAAS TENMILE, OR

START TO FINISH: 15 MIN. • **MAKES:** 6 SERVINGS

- ½ large sweet onion, thinly sliced
- 1 medium cucumber, sliced
- 2 cups grape tomatoes
- ½ cup loosely packed fresh basil leaves, sliced
- 4 ounces fresh mozzarella cheese, sliced
- ⅓ cup fat-free Italian salad dressing

Arrange the onion, cucumber, tomatoes, basil and mozzarella on six salad plates. Drizzle with salad dressing. Serve immediately..

PER SERVING *1 serving equals 85 cal., 4 g fat (3 g sat. fat), 15 mg chol., 224 mg sodium, 7 g carb., 1 g fiber, 5 g pro. Diabetic Exchanges: 1 lean meat, 1 vegetable.*

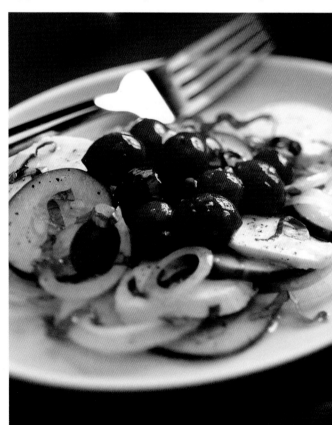

> "This program is great because the recipes are so family-friendly. My husband has loved all of those that I've made. It's not hard to make healthier choices with all the good things we can eat."

—ANDREA JOHNSON

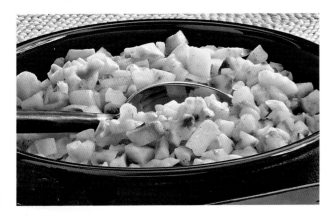

89 CALORIES Grilled Hash Browns

Since my husband and I love to grill meats, we're always looking for easy side dishes to cook on the grill, too. So I came up with a simple recipe for hash browns.

—KELLY CHASTAIN BEDFORD, IN

START TO FINISH: 20 MIN. • **MAKES:** 4 SERVINGS

- 3½ cups frozen cubed hash brown potatoes, thawed
- 1 small onion, chopped
- 1 tablespoon beef bouillon granules
   Dash seasoned salt
   Dash pepper
- 1 tablespoon butter, melted

1. Place potatoes on a piece of heavy-duty foil (about 20 in. x 18 in.) coated with cooking spray. Sprinkle with onion, bouillon, seasoned salt and pepper; drizzle with butter.
2. Fold foil around potatoes and seal tightly. Grill, covered, over indirect medium heat for 10-15 minutes or until potatoes are tender, turning once.
PER SERVING *¾ cup equals 89 cal., 3 g fat (2 g sat. fat), 8 mg chol., 652 mg sodium, 14 g carb., 1 g fiber, 2 g pro.*

45 CALORIES Balsamic Asparagus

Pretty spears of crisp-tender asparagus are drizzled with a balsamic vinegar mixture for a sensational side dish that's ready in no time.

—TASTE OF HOME TEST KITCHEN

START TO FINISH: 15 MIN. • **MAKES:** 4 SERVINGS

- 1 cup water
- 1 pound fresh asparagus, trimmed
- 2 tablespoons balsamic vinegar
- 1 tablespoon butter, melted
- 1 teaspoon minced garlic
- ¼ teaspoon salt
- ¼ teaspoon pepper

In a large skillet, bring the water to a boil. Add asparagus; cover and cook for 2-4 minutes or until crisp-tender. In a small bowl, combine the vinegar, butter, garlic, salt and pepper. Drain asparagus; drizzle with balsamic mixture.
PER SERVING *1 serving equals 45 cal., 3 g fat (2 g sat. fat), 8 mg chol., 185 mg sodium, 4 g carb., 1 g fiber, 2 g pro.* **Diabetic Exchanges::** *1 vegetable, ½ fat.*

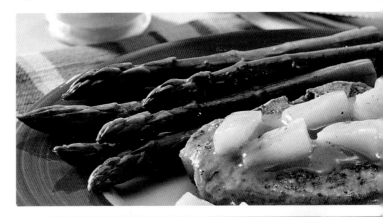

80 CALORIES

Greek-Style Squash

What a handy way to use up summer squash! You can almost taste the sunshine in this quick grilled dish, and the foil packet means easy cleanup.

—**BETTY WASHBURN** RENO, NV

PREP: 15 MIN. • **GRILL:** 30 MIN.
MAKES: 4 SERVINGS

- 2 **small yellow summer squash, thinly sliced**
- 2 **small zucchini, thinly sliced**
- 1 **medium tomato, seeded and chopped**
- ¼ **cup pitted ripe olives**
- 2 **tablespoons chopped green onion**
- 2 **teaspoons olive oil**
- 1 **teaspoon lemon juice**
- ¾ **teaspoon garlic salt**
- ¼ **teaspoon dried oregano**
- ⅛ **teaspoon pepper**
- 2 **tablespoons grated Parmesan cheese**

1. Place squash, zucchini, tomato, olives and onion on a double thickness of heavy-duty foil (about 17 in. x 18 in.). Combine oil, lemon juice, garlic salt, oregano and pepper; add to vegetables. Fold foil around mixture and seal tightly.
2. Grill, covered, over medium heat for 30-35 minutes or until vegetables are tender. Open foil carefully to allow steam to escape. Transfer vegetables to a serving bowl. Sprinkle with cheese.
PER SERVING *¾ cup equals 80 cal., 5 g fat (1 g sat. fat), 2 mg chol., 479 mg sodium, 8 g carb., 3 g fiber, 4 g pro. Diabetic Exchanges: 2 vegetable, ½ fat.*

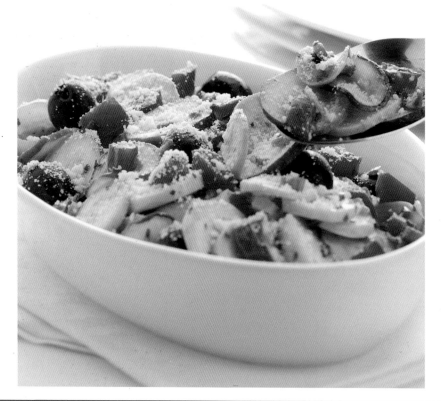

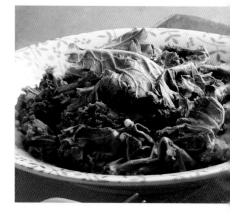

61 CALORIES # Steamed Kale

You'll find a wonderful accompaniment to almost any entree with good-for-you steamed kale, which is packed with vitamins. I use garlic, red pepper and balsamic vinegar to keep my family coming back for more!

—**MARY BILYEU** ANN ARBOR, MI

PREP: 15 MIN. • **COOK:** 25 MIN.
MAKES: 4 SERVINGS

- 1 **bunch kale**
- 1 **tablespoon olive oil**
- 3 **garlic cloves, minced**
- ⅔ **cup water**
- ¼ **teaspoon salt**
- ⅛ **teaspoon crushed red pepper flakes**
- 1 **tablespoon balsamic vinegar**

1. Trim kale, discarding the thick ribs and stems. Chop leaves. In a Dutch oven, saute kale leaves in oil until wilted. Add garlic; cook for 1 minute longer.
2. Stir in the water, salt and pepper flakes. Bring to a boil. Reduce heat; cover and simmer for 20-25 minutes or until kale is tender. Remove from the heat; stir in balsamic vinegar.
PER SERVING *¾ cup equals 61 cal., 4 g fat (1 g sat. fat), 0 chol., 171 mg sodium, 6 g carb., 1 g fiber, 2 g pro.*

55 CALORIES Italian Broccoli with Peppers

For a satisfying meal, we like to combine this zesty vegetable blend with pasta and grilled chicken or turkey breasts.

—MAUREEN MCCLANAHAN

ST. LOUIS, MO

START TO FINISH: 20 MIN.
MAKES: 6 SERVINGS

- 6 **cups water**
- 4 **cups fresh broccoli florets**
- 1 **medium sweet red pepper, julienned**
- 1 **medium sweet yellow pepper, julienned**
- 1 **tablespoon olive oil**
- 1 **garlic clove, minced**
- 1 **teaspoon dried oregano**
- ½ **teaspoon salt**
- ¼ **teaspoon pepper**
- 1 **medium ripe tomato, cut into wedges and seeded**
- 1 **tablespoon grated Parmesan cheese**

1. In a large saucepan, bring water to a boil. Add broccoli; cover and boil for 3 minutes. Drain and immediately place broccoli in ice water. Drain and pat dry.

2. In a large nonstick skillet, saute peppers in oil for 3 minutes or until crisp-tender. Add the broccoli, garlic, oregano, salt and pepper; cook 2 minutes longer. Add the tomato and heat through. Sprinkle with cheese.

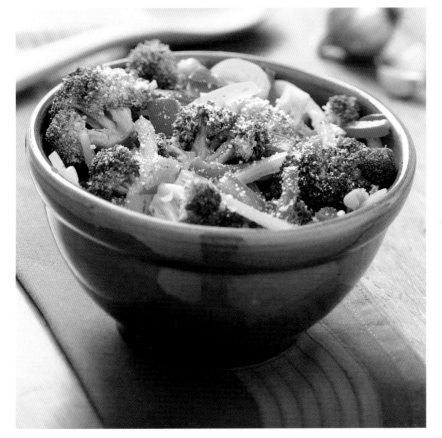

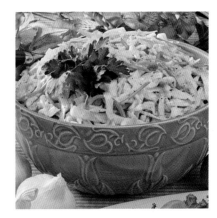

PER SERVING ¾ cup equals 55 cal., 3 g fat (1 g sat. fat), 1 mg chol., 228 mg sodium, 7 g carb., 2 g fiber, 2 g pro. *Diabetic Exchanges: 1 vegetable, ½ fat.*

88 CALORIES Home-Style Coleslaw

This recipe is a staple at our house. It even gets requested by the kids.

—JOY COCHRAN ROY, WA

PREP: 20 MIN. + CHILLING
MAKES: 7 SERVINGS

- 8 **cups finely shredded cabbage**
- ½ **cup shredded carrot**

DRESSING

- ⅓ **cup reduced-fat mayonnaise**
- ⅓ **cup fat-free sour cream**
- 1 **tablespoon sugar**
- 2 **teaspoons cider vinegar**
- ½ **teaspoon salt**
- ¼ **teaspoon pepper**

In a large bowl, combine cabbage and carrot. In a small bowl, combine the dressing ingredients. Pour over cabbage mixture; toss to coat. Chill 6-8 hours or overnight.

PER SERVING ⅔ cup equals 88 cal., 4 g fat (1 g sat. fat), 5 mg chol., 292 mg sodium, 12 g carb., 3 g fiber, 2 g pro. *Diabetic Exchanges: 1 vegetable, 1 fat, ½ starch.*

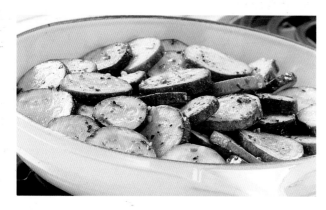

90 CALORIES Garlic Oregano Zucchini

I've found that this flavorful side dish complements almost any main course, from chicken to fish. If you like, use half yellow summer squash for a colorful variation.

—TERESA KRAUS CORTEZ, CO

START TO FINISH: 15 MIN. • **MAKES:** 4 SERVINGS

- 1 teaspoon minced garlic
- 2 tablespoons canola oil
- 4 medium zucchini, sliced
- 1 teaspoon dried oregano
- ½ teaspoon salt
- ⅛ teaspoon pepper

In a large skillet, cook and stir the garlic in oil over medium heat for 1 minute. Add the zucchini, oregano, salt and pepper. Cook and stir for 4-6 minutes or until zucchini is crisp-tender.

PER SERVING *1 cup equals 90 cal., 7 g fat (1 g sat. fat), 0 chol., 301 mg sodium, 6 g carb., 3 g fiber, 2 g pro. Diabetic Exchanges: 1½ fat, 1 vegetable.*

82 CALORIES Parmesan Roasted Carrots

Here's a baked side that turned my children on to eating carrots. This downsized version of the recipe is just right for two.

—PAM ION GAITHERSBURG, MD

START TO FINISH: 20 MIN. • **MAKES:** 2 SERVINGS

- 4 large carrots, cut diagonally into ¼-inch slices
- 2 tablespoons unsweetened applesauce
- 1 tablespoon finely chopped onion
- ¼ teaspoon salt
  Dash paprika
  Pepper to taste
- 1 tablespoon grated Parmesan cheese

1. In a small bowl, combine the first six ingredients. Transfer to a baking sheet coated with cooking spray.
2. Bake at 425° for 10-15 minutes or until golden brown. Sprinkle with Parmesan cheese. Serve immediately.

PER SERVING *½ cup equals 82 cal., 1 g fat (1 g sat. fat), 2 mg chol., 392 mg sodium, 17 g carb., 5 g fiber, 3 g pro. Diabetic Exchange: 1 starch.*

74 CALORIES Savory Asparagus

Fresh asparagus dresses up any weeknight meal with a touch of aromatic tarragon. Try substituting broccoli for the asparagus to create a new twist.

—TASTE OF HOME TEST KITCHEN

START TO FINISH: 15 MIN. • **MAKES:** 4 SERVINGS

- 1 pound fresh asparagus, trimmed
- 2 tablespoons olive oil
- ¼ to ½ teaspoon dried tarragon
- ¼ teaspoon onion powder
- ⅛ teaspoon pepper

1. In a large skillet, bring ½ in. of water to a boil. Add asparagus; cover and cook for 3-4 minutes or until crisp-tender.
2. Meanwhile, in a small bowl, combine the oil, tarragon, onion powder and pepper. Drain asparagus; drizzle with oil mixture and toss to coat.

PER SERVING *1 serving equals 74 cal., 7 g fat (1 g sat. fat), 0 chol., 6 mg sodium, 3 g carb., 1 g fiber, 1 g pro. Diabetic Exchanges: 1 vegetable, 1 fat.*

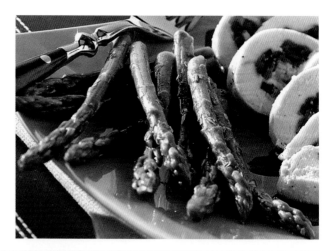

85 CALORIES Pineapple Cabbage Saute

This dish works best with thinly sliced cabbage, so it is best not to use a shredder. Try it with pork chops for a simple but satisfying dinner.
—**TASTE OF HOME TEST KITCHEN**

START TO FINISH: 20 MIN. • **MAKES:** 6 SERVINGS

- 1 **can (8 ounces) crushed pineapple**
- 6 **cups thinly sliced cabbage**
- 1 **tablespoon olive oil**
- 2 **tablespoons honey mustard salad dressing**
- ⅛ **teaspoon white pepper**

Drain pineapple, reserving 1 tablespoon juice; set aside. In a large skillet, saute cabbage in oil for 5-8 minutes or until crisp-tender. Add the salad dressing, pepper and reserved pineapple and juice. Cook for 1 minute or until heated through.
PER SERVING *¾ cup equals 85 cal., 4 g fat (1 g sat. fat), 0 chol., 48 mg sodium, 12 g carb., 2 g fiber, 1 g pro.*

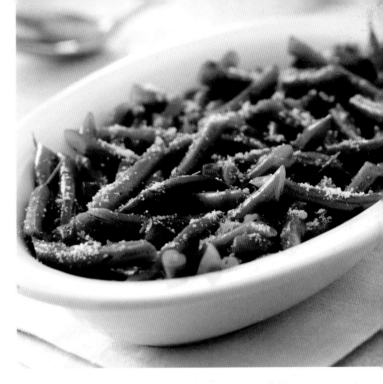

60 CALORIES Sesame Vegetable Medley

To save time, you can pick up many of the vegetables for my yummy medley at your store's salad bar. The side dish makes a great accompaniment to any menu.
—**TANYA LAMB** TALKING ROCK, GA

START TO FINISH: 10 MIN. • **MAKES:** 4 SERVINGS

- 1 **cup each baby carrots, broccoli florets and sliced fresh mushrooms**
- 1 **cup sliced zucchini (½ inch thick)**
- 1 **teaspoon minced garlic**
- 2 **tablespoons water**
- 1 **tablespoon butter**
- 2 **teaspoons sesame seeds, toasted**
- ⅛ **teaspoon salt**
- ⅛ **teaspoon pepper**

In a large microwave-safe bowl, combine the carrots, broccoli, mushrooms, zucchini, garlic and water. Cover and microwave on high for 3-5 minutes or until vegetables are tender, stirring twice; drain. Stir in the butter, sesame seeds, salt and pepper.
NOTE *This recipe was tested in a 1,100-watt microwave.*
PER SERVING *¾ cup equals 60 cal., 4 g fat (2 g sat. fat), 8 mg chol., 145 mg sodium, 6 g carb., 2 g fiber, 2 g pro.*
Diabetic Exchanges: 1 vegetable, ½ fat.

59 CALORIES Savory Green Beans

My mother always grew savory in her garden, and this was her favorite way to prepare green beans. Garden herbs give the crisp-tender vegetables a wonderfully fresh flavor.
—**CAROL ANN HAYDEN** EVERSON, WA

START TO FINISH: 30 MIN. • **MAKES:** 6 SERVINGS

- ¾ **cup chopped sweet red pepper**
- 1 **tablespoon canola oil**
- 1 **garlic clove, minced**
- 1½ **pounds fresh green beans, trimmed and cut into 2-inch pieces**
- ½ **cup water**
- 2 **tablespoons minced fresh savory or 2 teaspoons dried savory**
- 1 **tablespoon minced chives**
- ½ **teaspoon salt**

In a large skillet, saute red pepper in oil for 2-3 minutes or until tender. Add garlic; cook 1 minute longer. Stir in the green beans, water, savory, chives and salt. Bring to a boil. Reduce heat; cover and simmer for 8-10 minutes or until beans are crisp-tender.
PER SERVING *¾ cup equals 59 cal., 3 g fat (trace sat. fat), 0 chol., 203 mg sodium, 9 g carb., 4 g fiber, 2 g pro.*
Diabetic Exchanges: 2 vegetable, ½ fat.

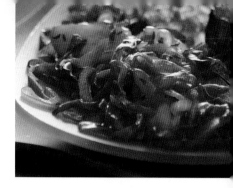

76 CALORIES
Savory Brussels Sprouts

Brussels sprouts are treated to a surprisingly guilt-free sauce in this delicious recipe.

—**PAULA MICHAUD** WATERBURY, CT

START TO FINISH: 30 MIN.
MAKES: 4 SERVINGS

- 1 **pound fresh brussels sprouts**

DIJON MUSTARD SAUCE
- ½ **cup fat-free plain yogurt**
- 1 **tablespoon reduced-fat mayonnaise**
- 1½ **teaspoons Dijon mustard**
- ¼ **teaspoon celery seed**

1. Cut an "X" in the core of each Brussels sprout. Place in a steamer basket; place in a large saucepan over 1 in. of water. Bring to a boil; cover and steam for 8-11 minutes or until tender.

2. Meanwhile, in a small saucepan, combine the yogurt, mayonnaise, mustard and celery seed. Cook and stir just until heated through. Serve with Brussels sprouts.

PER SERVING *¾ cup Brussels sprouts with 2 tablespoons sauce*

equals 76 cal., 2 g fat (trace sat. fat), 2 mg chol., 120 mg sodium, 13 g carb., 4 g fiber, 5 g pro. **Diabetic Exchange:** *2 vegetable.*

62 CALORIES
Veggie Tossed Salad

This simple salad delivers a dose of veggies and fresh flavors. Try it with a different low-fat dressing if you prefer.

—**EVELYN SLADE** FRUITA, CO

START TO FINISH: 10 MIN.
MAKES: 4 SERVINGS

- 1½ **cups torn romaine**
- 1½ **cups fresh baby spinach**
- ¾ **cup sliced fresh mushrooms**
- ¾ **cup grape tomatoes**
- ½ **cup sliced cucumber**
- ⅓ **cup sliced ripe olives**
- 1 **tablespoon grated Parmesan cheese**
- ¼ **cup reduced-fat Italian salad dressing**

In a large bowl, combine the first seven ingredients. Add salad dressing; toss to coat.

PER SERVING *1 cup equals 62 cal., 4 g fat (1 g sat. fat), 1 mg chol.,* 245 mg sodium, 5 g carb., 2 g fiber, 2 g pro. **Diabetic Exchanges:** *1 vegetable, 1 fat.*

62 CALORIES Red Cabbage with Apples

Looking for a tasty lower-in-sodium alternative to sauerkraut you can serve with pork? Try my colorful side dish with the slightly sweet flavor of apples.

—**MICHELLE DOUGHERTY**
LEWISTON, ID

START TO FINISH: 30 MIN.
MAKES: 4 SERVINGS

- 3 **cups shredded red cabbage**
- 1 **medium apple, peeled and thinly sliced**
- 1 **small onion, halved and sliced**
- 2 **tablespoons water**
- 2 **tablespoons thawed apple juice concentrate**
- ½ **teaspoon chicken bouillon granules**
- ¼ **teaspoon salt**
- ¼ **teaspoon caraway seeds**
- 1 **tablespoon red wine vinegar**

In a large saucepan, combine the first eight ingredients. Bring to a boil. Reduce heat; cover and simmer for 10-15 minutes or until cabbage is tender. Stir in vinegar.

PER SERVING *½ cup equals 62 cal., trace fat (trace sat. fat), trace chol., 261 mg sodium, 15 g carb., 2 g fiber, 1 g pro.* **Diabetic Exchanges:** *1 vegetable, ½ fruit.*

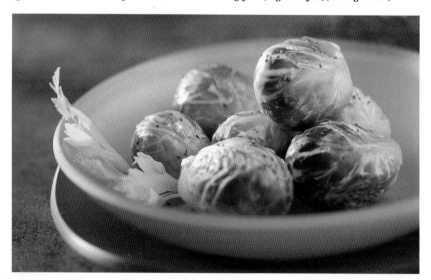

Vegetables in Dill Sauce

Creamy dill sauce makes for a decadent-tasting side dish that still lets you meet your calorie goals. Enjoy!

—EDIE DESPAIN LOGAN, UTAH

START TO FINISH: 30 MIN.
MAKES: 6 SERVINGS

- 4 **cups water**
- 1½ **cups pearl onions**
- 1 **medium carrot, sliced**
- 1 **tablespoon butter**
- ½ **pound sliced fresh mushrooms**
- 2 **small zucchini, sliced**
- 2 **teaspoons lemon juice**
- 1 **teaspoon dried marjoram**
- ¼ **teaspoon salt**

SAUCE

- 2 **tablespoons plus 2 teaspoons fat-free sour cream**
- 2 **tablespoons plus 2 teaspoons reduced-fat mayonnaise**
- 2 **tablespoons fat-free milk**
- 2¼ **teaspoons finely chopped onion**
- ½ **teaspoon snipped fresh dill Dash white pepper**

1. In a large saucepan, bring water to a boil. Add pearl onions; boil for 3 minutes. Drain and rinse in cold water; peel.

2. In a large nonstick skillet coated with cooking spray, saute onions and carrot in butter for 1 minute. Add mushrooms and zucchini; saute 6-8 minutes longer or until vegetables are tender. Stir in the lemon juice, marjoram and salt.

3. In a small microwave-safe bowl, combine the sauce ingredients. Cover and microwave on high until heated through, stirring once. Serve with vegetables.

PER SERVING *½ cup vegetables with 1 tablespoon sauce equals 80 cal., 4 g fat (2 g sat. fat), 9 mg chol., 186 mg sodium, 9 g carb., 2 g fiber, 3 g pro. Diabetic Exchanges: 1 vegetable, 1 fat.*

Mediterranean Summer Squash

I came up with this recipe when my garden was really producing and I had lots of fresh zucchini, yellow squash and tomatoes. I combined the three, added some herbs, garlic and feta and ended up with a flavorful dish that I love. My son eats it up like crazy, too!

—DAWN E. BRYANT THEDFORD, NE

START TO FINISH: 25 MIN.
MAKES: 4 SERVINGS

- ¼ **cup chopped onion**
- 1 **tablespoon olive oil**
- 1 **small yellow summer squash, thinly sliced**
- 1 **small zucchini, thinly sliced**
- 1 **garlic clove, minced**
- 1 **plum tomato, seeded and chopped**
- ½ **teaspoon dried oregano**
- ¼ **cup crumbled feta cheese**
- ¼ **teaspoon salt**
- ¼ **teaspoon pepper**

In a large skillet, saute onion in oil until tender. Add squash and zucchini; saute 6-8 minutes longer or until tender. Add garlic; cook 1 minute longer. Stir in the remaining ingredients; heat through.

PER SERVING *⅔ cup equals 69 cal., 5 g fat (1 g sat. fat), 4 mg chol., 220 mg sodium, 5 g carb., 2 g fiber, 3 g pro. Diabetic Exchanges: 1 vegetable, 1 fat.*

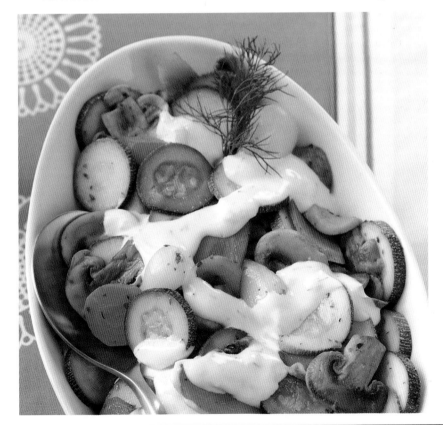

101-200 CALORIES

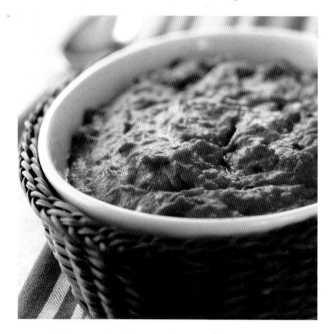

162 CALORIES Nutty Vegetable Rice

Here is a nutritious and delicious recipe that my family and guests love. We enjoy it alongside grilled meats.
—**KATHY RAIRIGH** MILFORD, IN

START TO FINISH: 30 MIN. • **MAKES:** 2 SERVINGS

- ⅔ cup water
- ½ teaspoon chicken bouillon granules
- ⅛ teaspoon salt
  Dash pepper
- ¼ cup uncooked long grain rice
- ¾ cup sliced fresh mushrooms
- 1 medium carrot, shredded
- ¼ cup minced fresh parsley
- 1 green onion, thinly sliced
- 2 tablespoons chopped pecans, toasted

1. In a small saucepan, bring the water, bouillon, salt and pepper to a boil. Stir in rice. Reduce heat; cover and simmer for 15 minutes.
2. Stir in the mushrooms, carrot, parsley and onion. Cover and cook for 5-10 minutes or until rice is tender and vegetables are crisp-tender. Sprinkle with pecans.
PER SERVING *¾ cup equals 162 cal., 6 g fat (1 g sat. fat), trace chol., 386 mg sodium, 25 g carb., 3 g fiber, 4 g pro. **Diabetic Exchanges:** 1 starch, 1 vegetable, 1 fat.*

189 CALORIES Sweet Potato Banana Bake

This yummy casserole makes what's good for you taste good, too! Pairing bananas with sweet potatoes unites two power foods in a change-of-pace side dish.
—**SUSAN MCCARTNEY** ONALASKA, WI

PREP: 10 MIN. • **BAKE:** 30 MIN. • **MAKES:** 6 SERVINGS

- 2 cups mashed sweet potatoes
- 1 cup mashed ripe bananas (2 to 3 medium)
- ½ cup reduced-fat sour cream
- 1 egg, lightly beaten
- ¾ teaspoon curry powder
- ½ teaspoon salt

1. In a large bowl, combine all ingredients until smooth. Transfer to a 1-qt. baking dish coated with cooking spray.
2. Cover and bake at 350° for 30-35 minutes or until a thermometer inserted near the center reads 160°.
PER SERVING *½ cup equals 189 cal., 3 g fat (2 g sat. fat), 42 mg chol., 235 mg sodium, 37 g carb., 3 g fiber, 5 g pro.*

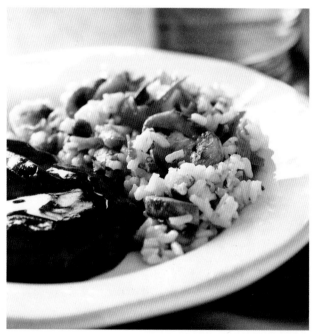

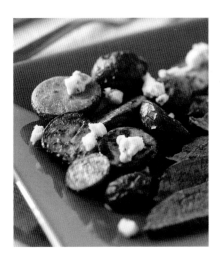

150 CALORIES

Roasted Potatoes with Thyme and Gorgonzola

Creamy Gorgonzola cheese turns my basic potato recipe into a spectacular side dish! Try it with all of your favorite entrees any time of year.
—**VIRGINIA STURM** SAN FRANCISCO, CA

START TO FINISH: 30 MIN.
MAKES: 2 SERVINGS

- ½ **pound small red potatoes, halved**
- 1½ **teaspoons olive oil**
- 1½ **teaspoons minced fresh thyme or**
  - ½ **teaspoon dried thyme**
- ⅛ **teaspoon salt**
- ⅛ **teaspoon pepper**
- 3 **tablespoons crumbled**
  - **Gorgonzola cheese**

1. Preheat oven to 425°. In a large bowl, combine first five ingredients. Place in a greased 15x10x1-in. baking pan.
2. Bake, uncovered, 20-25 minutes or until potatoes are tender, stirring once. Sprinkle with cheese.
PER SERVING ⅔ cup equals 150 cal., 7 g fat (3 g sat. fat), 9 mg chol., 297 mg sodium, 19 g carb., 2 g fiber, 4 g pro. **Diabetic Exchanges:** 1 starch, 1 fat.

Here are some typical **side dishes** and the calories they contain so you can determine how to stay within your goal of a **500-calorie dinner**.

- ½ cup cooked brown rice, **108 CALORIES**

- ½ cup cooked white rice, **103 CALORIES**

- 1 cup cooked egg noodles, **221 CALORIES**

- 1 cup cooked spaghetti, **200 CALORIES**

- 1 cup cooked whole wheat spaghetti, **176 CALORIES**

- ½ cup corn, **83 CALORIES**

- 1 small baked russet potato, **138 CALORIES**

- 1 small baked sweet potato, **128 CALORIES**

- 1 medium baked red potato, **154 CALORIES**

- ½ cup peas, **59 CALORIES**

- ½ cup cooked barley, **97 CALORIES**

- ½ cup cooked couscous, **90 CALORIES**

- ½ cup 1% cottage cheese, **81 CALORIES**

- ½ cup cooked lentils, **115 CALORIES**

- ½ cup cooked wild rice, **83 CALORIES**

- 1 piece of corn bread prepared from a dry mix, **188 CALORIES**

- 1 small breadstick (4¼" long), **21 CALORIES**

- 1 slice whole wheat bread, **69 CALORIES**

- 1 slice reduced-calorie white bread, **48 CALORIES**

- 1 flour tortilla (6" diameter), **90 CALORIES**

- 1 corn tortilla (6" diameter), **58 CALORIES**

- 1 whole wheat dinner roll, **76 CALORIES**

- 1 saltine cracker, **13 CALORIES**

For the calories of other side dish options, see the Free Foods List on page 41 and the Snacks Calorie List on pages 84 and 85. Also check the Nutrition Facts labels on packaged foods.

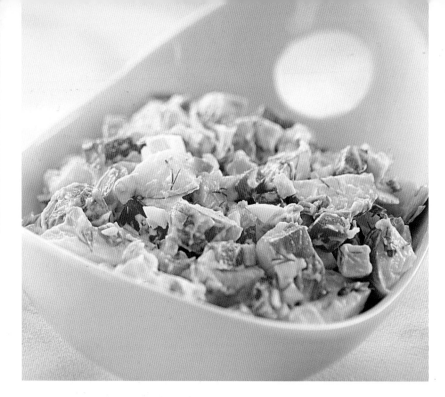

191 CALORIES

Creamed Peas and Carrots

This comforting dish features a simply seasoned cream sauce, which nicely complements the vegetables.
—**GAYLEEN GROTE** BATTLEVIEW, ND

START TO FINISH: 25 MIN.
MAKES: 4 SERVINGS

- 4 **medium carrots, sliced**
- 2 **cups frozen peas**
- 1 **tablespoon cornstarch**
- ¼ **teaspoon salt**
- ⅛ **teaspoon pepper**
- ½ **cup heavy whipping cream**

1. Place carrots in a large saucepan; add 1 in. of water. Bring to a boil. Reduce heat; cover and simmer for 5-8 minutes or until crisp-tender.
2. Add peas; return to a boil. Reduce heat; cover and simmer 5-10 minutes longer or until vegetables are tender. Drain, reserving ½ cup cooking liquid. Return vegetables and reserved liquid to the pan.
3. In a small bowl, combine the cornstarch, salt, pepper and cream until smooth. Stir into vegetables. Bring to a boil; cook and stir for 1-2 minutes or until thickened.
PER SERVING ⅔ *cup equals 191 cal., 11 g fat (7 g sat. fat), 41 mg chol., 282 mg sodium, 18 g carb., 5 g fiber, 5 g pro.*

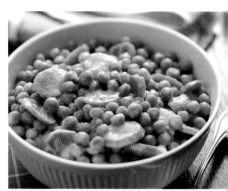

---

142 CALORIES

Herbed Potato Salad

Satisfying cheese and chopped egg, plus potatoes and peppers packed with vitamin C make this picnic favorite something to smile about!
—**JUDY GREBETZ** RACINE, WI

PREP: 40 MIN. + CHILLING
MAKES: 10 SERVINGS

- 3 **pounds small red potatoes, cubed**
- ½ **cup cubed reduced-fat cheddar cheese**
- ¼ **cup chopped dill pickle**
- ¼ **cup chopped red onion**
- ¼ **cup chopped green pepper**
- ¼ **cup chopped sweet red pepper**
- 1 **jalapeno pepper, seeded and minced**
- ¾ **cup fat-free mayonnaise**
- 1 **tablespoon minced fresh basil**
- 1 **tablespoon snipped fresh dill**
- 1 **tablespoon minced fresh tarragon**
- ½ **teaspoon salt**
- ½ **teaspoon pepper**
- 1 **hard-cooked egg, chopped**

1. Place potatoes in a large saucepan and cover with water. Bring to a boil. Reduce heat; cover and simmer for 10-15 minutes or until tender. Drain and cool to room temperature.
2. In a large bowl, combine the potatoes, cheese, pickle, onion and peppers. In a small bowl, combine the mayonnaise, basil, dill, tarragon, salt and pepper. Pour over salad and toss to coat. Cover and refrigerate until chilled. Garnish with chopped egg.
NOTE *Wear disposable gloves when cutting hot peppers; the oils can burn skin. Avoid touching your face.*
PER SERVING ¾ *cup equals 142 cal., 3 g fat (1 g sat. fat), 27 mg chol., 371 mg sodium, 25 g carb., 3 g fiber, 5 g pro.* **Diabetic Exchange:** *1½ starch.*

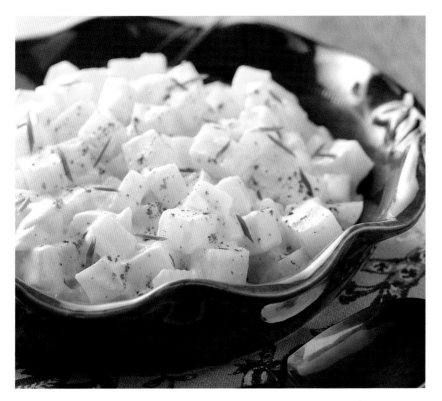

Oven French Fries

Perfect for two, these fries are crisp and offer a flavor you'll both enjoy. They go well with a variety of main courses.

—MARGARET TAYLOR SALEM, MO

PREP: 15 MIN. + CHILLING
BAKE: 30 MIN. • **MAKES:** 2 SERVINGS

- 1 tablespoon cornstarch
- 2 cups water
- 1 tablespoon reduced-sodium soy sauce
- 2 medium potatoes, peeled and cut into strips
- 2 teaspoons olive oil
- ⅛ teaspoon salt

1. In a large bowl, combine the cornstarch, water and soy sauce until smooth. Add potatoes; cover and refrigerate for 1 hour.
2. Drain potatoes and pat dry on paper towels. Toss potatoes with oil and sprinkle with salt. Place on a baking sheet coated with cooking spray.
3. Bake at 375° for 15-20 minutes on each side or until tender and golden brown.
PER SERVING ¾ cup equals 167 cal., 5 g fat (1 g sat. fat), 0 chol., 457 mg sodium, 29 g carb., 2 g fiber, 3 g pro. *Diabetic Exchanges: 2 starch, 1 fat.*

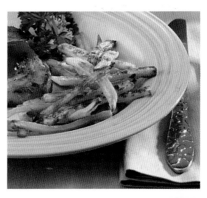

125 CALORIES

Creamed Kohlrabi

This might look like potato salad, but it's actually kohlrabi cubes covered in a velvety white sauce and accented with chives. A lovely change of pace, kohlrabi is a favorite vegetable of mine.

—LORRAINE FOSS PUYALLUP, WA

START TO FINISH: 30 MIN.
MAKES: 6 SERVINGS

- 4 cups cubed peeled kohlrabies (about 6 medium)
- 2 tablespoons butter
- 2 tablespoons all-purpose flour
- 2 cups milk
- ½ teaspoon salt
- ¼ teaspoon pepper
  Dash paprika
- 1 egg yolk, lightly beaten
  Minced chives and additional paprika

1. Place kohlrabies in a large saucepan; add 1 in. of water. Bring to a boil. Reduce heat; cover and simmer for 6-8 minutes or until crisp-tender.
2. Meanwhile, in a small saucepan, melt butter. Stir in flour until smooth; gradually add milk. Bring to a boil. Stir in the salt, pepper and paprika. Gradually stir a small amount of hot mixture into egg yolk; return all to the pan, stirring constantly. Bring to a gentle boil; cook and stir for 2 minutes.
3. Drain kohlrabies and place in a serving bowl; add sauce and stir to coat. Sprinkle with chives and additional paprika.
PER SERVING ⅔ cup equals 125 cal., 7 g fat (4 g sat. fat), 52 mg chol., 276 mg sodium, 11 g carb., 3 g fiber, 5 g pro. *Diabetic Exchanges: 1½ fat, 1 vegetable, ½ starch.*

193 CALORIES Gruyere Mashed Potatoes

Here, Gruyere cheese and chives take mashed potatoes to a whole new level! Don't have Gruyere? Swap in Swiss cheese instead. Missing chives? Try using extra green onion.
—**PRECI D'SILVA** DUBAI, UAE

START TO FINISH: 25 MIN. • **MAKES:** 8 SERVINGS

- 2 **pounds potatoes, peeled and cubed**
- ½ **cup sour cream**
- ⅓ **cup milk**
- ¼ **cup butter, cubed**
- ¼ **cup shredded Gruyere or Swiss cheese**
- ¼ **cup chopped green onions**
- ¼ **cup minced chives**
- 1 **teaspoon minced garlic**
- ½ **teaspoon garlic salt**
- ¼ **teaspoon pepper**

1. Place potatoes in a Dutch oven and cover with water. Bring to a boil. Reduce heat; cover and cook for 10-15 minutes or until tender. Drain.
2. In a large bowl, mash potatoes with remaining ingredients.
PER SERVING *¾ cup equals 193 cal., 9 g fat (6 g sat. fat), 29 mg chol., 175 mg sodium, 23 g carb., 2 g fiber, 4 g pro.*

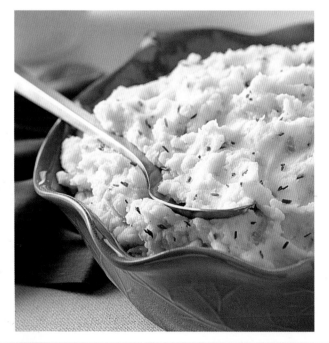

114 CALORIES Peas in Cheese Sauce

My mom's creamed peas were part of a special meal she used to serve and one that my family still has fond memories of.
—**JUNE BLOMQUIST** EUGENE, OR

START TO FINISH: 20 MIN. • **MAKES:** 8 SERVINGS

- 4½ **teaspoons butter**
- 4½ **teaspoons all-purpose flour**
- ¼ **teaspoon salt**
- ⅛ **teaspoon white pepper**
- 1½ **cups 2% milk**
- ¾ **cup cubed process cheese (Velveeta)**
- 2 **packages (10 ounces each) frozen peas, thawed**

In a large saucepan, melt butter over low heat. Stir in the flour, salt and pepper until smooth. Gradually add milk. Bring to a boil; cook and stir for 2 minutes or until thickened. Add the cheese; stir until melted. Stir in peas; cook 1-2 minutes longer or until heated through.
PER SERVING *⅔ cup equals 114 cal., 6 g fat (4 g sat. fat), 19 mg chol., 284 mg sodium, 9 g carb., 2 g fiber, 6 g pro.*

132 CALORIES Glazed Orange Carrots

Want your kids to eat more carrots? This tender dish has a pleasant citrus flavor and a pretty orange glaze. It's a must at our family gatherings.
—**MARILYN HASH** ENUMCLAW, WA

START TO FINISH: 25 MIN. • **MAKES:** 6 SERVINGS

- 2 **pounds fresh carrots, sliced**
- 2 **tablespoons butter**
- ¼ **cup thawed orange juice concentrate**
- 2 **tablespoons brown sugar**
- 2 **tablespoons minced fresh parsley**

1. Place 1 in. of water in a saucepan; add carrots. Bring to a boil. Reduce heat; cover and simmer for 7-9 minutes or until crisp-tender. Drain.
2. Melt butter in a large skillet; stir in orange juice concentrate and brown sugar. Add carrots and parsley; stir to coat. Cook and stir for 1-2 minutes or until glaze is thickened.
PER SERVING *⅔ cup equals 132 cal., 4 g fat (2 g sat. fat), 10 mg chol., 134 mg sodium, 24 g carb., 4 g fiber, 2 g pro.* **Diabetic Exchanges:** *1 vegetable, 1 fat, ½ starch.*

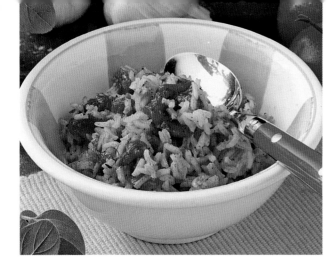

156 CALORIES Spanish Rice

This rice recipe has been in our family for years. It's handy when you're in a hurry for a side dish to complement almost any main dish, not just Tex-Mex fare.

—SHARON DONAT KALISPELL, MT

START TO FINISH: 30 MIN. • **MAKES:** 6 SERVINGS

- 1 can (14½ ounces) vegetable broth
- 1 can (14½ ounces) stewed tomatoes
- 1 cup uncooked long grain rice
- 1 teaspoon olive oil
- 1 teaspoon chili powder
- ¼ teaspoon dried oregano
- ¼ teaspoon garlic salt

In a large saucepan, combine all ingredients. Bring to a boil. Reduce heat; cover and simmer for 20-25 minutes or until rice is tender and liquid is absorbed.

PER SERVING ⅔ *cup equals 156 cal., 1 g fat (trace sat. fat), 0 chol., 350 mg sodium, 32 g carb., 1 g fiber, 4 g pro. Diabetic Exchange: 2 starch.*

186 CALORIES Sweet Potato Casserole

I'm always looking for ways to use our abundant sweet potatoes. This recipe is my own creation, and I've made it many times. When I take the casserole to family potlucks, it never fails to get compliments.

—KATHY RAIRIGH MILFORD, IN

PREP: 30 MIN. • **BAKE:** 35 MIN. • **MAKES:** 8 SERVINGS

- 2¼ pounds sweet potatoes (about 3 large), peeled and cubed
- 3 egg whites, lightly beaten
- 3 tablespoons maple syrup
- 1 teaspoon vanilla extract

TOPPING
- ¼ cup chopped pecans
- 1 tablespoon brown sugar
- 1 tablespoon butter, melted
- ⅛ teaspoon ground cinnamon
- ⅓ cup dried apricots, chopped
- ⅓ cup dried cherries, chopped

1. Place sweet potatoes in a Dutch oven and cover with water. Bring to a boil. Reduce heat; cover and simmer for 15-20 minutes or until tender. Drain and place in a large bowl; mash. Cool slightly. Stir in the egg whites, syrup and vanilla.

2. Transfer to an 8-in. square baking dish coated with cooking spray. Combine the pecans, brown sugar, butter and cinnamon; sprinkle over the top.

3. Bake, uncovered, at 350° for 30 minutes. Sprinkle with apricots and cherries. Bake 5-7 minutes longer or until a thermometer reads 160° and the fruits are heated through.

PER SERVING ½ *cup equals 186 cal., 4 g fat (1 g sat. fat), 4 mg chol., 40 mg sodium, 34 g carb., 3 g fiber, 3 g pro. Diabetic Exchanges: 1½ starch, 1 fat, ½ fruit.*

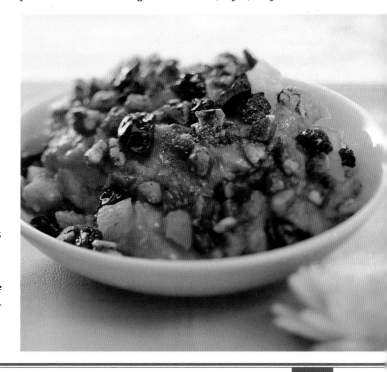

Alfresco Bean Salad

Bored with the usual greens? Try this super-healthy version of three-bean salad. It's terrific as a side, but I've been known to fill my plate and make it a meal!

—CRISTINA VIVES
PALM BEACH GARDENS, FL

START TO FINISH: 25 MIN.
MAKES: 12 SERVINGS

- ¼ cup lime juice
- 4½ teaspoons olive oil
- ½ teaspoon chili powder
   Dash salt and pepper
- 1 can (16 ounces) red beans, rinsed and drained
- 1 can (15¼ ounces) whole kernel corn, drained
- 1 can (15 ounces) garbanzo beans or chickpeas, rinsed and drained
- 1 can (15 ounces) black beans, rinsed and drained
- 2 medium tomatoes, seeded and chopped
- 1 cup coarsely chopped fresh cilantro
- 1 small yellow onion, chopped
- 1 small red onion, chopped
- 1 jalapeno pepper, seeded and chopped

In a large bowl, whisk the lime juice, oil, chili powder, salt and pepper. Add the remaining ingredients and toss to coat. Chill until serving.
NOTE *Wear disposable gloves when cutting hot peppers; the oils can burn skin. Avoid touching your face.*
PER SERVING ⅔ *cup equals 146 cal., 3 g fat (trace sat. fat), 0 chol., 360 mg sodium, 23 g carb., 6 g fiber, 6 g pro.* **Diabetic Exchanges:** *1½ starch, 1 lean meat.*

Seasoned Yukon Gold Wedges

These zesty potatoes are a snap to make. My two boys and husband just love them. They're good with roast or chops, but can also double as an appetizer when served with a dip.

—JANE LYNCH SCARBOROUGH, ON

PREP: 10 MIN. • **BAKE:** 40 MIN.
MAKES: 6 SERVINGS

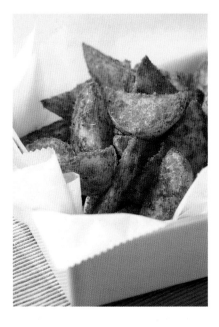

- 1½ pounds Yukon Gold potatoes (about 3 medium), cut into wedges
- 1 tablespoon olive oil
- ¼ cup dry bread crumbs
- 1½ teaspoons paprika
- ¾ teaspoon salt
- ¼ teaspoon dried oregano
- ¼ teaspoon dried thyme
- ¼ teaspoon ground cumin
- ⅛ teaspoon pepper
- ⅛ teaspoon cayenne pepper

1. In a large bowl, toss potatoes with oil. Combine the remaining ingredients; sprinkle over potatoes and toss to coat.
2. Arrange potatoes in a single layer in a 15-in. x 10-in. x 1-in. baking pan coated with cooking spray.
3. Bake, uncovered, at 425° for 40-45 minutes or until tender, stirring once.
PER SERVING ¾ *cup equals 121 cal., 3 g fat (trace sat. fat), 0 chol., 339 mg sodium, 21 g carb., 2 g fiber, 3 g pro.* **Diabetic Exchanges:** *1½ starch, ½ fat.*

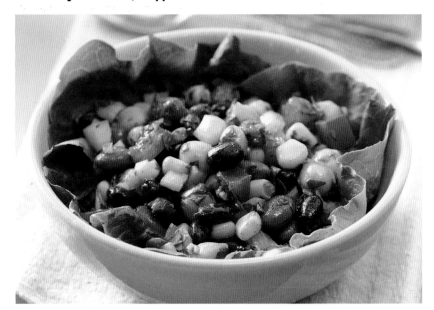

196 CALORIES Never-Fail Scalloped Potatoes

Take the chill off any blustery day and make something special to accompany meaty entrees. This creamy, stick-to-the-ribs, potato-and-onion side dish is one you'll turn to often.

—AGNES WARD STRATFORD, ON

PREP: 30 MIN. • **BAKE:** 1 HOUR
MAKES: 6 SERVINGS

- 2 **tablespoons butter**
- 3 **tablespoons all-purpose flour**
- 1 **teaspoon salt**
- ¼ **teaspoon pepper**
- 1½ **cups fat-free milk**
- ½ **cup shredded reduced-fat cheddar cheese**
- 1¾ **pounds potatoes, peeled and thinly sliced (about 5 medium)**
- 1 **medium onion, halved and thinly sliced**

1. In a small nonstick skillet, melt butter. Stir in the flour, salt and pepper until smooth; gradually add milk. Bring to a boil. Cook and stir for 2 minutes or until thickened. Remove from the heat; stir in cheese until blended.

2. Place half of the potatoes in a 1½-qt. baking dish coated with cooking spray; layer with half of the onion and cheese sauce. Repeat the layers.

3. Cover and bake at 350° for 50 minutes. Uncover; bake 10-15 minutes longer or until bubbly and potatoes are tender.

PER SERVING *¾ cup equals 196 cal., 6 g fat (4 g sat. fat), 18 mg chol., 530 mg sodium, 29 g carb., 3 g fiber, 7 g pro.* **Diabetic Exchanges:** *2 starch, 1 fat.*

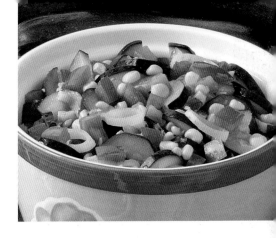

113 CALORIES Summer Garden Medley

This colorful side brings back sweet memories of the corn-and-tomato dish my mother often prepared in the summer. Farmers in our area supply us with delicious eggplant...so I sometimes substitute them for the zucchini in veggie recipes like this one.

—ELAINE NELSON FRESNO, CA

START TO FINISH: 15 MIN.
MAKES: 4 SERVINGS

- 2 **medium zucchini, halved lengthwise and cut into ¼-inch slices**
- 1 **cup fresh or frozen corn, thawed**
- ¾ **cup diced green pepper**
- 1 **medium leek (white portion only), sliced**
- ½ **teaspoon seasoned salt**
- 1 **tablespoon olive oil**
- 2 **medium tomatoes, seeded and diced**

In a large nonstick skillet, saute the zucchini, corn, green pepper, leek and seasoned salt in oil until vegetables are tender. Stir in the tomatoes; heat through.

PER SERVING *1 cup equals 113 cal., 4 g fat (1 g sat. fat), 0 chol., 202 mg sodium, 19 g carb., 3 g fiber, 3 g pro.* **Diabetic Exchanges:** *2 vegetable, ½ starch, ½ fat.*

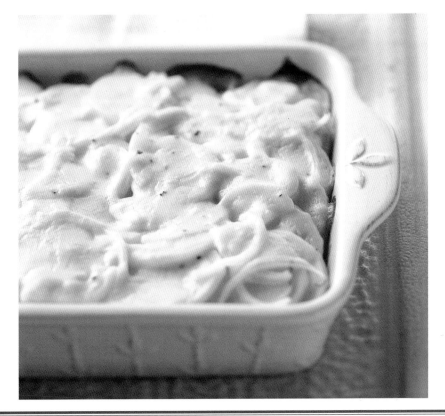

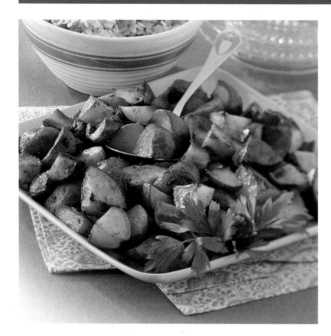

honey. Sprinkle with the chili powder, salt, garlic powder and pepper; toss to coat.

2. Bake, uncovered, at 450° for 25-30 minutes or until potatoes are tender and golden brown, stirring once.

PER SERVING *1 cup equals 158 cal., 4 g fat (2 g sat. fat), 10 mg chol., 258 mg sodium, 28 g carb., 3 g fiber, 3 g pro.* **Diabetic Exchange:** *2 starch.*

160 CALORIES Savory Skillet Noodles

My daughter is a vegetarian, so I created this colorful side to serve with main-course veggie dishes. She asks for it at least once a week! Chopped sweet peppers, onion and almonds accent the mild buttery noodles.

—LUCILLE GOERS SEMINOLE, FL

START TO FINISH: 20 MIN. • **MAKES:** 8 SERVINGS

- 8 ounces uncooked yolk-free noodles
- 1 cup sliced fresh mushrooms
- ¼ cup chopped sweet red pepper
- ¼ cup chopped green pepper
- 2 tablespoons chopped onion
- 2 tablespoons butter
- ⅓ cup sliced almonds
- 1 teaspoon chicken bouillon granules or ½ vegetable bouillon cube, crushed
- 2 tablespoons minced fresh parsley

Cook noodles according to package directions. Meanwhile, in a large nonstick skillet, saute the mushrooms, peppers and onion in butter until tender. Drain noodles; add to skillet. Sprinkle with almonds and bouillon; toss gently to combine. Heat through. Garnish with parsley.

PER SERVING *⅔ cup equals 160 cal., 5 g fat (2 g sat. fat), 8 mg chol., 189 mg sodium, 22 g carb., 2 g fiber, 5 g pro.* **Diabetic Exchanges:** *1½ starch, 1 fat.*

158 CALORIES Barbecued Potato Wedges

So easy to prepare, these toasty, roasted potatoes go well with just about any meat entree, and they are a year-round favorite at our house.

—KAREN MCROWE AVON, OH

PREP: 10 MIN. • **BAKE:** 25 MIN. • **MAKES:** 6 SERVINGS

- 2 pounds small red potatoes, cut into wedges
- 2 tablespoons butter, melted
- 1 tablespoon honey
- 3 teaspoons chili powder
- ½ teaspoon salt
- ¼ teaspoon garlic powder
- ¼ teaspoon pepper

1. Place the potatoes in a 15-in. x 10-in. x 1-in. baking pan coated with cooking spray. Drizzle with butter and

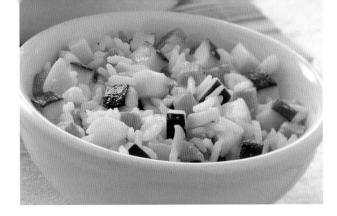

Rice with Summer Squash

I don't usually create my own recipes, but this one passed my palate test. It offers a wonderfully buttery flavor.
—**HEATHER RATIGAN** KAUFMAN, TX

PREP: 15 MIN. • **COOK:** 25 MIN. • **MAKES:** 4 SERVINGS

- 1 cup chopped carrots
- ½ cup chopped onion
- 1 tablespoon butter
- 1 cup reduced-sodium chicken broth or vegetable broth
- ⅓ cup uncooked long grain rice
- ¼ teaspoon salt
- ¼ teaspoon pepper
- 1 medium yellow summer squash, chopped
- 1 medium zucchini, chopped

1. In a large saucepan coated with cooking spray, cook carrots and onion in butter until tender. Stir in the broth, rice, salt and pepper. Bring to a boil. Reduce heat; cover and simmer for 13 minutes.

2. Stir in yellow squash and zucchini. Cover and simmer 6-10 minutes longer or until the rice and vegetables are tender.

PER SERVING *¾ cup equals 123 cal., 3 g fat (2 g sat. fat), 8 mg chol., 346 mg sodium, 21 g carb., 3 g fiber, 4 g pro.* **Diabetic Exchanges:** *1 starch, 1 vegetable, ½ fat.*

167 CALORIES Golden au Gratin Potatoes

With its crunchy, golden topping and cheesy interior, this comforting spin on a classic side dish is brimming with robust flavors. Horseradish and nutmeg add that extra-special touch.
—**JANICE ELDER** CHARLOTTE, NC

PREP: 35 MIN. • **BAKE:** 1½ HOURS • **MAKES:** 15 SERVINGS

- 2 large onions, thinly sliced
- 2 tablespoons butter
- 1 cup half-and-half cream
- 1 cup canned pumpkin
- 1 tablespoon prepared horseradish
- ½ teaspoon ground nutmeg
- 1 teaspoon salt
- ½ teaspoon pepper
- 2¼ pounds potatoes, peeled and cut into ¼-inch slices
- 2 cups soft bread crumbs
- 8 ounces Gruyere or Swiss cheese, shredded
- 2 tablespoons chopped fresh sage

1. In a large skillet, cook onions in butter over medium heat for 15-20 minutes or until onions are golden brown, stirring frequently.

2. In a large bowl, combine the cream, pumpkin, horseradish, nutmeg, salt and pepper. In a greased 13-in. x 9-in. baking pan, layer potato slices and onions. Spread with pumpkin mixture. Cover and bake at 350° for 1¼ hours.

3. Increase temperature to 400°. In a large bowl, combine the bread crumbs, cheese and sage. Sprinkle over top. Bake, uncovered, 15-20 minutes longer or until golden brown.

PER SERVING *1 serving equals 167 cal., 8 g fat (5 g sat. fat), 29 mg chol., 274 mg sodium, 16 g carb., 2 g fiber, 7 g pro.* **Diabetic Exchanges:** *1 starch, 1 lean meat, 1 fat.*

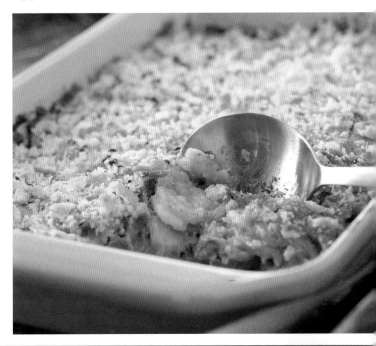

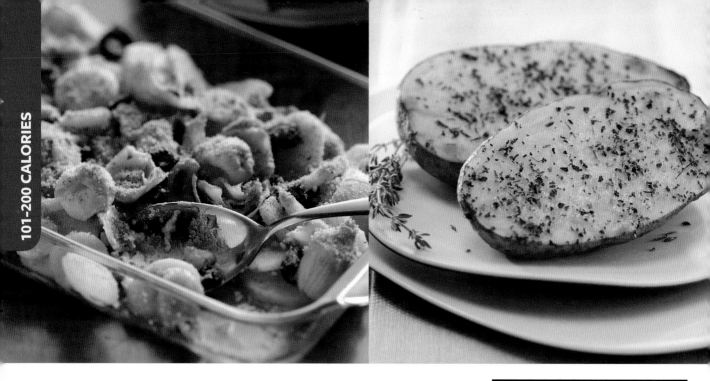

Antipasto Potato Bake

This hearty side dish has a surprising Mediterranean flavor. Red peppers and black olives give a pop of color, making the casserole a pretty addition to any party buffet.

—KELLEY BUTLER-LUDINGTON
EAST HAVEN, CT

PREP: 15 MIN. • **BAKE:** 20 MIN.
MAKES: 10 SERVINGS

- 2 **cans (14½ ounces each) sliced potatoes, drained**
- 2 **cans (14 ounces each) water-packed artichoke hearts, rinsed and drained**
- 2 **jars (7 ounces each) roasted sweet red peppers, drained**
- 1 **can (3.8 ounces) sliced ripe olives, drained**
- ¼ **cup grated Parmesan cheese**
- 1½ **teaspoons minced garlic**
- ⅓ **cup olive oil**
- ½ **cup seasoned bread crumbs**
- 1 **tablespoon butter, melted**

1. In a large bowl, combine potatoes, artichokes, peppers, olives, cheese and garlic. Drizzle with oil; toss gently to coat. Transfer to a greased 3-qt. baking dish. Toss bread crumbs and butter; sprinkle over top.

2. Bake, uncovered, at 375° for 20-25 minutes or until lightly browned.

PER SERVING *¾ cup equals 152 cal., 10 g fat (2 g sat. fat), 5 mg chol., 484 mg sodium, 12 g carb., 1 g fiber, 3 g pro.*

Seasoned Baked Potatoes

My friends still remember these crisp, delicious potatoes brushed with basil, garlic and onion salt that I used to make. Now they happily pass on my recipe to their friends.

—RUTH ANDREWSON
LEAVENWORTH, WA

PREP: 5 MIN. • **BAKE:** 35 MIN.
MAKES: 4 SERVINGS

- 4 **medium baking potatoes**
- 1 **tablespoon olive oil**
- 1½ **teaspoons dried basil**
- ½ **teaspoon onion salt**
- ½ **teaspoon garlic powder**

1. Scrub potatoes and cut in half lengthwise; place cut side up on an ungreased baking sheet. Brush with oil. Sprinkle with basil, onion salt and garlic powder.

2. Bake at 400° for 35-40 minutes or until tender.

PER SERVING *2 potato halves equals 167 cal., 4 g fat (1 g sat. fat), 0 chol., 237 mg sodium, 31 g carb., 3 g fiber, 4 g pro.* **Diabetic Exchanges:** *2 starch, ½ fat.*

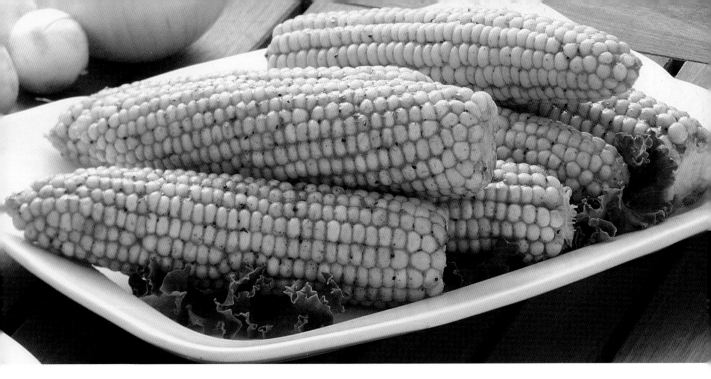

Cajun Buttered Corn

I like to spice up summer meals with this seasoned butter. Garlic and chili powders make it the perfect complement to fresh corn on the cob.
—ANNE-LISE BOTTING DULUTH, GA

START TO FINISH: 20 MIN.
MAKES: 8 SERVINGS

- 8 **medium ears sweet corn**
- 2 **tablespoons butter**
- ¼ **teaspoon chili powder**
- ¼ **teaspoon coarsely ground pepper**
- ⅛ **teaspoon garlic powder**
- ⅛ **teaspoon cayenne pepper**
- 1 **teaspoon cornstarch**
- ¼ **cup reduced-sodium chicken or vegetable broth**

1. In a large kettle, bring 3 qts. of water to a boil; add corn. Return to a boil; cook for 3-5 minutes or until tender.
2. Meanwhile, in a small saucepan, melt butter. Stir in chili powder, pepper, garlic powder and cayenne; cook and stir for 1 minute. Combine cornstarch and broth until smooth; gradually whisk into butter mixture. Bring to a boil; cook and stir for 1-2 minutes or until slightly thickened. Drain corn; serve with butter.
PER SERVING *1 ear equals 105 cal., 4 g fat (2 g sat. fat), 8 mg chol., 63 mg sodium, 18 g carb., 2 g fiber, 3 g pro.*

Parmesan Cauliflower

Need a last-minute side dish? This quick and cheesy recipe can be table-ready in minutes! It's also yummy with broccoli.
—BRENDA BIRON SYDNEY, NS

START TO FINISH: 15 MIN.
MAKES: 2 SERVINGS

- 1½ **cups fresh cauliflowerets**
- 5 **teaspoons reduced-fat butter**
- 2 **teaspoons all-purpose flour**
- 3 **tablespoons reduced-fat sour cream**
- 2 **tablespoons shredded Parmesan cheese**
- ¼ **teaspoon salt**
- ⅛ **teaspoon white pepper**
  Minced fresh parsley, optional

1. Place cauliflower in a steamer basket; place in a small saucepan over 1 in. of water. Bring to a boil; cover and steam for 4-5 minutes or until crisp-tender.
2. Meanwhile, in another small saucepan, melt butter. Stir in flour until smooth. Remove from the heat; stir in the sour cream, Parmesan cheese, salt and pepper.
3. Add cauliflower to cream sauce. Cook and stir over low heat for 1-2 minutes or until heated through. Sprinkle with parsley if desired.
PER SERVING *¾ cup equals 121 cal., 8 g fat (6 g sat. fat), 28 mg chol., 476 mg sodium, 8 g carb., 2 g fiber, 6 g pro.* **Diabetic Exchanges:** *1½ fat, 1 vegetable.*

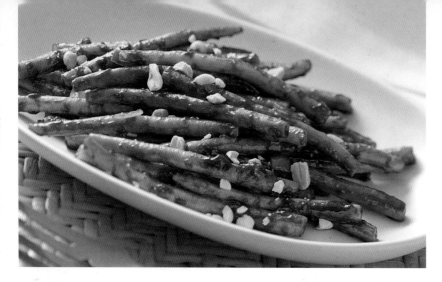

168 CALORIES
Thai-Style Green Beans

Two for Thai, anyone? Peanut butter, soy and hoisin sauces flavor this quick and fabulous bean dish.

—CANDACE MCMENAMIN
LEXINGTON, SC

START TO FINISH: 20 MIN.
MAKES: 2 SERVINGS

- 1 tablespoon reduced-sodium soy sauce
- 1 tablespoon hoisin sauce
- 1 tablespoon creamy peanut butter
- ⅛ teaspoon crushed red pepper flakes
- 1 tablespoon chopped shallot
- 1 teaspoon minced fresh gingerroot
- 1 tablespoon canola oil
- ½ pound fresh green beans, trimmed
  Minced fresh cilantro and chopped dry roasted peanuts, optional

1. In a small bowl, combine the soy sauce, hoisin sauce, peanut butter and red pepper flakes; set aside.
2. In a small skillet, saute shallot and ginger in oil over medium heat for 2 minutes or until crisp-tender.

Add green beans; cook and stir for 3 minutes or until crisp-tender. Add reserved sauce; toss to coat. Sprinkle with cilantro and peanuts if desired.
PER SERVING *1 serving (calculated without peanuts) equals 168 cal., 12 g fat (1 g sat. fat), trace chol., 476 mg sodium, 14 g carb., 4 g fiber, 5 g pro.*

103 CALORIES
Grandma's Stuffed Yellow Squash

My grandma, who raised me, was an awesome cook. This is a recipe she fixed every summer when our garden overflowed with yellow squash. My family still enjoys it!

—JANIE MCGRAW SALLISAW, OK

PREP: 25 MIN. • **BAKE:** 25 MIN.
MAKES: 2 SERVINGS

- 1 medium yellow summer squash
- ¼ cup egg substitute
- 2 tablespoons finely chopped onion
- ¼ teaspoon salt
- ⅛ teaspoon pepper
- 2 slices bread, toasted and diced

1. Place squash in a large saucepan; cover with water. Bring to a boil; cover and cook for 7-9 minutes or until crisp-tender. Drain.
2. When cool enough to handle, cut squash in half lengthwise; scoop out and reserve pulp, leaving a ⅜-in. shell. Invert shells on paper towel.
3. In a small bowl, combine the egg substitute, onion, salt and pepper. Stir in toasted bread cubes and squash pulp. Spoon into squash shells.
4. Place in an 8-in. square baking dish coated with cooking spray. Cover and bake at 375° for 20 minutes. Uncover; bake 5-10 minutes longer or until lightly browned.
PER SERVING *½ squash equals 103 cal., 1 g fat (trace sat. fat), trace chol., 490 mg sodium, 18 g carb., 3 g fiber, 6 g pro.* **Diabetic Exchanges:** *1 starch, 1 vegetable.*

159 CALORIES
Chive 'n' Garlic Corn

We created this fresh-tasting side dish as a great way to dress up quick, convenient frozen corn.

—TASTE OF HOME TEST KITCHEN

START TO FINISH: 15 MIN.
MAKES: 4 SERVINGS

- 1 package (16 ounces) frozen corn, thawed
- ½ cup finely chopped onion
- 2 tablespoons butter
- ¼ cup minced chives
- ½ teaspoon minced garlic
- ⅛ teaspoon salt
  Pepper to taste

In a large skillet, saute corn and onion in butter for 5-7 minutes or until tender. Stir in the chives, garlic, salt and pepper.
PER SERVING *½ cup equals 159 cal., 7 g fat (4 g sat. fat), 15 mg chol., 136 mg sodium, 26 g carb., 3 g fiber, 4 g pro.* **Diabetic Exchanges:** *1½ starch, 1½ fat.*

154 CALORIES Sweet Pepper Wild Rice Salad

This wild rice salad is packed with nutrients and fun flavors in every bite.

—SHERRYL LUDLOW ROLLA, MO

PREP: 20 MIN. • **COOK:** 1 HOUR
MAKES: 8 SERVINGS

- ½ cup uncooked wild rice
- 1 can (14½ ounces) reduced-sodium chicken broth, divided
- 1¼ cups water, divided
- ¾ cup uncooked long grain rice
- 1 medium sweet red pepper, chopped
- 1 medium sweet yellow pepper, chopped
- 1 medium zucchini, chopped
- 2 tablespoons olive oil, divided
- 4 green onions, chopped
- ½ teaspoon salt
- ¼ teaspoon pepper
- 2 tablespoons lemon juice

1. In a small saucepan, combine the wild rice, 1 cup broth and ½ cup water. Bring to a boil. Reduce heat; cover and simmer for 50-60 minutes or until rice is tender.

2. Meanwhile, in a large saucepan, combine the long grain rice and remaining broth and water. Bring to a boil. Reduce heat; cover and simmer for 15-18 minutes or until rice is tender.

3. In a large nonstick skillet, saute the peppers and zucchini in 1 tablespoon oil for 3 minutes. Add onions; saute 1-2 minutes longer or until the vegetables are tender. Transfer to a large bowl.

4. Drain wild rice if necessary; stir into vegetable mixture. Stir in white rice. Sprinkle with salt and pepper. Drizzle with lemon juice and remaining oil; toss to coat. Serve warm or at room temperature.

PER SERVING *¾ cup equals 154 cal., 4 g fat (1 g sat. fat), 0 chol., 287 mg sodium, 26 g carb., 2 g fiber, 4 g pro.* **Diabetic Exchanges:** *1½ starch, 1 fat.*

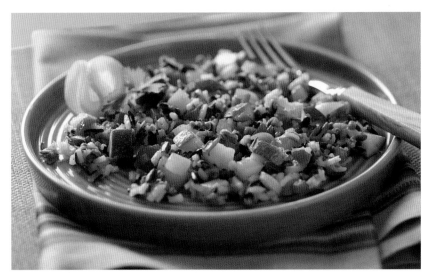

112 CALORIES

Peas a la Francaise

I adore peas, and this recipe is a favorite. It features tiny pearl onions touched with thyme and chervil, and its presentation is lovely.

—CHRISTINE FRAZIER AUBURNDALE, FL

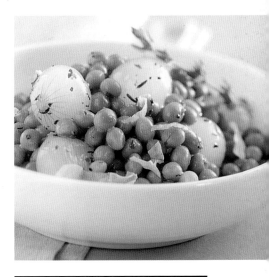

START TO FINISH: 30 MIN.
MAKES: 12 SERVINGS (½ CUP EACH)

- 1½ cups pearl onions, trimmed
- ¼ cup butter, cubed
- ¼ cup water
- 1 tablespoon sugar
- 1 teaspoon salt
- ¼ teaspoon dried thyme
- ¼ teaspoon dried chervil
- ¼ teaspoon pepper
- 2 packages (16 ounces each) frozen peas, thawed
- 2 cups shredded lettuce

1. In a Dutch oven, bring 6 cups water to a boil. Add pearl onions; boil for 3 minutes. Drain and rinse in cold water; peel and set aside.

2. In the same saucepan, melt butter over medium heat. Stir in the onions, water, sugar and seasonings. Add peas and lettuce; stir until blended. Cover and cook for 6-8 minutes or until the vegetables are tender. Serve with a slotted spoon.

PER SERVING *½ cup equals 112 cal., 4 g fat (2 g sat. fat), 10 mg chol., 315 mg sodium, 15 g carb., 4 g fiber, 4 g pro.* **Diabetic Exchanges:** *1 starch, 1 fat.*

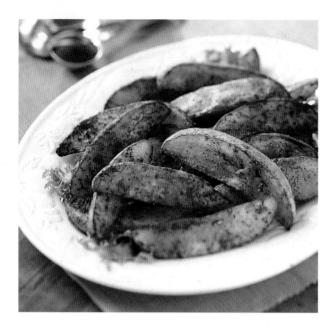

164 CALORIES Vegetable Rice Skillet

This is a favorite vegetable casserole of ours. It's very filling served over rice, and the cheese gives the veggies extra flavor. It's great the next day—if any is left!
—**ARLENE LEE** HOLLAND, MB

PREP: 10 MIN. • **COOK:** 30 MIN. • **MAKES:** 8 SERVINGS

- 1 **medium onion, chopped**
- 1 **tablespoon butter**
- 2 **medium carrots, sliced**
- 1½ **cups cauliflowerets**
- 1½ **cups broccoli florets**
- 1 **cup uncooked long grain rice**
- 2 **garlic cloves, minced**
- 1½ **cups reduced-sodium chicken broth**
- 1 **cup (4 ounces) shredded reduced-fat cheddar cheese**
- 1 **tablespoon minced fresh parsley**
- ¾ **teaspoon salt**
- ¼ **teaspoon pepper**

1. In a large nonstick skillet over medium heat, cook onion in butter until tender. Add carrots; cook for 5 minutes longer. Stir in the cauliflower, broccoli, rice and garlic. Add broth; bring mixture to a boil.
2. Reduce heat; cover and simmer for 20-25 minutes or until rice is tender. Remove from the heat; stir in the cheese, parsley, salt and pepper.
PER SERVING *¾ cup equals 164 cal., 5 g fat (3 g sat. fat), 14 mg chol., 459 mg sodium, 24 g carb., 2 g fiber, 7 g pro.* **Diabetic Exchanges:** *1 starch, 1 vegetable, 1 fat.*

182 CALORIES

Chili-Seasoned Potato Wedges

When I tried out these roasted potato wedges on my family, it was love at first taste! Since I generally have the soup mix and seasonings on hand, this recipe couldn't be easier. Alter the spices to your liking.
—**IRENE MARSHALL** NAMPA, ID

PREP: 10 MIN. • **BAKE:** 35 MIN. • **MAKES:** 8 SERVINGS

- 1 **tablespoon onion soup mix**
- 1 **tablespoon chili powder**
- ¼ **teaspoon salt**
- ¼ **teaspoon garlic powder**
- ¼ **teaspoon pepper**
- 4 **large baking potatoes**
- 2 **tablespoons canola oil**

1. In a large resealable plastic bag, combine the soup mix, chili powder, salt, garlic powder and pepper. Cut each potato into eight wedges; place in the bag and shake to coat.
2. Arrange in a single layer in a greased 15-in. x 10-in. x 1-in. baking pan. Drizzle with oil.
3. Bake, uncovered, at 425° for 12-20 minutes on each side or until crisp.
PER SERVING *4 pieces equals 182 cal., 4 g fat (1 g sat. fat), 0 chol., 172 mg sodium, 34 g carb., 3 g fiber, 4 g pro.*

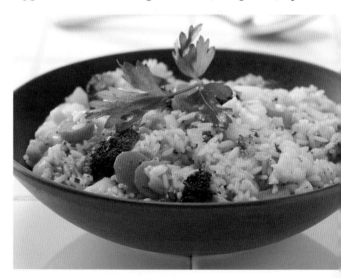

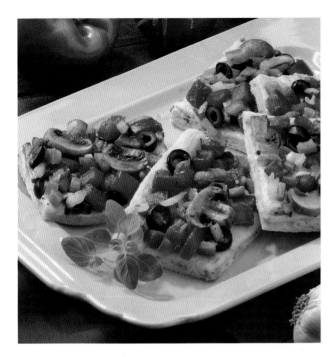

1. In a large bowl, combine 2 cups flour, yeast and salt. Add water and oil; beat until smooth. Stir in enough remaining flour to form a soft dough.

2. Turn onto a floured surface; knead until smooth and elastic, about 4 minutes. Cover and let rest for 15 minutes. Meanwhile, in a bowl, combine the tomatoes, mushrooms, green pepper, olives, onion, oil, vinegar and seasonings.

3. Coat a 15-in. x 10-in. x 1-in. baking pan with cooking spray; sprinkle with cornmeal. Press dough into pan. Prick dough generously with a fork.

4. Bake at 475° for 5 minutes or until lightly browned. Cover with vegetable mixture. Bake 8-10 minutes longer or until edges of crust are golden brown.

PER SERVING *1 piece equals 121 cal., 5 g fat (1 g sat. fat), 0 chol., 376 mg sodium, 17 g carb., 1 g fiber, 3 g protein.* **Diabetic Exchanges:** *1 starch, 1 fat.*

186 CALORIES Baked Corn Pudding

Here's a comforting side dish that can turn even ordinary meals into something to celebrate. Often requested by our entire family, it spoons up as sweet and creamy as custard. Guests give it rave reviews and always ask for the recipe.
—**PEGGY WEST** GEORGETOWN, DE

PREP: 10 MIN. • **BAKE:** 45 MIN. • **MAKES:** 10 SERVINGS

- ½ cup sugar
- 3 tablespoons all-purpose flour
- 3 eggs
- 1 cup milk
- ¼ cup butter, melted
- ½ teaspoon salt
- ½ teaspoon pepper
- 1 can (15¼ ounces) whole kernel corn, drained
- 1 can (14¾ ounces) cream-style corn

1. In a large bowl, combine sugar and flour. Whisk in the eggs, milk, butter, salt and pepper. Stir in the corn and cream-style corn.

2. Pour into a greased 1½-qt. baking dish. Bake, uncovered, at 350° for 45-50 minutes or until a knife inserted near the center comes out clean.

PER SERVING *½ cup equals 186 cal., 7 g fat (4 g sat. fat), 79 mg chol., 432 mg sodium, 26 g carb., 1 g fiber, 4 g pro.*

121 CALORIES Vegetable Focaccia

This from-scratch recipe began as herb focaccia but gradually came to include our favorite vegetables as well. It's on the light side because the recipe doesn't call for cheese...something that most people don't even notice!
—**MICHELE FAIRCHOK** GROVE CITY, OH

PREP: 15 MIN. + RISING • **BAKE:** 15 MIN. • **MAKES:** 12 SERVINGS

- 2 to 2¼ cups bread flour
- 1 package (¼ ounce) quick-rise yeast
- 1 teaspoon salt
- 1 cup warm water (120° to 130°)
- 1 tablespoon olive oil

TOPPING

- 3 plum tomatoes, chopped
- 5 medium fresh mushrooms, sliced
- ½ cup chopped green pepper
- ½ cup sliced ripe olives
- ¼ cup chopped onion
- 3 tablespoons olive oil
- 2 teaspoons red wine vinegar
- ¾ teaspoon salt
- ¼ teaspoon garlic powder
- ¼ teaspoon dried oregano
- ¼ teaspoon pepper
- 2 teaspoons cornmeal

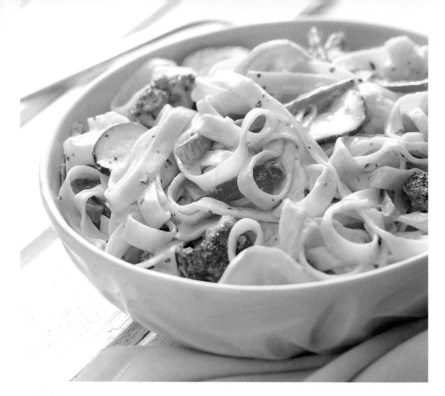

2 cups fresh corn
1 tablespoon olive oil
2 large sweet red peppers, chopped
½ cup chopped onion
1 garlic clove, minced
¼ cup minced fresh parsley
½ teaspoon chili powder
½ teaspoon salt
¼ teaspoon pepper

In a large nonstick skillet, cook corn in oil for 2 minutes. Add the red peppers, onion and garlic; cook and stir for 4-6 minutes or until peppers are crisp-tender. Stir in the parsley, chili powder, salt and pepper; cook 1-2 minutes longer.

PER SERVING *¾ cup equals 130 cal., 5 g fat (1 g sat. fat), 0 chol., 314 mg sodium, 22 g carb., 4 g fiber, 4 g pro.* **Diabetic Exchanges:** *1 starch, 1 vegetable, 1 fat.*

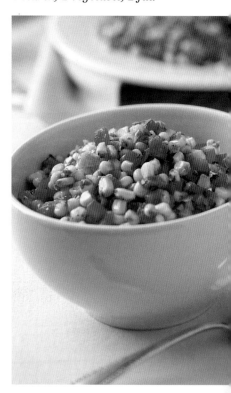

165 CALORIES Garden Primavera Fettuccine

I created this side while trying to make broccoli Alfredo. I kept adding fresh vegetables, and the result was this creamy pasta dish!

—**TAMMY PERRAULT** LANCASTER, OH

START TO FINISH: 30 MIN.
MAKES: 10 SERVINGS

1 package (12 ounces) fettuccine
1 cup fresh cauliflowerets
1 cup fresh broccoli florets
½ cup julienned carrot
1 small sweet red pepper, julienned
½ small yellow summer squash, sliced
½ small zucchini, sliced
1 cup Alfredo sauce
1 teaspoon dried basil
Shredded Parmesan cheese, optional

1. In a large saucepan, cook fettuccine according to package directions, adding vegetables during the last 4 minutes. Drain and return to the pan.
2. Add Alfredo sauce and basil; toss to coat. Cook over low heat for 1-2 minutes or until heated through. Sprinkle with cheese if desired.

PER SERVING *¾ cup (calculated without cheese) equals 165 cal., 3 g fat (2 g sat. fat), 7 mg chol., 121 mg sodium, 28 g carb., 3 g fiber, 7 g pro.* **Diabetic Exchanges:** *2 starch, ½ fat.*

130 CALORIES Corn 'n' Red Pepper Medley

This fresh-tasting side dish is a fun treatment for corn. It's colorful, comes together quickly on the stovetop and goes well with just about any main course—particularly grilled foods.

—**LILY JULOW** GAINESVILLE, FL

START TO FINISH: 25 MIN.
MAKES: 4 SERVINGS

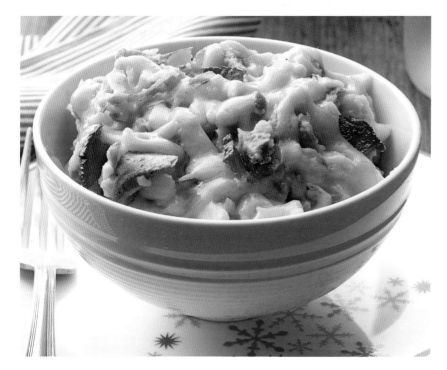

528 mg sodium, 25 g carb.,
3 g fiber, 7 g pro. *Diabetic
Exchanges:* 1½ starch, 1½ fat.

Quick Mashed Potato Cakes

Here's a great way to use up any remaining mashed potatoes! These light cakes cook up golden brown and have a wonderful butter-and-onion flavor. Kids and adults alike will love this healthy spin on a classic!
—**TASTE OF HOME TEST KITCHEN**

START TO FINISH: 25 MIN.
MAKES: 2 SERVINGS

- 1 **egg white, lightly beaten**
- 1 **cup mashed potatoes (with added milk and butter)**
- 1 **tablespoon all-purpose flour**
- 2½ **teaspoons finely chopped green onion**
- ½ **teaspoon minced fresh parsley**
- ⅛ **teaspoon salt**
- ⅛ **teaspoon pepper**
  Butter-flavored cooking spray
- 1 **teaspoon butter**

1. In a small bowl, combine the first seven ingredients. In a large nonstick skillet coated with butter-flavored cooking spray, melt butter over medium heat.
2. Drop the potato mixture by ¼ cupfuls into skillet; press lightly to flatten. Cook over medium heat for 4-5 minutes on each side or until golden brown. Serve warm.
PER SERVING *2 potato cakes equals 155 cal., 6 g fat (3 g sat. fat), 14 mg chol., 525 mg sodium, 21 g carb., 2 g fiber, 4 g pro.* ***Diabetic Exchanges:*** *1½ starch, 1 fat.*

Caramelized Onion Mashed Potatoes

Caramelized onions give a sweet and savory taste to this side dish. Prepared with red potatoes, reduced-fat cheese and bacon, it makes a heartwarming accompaniment to any entree.
—**TASTE OF HOME TEST KITCHEN**

PREP: 15 MIN. • **COOK:** 45 MIN.
MAKES: 6 SERVINGS

- 1 **tablespoon canola oil**
- 2 **large onions, thinly sliced**
- 1 **teaspoon salt, divided**
- 1½ **pounds medium red potatoes, quartered**
- 3 **garlic cloves, peeled and halved**
- ⅓ **cup reduced-fat sour cream**
- 3 **tablespoons fat-free milk**
- ¼ **teaspoon pepper**
- 1 **tablespoon butter, melted**
- ½ **cup shredded reduced-fat cheddar cheese**
- 2 **bacon strips, cooked and crumbled**

1. Heat oil in a large nonstick skillet over medium heat; add onions and ½ teaspoon salt. Cook and stir for 15 minutes or until moisture has evaporated and onions are completely wilted. Reduce heat to medium-low. Cook and stir for 30-40 minutes or until onions are caramelized. (If necessary, add water, 1 tablespoon at a time, if onions begin to stick to the pan.)
2. Meanwhile, place potatoes and garlic in a large saucepan; cover with water. Bring to a boil. Reduce heat; cover and cook for 18-22 minutes or until tender.
3. Drain potatoes; place in a large bowl and mash. Add the sour cream, milk, pepper and remaining salt; mash until blended. Stir in caramelized onions. Transfer to a serving bowl. Drizzle with butter; sprinkle with cheese and bacon.
PER SERVING ⅔ *cup equals 200 cal., 9 g fat (4 g sat. fat), 18 mg chol.,*

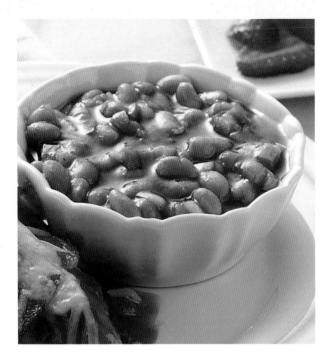

129 CALORIES In-a-Flash Beans

No one will guess this recipe begins with a can. Chopped onion and green pepper lend a little crunch, while barbecue sauce delivers lots of home-cooked flavor.

—LINDA COLEMAN CEDAR RAPIDS, IA

START TO FINISH: 10 MIN. • **MAKES:** 4 SERVINGS

- 1 can (15¾ ounces) pork and beans
- ½ cup barbecue sauce
- ½ cup chopped onion
- ¼ cup chopped green pepper, optional

In a large saucepan, combine the beans, barbecue sauce, onion and green pepper if desired. Cook and stir over medium heat until heated through.

PER SERVING ⅔ cup equals 129 cal., 2 g fat (trace sat. fat), 0 chol., 647 mg sodium, 26 g carb., 6 g fiber, 6 g pro.

180 CALORIES Corn Potato Pancakes

I love combining different foods to see what I can come up with. In this case, I used leftover mashed potatoes to make slightly crisp, golden brown cakes.

—CAROLYN WILSON LYNDON, KS

START TO FINISH: 20 MIN. • **MAKES:** ABOUT 1 DOZEN

- 2 cups mashed potatoes (with added milk and butter)
- ¼ cup all-purpose flour
- ¼ cup cream-style corn
- 1 egg, beaten
- 3 tablespoons finely chopped onion
- 1 teaspoon minced fresh parsley
- ½ teaspoon salt
- ½ teaspoon minced garlic
- ⅛ teaspoon pepper
- 3 tablespoons canola oil, divided

In a large bowl, combine the first nine ingredients. In a large skillet, heat 1 tablespoon oil; drop four ¼ cupfuls of batter into skillet. Cook for 1-2 minutes on each side or until golden brown. Repeat with the remaining oil and batter.

PER SERVING 2 pancakes equals 180 cal., 11 g fat (3 g sat. fat), 43 mg chol., 461 mg sodium, 18 g carb., 1 g fiber, 3 g pro.

106 CALORIES Stir-Fried Carrots

For a colorful side dish that's as good as it is good for you, I cook up these fast and fail-proof carrots with rosemary fresh from my garden. It's my hubby Tom's favorite way to do carrots, and it just happens to be healthy, too!

—GRACE YASKOVIC BRANCHVILLE, NJ

START TO FINISH: 20 MIN. • **MAKES:** 4 SERVINGS

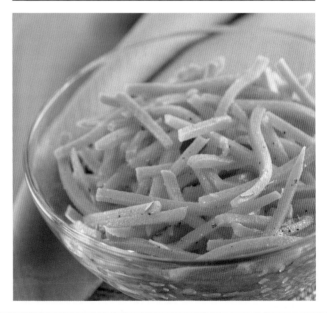

1½ pounds fresh carrots, julienned
1 tablespoon olive oil
½ cup chicken broth
1 teaspoon dried rosemary, crushed
¼ teaspoon pepper

In a large skillet or wok, stir-fry carrots in oil until crisp-tender. Stir in the broth, rosemary and pepper. Bring to a boil. Reduce heat; simmer, uncovered, for 2-3 minutes or until liquid is reduced.
PER SERVING *¾ cup equals 106 cal., 4 g fat (1 g sat. fat), 0 chol., 176 mg sodium, 18 g carb., 5 g fiber, 2 g pro.* **Diabetic Exchanges:** *1 starch, ½ fat.*

131 CALORIES Quick Creamed Spinach

The inspiration for this creamy side dish came from a local restaurant. I lightened up the original recipe by using fat-free half-and-half and fat-free cream cheese. It goes great with most any meal.

—SUSAN GEDDIE HARKER HEIGHTS, TX

START TO FINISH: 15 MIN. • **MAKES:** 5 SERVINGS

¼ cup diced onion
1 garlic clove, minced
1 tablespoon butter
1 tablespoon all-purpose flour
1¼ cups fat-free half-and-half
4 ounces fat-free cream cheese, cubed
¾ teaspoon salt
⅛ teaspoon ground nutmeg
⅛ teaspoon pepper
1 package (16 ounces) frozen leaf spinach, thawed and squeezed dry
¼ cup plus 1 tablespoon shredded Parmesan cheese, divided

1. In a large nonstick skillet, saute onion and garlic in butter until tender. Stir in flour until blended. Gradually whisk in half-and-half until blended. Bring to a boil over medium-low heat; cook and stir for 2 minutes or until slightly thickened.
2. Add the cream cheese, salt, nutmeg and pepper, stirring until cream cheese is melted. Stir in spinach and ¼ cup Parmesan cheese; heat through. Sprinkle with remaining Parmesan cheese. Serve immediately.
PER SERVING *½ cup equals 131 cal., 4 g fat (3 g sat. fat), 12 mg chol., 704 mg sodium, 13 g carb., 2 g fiber, 10 g pro.*

121 CALORIES Spiced Polenta Steak Fries

Adults and kids alike will delight in these steak-fry substitutes with a crisp, spicy exterior and a creamy, sweet interior.
—TASTE OF HOME TEST KITCHEN

START TO FINISH: 30 MIN. • **MAKES:** 4 SERVINGS

1 tube (1 pound) polenta
1 tablespoon olive oil
¼ teaspoon onion powder
¼ teaspoon garlic powder
¼ teaspoon chili powder
⅛ teaspoon paprika
⅛ teaspoon pepper

1. Cut polenta in half widthwise; cut each portion in half lengthwise. Cut each section into eight strips. Arrange strips in a single layer in a 15-in. x 10-in. x 1-in. baking pan coated with cooking spray.
2. Combine the oil and seasonings; drizzle over polenta strips and gently toss to coat. Bake at 425° for 7-10 minutes on each side or until golden brown.
PER SERVING *8 fries equals 121 cal., 3 g fat (trace sat. fat), 0 chol., 383 mg sodium, 20 g carb., 1 g fiber, 2 g pro.* **Diabetic Exchanges:** *1 starch, ½ fat.*

201-250 CALORIES

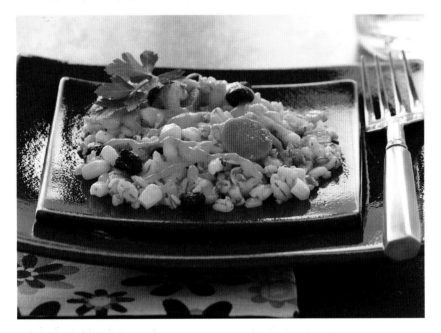

226 CALORIES Go for the Grains Casserole

A friend of mine gave me the recipe for her hearty and delicious casserole when I was compiling some healthy recipes. The colorful medley has "good for you" written all over it.

—MELANIE BLAIR WARSAW, IN

PREP: 25 MIN. • **BAKE:** 55 MIN.
MAKES: 10 SERVINGS

- 5 **medium carrots, thinly sliced**
- 2 **cups frozen corn, thawed**
- 1 **medium onion, diced**
- 1 **cup quick-cooking barley**
- ½ **cup bulgur**
- ⅓ **cup minced fresh parsley**
- 1 **teaspoon salt**
- ½ **teaspoon pepper**
- 3 **cups vegetable broth**
- 1 **can (15 ounces) black beans, rinsed and drained**
- 1½ **cups (6 ounces) shredded reduced-fat cheddar cheese**

1. In a large bowl, combine the carrots, corn, onion, barley, bulgur, parsley, salt and pepper. Stir in broth and beans. Transfer to a 13-in. x 9-in. baking dish coated with cooking spray.
2. Cover and bake at 350° for 50-55 minutes or until grains are tender, stirring once. Sprinkle with cheese. Bake, uncovered, 3-5 minutes longer or until cheese is melted.
PER SERVING ¾ cup equals 226 cal., 5 g fat (3 g sat. fat), 12 mg chol., 741 mg sodium, 38 g carb., 8 g fiber, 12 g pro.

216 CALORIES
Brown Sugar Squash

With brown sugar, butter and honey, what's not to love about this sweet and yummy side dish? It's ready in no time from the microwave.

—KARA DE LA VEGA SANTA ROSA, CA

START TO FINISH: 20 MIN.
MAKES: 4 SERVINGS

- 2 **medium acorn squash**
- ¼ **cup packed brown sugar**
- 2 **tablespoons butter**
- 4 **teaspoons honey**
- ¼ **teaspoon salt**
- ¼ **teaspoon pepper**

1. Cut squash in half; discard seeds. Place squash cut side down in a microwave-safe dish. Cover and microwave on high for 10-12 minutes or until tender.
2. Turn squash cut side up. Fill centers of squash with brown sugar, butter and honey; sprinkle with salt and pepper. Cover and microwave on high for 2-3 minutes or until heated through.
NOTE This recipe was tested in a 1,100-watt microwave.
PER SERVING 1 squash half equals 216 cal., 6 g fat (4 g sat. fat), 15 mg chol., 200 mg sodium, 43 g carb., 3 g fiber, 2 g pro.

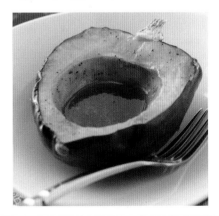

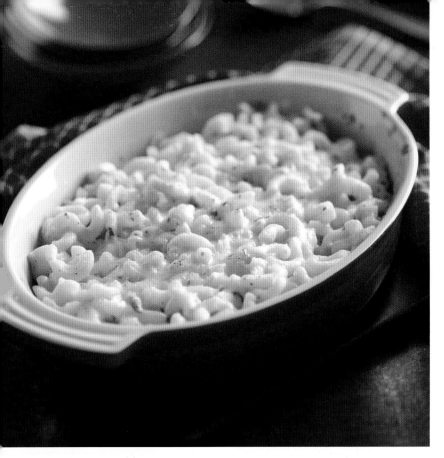

Light Rosemary Rice

This quick dish is a favorite with my family. It's low in fat because it gets flavor from herbs, not butter.
—**CONNIE REGALADO** EL PASO, TX

START TO FINISH: 25 MIN.
MAKES: 4 SERVINGS

- ¼ **cup chopped onion**
- 1 **garlic clove, minced**
- 1 **tablespoon olive oil**
- 1 **can (14½ ounces) reduced-sodium chicken broth or vegetable broth**
- ¼ **cup water**
- 1 **cup uncooked long grain rice**
- 1 **tablespoon minced fresh rosemary or 1 teaspoon dried rosemary, crushed**
- ¼ **teaspoon pepper**
- ¼ **cup shredded Parmesan cheese**

In a saucepan, saute onion and garlic in oil until tender. Add broth and water; bring to a boil. Stir in rice, rosemary and pepper. Reduce heat; cover and simmer for 15-18 minutes or until rice is tender. Remove from heat; stir in cheese.
PER SERVING *¾ cup equals 250 cal., 5 g fat (1 g sat. fat), 4 mg chol., 367 mg sodium, 42 g carb., 1 g fiber, 7 g pro.*

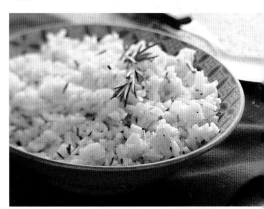

Creamy Macaroni 'n' Cheese

I prepare this cheesy recipe when I'm craving comfort food but trying to eat a little lighter. A hint of mustard adds zip to the creamy side dish.
—**DAWN ROYER** ALBANY, OR

PREP: 15 MIN. • **BAKE:** 20 MIN.
MAKES: 8 SERVINGS

- ⅓ **cup finely chopped onion**
- 3½ **cups cooked elbow macaroni**
- 1¾ **cups shredded reduced-fat cheddar cheese**
- 2 **tablespoons minced fresh parsley**
- ½ **cup fat-free evaporated milk**
- 1¾ **cups 2% cottage cheese**
- 1 **teaspoon Dijon mustard**
- ½ **teaspoon salt**
- ¼ **teaspoon pepper**

1. In a large microwave-safe bowl, cover and microwave onion on high for 1 minute or until tender; drain. Add the macaroni, cheddar cheese and parsley; set aside.
2. In a blender, combine the milk, cottage cheese, mustard, salt and pepper; cover and process until smooth. Stir into macaroni mixture.
3. Pour into a 1½-qt. baking dish coated with cooking spray. Bake, uncovered, at 350° for 20-25 minutes or until lightly browned.
NOTE *This recipe was tested in a 1,100-watt microwave.*
PER SERVING *⅔ cup equals 229 cal., 6 g fat (4 g sat. fat), 19 mg chol., 491 mg sodium, 24 g carb., 1 g fiber, 20 g pro.* **Diabetic Exchanges:** *2 lean meat, 1½ starch.*

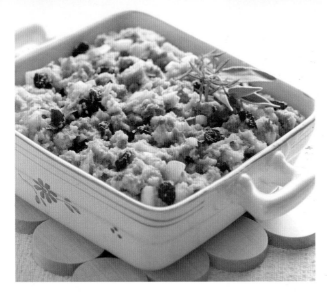

205 CALORIES

Cranberry Cornmeal Dressing

This home-style dressing is perfect with poultry or even roasted pork. The sweet-tart flavor of dried cranberries really complements the dish's turkey sausage.
—**CORINNE PORTTEUS** ALBUQUERQUE, NM

PREP: 30 MIN. • **BAKE:** 40 MIN. • **MAKES:** 8 SERVINGS

- 3 cups reduced-sodium chicken broth, divided
- ½ cup yellow cornmeal
- ½ teaspoon salt
- ½ teaspoon white pepper
- ½ pound Italian turkey sausage links, casings removed
- 1 large onion, diced
- 1 large fennel bulb, diced (about 1 cup)
- 1 garlic clove, minced
- 1 egg yolk, beaten
- 4 cups soft French or Italian bread crumbs
- ¾ cup dried cranberries
- 2 tablespoons minced fresh parsley
- 1 tablespoon balsamic vinegar
- 1 teaspoon minced fresh sage
- 1 teaspoon minced fresh savory
- ¼ teaspoon ground nutmeg

1. In a small bowl, whisk 1 cup broth, cornmeal, salt and pepper until smooth. In a large saucepan, bring remaining broth to a boil. Add cornmeal mixture, stirring constantly. Return to a boil; cook and stir for 3 minutes or until thickened. Remove from the heat; set aside.

2. Crumble sausage into a large nonstick skillet; add onion and fennel. Cook over medium heat until sausage is no longer pink. Add garlic; cook 1 minute longer. Drain. Stir in egg yolk and cornmeal mixture. Add bread crumbs, cranberries, parsley, vinegar, sage, savory and nutmeg.

3. Transfer to a 1½-qt. baking dish coated with cooking spray. Cover and bake at 350° for 40-45 minutes or until a thermometer reads 160°.

PER SERVING *⅔ cup equals 205 cal., 4 g fat (1 g sat. fat), 42 mg chol., 695 mg sodium, 33 g carb., 3 g fiber, 9 g pro.* **Diabetic Exchanges:** *2 starch, 1 lean meat.*

224 CALORIES ## Chipotle Sweet Potato and Spiced Apple Purees

I used to make the same dish with lots of butter, brown sugar and cream. I slimmed it down, and my low-fat version is just as delicious! My family loves it.
—**SHANNON ABDOLLMOHAMMADI** WOODINVILLE, WA

PREP: 30 MIN. • **BAKE:** 35 MIN. • **MAKES:** 8 SERVINGS

- 2 large tart apples, peeled and quartered
- ¼ cup lemon juice
- ¼ cup honey
- 2 tablespoons butter, melted
- 1½ teaspoons salt, divided
- ¼ teaspoon Chinese five-spice powder
- 4 pounds sweet potatoes (about 6 large), peeled and quartered

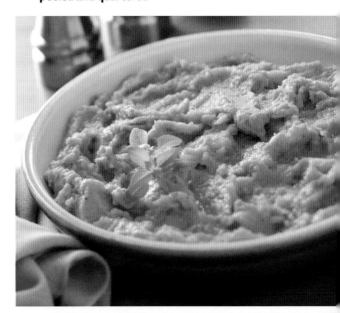

¼ cup fat-free milk, warmed
2 teaspoons minced chipotle pepper in adobo sauce
¼ teaspoon pepper

1. In an ungreased 11-in. x 7-in. baking dish, toss the apples, lemon juice, honey, butter, ½ teaspoon salt and five-spice powder. Bake, uncovered, at 400° for 35-40 minutes or until apples are tender, turning once.
2. Meanwhile, place sweet potatoes in a Dutch oven and cover with water. Bring to a boil. Reduce heat; cover and cook for 15-20 minutes or until tender. Drain well. Over very low heat, stir potatoes for 1-2 minutes or until steam has evaporated.
3. Place potatoes in a food processor; add the milk, chipotle, pepper and remaining salt. Cover and process until smooth. Transfer mixture to a serving bowl and keep warm.
4. Place apples and cooking juices in a clean food processor; cover and process until smooth. Spoon over sweet potato puree.
PER SERVING ¾ cup sweet potato puree with 4 teaspoons apple puree equals 224 cal., 3 g fat (2 g sat. fat), 8 mg chol., 498 mg sodium, 49 g carb., 5 g fiber, 3 g pro.

204 CALORIES Oven Fries

Jazz up potato fries with paprika and garlic powder. Something about that combination of spices packs a heck of a punch. Everyone loves these—we even enjoy the leftovers cold!
—**HEATHER BYERS** PITTSBURGH, PA

PREP: 10 MIN. • **BAKE:** 40 MIN. • **MAKES:** 4 SERVINGS

4 medium potatoes
1 tablespoon olive oil
2½ teaspoons paprika
¾ teaspoon salt
¾ teaspoon garlic powder

1. Preheat oven to 400°. Cut each potato into 12 wedges. In a large bowl, combine oil, paprika, salt and garlic powder. Add potatoes; toss to coat.
2. Transfer to a 15x10x1-in. baking pan coated with cooking spray. Bake 40-45 minutes or until tender, turning once.
PER SERVING 12 potato wedges equals 204 cal., 4 g fat (1 g sat. fat), 0 chol., 456 mg sodium, 39 g carb., 4 g fiber, 5 g pro.

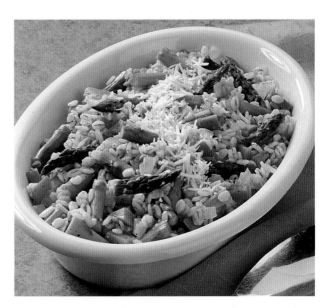

226 CALORIES Springtime Barley

While working as a sorority housemother, I occasionally filled in for the cook. The girls really liked nutritious low-fat dishes, including this attractive medley.
—**SHARON HELMICK** COLFAX, WA

START TO FINISH: 30 MIN. • **MAKES:** 4 SERVINGS

1 small onion, chopped
1 medium carrot, chopped
1 tablespoon butter
1 cup quick-cooking barley
2 cups reduced-sodium chicken broth, divided
½ pound fresh asparagus, trimmed and cut into 1-inch pieces
¼ teaspoon dried marjoram
⅛ teaspoon pepper
2 tablespoons shredded Parmesan cheese

1. In a large skillet, saute onion and carrot in butter until crisp-tender. Add barley; cook and stir 1 minute. Stir in 1 cup broth. Bring to a boil. Reduce heat; cook and stir until most of the liquid is absorbed.
2. Add asparagus. Cook for 15-20 minutes or until barley is tender and liquid is absorbed, stirring occasionally and adding more broth as needed. Stir in marjoram and pepper; sprinkle with cheese.
PER SERVING ¾ cup equals 226 cal., 5 g fat (2 g sat. fat), 9 mg chol., 396 mg sodium, 39 g carb., 9 g fiber, 9 g pro. *Diabetic Exchanges:* 2 starch, 1 vegetable, ½ fat.

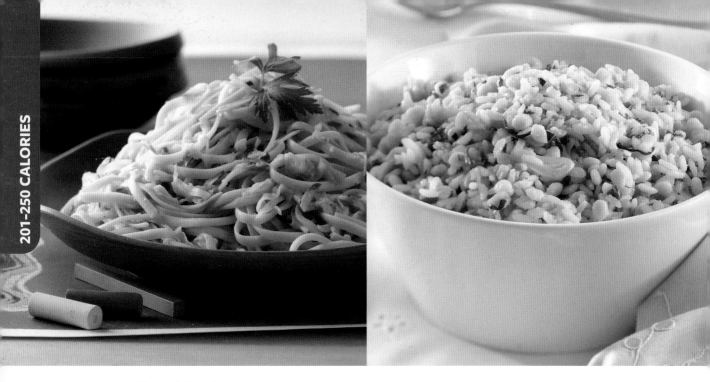

219 CALORIES Zucchini Pasta

The taste of this rich and creamy dish will have people convinced it's not low in fat, but it is! Garlicky and fresh-flavored, it's sure to be a hit.

—MARIA REGAKIS SOMERVILLE, MA

START TO FINISH: 25 MIN.
MAKES: 6 SERVINGS

- 8 **ounces uncooked linguine**
- 4 **cups coarsely shredded zucchini (about 3 medium)**
- 4 **teaspoons olive oil**
- 2 **garlic cloves, thinly sliced**
- ¼ **cup fat-free plain yogurt**
- ¾ **cup shredded reduced-fat cheddar cheese**
- ¾ **teaspoon salt**
- ¼ **teaspoon pepper**

1. Cook linguine according to package directions. In a sieve or colander, drain zucchini, squeezing to remove excess liquid. Pat dry.
2. In a large nonstick skillet, saute zucchini in oil for 2 minutes. Add garlic; saute 1-2 minutes longer or until zucchini is tender. Transfer to a large bowl. Add the yogurt, cheese, salt and pepper. Drain linguine; add to zucchini mixture and toss to coat.

PER SERVING *¾ cup equals 219 cal., 7 g fat (3 g sat. fat), 10 mg chol., 395 mg sodium, 32 g carb., 2 g fiber, 10 g pro.* **Diabetic Exchanges:** *1½ starch, 1½ fat, 1 vegetable.*

227 CALORIES
Garlic-Herb Orzo Pilaf

Mildly flavored and flecked with herbs, this side dish can accompany a wide variety of entrees. Plus, it's a cinch to put together.

—MARY RELYEA CANASTOTA, NY

PREP: 10 MIN. • **COOK:** 30 MIN.
MAKES: 4 SERVINGS

- 8 **garlic cloves, peeled and thinly sliced**
- 1 **tablespoon olive oil**
- ½ **cup uncooked orzo pasta**
- ½ **cup uncooked long grain rice**
- 1 **can (14½ ounces) reduced-sodium chicken broth or vegetable broth**
- ⅓ **cup water**
- 3 **green onions, thinly sliced**
- ⅓ **cup thinly sliced fresh basil leaves**
- ¼ **cup minced fresh parsley**
- ¼ **teaspoon salt**

1. In a large nonstick skillet coated with cooking spray, cook garlic in oil over medium-high heat for 1 minute. Add orzo and rice; cook 4-6 minutes longer or until lightly browned.
2. Stir in broth and water. Bring to a boil. Reduce heat; cover and simmer for 15-20 minutes or until rice is tender and liquid is absorbed.
3. Stir in the onions, basil, parsley and salt.

PER SERVING *¾ cup equals 227 cal., 4 g fat (1 g sat. fat), 0 chol., 426 mg sodium, 40 g carb., 1 g fiber, 7 g pro.* **Diabetic Exchanges:** *2½ starch, ½ fat.*

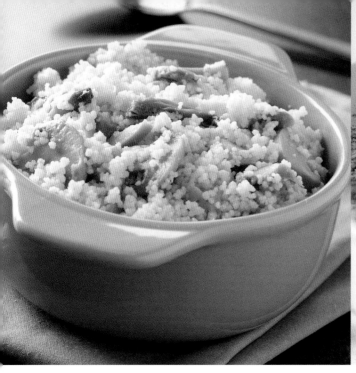
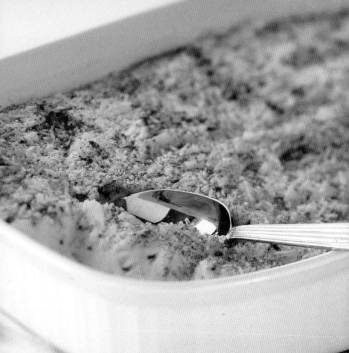

Couscous with Mushrooms

Fluffy and flavorful couscous takes only minutes to prepare. I use the versatile pasta a lot because it cooks quickly and you can add almost any vegetable to it.

—CLAUDIA RUISS MASSAPEQUA, NY

START TO FINISH: 15 MIN.
MAKES: 4 SERVINGS

- 1¼ cups water
- 2 tablespoons butter
- 2 teaspoons chicken bouillon granules
- ¼ teaspoon salt
- ¼ teaspoon pepper
- 1 cup uncooked couscous
- 1 can (7 ounces) mushroom stems and pieces, drained

1. In a small saucepan, combine the first five ingredients; bring to a boil. Stir in couscous and mushrooms.
2. Remove from the heat; let stand, covered, for 5-10 minutes or until the liquid is absorbed. Fluff with a fork before serving.

PER SERVING *¾ cup equals 230 cal., 6 g fat (4 g sat. fat), 15 mg chol., 794 mg sodium, 37 g carb., 3 g fiber, 8 g pro.*

Makeover Patrician Potatoes

The Thanksgiving table just isn't complete without a steaming side of mashed potatoes. This light version feels holiday-special without all of the calories and fat.

—KATHY FLEMING LISLE, IL

PREP: 45 MIN. • **BAKE:** 20 MIN.
MAKES: 12 SERVINGS

- 5 pounds medium potatoes, peeled and quartered
- 2 tablespoons butter, melted
- 1 package (8 ounces) fat-free cream cheese
- 1 cup (8 ounces) reduced-fat sour cream
- 2 teaspoons salt
- 2 teaspoons minced chives
- ¼ cup shredded Parmesan cheese
- 1 teaspoon paprika

1. Place potatoes in a Dutch oven and cover with water. Bring to a boil. Reduce heat; cover and simmer for 15-20 minutes or until tender.
2. Drain potatoes and place in a large bowl; mash with butter. In a small bowl, beat cream cheese, sour cream and salt until light and fluffy; add to potatoes. Stir in chives.
3. Transfer to a 13-in. x 9-in. baking dish coated with cooking spray. Sprinkle with cheese and the paprika.
4. Bake the potatoes, uncovered, at 350° for 20-25 minutes or until heated through.

PER SERVING *1 cup equals 207 cal., 4 g fat (3 g sat. fat), 14 mg chol., 563 mg sodium, 35 g carb., 3 g fiber, 8 g pro.* **Diabetic Exchanges:** *2 starch, 1 fat.*

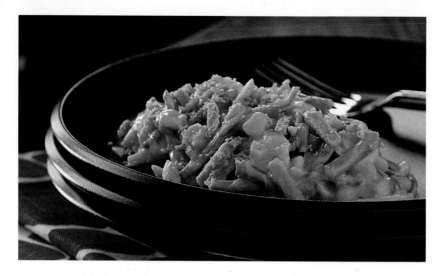

213 CALORIES Makeover Fancy Bean Casserole

My daughter gave me this wonderful recipe, and I've since shared it with many of my friends. The lightened-up version retains all of the original's crunchy, creamy goodness.

—VENOLA SHARPE

CAMPBELLSVILLE, KY

PREP: 15 MIN. • **BAKE:** 35 MIN.
MAKES: 6 SERVINGS

- 3 **cups frozen French-style green beans, thawed**
- 1 **can (10¾ ounces) reduced-fat reduced-sodium condensed cream of chicken soup, undiluted**
- 1½ **cups frozen corn, thawed**
- 1 **can (8 ounces) sliced water chestnuts, drained**
- 1 **medium onion, chopped**
- ½ **cup reduced-fat sour cream**
- ¼ **cup cubed reduced-fat process cheese (Velveeta)**
- 5 **teaspoons reduced-fat butter**
- ⅓ **cup crushed butter-flavored crackers**
- 2 **tablespoons slivered almonds**

1. In a large bowl, combine the first seven ingredients. Transfer to an 11-in. x 7-in. baking dish coated with cooking spray.
2. In a small skillet, melt butter. Add cracker crumbs and almonds; cook and stir until lightly browned. Sprinkle over the top.
3. Bake casserole, uncovered, at 350° for 35-40 minutes or until heated through and the topping is golden brown.
NOTE *This recipe was tested with Land O'Lakes light stick butter.*
PER SERVING *⅔ cup equals 213 cal., 8 g fat (3 g sat. fat), 17 mg chol., 355 mg sodium, 32 g carb., 5 g fiber, 7 g pro.* **Diabetic Exchanges:** *1½ starch, 1 vegetable, 1 fat.*

226 CALORIES Broccoli-Cheddar Baked Potatoes

This hearty side dish will bring good taste to any holiday table. It's great with almost any entree. Adding a cup of leftover diced chicken to the vegetables can turn it into a simple lunch.

—MARY BAUER WICHITA, KS

PREP: 70 MIN. • **BAKE:** 10 MIN.
MAKES: 2 SERVINGS

- 1 **large baking potato**
- ¼ **cup chopped fresh broccoli**
- ¼ **cup sliced fresh mushrooms**
- 1 **tablespoon diced pimientos**
- 1 **teaspoon canola oil**
- ¼ **cup shredded reduced-fat cheddar cheese, divided**
- ¼ **cup fat-free plain yogurt**
- ¼ **teaspoon salt**
- ⅛ **teaspoon garlic powder**
- ⅛ **teaspoon paprika**
  Pepper to taste

1. Scrub and pierce potato. Bake at 375° for 1 hour or until tender. Meanwhile, in a small skillet, saute the broccoli, mushrooms and pimientos in oil until vegetables are tender; set aside.
2. When potato is cool enough to handle, cut in half lengthwise. Scoop out pulp, leaving a thin shell.
3. In a small bowl, mash the pulp. Stir in 2 tablespoons cheese, yogurt, salt, garlic powder, paprika and pepper. Stir in broccoli mixture. Spoon into potato shells. Sprinkle with remaining cheese. Place on a baking sheet.
4. Bake at 375° for 10 minutes or until cheese is melted.
PER SERVING *1 stuffed potato half equals 226 cal., 6 g fat (2 g sat. fat), 11 mg chol., 417 mg sodium, 37 g carb., 3 g fiber, 9 g pro.*

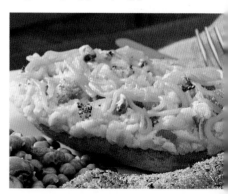

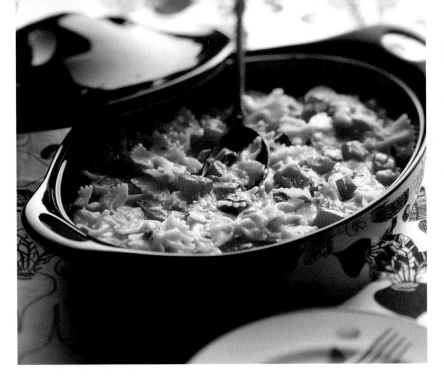

Rice and Mushrooms

Don't count on having any leftovers with this tasty, yet simple, dish. A friend gave me the recipe more than a decade ago, and it's been a family favorite ever since.

—BETH MCCAW NASHVILLE, TN

START TO FINISH: 25 MIN.
MAKES: 8 SERVINGS

- 1 **small onion, finely chopped**
- 1 **celery rib, chopped**
- ½ **cup chopped celery leaves**
- 2 **tablespoons butter**
- 1 **pound sliced fresh mushrooms**
- 3 **cups uncooked instant rice**
- 3 **cups water**
- 4 **teaspoons Greek seasoning**
- ½ **cup chopped pecans, toasted**

1. In a large nonstick skillet coated with cooking spray, saute the onion, celery and celery leaves in butter for 4 minutes. Add mushrooms; cook 4 minutes longer.

2. Add rice; cook for 4-5 minutes or until lightly browned. Stir in the water and Greek seasoning. Bring to a boil. Remove from the heat; cover and let stand for 5 minutes. Fluff with a fork. Sprinkle with pecans.

PER SERVING *1 cup equals 232 cal., 9 g fat (2 g sat. fat), 8 mg chol., 529 mg sodium, 35 g carb., 2 g fiber, 5 g pro.* **Diabetic Exchanges:** *2 starch, 1½ fat, 1 vegetable.*

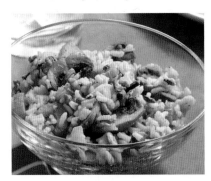

Southwestern Pasta & Cheese

I decided to give my old mac 'n' cheese recipe a new twist by including some of my favorite Southwestern ingredients. I especially like the smoky flavors of chipotle and bacon...and my family loves every spoonful!

—NAOMI REED MCMINNVILLE, OR

PREP: 30 MIN. • **BAKE:** 20 MIN.
MAKES: 8 SERVINGS

- 3⅓ **cups uncooked bow tie pasta**
- 1 **medium sweet red pepper, chopped**
- 8 **green onions, chopped**
- 1 **tablespoon olive oil**
- ¼ **cup all-purpose flour**
- 1 **teaspoon chili powder**
- 1 **teaspoon minced chipotle pepper in adobo sauce**
- ½ **teaspoon salt**
- ½ **teaspoon ground cumin**
- 2¼ **cups fat-free milk**
- 1 **cup (4 ounces) shredded sharp cheddar cheese, divided**
- 4 **center-cut bacon strips, cooked and crumbled**
- 2 **tablespoons minced fresh cilantro**

1. Cook pasta according to package directions.

2. Meanwhile, in a large skillet, saute pepper and onions in oil until tender. Stir in flour, chili powder, chipotle pepper, salt and cumin until blended. Gradually stir in milk. Bring to a boil; cook and stir for 2 minutes or until thickened. Stir in ¼ cup cheese until melted.

3. Drain pasta; toss with sauce. Stir in bacon and cilantro. Transfer to a 2-qt. baking dish coated with cooking spray. Sprinkle with remaining cheese. Bake, uncovered, at 400° for 20-25 minutes or until bubbly.

PER SERVING *¾ cup equals 240 cal., 8 g fat (4 g sat. fat), 20 mg chol., 327 mg sodium, 32 g carb., 2 g fiber, 12 g pro.* **Diabetic Exchanges:** *2 starch, 1 medium-fat meat, ½ fat.*

Desserts

There's always room for dessert...especially classics like **cupcakes, cookies, bars, pudding** and more! When planning your daily meals, remember to **set aside some calories** so you can **treat yourself to a sweet bite** and still land within the **1,400-calorie daily guideline**.

CONTENTS

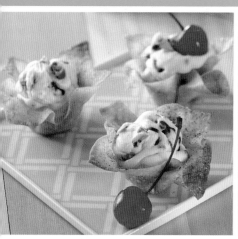

WONTON SUNDAES PAGE 402

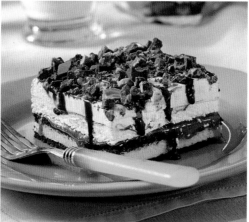

ICE CREAM SANDWICH DESSERT PAGE 428

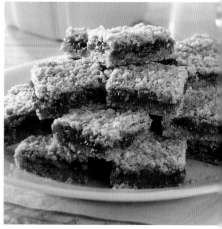

APRICOT DATE SQUARES PAGE 410

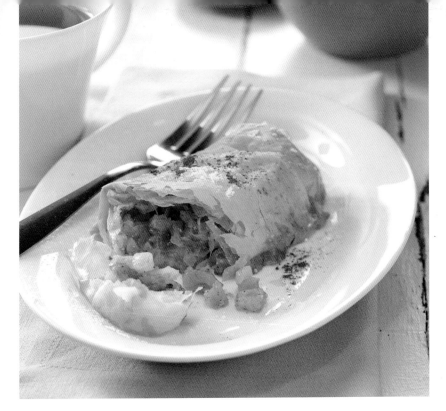

Broiled Fruit Dessert

This yummy dessert is a quick guilt-free treat. It's perfect for enjoying the fruits of summer.
—**JIM GALES** GLENDALE, WI

START TO FINISH: 15 MIN.
MAKES: 2 SERVINGS

- 1 **medium peach**
- 1 **medium fresh nectarine**
- 1 **tablespoon brown sugar**
  Whipped cream or vanilla ice cream, optional

1. Halve and pit the peach and nectarine. Line a shallow baking dish with foil; coat foil with cooking spray. Place fruit cut side down in prepared dish.
2. Broil 6 in. from the heat for 3 minutes; turn fruit over and sprinkle with brown sugar. Broil 2-3 minutes longer or until sugar is melted and bubbly. Serve warm with whipped cream or ice cream if desired.

PER SERVING *1 serving (calculated without whipped cream or ice cream) equals 80 cal., trace fat (trace sat. fat), 0 chol., 3 mg sodium, 20 g carb., 2 g fiber, 1 g pro.* **Diabetic Exchange:** *1 fruit.*

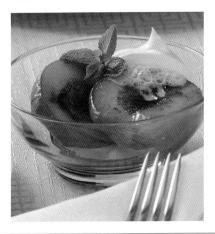

Mini Apple Strudels

Crisp sheets of phyllo dough surround tender slices of apple in this easy play on strudel. Walnuts and cinnamon enhance the traditional apple flavor.
—**TASTE OF HOME TEST KITCHEN**

PREP: 30 MIN. • **BAKE:** 20 MIN.
MAKES: 6 SERVINGS

- 1½ **cups chopped peeled tart apples**
- 2 **tablespoons plus 2 teaspoons sugar**
- 2 **tablespoons chopped walnuts**
- 1 **tablespoon all-purpose flour**
- ¼ **teaspoon ground cinnamon**
- 6 **sheets phyllo dough (14 inches x 9 inches)**
  Butter-flavored cooking spray
  Confectioners' sugar, optional

1. In a small bowl, combine the apples, sugar, walnuts, flour and cinnamon. Set aside.

2. Place one sheet of phyllo dough on a work surface (keep remaining dough covered with plastic wrap and a damp towel to prevent it from drying out). Spray sheet with butter-flavored spray.
3. Fold in half widthwise; spray again with butter-flavored spray. Spoon a scant ⅓ cup filling onto phyllo about 2 in. from a short side. Fold side and edges over filling and roll up. Place seam side down on a baking sheet coated with cooking spray. Repeat.
4. With a sharp knife, cut diagonal slits in tops of strudels. Spray strudels with butter-flavored spray. Bake at 350° for 20-22 minutes or until golden brown. Sprinkle with confectioners' sugar if desired.

PER SERVING *1 strudel equals 100 cal., 3 g fat (trace sat. fat), 0 chol., 45 mg sodium, 17 g carb., 1 g fiber, 2 g pro.*

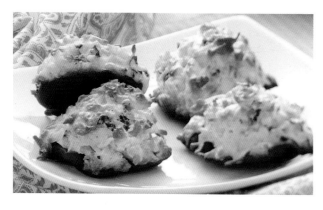

Yellow cake mix, applesauce and raisins make this tender spiced loaf a no-fuss favorite. It's a great go-to recipe because I usually have all the ingredients in my pantry. For a special occasion, top the slices with fresh fruit.

—LUELLEN SPAULDING CARO, MI

PREP: 10 MIN. • **BAKE:** 45 MIN.
MAKES: 2 LOAVES (16 SLICES EACH)

- 1 **package yellow cake mix (regular size)**
- 1 **cup applesauce**
- ½ **cup water**
- ¼ **cup canola oil**
- 3 **eggs**
- ½ **teaspoon ground cinnamon**
- ¼ **teaspoon ground nutmeg**
- ¼ **teaspoon ground allspice**
- ½ **cup raisins**

1. In a large bowl, combine cake mix, applesauce, water, oil, eggs, cinnamon, nutmeg and allspice. Beat on medium speed for 2 minutes. Stir in raisins. Pour into two greased 8x4-in. loaf pans.
2. Bake at 350° for 45-50 minutes or until a toothpick inserted near the center comes out clean. Cool for 5-10 minutes before removing from pans to wire racks.
PER SERVING *1 slice equals 100 cal., 4 g fat (1 g sat. fat), 20 mg chol., 108 mg sodium, 16 g carb., 1 g fiber, 1 g pro.* **Diabetic Exchanges:** *1 starch, 1 fat.*

91 CALORIES
Cranberry Almond Macaroons

You'll relish my lower-calorie take on a classic cookie. It's enhanced with cranberries and luscious dark chocolate. My son is diabetic and loves these. A co-worker calls them a piece of coconut heaven.

—RAMONA CORNELL LEVITTOWN, NY

PREP: 15 MIN. • **BAKE:** 10 MIN. + COOLING • **MAKES:** 11 COOKIES

- 2 **egg whites**
- ¼ **teaspoon almond extract**
  Sugar substitute equivalent to
  2 tablespoons sugar
- 1 **cup flaked coconut**
- ¼ **cup dried cranberries, chopped**
- ¼ **cup chopped almonds**
- ¼ **cup semisweet chocolate chips, melted**

1. Place egg whites in a small bowl; let stand at room temperature for 30 minutes. Add extract; beat on medium speed until soft peaks form. Gradually beat in sugar substitute on high until stiff glossy peaks form. Fold in the coconut, cranberries and almonds.
2. Drop by rounded tablespoonfuls 2 in. apart onto a baking sheet coated with cooking spray. Bake at 325° for 10-15 minutes or until set. Cool for 15 minutes before carefully removing from pan to a wire rack.
3. Spread about 1 teaspoon melted chocolate on the bottom of each cookie. Place on waxed paper with chocolate side up; let stand until set.
NOTE *This recipe was tested with Splenda no-calorie sweetener.*
PER SERVING *1 cookie equals 91 cal., 6 g fat (3 g sat. fat), 0 chol., 33 mg sodium, 10 g carb., 1 g fiber, 2 g pro.* **Diabetic Exchanges:** *1 fat, ½ starch.*

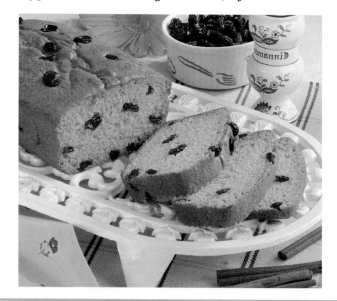

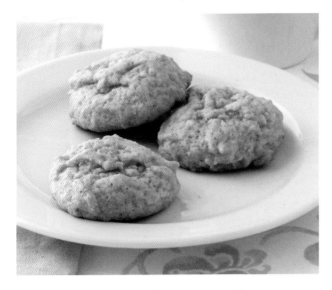

Soft Honey Cookies

My old-fashioned cookie has a pleasant honey-cinnamon flavor and a tender texture that resembles cake. It has been a family favorite for years, and I love sharing the recipe.
—ROCHELLE FRIEDMAN BROOKLYN, NY

PREP: 15 MIN. + CHILLING • **BAKE:** 10 MIN. • **MAKES:** 16 COOKIES

- ¼ **cup sugar**
- 2 **tablespoons canola oil**
- 1 **egg**
- 3 **tablespoons honey**
- ¾ **teaspoon vanilla extract**
- 1 **cup plus 2 tablespoons all-purpose flour**
- ¼ **teaspoon baking powder**
- ¼ **teaspoon ground cinnamon**
- ⅛ **teaspoon salt**

1. In a small bowl, beat sugar and oil until blended. Beat in egg until blended; beat in honey and vanilla. Combine the flour, baking powder, cinnamon and salt; gradually add to sugar mixture and mix well (dough will be stiff). Cover and refrigerate for at least 2 hours.

2. Drop dough by tablespoonfuls 2 in. apart onto a greased baking sheet. Bake at 350° for 8-10 minutes or until bottoms are lightly browned. Cool for 1 minute before removing from pan to a wire rack. Store in an airtight container.

PER SERVING *1 cookie equals 77 cal., 2 g fat (trace sat. fat), 13 mg chol., 29 mg sodium, 13 g carb., trace fiber, 1 g pro.* **Diabetic Exchange: 1 starch.**

96 CALORIES Jellied Champagne Dessert

We've fashioned this refreshing dessert to look just like a glass of bubbling champagne, making it perfect for New Year's Eve!
—TASTE OF HOME TEST KITCHEN

PREP: 20 MIN. + CHILLING • **MAKES:** 8 SERVINGS

- 1 **tablespoon unflavored gelatin**
- 2 **cups cold white grape juice, divided**
- 2 **tablespoons sugar**
- 2 **cups champagne or club soda**
- 8 **fresh strawberries, hulled**

1. In a small saucepan, sprinkle gelatin over 1 cup cold grape juice; let stand for 1 minute. Heat over low heat, stirring until gelatin is completely dissolved. Stir in sugar. Remove from the heat; stir in remaining grape juice. Cool to room temperature.

2. Transfer gelatin mixture to a large bowl. Slowly stir in champagne. Pour half of the mixture into eight champagne or parfait glasses. Add one strawberry to each glass. Chill glasses and remaining gelatin mixture until almost set, about 1 hour.

3. Place the reserved gelatin mixture in a blender; cover and process until foamy. Pour into glasses. Chill for 3 hours or until set.

PER SERVING *½ cup equals 96 cal., trace fat (trace sat. fat), 0 chol., 9 mg sodium, 13 g carb., trace fiber, 1 g pro.* **Diabetic Exchange: 1 starch.**

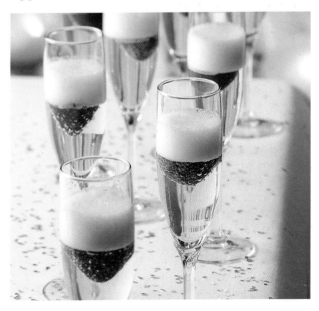

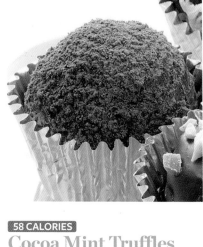

75 CALORIES
Chocolate-Dipped Phyllo Sticks

Looking for a little something special? Try these elegant crunchy treats. They're great with coffee or alongside sorbet.
—**TASTE OF HOME TEST KITCHEN**

PREP: 35 MIN. • **BAKE:** 5 MIN.
MAKES: 20 STICKS

- 4 **sheets phyllo dough (14 inches x 9 inches)**
- 2 **tablespoons butter, melted**
- 1 **tablespoon sugar**
- ¼ **teaspoon ground cinnamon**
  Cooking spray
- 2 **ounces semisweet chocolate, finely chopped**
- ½ **teaspoon shortening**
- ½ **ounce white baking chocolate, melted**

1. Place one sheet of phyllo dough on a work surface; brush with butter. Cover with a second sheet of phyllo; brush with butter. (Keep remaining phyllo dough covered with plastic wrap and a damp towel to prevent it from drying out.) Cut phyllo in half lengthwise. Cut each half into five 4½-in. x 2¾-in. rectangles. Tightly roll each rectangle from one long side, forming a 4½-in.-long stick. Combine sugar and cinnamon. Coat sticks with cooking spray; sprinkle with cinnamon-sugar.

2. Place on an ungreased baking sheet. Bake at 425° for 3-5 minutes or until lightly browned. Remove to a wire rack to cool. Repeat with remaining phyllo dough, butter and cinnamon-sugar.

3. In a microwave, melt semisweet chocolate and shortening; stir until smooth. Dip one end of phyllo sticks in chocolate; allow extra to drip off. Place on waxed paper; let stand until set. Drizzle with white chocolate.

PER SERVING *2 sticks equals 75 cal., 5 g fat (3 g sat. fat), 6 mg chol., 43 mg sodium, 8 g carb., 1 g fiber, 1 g pro. Diabetic Exchanges: 1 fat, ½ starch.*

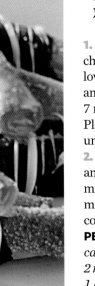

58 CALORIES
Cocoa Mint Truffles

Wow! These easy chocolate truffles will be a hit at parties. Moist with a rich minty flavor inside, the candies have a powdered cocoa outer layer. Best of all, they're oh-so-simple to do!
—**TASTE OF HOME TEST KITCHEN**

PREP: 30 MIN. + FREEZING
MAKES: 16 TRUFFLES

- ¾ **cup semisweet chocolate chips**
- 6 **mint Andes candies**
- ¾ **cup whipped topping**
- 2 **tablespoons baking cocoa**
- ⅛ **teaspoon instant coffee granules**

1. In a small saucepan, melt chocolate chips and candies over low heat. Transfer to a small bowl and cool to lukewarm, about 7 minutes. Beat in whipped topping. Place in freezer for 15 minutes or until firm enough to form into balls.

2. In a small bowl, combine cocoa and coffee granules. Shape chocolate mixture into 1-in. balls; roll in cocoa mixture. Store in an airtight container in the refrigerator.

PER SERVING *1 truffle equals 58 cal., 4 g fat (2 g sat. fat), 0 chol., 2 mg sodium, 7 g carb., 1 g fiber, 1 g pro.*

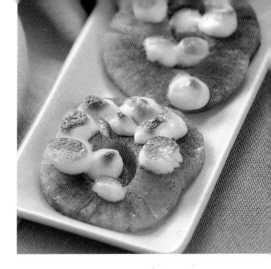

66 CALORIES Banana Chocolate Chip Cookies

These soft cookies have a cakelike texture and lots of banana flavor that folks just seem to love.
—**VICKI RAATZ** WATERLOO, WI

PREP: 20 MIN. • **BAKE:** 10 MIN./BATCH
MAKES: 3 DOZEN

- ⅓ **cup butter, softened**
- ½ **cup sugar**
- 1 **egg**
- ½ **cup mashed ripe banana**
- ½ **teaspoon vanilla extract**
- 1 **cup all-purpose flour**
- 1 **teaspoon baking powder**
- ¼ **teaspoon salt**
- ⅛ **teaspoon baking soda**
- 1 **cup (6 ounces) semisweet chocolate chips**

1. In a small bowl, cream butter and sugar until light and fluffy. Beat in the egg, banana and vanilla. Combine the flour, baking powder, salt and baking soda; gradually add to creamed mixture and mix well. Stir in chocolate chips.
2. Drop by tablespoonfuls 2 in. apart onto baking sheets coated with cooking spray. Bake at 350° for 9-11 minutes or until edges are lightly browned. Remove to wire racks to cool.

PER SERVING *1 cookie equals 66 cal., 3 g fat (2 g sat. fat), 10 mg chol., 51 mg sodium, 9 g carb., trace fiber, 1 g pro.* **Diabetic Exchanges:** *½ starch, ½ fat.*

98 CALORIES Broiled Pineapple Dessert

For that little something sweet after a filling meal, try our scrumptious cinnamon-sprinkled dessert. It couldn't be much easier.
—**TASTE OF HOME TEST KITCHEN**

START TO FINISH: 10 MIN.
MAKES: 2 SERVINGS

- 1 **can (8 ounces) unsweetened sliced pineapple, drained and patted dry**
- 2 **teaspoons brown sugar**
- ¼ **teaspoon ground cinnamon**
- ¼ **cup miniature marshmallows**

1. In an ungreased 9-in. square baking pan, overlap pineapple in two stacks of two slices each. Combine brown sugar and cinnamon; sprinkle over pineapple.
2. Broil 4-6 in. from the heat for 1 to 1½ minutes or until sugar is melted. Top with miniature marshmallows and broil for 1 to 1½ minutes more or until marshmallows are golden brown.

PER SERVING *1 serving equals 98 cal., trace fat (trace sat. fat), 0 chol., 15 mg sodium, 25 g carb., 1 g fiber, trace pro.* **Diabetic Exchanges:** *1 fruit, ½ starch.*

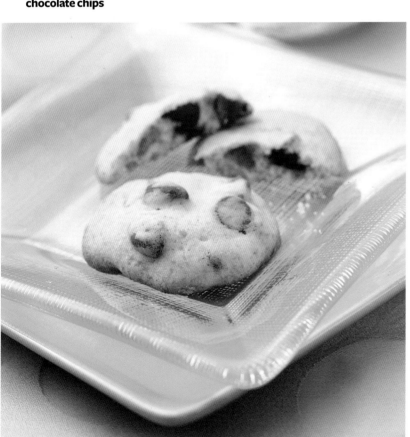

❝ I have learned to love eating lighter because I love how my weight loss has made me feel: fit, strong, proud and healthy! ❞

—JESSICA SANTISTEVAN MARTINEZ

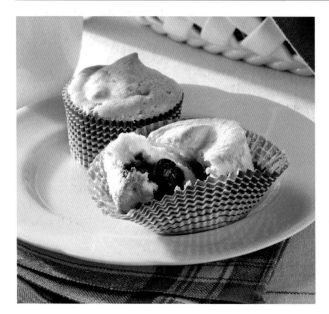

76 CALORIES Blueberry Angel Cupcakes

Like angel food cake, these special cupcakes don't last long at my house. They're so light and airy, they melt in your mouth.
—**KATHY KITTELL** LENEXA, KS

PREP: 25 MIN. • **BAKE:** 15 MIN./BATCH + COOLING
MAKES: 2½ DOZEN

- 11 egg whites
- 1 cup plus 2 tablespoons cake flour
- 1½ cups sugar, divided
- 1¼ teaspoons cream of tartar
- 1 teaspoon vanilla extract
- ½ teaspoon salt
- 1½ cups fresh or frozen blueberries
- 1 teaspoon grated lemon peel
GLAZE
- 1 cup confectioners' sugar
- 3 tablespoons lemon juice

1. Place egg whites in a large bowl; let stand at room temperature for 30 minutes. Sift together flour and ½ cup sugar three times; set aside.
2. Add cream of tartar, vanilla and salt to egg whites; beat on medium speed until soft peaks form. Gradually add remaining sugar, about 2 tablespoons at a time, beating on high until stiff glossy peaks form and sugar is dissolved. Gradually fold in flour mixture, about ½ cup at a time. Fold in blueberries and lemon peel.
3. Fill paper-lined muffin cups three-fourths full. Bake at 375° for 14-17 minutes or until cupcakes spring back when lightly touched. Immediately remove from pans to wire racks to cool completely.
4. In a small bowl, whisk confectioners' sugar and lemon juice until smooth. Brush over cupcakes. Let stand until set.

NOTE *If using frozen blueberries, use without thawing to avoid discoloring the batter.*

PER SERVING *1 cupcake equals 76 cal., trace fat (trace sat. fat), 0 chol., 60 mg sodium, 18 g carb., trace fiber, 2 g pro.* **Diabetic Exchange:** *1 starch.*

65 CALORIES Banana-Chip Mini Cupcakes

These cute little minis are packed with banana flavor, chocolate chips and topped off with a creamy frosting. They make a fast snack when the kids come home from school.
—**BEVERLY COYDE** GASPORT, NY

PREP: 30 MIN. • **BAKE:** 15 MIN. + COOLING • **MAKES:** 3½ DOZEN

- 1 package (14 ounces) banana quick bread and muffin mix
- ¾ cup water
- ⅓ cup sour cream
- 1 egg
- 1 cup miniature semisweet chocolate chips, divided
- 1 tablespoon shortening

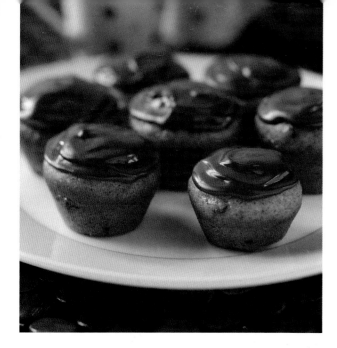

1. In a large bowl, combine the muffin mix, water, sour cream and egg; stir just until moistened. Fold in ½ cup chocolate chips.

2. Fill greased or paper-lined miniature muffin cups two-thirds full. Bake at 375° for 12-15 minutes or until a toothpick inserted near the center comes out clean. Cool for 5 minutes before removing from pans to wire racks to cool completely.

3. For frosting, in a microwave-safe bowl, melt the shortening and remaining chocolate chips; stir until smooth. Frost cupcakes.

PER SERVING *1 cupcake equals 65 cal., 2 g fat (1 g sat. fat), 6 mg chol., 57 mg sodium, 10 g carb., trace fiber, 1 g pro.*

92 CALORIES Chunky Fruit 'n' Nut Fudge

Variations on this fudge are endless, but this recipe is my own favorite. Besides five types of chips, it includes everything from dried fruit to nuts. Every bite is packed with flavor and crunch.
—ALLENE BARY-COOPER WICHITA FALLS, TX

PREP: 30 MIN. + STANDING • **MAKES:** 6¾ POUNDS

- 1 package (11 ounces) dried cherries
- 1 cup dried cranberries
- 1½ teaspoons plus ¾ cup butter, softened, divided
- 1 can (14 ounces) sweetened condensed milk
- 1 package (12 ounces) miniature semisweet chocolate chips
- 1 package (11½ ounces) milk chocolate chips
- 1 package (10 to 11 ounces) butterscotch chips
- 1 package (10 ounces) peanut butter chips
- 3 tablespoons heavy whipping cream
- 1 jar (7 ounces) marshmallow creme
- ½ teaspoon almond or rum extract
- 1½ cups unsalted cashew halves
- 1 package (11½ ounces) semisweet chocolate chunks

1. In a large bowl, combine cherries and cranberries. Add enough warm water to cover; set aside. Line a 15-in. x 10-in. x 1-in. pan with foil and grease the foil with 1½ teaspoons butter; set aside.

2. In a large heavy saucepan, melt remaining butter. Stir in the milk, chips and cream. Cook and stir over low heat for 15-20 minutes or until chips are melted and mixture is smooth and blended (mixture will first appear separated, but continue stirring until fully blended). Remove from the heat; stir in marshmallow creme and extract.

3. Drain cherries and cranberries; pat dry with paper towels. Stir the fruit, cashews and chocolate chunks into chocolate mixture. Spread into prepared pan. Let stand at room temperature until set.

4. Using foil, lift fudge out of pan. Discard foil; cut fudge into 1-in. squares.

PER SERVING *1 piece equals 92 cal., 5 g fat (3 g sat. fat), 4 mg chol., 23 mg sodium, 12 g carb., 1 g fiber, 1 g pro.*

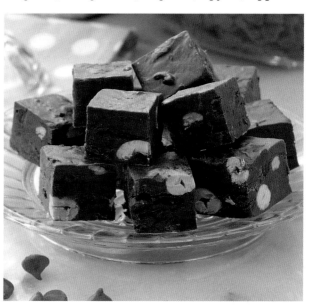

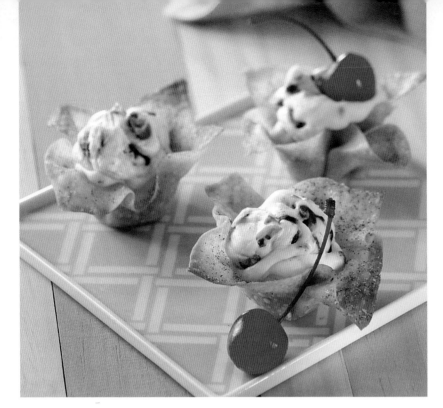

96 CALORIES

Pumpkin Mousse

I guarantee that guests will savor every creamy, smooth spoonful of this spiced autumn dessert. It tastes so good, no one guesses that it's actually low in fat.

—PATRICIA SIDLOSKAS ANNISTON, AL

START TO FINISH: 15 MIN.
MAKES: 4 SERVINGS

- 1½ cups cold fat-free milk
- 1 package (1 ounce) sugar-free instant butterscotch pudding mix
- ½ cup canned pumpkin
- ½ teaspoon ground cinnamon
- ¼ teaspoon ground ginger
- ¼ teaspoon ground allspice
- 1 cup fat-free whipped topping, divided

1. In a large bowl, whisk milk and pudding mix for 2 minutes. Let stand for 2 minutes or until soft-set. Combine the pumpkin, cinnamon, ginger and allspice; fold into pudding. Fold in ½ cup whipped topping.
2. Transfer to individual serving dishes. Refrigerate until serving. Garnish with the remaining whipped topping.

PER SERVING *⅔ cup mousse with 2 tablespoons whipped topping equals 96 cal., trace fat (trace sat. fat), 2 mg chol., 360 mg sodium, 18 g carb., 1 g fiber, 4 g pro.*

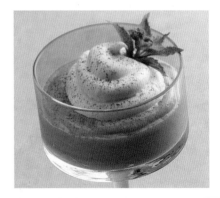

83 CALORIES

Wonton Sundaes

Whether set on appetizer trays or dessert buffets, these irresistible little bites will disappear in no time. I created the recipe by combining two of my favorite treats.

—BETTY JO MORRIS LITTLE ROCK, AR

PREP: 25 MIN. • **BAKE:** 10 MIN. + COOLING
MAKES: 2 DOZEN

- 24 wonton wrappers
  Refrigerated butter-flavored spray
- 1 tablespoon plus ¼ cup sugar, divided
- 1 teaspoon ground cinnamon
- 1 package (8 ounces) reduced-fat cream cheese
- 1 teaspoon vanilla extract
- ¼ cup miniature semisweet chocolate chips
- ¼ cup chopped pecans
- 24 maraschino cherries with stems

1. Place wonton wrappers on a work surface; spritz with the butter-flavored spray. Combine 1 tablespoon sugar and cinnamon; sprinkle over wrappers. Press into miniature muffin cups coated with cooking spray.
2. Bake at 350° for 4-5 minutes or until lightly browned. Immediately remove wonton cups to an ungreased baking sheet. Bake 2-3 minutes longer until bottoms of cups are lightly browned. Remove to a wire rack to cool completely.
3. In a small bowl, beat the cream cheese, vanilla and remaining sugar until smooth. Stir in chocolate chips and pecans. Spoon into wonton cups. Top each with a cherry.

PER SERVING *1 sundae equals 83 cal., 3 g fat (1 g sat. fat), 6 mg chol., 74 mg sodium, 12 g carb., trace fiber, 2 g pro.* **Diabetic Exchanges:** *1 starch, ½ fat.*

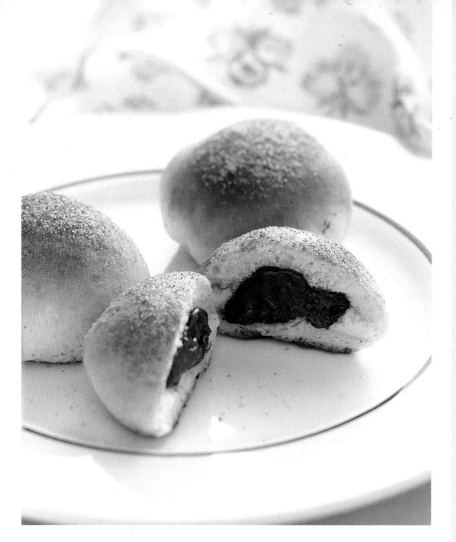

Check out these simple solutions! For other satisfying ideas, see the list of low-calorie snacks—all have 100 calories or less—on pages 84 and 85.

- ½ cup fat-free, sugar-free chocolate frozen yogurt, **100 CALORIES**
- Quaker Chewy Chocolate Chunk Granola Bar, **90 CALORIES**
- 2 Twizzlers strawberry twists, **66 CALORIES**
- Hunt's Fat-Free Snack Pack Tapioca Pudding, **80 CALORIES**
- ⅓ cup Cracker Jack Original Caramel-Coated Popcorn & Peanuts, **79 CALORIES**
- Skinny Cow Mini Fudge Pop, **50 CALORIES**
- McDonald's Kiddie Cone, **45 CALORIES**
- 20 small jelly beans, **82 CALORIES**
- 2 Dove Promises dark chocolate candies, **84 CALORIES**

78 CALORIES

Chocolate Biscuit Puffs

I know my favorite snack is fun for kids to make and eat because I dreamed it up at age 9! The puffs are shaped to hide chocolate inside for a tasty surprise.
—**JOY CLARK** SEABECK, WA

START TO FINISH: 20 MIN.
MAKES: 10 SERVINGS

- 1 **tube (12 ounces) refrigerated flaky buttermilk biscuits**
- 1 **milk chocolate candy bar (1.55 ounces)**
- 2 **teaspoons cinnamon-sugar**

1. Flatten each biscuit into a 3-in. circle. Break candy bar into 10 pieces; place a piece on each biscuit. Bring up edges to enclose candy and pinch to seal.
2. Place on an ungreased baking sheet. Sprinkle with the cinnamon-sugar. Bake at 450° for 8-10 minutes or until golden brown.
PER SERVING *1 puff equals 100 cal., 2 g fat (1 g sat. fat), 1 mg chol., 274 mg sodium, 18 g carb., trace fiber, 3 g pro.*

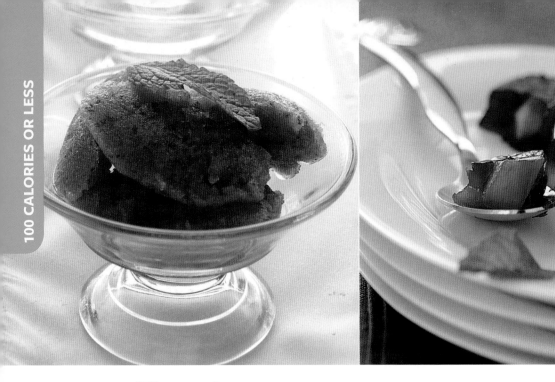

95 CALORIES Watermelon Berry Sorbet

Strawberries, watermelon and fresh mint are practically all you need for this low-fat freezer treat. A friend gave me the recipe, promising it was the ultimate in refreshing summer desserts. I couldn't agree more.

—**JILL SWAVELY** GREEN LANE, PA

PREP: 30 MIN. + FREEZING
MAKES: 6 SERVINGS

- 1 **cup water**
- ½ **cup sugar**
- 2 **cups cubed seedless watermelon**
- 2 **cups fresh strawberries, hulled**
- 1 **tablespoon minced fresh mint**

1. In a small heavy saucepan, bring the water and sugar to a boil. Cook and stir until sugar is dissolved. Remove from the heat; cool slightly.
2. Place the watermelon and strawberries in a blender; add sugar syrup. Cover and process for 2-3 minutes or until smooth. Strain and discard seeds and pulp. Transfer the puree to a 13-in. x 9-in. dish. Freeze for 1 hour or until edges begin to firm.
3. Stir in mint. Freeze 2 hours longer or until firm. Just before serving, transfer to a blender; cover and process for 2-3 minutes or until smooth.
PER SERVING ½ *cup equals 95 cal., trace fat (trace sat. fat), 0 chol., 3 mg sodium, 25 g carb., 2 g fiber, 1 g pro.* **Diabetic Exchanges:** *1 starch, ½ fruit.*

70 CALORIES Apple Cranberry Delight

My husband and I went to a cranberry festival, and I came home with 5 pounds of the berries! Luckily they freeze well and taste great in this sweet and tempting dessert.

—**BEVERLY KOESTER** APPLETON, WI

PREP: 25 MIN. + CHILLING
MAKES: 6 SERVINGS

- 1½ **cups fresh or frozen cranberries**
- 1¾ **cups unsweetened apple juice, divided**
- 1 **package (.3 ounce) sugar-free cranberry gelatin**
- 2 **cups chopped peeled Golden Delicious apples**

1. In a small saucepan, combine cranberries and 1 cup apple juice. Bring to a boil. Reduce heat; cover and simmer for 10-15 minutes or until the berries pop. Stir in gelatin until dissolved. Remove from the heat; stir in apples and remaining apple juice.
2. Pour into a 4-cup mold coated with cooking spray. Refrigerate for 4 hours or until firm. Unmold onto a serving plate.
PER SERVING ½ *cup equals 70 cal., trace fat (trace sat. fat), 0 chol., 42 mg sodium, 16 g carb., 2 g fiber, 1 g pro.* **Diabetic Exchange:** *1 fruit.*

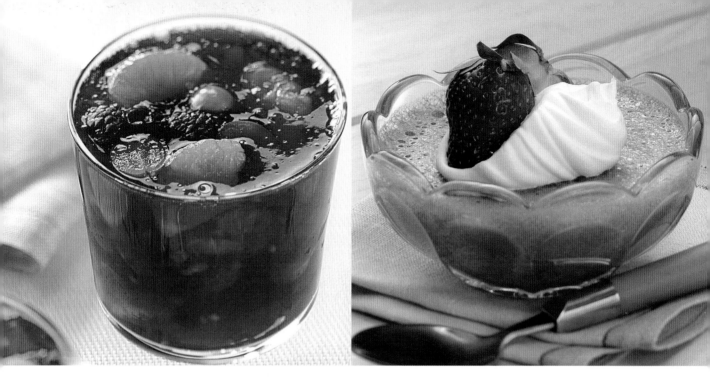

95 CALORIES Sangria Gelatin Dessert

A splash of white wine gives this festive finale a refreshing twist, and the vibrant color dresses up dinners.

—TASTE OF HOME TEST KITCHEN

PREP: 15 MIN. + CHILLING
MAKES: 6 SERVINGS

> 1 package (.3 ounce) sugar-free lemon gelatin
> 1 package (.3 ounce) sugar-free raspberry gelatin
> 1½ cups boiling water
> 1 cup cold water
> 1 cup white wine
> 1 can (11 ounces) mandarin oranges, drained
> 1 cup fresh raspberries
> 1 cup green grapes, halved

In a large bowl, dissolve gelatins in the boiling water. Let stand for 10 minutes. Stir in cold water and wine; refrigerate for 45 minutes or until partially set. Fold in the oranges, raspberries and grapes. Transfer to six large wine glasses, 1 cup in each. Refrigerate for 4 hours or until set.

PER SERVING *1 serving equals 95 cal., trace fat (trace sat. fat), 0 chol., 83 mg sodium, 13 g carb., 2 g fiber, 2 g pro.* **Diabetic Exchange:** *1 fruit.*

78 CALORIES Strawberry Banana Delight

With a classic pairing of fruity flavors, my whipped gelatin is light and refreshing.

—MARY BLACKLEDGE
NORTH PLATTE, NE

PREP: 15 MIN. + CHILLING
MAKES: 4 SERVINGS

> 1 package (.3 ounce) sugar-free strawberry gelatin
> 1 cup boiling water
> 6 ice cubes
> 2 medium ripe bananas, cut into chunks
> 4 tablespoons whipped topping
> 4 fresh strawberries

1. In a small bowl, dissolve the gelatin in boiling water; cool for 10 minutes.

2. Add enough water to ice cubes to measure 1 cup. In a blender, combine gelatin and ice mixture; cover and process for 1 minute or until ice cubes are dissolved. Add bananas; process 1-2 minutes longer or until blended.

3. Pour into four dessert dishes. Refrigerate for at least 30 minutes or until set.

4. Garnish each with 1 tablespoon whipped topping and a strawberry.

PER SERVING *1 serving equals 78 cal., 1 g fat (1 g sat. fat), 0 chol., 48 mg sodium, 16 g carb., 2 g fiber, 2 g pro.* **Diabetic Exchange:** *1 fruit.*

95 CALORIES

Marbled Chocolate Cheesecake Bars

Chocolate and cream cheese are swirled in these yummy bars to create a sensation that's sure to please your sweet tooth and fool it at the same time! This dessert tastes so rich, it's hard to believe it's low in fat.

—JEAN KOMLOS PLYMOUTH, MI

PREP: 20 MIN. • **BAKE:** 20 MIN. + COOLING
MAKES: ABOUT 4 DOZEN

- ¾ cup water
- ⅓ cup butter
- 1½ ounces unsweetened chocolate
- 2 cups all-purpose flour
- 1½ cups packed brown sugar
- 1 teaspoon baking soda
- ½ teaspoon salt
- 1 egg
- 1 egg white
- ½ cup reduced-fat sour cream

CREAM CHEESE MIXTURE

- 1 package (8 ounces) reduced-fat cream cheese
- ⅓ cup sugar
- 1 egg white
- 1 tablespoon vanilla extract
- 1 cup (6 ounces) miniature semisweet chocolate chips

1. In a small saucepan, combine the water, butter and chocolate. Cook and stir over low heat until melted; stir until smooth. Cool.

2. In a large bowl, combine the flour, brown sugar, baking soda and salt. Beat in the egg, egg white and sour cream on low speed just until combined. Beat in chocolate mixture until smooth. In another bowl, beat the cream cheese, sugar, egg white and vanilla until smooth; set aside.

3. Spread chocolate batter into a 15-in. x 10-in. x 1-in. baking pan coated with cooking spray. Drop the cream cheese mixture by tablespoonfuls over batter; cut through batter with a knife to swirl. Sprinkle with chocolate chips.

4. Bake at 375° for 20-25 minutes or until a toothpick inserted near the center comes out clean. Cool on a wire rack.

PER SERVING *1 bar equals 95 cal., 4 g fat (2 g sat. fat), 10 mg chol., 90 mg sodium, 15 g carb., trace fiber, 2 g pro.* **Diabetic Exchanges:** *1 starch, ½ fat.*

84 CALORIES Lemon Pudding Cups

This make-ahead recipe is a favorite from my mother's church cookbook. The texture is so light and satisfying, and a touch of tart lemon is always wonderful after dinner.

—DOLLY JONES HIGHLAND, IN

PREP: 10 MIN. + CHILLING • **MAKES:** 6 SERVINGS

- 1 package (.3 ounce) sugar-free lemon gelatin
- 2 cups boiling water
- 1 pint lemon sherbet, softened
- 1 tablespoon lemon juice
- 1 tablespoon grated lemon peel
- 6 tablespoons reduced-fat whipped topping

In a large bowl, dissolve gelatin in boiling water. Slowly stir in the sherbet, lemon juice and lemon peel. Pour into six dessert cups. Cover and refrigerate overnight. Garnish with whipped topping.

PER SERVING *½ cup with 1 tablespoon whipped topping equals 84 cal., 1 g fat (1 g sat. fat), 3 mg chol., 56 mg sodium, 16 g carb., 0.55 g fiber, 1 g pro.* **Diabetic Exchange:** *1 starch.*

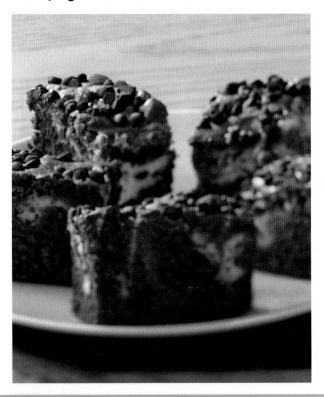

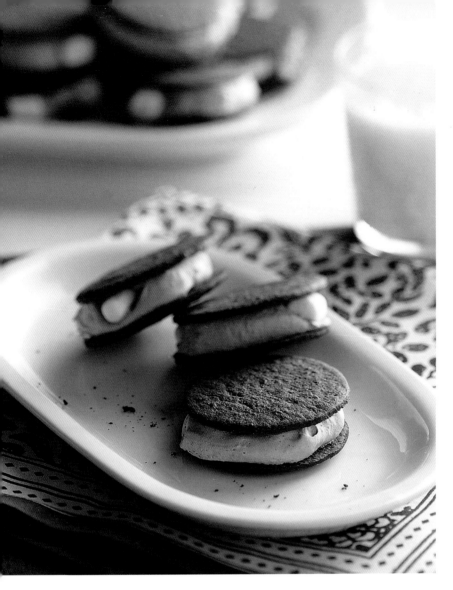

2 tablespoons of pudding mixture on the bottom of a chocolate wafer; top with another wafer. Stack sandwiches in an airtight container.

3. Freeze until firm, about 3 hours. Remove from the freezer 5 minutes before serving.

PER SERVING *1 sandwich equals 73 cal., 2 g fat (1 g sat. fat), 1 mg chol., 114 mg sodium, 12 g carb., 1 g fiber, 1 g pro.* **Diabetic** **Exchange:** *1 starch.*

87 CALORIES Cookout Caramel S'mores

These gooey treats make a great finish to an informal meal. Toasting the marshmallows extends our after-dinner time together, giving us something fun to do as a family.

—**MARTHA HASEMAN** HINCKLEY, IL

START TO FINISH: 10 MIN.
MAKES: 4 SERVINGS

- 8 **large marshmallows**
- 2 **teaspoons fat-free chocolate syrup**
- 4 **whole reduced-fat graham crackers, halved**
- 2 **teaspoons fat-free caramel ice cream topping**

Using a long-handled fork, toast marshmallows 6 in. from medium-hot heat until golden brown, turning occasionally. Drizzle chocolate syrup over four graham crackers; top each with two toasted marshmallows. Drizzle with caramel topping. Cover with remaining graham crackers.

PER SERVING *1 s'more equals 87 cal., 1 g fat (1 g sat. fat), 1 mg chol., 82 mg sodium, 20 g carb., 1 g fiber, 1 g pro.* **Diabetic Exchange:** *1 starch.*

73 CALORIES Chocolate Pudding Sandwiches

Frozen cookie sandwiches are one of my kids' favorite desserts and after-school snacks...and even my diabetic husband enjoys one now and then!

—**JAN THOMAS** RICHMOND, VA

PREP: 15 MIN. + FREEZING
MAKES: 43 SANDWICHES

- 1½ **cups cold fat-free milk**
- 1 **package (1.4 ounces) sugar-free instant chocolate pudding mix**
- 1 **carton (8 ounces) frozen reduced-fat whipped topping, thawed**
- 1 **cup miniature marshmallows**
- 2 **packages (9 ounces each) chocolate wafers**

1. In a large bowl, whisk milk and pudding mix for 2 minutes; let stand for 2 minutes or until slightly thickened. Fold in whipped topping, then marshmallows.

2. For each sandwich, spread about

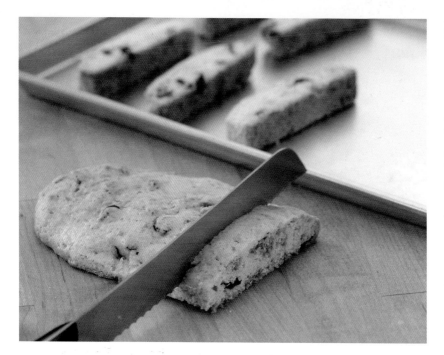

60 CALORIES

Frozen Fruit Pops

My grandson, Patrick, has been Grammy's Helper for years. Recently, we made these fun little pops for company and everyone, including the adults, loved them. They're as delicious as they are good for you!

—**JUNE DICKENSON** PHILIPPI, WV

PREP: 15 MIN. + FREEZING
MAKES: 1 DOZEN

- 2¼ cups (18 ounces) raspberry yogurt
- 2 tablespoons lemon juice
- 2 medium ripe bananas, cut into chunks
- 12 Popsicle molds or paper cups (3 ounces each) and Popsicle sticks

1. In a blender, combine the yogurt, lemon juice and bananas; cover and process for 45 seconds or until smooth. Stir if necessary.

2. Fill molds or cups with ¼ cup yogurt mixture; top with holders or insert sticks into cups. Freeze.

PER SERVING *1 fruit pop equals 60 cal., 1 g fat (trace sat. fat), 2 mg chol., 23 mg sodium, 13 g carb., 1 g fiber, 2 g pro.* ***Diabetic Exchange:*** *1 starch.*

66 CALORIES

Lemon Anise Biscotti

With the growing popularity of gourmet coffees, cappuccino and espresso, I'm finding that lots of people enjoy these classic Sicilian dippers.

—**CARRIE SHERRILL** FORESTVILLE, WI

PREP: 25 MIN. • **BAKE:** 40 MIN. + COOLING
MAKES: 3 DOZEN

- 2 eggs
- 1 cup sugar
- ¼ cup canola oil
- ½ teaspoon lemon extract
- ¼ teaspoon vanilla extract
- 2 cups all-purpose flour
- 1 teaspoon baking powder
- ½ teaspoon salt
- 4 teaspoons grated lemon peel
- 2 teaspoons aniseed, crushed

1. In a small bowl, beat eggs and sugar for 2 minutes or until thickened. Add oil and extracts; mix well. Combine the flour, baking powder and salt; beat into egg mixture. Beat in lemon peel and aniseed.

2. Divide dough in half. On a lightly floured surface, shape each portion into a 12-in. x 2-in. rectangle. Transfer to a baking sheet lined with parchment paper. Flatten to ½-in. thickness.

3. Bake at 350° for 30-35 minutes or until golden and tops begin to crack. Carefully remove to wire racks; cool for 5 minutes.

4. Transfer to a cutting board; cut with a serrated knife into scant ¾-in. slices. Place cut side down on ungreased baking sheets. Bake for 5 minutes. Turn and bake 5-7 minutes longer or until firm and golden brown. Remove biscotti to wire racks to cool. Store in an airtight container.

PER SERVING *1 cookie equals 66 cal., 2 g fat (trace sat. fat), 12 mg chol., 48 mg sodium, 11 g carb., trace fiber, 1 g pro.* ***Diabetic Exchanges:*** *½ starch, ½ fat.*

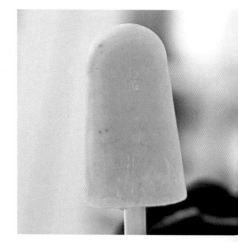

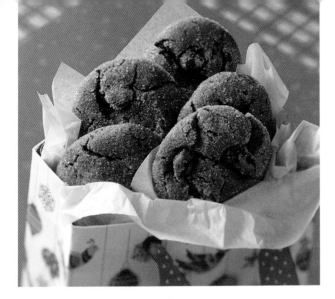

69 CALORIES Chocolate Gingersnaps

When my daughter, Jennifer, was 15 years old, she created this recipe as a way to combine two of her favorite flavors. They're great with a glass of milk.
—**PAULA ZSIRAY** LOGAN, UTAH

PREP: 45 MIN. + CHILLING • **BAKE:** 10 MIN./BATCH
MAKES: 3 DOZEN

- ½ **cup butter, softened**
- ½ **cup packed dark brown sugar**
- ¼ **cup molasses**
- 1 **tablespoon water**
- 2 **teaspoons minced fresh gingerroot**
- 1½ **cups all-purpose flour**
- 1 **tablespoon baking cocoa**
- 1¼ **teaspoons ground ginger**
- 1 **teaspoon baking soda**
- 1 **teaspoon ground cinnamon**
- ¼ **teaspoon ground nutmeg**
- ¼ **teaspoon ground cloves**
- 7 **ounces semisweet chocolate, finely chopped**
- ¼ **cup sugar**

1. In a large bowl, cream butter and brown sugar until light and fluffy. Beat in the molasses, water and gingerroot. Combine the flour, cocoa, ginger, baking soda, cinnamon, nutmeg and cloves; gradually add to creamed mixture and mix well. Stir in chocolate. Cover and refrigerate for 2 hours or until easy to handle.
2. Shape dough into 1-in. balls; roll in sugar. Place 2 in. apart on greased baking sheets.

3. Bake at 350° for 10-12 minutes or until tops begin to crack. Cool for 2 minutes before removing to wire racks.
PER SERVING *1 cookie equals 69 cal., 3 g fat (2 g sat. fat), 7 mg chol., 63 mg sodium, 11 g carb., trace fiber, 1 g pro.*

80 CALORIES Sangria Gelatin Ring

This refreshing gelatin is enjoyed by everyone because you just can't go wrong with so many luscious berries!
—**NICOLE NEMETH** KOMOKA, ON

PREP: 15 MIN. + CHILLING • **MAKES:** 10 SERVINGS

- 2 **packages (3 ounces each) lemon gelatin**
- 1½ **cups boiling white wine or white grape juice**
- 2 **cups club soda, chilled**
- 1 **cup sliced fresh strawberries**
- 1 **cup fresh or frozen blueberries**
- 1 **cup fresh or frozen raspberries**
- ½ **cup green grapes, halved**

1. In a large bowl, dissolve gelatin in boiling wine or grape juice; cool for 10 minutes. Stir in club soda; refrigerate until set but not firm, about 45 minutes.
2. Fold in the berries and grapes. Pour into a 6-cup ring mold coated with cooking spray. Refrigerate for 4 hours or until set. Invert and unmold onto a serving platter.
PER SERVING *1 slice equals 80 cal., trace fat (trace sat. fat), 0 chol., 32 mg sodium, 14 g carb., 2 g fiber, 1 g pro.*

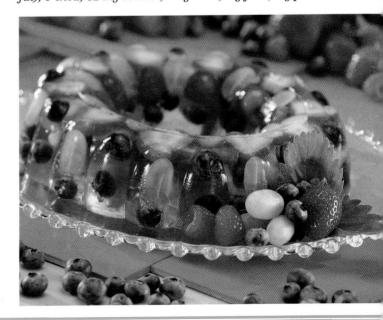

101-150 CALORIES

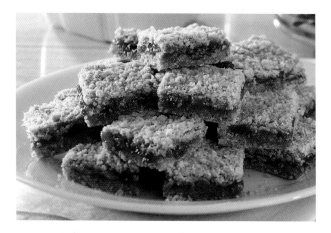

147 CALORIES Apricot Date Squares

Memories of my mom's fruity date bars inspired me to devise this wonderful treat. I've had great results replacing the apricot jam with orange marmalade, too.
—**SHANNON KOENE** BLACKSBURG, VA

PREP: 45 MIN. • **BAKE:** 20 MIN. + COOLING • **MAKES:** 3 DOZEN

- 1 cup water
- 1 cup sugar
- 1 cup chopped dates
- ½ cup 100% apricot spreadable fruit or jam
- 1¾ cups old-fashioned oats
- 1½ cups all-purpose flour
- 1 cup flaked coconut
- 1 cup packed brown sugar
- 1 teaspoon ground cinnamon
- ¼ teaspoon salt
- ¾ cup cold butter, cubed

1. In a small saucepan, combine the water, sugar and dates. Bring to a boil. Reduce heat; simmer, uncovered, for 30-35 minutes or until mixture is reduced to 1⅓ cups and is slightly thickened, stirring occasionally.
2. Remove from the heat. Stir in spreadable fruit until blended; set aside. In a food processor, combine the oats, flour, coconut, brown sugar, cinnamon and salt.

Add butter; cover and process until mixture resembles coarse crumbs.
3. Press 3 cups crumb mixture into a 13-in. x 9-in. baking dish coated with cooking spray. Spread date mixture to within ½ in. of edges. Sprinkle with remaining crumb mixture; press down gently.
4. Bake at 350° for 20-25 minutes or until edges are lightly browned. Cool on a wire rack. Cut into squares.
PER SERVING *1 bar equals 147 cal., 5 g fat (3 g sat. fat), 10 mg chol., 65 mg sodium, 25 g carb., 1 g fiber, 1 g pro.* **Diabetic Exchanges:** *1½ starch, 1 fat.*

114 CALORIES Granola Fudge Clusters

Short and sweet, my recipe for these tasty little bites uses only four ingredients. I always make a double batch because no one can eat just one.
—**LORAINE MEYER** BEND, OR

START TO FINISH: 25 MIN. • **MAKES:** ABOUT 2½ DOZEN

- 1 cup (6 ounces) semisweet chocolate chips
- 1 cup butterscotch chips
- 1¼ cups granola cereal without raisins
- 1 cup chopped walnuts

1. In a microwave-safe bowl, melt the chocolate and butterscotch chips; stir until smooth. Stir in granola and walnuts.
2. Drop by tablespoonfuls onto waxed paper-lined baking sheets. Refrigerate for 15 minutes or until firm.
PER SERVING *1 fudge cluster equals 114 cal., 7 g fat (3 g sat. fat), trace chol., 9 mg sodium, 12 g carb., 1 g fiber, 2 g pro.*

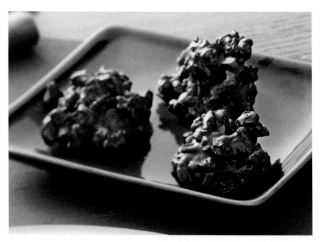

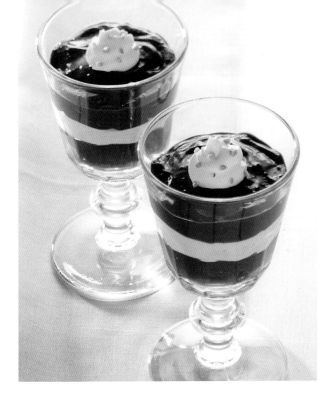

146 CALORIES

Chocolate Peanut Butter Parfaits

When a friend gave me this dessert and recipe, I knew it was a keeper. It's easy, low-calorie, low-fat, and it's pretty, to boot! You absolutely won't believe that this sweet is light.
—**PAT SOLOMAN** CASPER, WY

PREP: 20 MIN. + CHILLING • **MAKES:** 6 SERVINGS

- 2 **tablespoons reduced-fat chunky peanut butter**
- 2 **tablespoons plus 2 cups cold fat-free milk, divided**
- 1 **cup plus 6 tablespoons reduced-fat whipped topping, divided**
- 1 **package (1.4 ounces) sugar-free instant chocolate fudge pudding mix**
- 3 **tablespoons finely chopped salted peanuts**

1. In a small bowl, combine the peanut butter and 2 tablespoons milk. Fold in 1 cup whipped topping; set aside. In another small bowl, whisk remaining milk with the pudding mix for 2 minutes. Let stand for 2 minutes or until soft-set.

2. Spoon half of the pudding into six parfait glasses or dessert dishes. Layer with reserved peanut butter mixture and remaining pudding. Refrigerate for at least 1 hour. Refrigerate remaining whipped topping.

3. Just before serving, garnish each parfait with 1 tablespoon of whipped topping and 1½ teaspoons of chopped peanuts.

PER SERVING *1 parfait equals 146 cal., 6 g fat (3 g sat. fat), 2 mg chol., 300 mg sodium, 16 g carb., 1 g fiber, 6 g pro.* **Diabetic Exchanges:** *1 fat, ½ starch, ½ fat-free milk.*

105 CALORIES # Fruity Cereal Bars

With dried apple and cranberries, these crispy cereal bars are ideal for snacks or brown-bag lunches.
—**GIOVANNA KRANENBERG** CAMBRIDGE, MN

START TO FINISH: 30 MIN. • **MAKES:** 20 SERVINGS

- 3 **tablespoons butter**
- 1 **package (10 ounces) large marshmallows**
- 6 **cups crisp rice cereal**
- ½ **cup chopped dried apple**
- ½ **cup dried cranberries**

1. In a large saucepan, combine the butter and marshmallows. Cook and stir over medium-low heat until melted. Remove from the heat; stir in the cereal, apple and cranberries.

2. Pat into a 13-in. x 9-in. pan coated with cooking spray; cool. Cut into squares.

PER SERVING *1 bar equals 105 cal., 2 g fat (1 g sat. fat), 5 mg chol., 102 mg sodium, 22 g carb., trace fiber, 1 g pro.* **Diabetic Exchanges:** *1½ starch, ½ fat.*

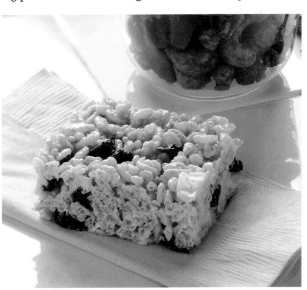

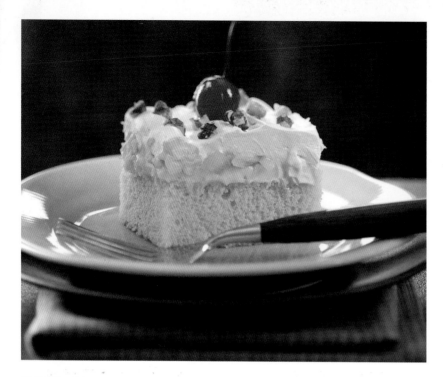

Vanilla Tapioca Pudding

As a widower, I've recently started to learn how to cook. I created this tapioca pudding that's not only low in fat, but easy to make, too.

—ROBERT DAGGIT SHOREVIEW, MN

PREP: 10 MIN. + CHILLING
MAKES: 4 SERVINGS

- 3¼ cups fat-free milk
- 2 tablespoons quick-cooking tapioca
- 2 tablespoons sugar
- 1 package (.8 ounce) cook-and-serve vanilla pudding mix
- ¼ teaspoon vanilla extract

1. In a large saucepan, combine the milk, tapioca, sugar and pudding mix. Bring to a boil, stirring constantly. Remove from the heat; stir in vanilla.
2. Spoon into four dessert dishes. Cover and refrigerate for 2 hours before serving.
PER SERVING *¾ cup equals 133 cal., trace fat (trace sat. fat), 4 mg chol., 118 mg sodium, 26 g carb., trace fiber, 7 g pro.* **Diabetic Exchanges:** *1 starch, 1 fat-free milk.*

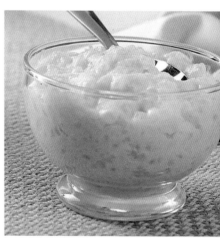

Pineapple Pudding Cake

My mother used to love making this easy dessert in the summertime. It's so cool and refreshing that it never lasts long!

—KATHLEEN WORDEN
NORTH ANDOVER, MA

PREP: 25 MIN. • **BAKE:** 15 MIN. + CHILLING
MAKES: 20 SERVINGS

- 1 package (9 ounces) yellow cake mix
- 1½ cups cold fat-free milk
- 1 package (1 ounce) sugar-free instant vanilla pudding mix
- 1 package (8 ounces) fat-free cream cheese
- 1 can (20 ounces) unsweetened crushed pineapple, well drained
- 1 carton (8 ounces) frozen fat-free whipped topping, thawed
- ¼ cup chopped walnuts, toasted
- 20 maraschino cherries, well drained

1. Prepare the cake mix batter according to package directions; pour into a 13-in. x 9-in. baking pan coated with cooking spray.
2. Bake at 350° for 15-20 minutes or until a toothpick inserted near the center comes out clean. Cool completely on a wire rack.
3. In a large bowl, whisk milk and pudding mix for 2 minutes. Let stand for 2 minutes or until soft-set.
4. In a small bowl, beat the cream cheese until smooth. Beat in the pudding mixture until blended. Spread evenly over cake. Sprinkle with pineapple; spread with the whipped topping. Sprinkle with walnuts and garnish with cherries. Refrigerate until serving.
PER SERVING *1 piece equals 131 cal., 2 g fat (1 g sat. fat), 1 mg chol., 217 mg sodium, 24 g carb., 1 g fiber, 3 g pro.* **Diabetic Exchange:** *1½ starch.*

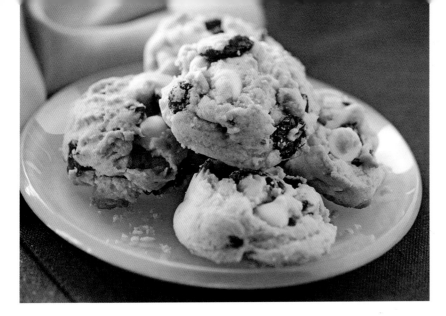

White Chocolate Cranberry Cookies

The red and white coloring in these sweet cookies makes them a festive addition to any cookie tray. The pairing of tart cranberry with rich, buttery white chocolate is a real classic.
—**DONNA BECK** SCOTTDALE, PA

PREP: 20 MIN. • **BAKE:** 10 MIN./BATCH
MAKES: 2 DOZEN

- ⅓ cup butter, softened
- ½ cup packed brown sugar
- ⅓ cup sugar
- 1 egg
- 1 teaspoon vanilla extract
- 1½ cups all-purpose flour
- ½ teaspoon salt
- ½ teaspoon baking soda
- ¾ cup dried cranberries
- ½ cup white baking chips

1. In a large bowl, beat butter and sugars until crumbly, about 2 minutes. Beat in egg and vanilla. Combine the flour, salt and baking soda; gradually add to the butter mixture and mix well. Stir in the cranberries and chips.

2. Drop by heaping tablespoonfuls 2 in. apart onto baking sheets coated with cooking spray. Bake at 375° for 8-10 minutes or until lightly browned. Cool for 1 minute before removing to wire racks.
PER SERVING *1 cookie equals 113 cal., 4 g fat (2 g sat. fat), 16 mg chol., 109 mg sodium, 18 g carb., trace fiber, 1 g pro.* ***Diabetic Exchanges:*** *1 starch, ½ fat.*

Lemon Fluff Dessert

This came from my grandmother, whose family owned a bakery. Since Grandma's version was full-fat and I didn't want to mess with perfection too much, I only made a few healthier substitutions. Now it's sweet, lemony, light and wonderful!
—**NANCY BROWN** DAHINDA, IL

PREP: 15 MIN. + CHILLING
MAKES: 20 SERVINGS

- 1 can (12 ounces) evaporated milk
- 1½ cups graham cracker crumbs
- ⅓ cup butter, melted
- 1 package (.3 ounce) sugar-free lemon gelatin
- 1 cup boiling water
- 3 tablespoons lemon juice
- 1 package (8 ounces) reduced-fat cream cheese
- ¾ cup sugar
- 1 teaspoon vanilla extract

1. Pour milk into a large metal bowl; place mixer beaters in the bowl. Cover and refrigerate for at least 2 hours.

2. In a small bowl, combine graham cracker crumbs and butter; set aside 1 tablespoon for topping. Press the remaining crumb mixture into a 13-in. x 9-in. baking dish. Refrigerate until set.

3. Meanwhile, in a small bowl, dissolve gelatin in boiling water. Stir in lemon juice; cool.

4. In another bowl, beat the cream cheese, sugar and vanilla until smooth. Add gelatin mixture and mix well. Beat evaporated milk until soft peaks form; fold into the cream cheese mixture. Pour over crust. Sprinkle with reserved crumbs. Refrigerate for at least 2 hours before serving.
PER SERVING *1 piece equals 135 cal., 7 g fat (4 g sat. fat), 21 mg chol., 136 mg sodium, 15 g carb., trace fiber, 3 g pro.* ***Diabetic Exchanges:*** *1 starch, 1 fat.*

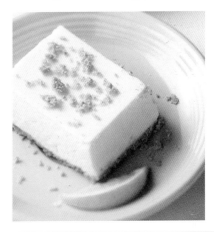

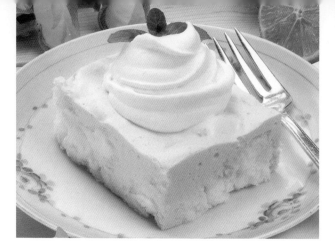

138 CALORIES Lemon Sorbet

Whether you serve it in chilled bowls or scooped into cut lemon halves, this creamy four-ingredient sorbet is both sweet and tart. It makes a delightful finish to any meal.

—**GOLDENE PETERSEN** BRIGHAM CITY, UTAH

PREP: 15 MIN. + COOLING • **PROCESS:** 20 MIN. + FREEZING
MAKES: 2 CUPS

- 1 cup sugar
- 1 cup water
- ¾ cup lemon juice
- 3 tablespoons grated lemon peel

1. In a small saucepan over medium heat, cook and stir sugar and water until mixture comes to a boil. Reduce heat; simmer, uncovered, for 2 minutes. Remove from the heat; cool to room temperature.

2. Stir in lemon juice and lemon peel. Freeze in an ice cream freezer according to manufacturer's directions. Transfer to a freezer container; freeze for at least 4 hours before serving.

PER SERVING ⅓ cup equals 138 cal., trace fat (trace sat. fat), 0 chol., 1 mg sodium, 36 g carb., trace fiber, trace pro. **Diabetic Exchange:** 2 starch.

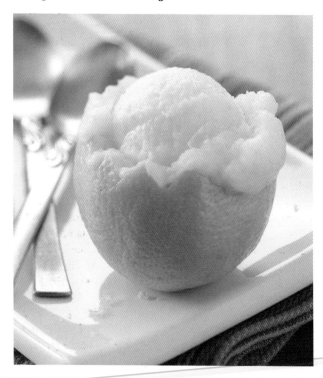

139 CALORIES

Luscious Lime Angel Squares

A creamy lime topping turns angel food cake into these yummy squares that are perfect for potlucks or picnics. You can eat a piece without feeling one bit guilty! I adapted this luscious treat from another recipe. It's super-easy to make.

—**BEVERLY MARSHALL** ORTING, WA

PREP: 15 MIN. + CHILLING • **MAKES:** 15 SERVINGS

- 1 package (.3 ounce) sugar-free lime gelatin
- 1 cup boiling water
- 1 prepared angel food cake (8 inches), cut into 1-inch cubes
- 1 package (8 ounces) reduced-fat cream cheese, cubed
- ½ cup sugar
- 2 teaspoons lemon juice
- 1½ teaspoons grated lemon peel
- 1 carton (8 ounces) reduced-fat whipped topping, thawed, divided

1. In a small bowl, dissolve gelatin in boiling water. Refrigerate until mixture just begins to thicken, about 35 minutes. Place cake cubes in a 13-in. x 9-in. dish coated with cooking spray; set aside.

2. In a small bowl, beat cream cheese until smooth. Beat in the sugar, lemon juice and peel. Add gelatin mixture; beat until combined. Fold in 1½ cups of whipped topping.

3. Spread over top of cake, covering completely. Refrigerate for at least 2 hours or until firm. Cut into squares; top with remaining whipped topping.

PER SERVING 1 piece equals 139 cal., 4 g fat (3 g sat. fat), 8 mg chol., 145 mg sodium, 21 g carb., trace fiber, 3 g pro. **Diabetic Exchanges:** 1½ starch, 1 fat.

110 CALORIES Mixed Berry Pizza

The fresh fruit shines through in this colorful dessert pizza. It's also a tempting appetizer at parties because it's a nice change of pace from the usual savory options.
—GRETCHEN WIDNER SUN CITY WEST, AZ

PREP: 10 MIN. • **BAKE:** 10 MIN. + CHILLING • **MAKES:** 20 SERVINGS

- 1 tube (8 ounces) refrigerated reduced-fat crescent rolls
- 11 ounces reduced-fat cream cheese
- ½ cup apricot preserves
- 2 tablespoons confectioners' sugar
- 2 cups sliced fresh strawberries
- 1 cup fresh blueberries
- 1 cup fresh raspberries

1. Unroll crescent roll dough and place in a 15-in. x 10-in. x 1-in. baking pan coated with cooking spray. Press onto the bottom and 1 in. up the sides of pan to form a crust; seal seams and perforations. Bake at 375° for 8-10 minutes or until golden. Cool completely.
2. In a large bowl, beat cream cheese until smooth. Beat in the preserves and confectioners' sugar; spread over crust. Cover and refrigerate for 1-2 hours.
3. Just before serving, arrange berries on top. Cut into 20 pieces.
PER SERVING *1 piece equals 110 cal., 5 g fat (2 g sat. fat), 9 mg chol., 143 mg sodium, 15 g carb., 1 g fiber, 3 g pro.* **Diabetic Exchanges:** *1 fruit, ½ starch.*

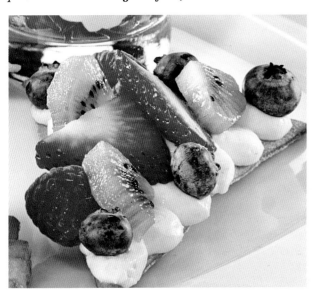

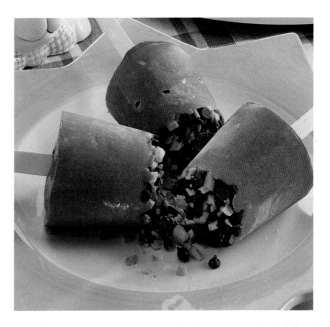

145 CALORIES Rocky Road Treat

On a hot day, these refreshing frozen pops are simple to prepare and guaranteed to bring out the kid in anyone. You won't be able to resist the chocolate and peanut topping!
—KAREN GRANT TULARE, CA

PREP: 15 MIN. + FREEZING • **MAKES:** 12 SERVINGS

- 1 package (3.4 ounces) cook-and-serve chocolate pudding mix
- 2½ cups whole milk
- ½ cup chopped peanuts
- ½ cup miniature semisweet chocolate chips
- 12 disposable plastic cups (3 ounces each)
- ½ cup marshmallow creme
- 12 Popsicle sticks

1. In a large microwave-safe bowl, combine pudding mix and milk. Microwave, uncovered, on high for 4-6 minutes or until bubbly and slightly thickened, stirring every 2 minutes. Cool for 20 minutes, stirring often.
2. Meanwhile, combine peanuts and chocolate chips; place about 2 tablespoons in each plastic cup. Stir marshmallow creme into pudding; spoon into cups. Insert Popsicle sticks; freeze.
NOTE *This recipe was tested in a 1,100-watt microwave.*
PER SERVING *1 pop equals 145 cal., 7 g fat (3 g sat. fat), 7 mg chol., 89 mg sodium, 19 g carb., 1 g fiber, 4 g pro.* **Diabetic Exchanges:** *1 starch, 1 fat.*

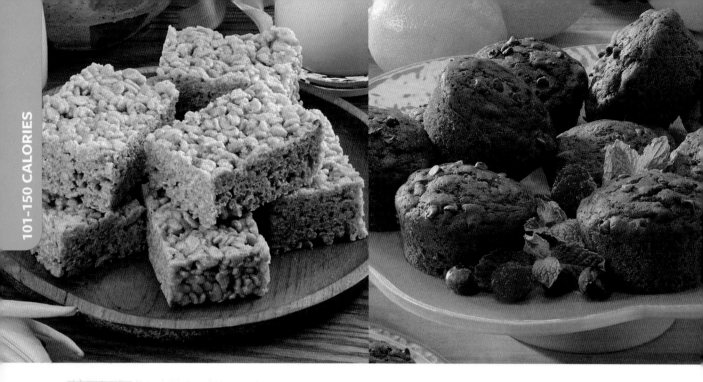

144 CALORIES
Honey-Peanut Crispy Bars

My daughters have loved these healthy snacks since they were in grade school. Now, both are adults and still make these bars when they want a quick treat.
—**URSULA MAURER** WAUWATOSA, WI

START TO FINISH: 30 MIN.
MAKES: 1 DOZEN

- ½ cup honey
- ½ cup reduced-fat chunky peanut butter
- ½ cup nonfat dry milk powder
- 4 cups Rice Krispies

1. In a large saucepan, combine the honey, peanut butter and milk powder. Cook and stir over low heat until blended.

2. Remove from the heat; stir in cereal. Press into an 8-in. square dish coated with cooking spray. Let stand until set. Cut into bars.

PER SERVING *1 bar equals 144 cal.,* 4 g fat (1 g sat. fat), 1 mg chol., 144 mg sodium, 25 g carb., 1 g fiber, 5 g pro. *Diabetic Exchanges: 1½ starch, ½ fat.*

139 CALORIES
Double Chocolate Cupcakes

These tender little cupcakes are chock-full of sweet flavor, yet each has only 139 calories and 2 grams of fat.
—**LINDA UTTER** SIDNEY, MT

PREP: 20 MIN. • **BAKE:** 15 MIN. + COOLING
MAKES: 14 CUPCAKES

- 2 tablespoons butter, softened
- ¾ cup sugar
- 1 egg
- 1 egg white
- ½ cup plus 2 tablespoons buttermilk
- ⅓ cup water
- 1 tablespoon white vinegar
- 1 teaspoon vanilla extract
- 1½ cups all-purpose flour
- ¼ cup baking cocoa
- 1 teaspoon baking soda
- ½ teaspoon salt
- ⅓ cup miniature semisweet chocolate chips

1. In a large bowl, beat butter and sugar until crumbly, about 2 minutes. Add egg, then egg white, beating well after each addition. Beat on high speed until light and fluffy. Beat in the buttermilk, water, vinegar and vanilla. Combine flour, cocoa, baking soda and salt; beat into batter just until moistened. Stir in chocolate chips.

2. Fill muffin cups coated with cooking spray three-fourths full. Bake at 375° for 15-18 minutes or until a toothpick inserted in the muffin comes out clean. Cool for 5 minutes before removing from pans to wire racks.

PER SERVING *1 cupcake equals 139 cal., 2 g fat (1 g sat. fat), 1 mg chol., 221 mg sodium, 29 g carb., 1 g fiber, 3 g pro. Diabetic Exchanges: 1½ starch, ½ fat.*

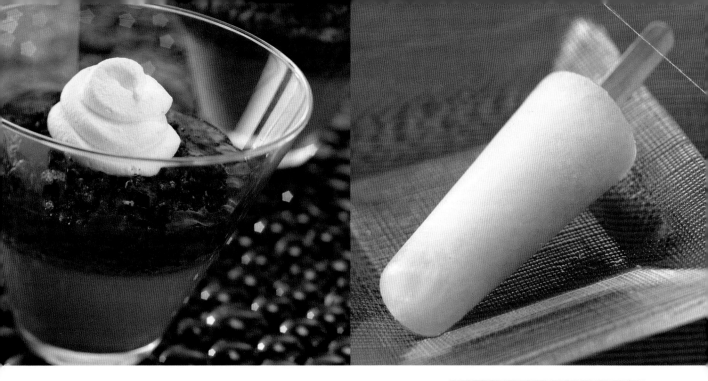

146 CALORIES Cherry Chocolate Parfaits

Here's a refreshing layered dessert that looks and tastes special. Families will go for this budget-friendly blend of chocolate cookies, cherry gelatin and creamy topping.

—TASTE OF HOME TEST KITCHEN

PREP: 15 MIN. + CHILLING
MAKES: 4 SERVINGS

- 1 package (.3 ounce) sugar-free cherry gelatin
- 1 cup boiling water
- ½ cup reduced-fat sour cream
- ¼ teaspoon almond extract
- ½ cup diet lemon-lime soda
- 8 reduced-fat Oreo cookies, crushed
- ¼ cup reduced-fat whipped topping

1. In a small bowl, dissolve gelatin in boiling water. Transfer ½ cup to another bowl; stir in sour cream and extract. Divide among four parfait glasses or dessert dishes.

Refrigerate until firm, about 35 minutes. Stir soda into the remaining gelatin; cover and refrigerate until partially set.
2. To assemble, sprinkle half of the cookies over cherry layer. Top with soda mixture and the remaining cookies. Refrigerate until firm. Just before serving, dollop each serving with whipped topping.

PER SERVING *1 parfait equals 146 cal., 5 g fat (3 g sat. fat), 10 mg chol., 207 mg sodium, 20 g carb., 1 g fiber, 4 g pro.* **Diabetic Exchanges:** *1 starch, 1 fat.*

149 CALORIES Fruit Juice Pops

I found that my children enjoyed these pops more than any store-bought ones I ever brought home. They taste great with either pineapple or orange juice. Try freezing and serving in cups made from hollowed-out oranges.

—BARBARA STEWART GARLAND, TX

PREP: 25 MIN. + FREEZING
MAKES: 1 DOZEN

- 2 cups water
- 1½ cups sugar
- 4 cups unsweetened apple juice
- 1 cup unsweetened pineapple or orange juice
- ½ cup lemon juice
- 12 Popsicle molds or paper cups (3 ounces each) and Popsicle sticks

1. In a large saucepan, combine water and sugar; bring to a boil. Reduce heat; simmer, uncovered, for 3-4 minutes or until sugar is dissolved, stirring occasionally. Remove from the heat; stir in juices.
2. Fill molds or cups with ¼ cup juice mixture; top with holders or insert sticks into cups. Freeze.

PER SERVING *1 juice pop equals 149 cal., trace fat (trace sat. fat), 0 chol., 3 mg sodium, 38 g carb., trace fiber, trace pro.*

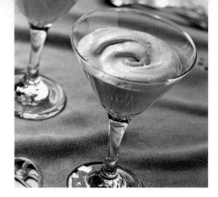

133 CALORIES

Chunky Pecan Bars

The first time I made these bars, I was so surprised by how quickly they vanished! Most folks can't eat just one of the rich and gooey treats. They taste a lot like chocolate pecan pie.

—HAZEL BALDNER AUSTIN, MN

PREP: 15 MIN. • **BAKE:** 20 MIN. + COOLING
MAKES: 4 DOZEN

- 1½ cups all-purpose flour
- ½ cup packed brown sugar
- ½ cup cold butter, cubed
FILLING
- 3 eggs
- ¾ cup sugar
- ¾ cup dark corn syrup
- 2 tablespoons butter, melted
- 1 teaspoon vanilla extract
- 1¾ cups semisweet chocolate chunks
- 1½ cups coarsely chopped pecans

1. In a small bowl, combine flour and brown sugar; cut in butter until crumbly. Press into a greased 13-in. x 9-in. baking pan. Bake at 350° for 10-15 minutes or until golden brown.
2. Meanwhile, in a large bowl, whisk eggs, sugar, corn syrup, butter and vanilla until blended. Stir in chocolate chunks and pecans. Pour over crust.
3. Bake for 20-25 minutes or until set. Cool completely on a wire rack. Cut into bars. Store in an airtight container in the refrigerator.
PER SERVING *1 bar equals 133 cal., 7 g fat (3 g sat. fat), 19 mg chol., 31 mg sodium, 17 g carb., 1 g fiber, 1 g pro.*

125 CALORIES

Cappuccino Mousse

We dreamed up this rich mousse with a pleasantly creamy texture and a hint of coffee flavor. Make it ahead for a delightful meal finale.

—TASTE OF HOME TEST KITCHEN

PREP: 15 MIN. + CHILLING
MAKES: 2 SERVINGS

- ½ teaspoon unflavored gelatin
- ¼ cup fat-free milk
- 1½ teaspoons baking cocoa
- ¼ teaspoon instant coffee granules
- ⅓ cup fat-free coffee-flavored yogurt
- 2 tablespoons sugar
- ½ cup reduced-fat whipped topping

1. In a small saucepan, sprinkle gelatin over milk; let stand for 1 minute. Heat over low heat, stirring until gelatin is completely dissolved. Add cocoa and coffee; stir until dissolved. Transfer to a small bowl; chill until mixture begins to thicken.
2. Beat mixture until light and fluffy. Combine yogurt and sugar; beat into gelatin mixture. Fold in whipped topping. Divide between two dessert dishes. Chill until firm.
PER SERVING *¾ cup equals 125 cal., 2 g fat (2 g sat. fat), 1 mg chol., 40 mg sodium, 22 g carb., trace fiber, 3 g pro.* **Diabetic Exchange:** *1½ starch.*

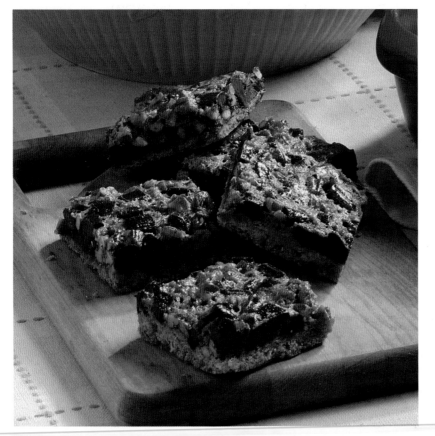

142 CALORIES
Coconut-Cherry Cream Squares

You'll be wowed by these cherry-topped delights! One delectable square will satisfy just about any sweet tooth.
—**TASTE OF HOME TEST KITCHEN**

PREP: 30 MIN. + CHILLING
MAKES: 16 SERVINGS

- ¾ **cup all-purpose flour**
- ⅓ **cup flaked coconut**
- 3 **tablespoons brown sugar**
- 3 **tablespoons cold reduced-fat butter**

FILLING

- ⅓ **cup all-purpose flour**
- ¼ **cup sugar**
  Sugar substitute equivalent to ¼ cup sugar
- ¼ **teaspoon salt**
- 2½ **cups fat-free milk**
- 2 **eggs, lightly beaten**
- ½ **cup flaked coconut**
- 2 **teaspoons coconut extract**
- 1 **can (20 ounces) reduced-sugar cherry pie filling**

1. In a small bowl, combine the flour, coconut and brown sugar; cut in butter until crumbly. Press into a 9-in. square baking pan coated with cooking spray. Bake at 400° for 7-10 minutes or until lightly browned. Cool on a wire rack.

2. In a small saucepan, combine the flour, sugar, sugar substitute and salt. Stir in milk until smooth. Cook and stir over medium-high heat until thickened and bubbly. Reduce heat; cook and stir 2 minutes longer. Remove from the heat.

3. Stir a small amount of hot filling into eggs; return all to the pan, stirring constantly. Bring to a gentle boil; cook and stir 2 minutes longer. Remove from the heat.

4. Gently stir in coconut and extract. Pour over crust. Refrigerate until set. Top with pie filling. Refrigerate for at least 2 hours before cutting.

NOTE *This recipe was tested with Splenda No Calorie Sweetener and Land O'Lakes stick light butter. Look for Splenda in the baking aisle.*

PER SERVING *1 square equals 142 cal., 4 g fat (3 g sat. fat), 31 mg chol., 95 mg sodium, 24 g carb., 1 g fiber, 3 g pro.* **Diabetic Exchanges:** *1½ starch, ½ fat.*

141 CALORIES No-Bake Cheesecake Pie

You won't miss the traditional graham cracker crust with this fluffy lemon dessert. The texture is wonderful and the citrus taste is great...plus it's easy as pie to prepare!
—**NORMA JO REYNOLDS** GOLDWAITE, TX

PREP: 20 MIN. + CHILLING
MAKES: 8 SERVINGS

- 2 **tablespoons graham cracker crumbs, divided**
- 1 **package (.3 ounce) sugar-free lemon gelatin**
- ⅔ **cup boiling water**
- 1 **package (8 ounces) reduced-fat cream cheese, cubed**
- 1 **cup (8 ounces) 1% cottage cheese**
- 2 **cups reduced-fat whipped topping**

1. Coat the bottom and sides of a 9-in. pie plate with cooking spray. Sprinkle with 1 tablespoon cracker crumbs; set aside.

2. In a small bowl, dissolve gelatin in boiling water; cool slightly. Pour into a blender; add cream cheese and cottage cheese. Cover and process until smooth. Transfer to a large bowl. Fold in whipped topping. Pour into prepared pie plate. Sprinkle with remaining cracker crumbs. Cover and refrigerate until set.

PER SERVING *1 slice equals 141 cal., 8 g fat (6 g sat. fat), 21 mg chol., 272 mg sodium, 9 g carb., trace fiber, 7 g pro.* **Diabetic Exchanges:** *1½ fat, ½ starch.*

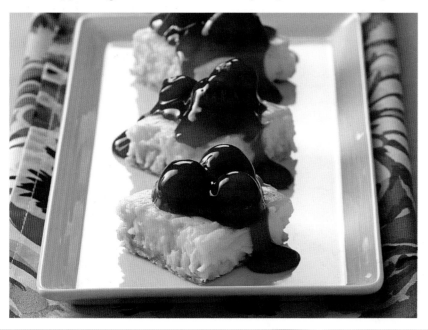

140 CALORIES Oatmeal Chip Cookies

My mom liked to experiment with different spices in traditional recipes to create unique and unexpected flavors. Molasses and cinnamon make these cookies stand out from ordinary oatmeal cookies.

—**SUSAN HENRY** BULLHEAD CITY, AZ

PREP: 20 MIN. • **BAKE:** 10 MIN. • **MAKES:** ABOUT 1½ DOZEN

- ½ **cup shortening**
- 1 **cup sugar**
- 1 **tablespoon molasses**
- 1 **egg**
- 1 **teaspoon vanilla extract**
- 1 **cup all-purpose flour**
- 1 **cup quick-cooking oats**
- 1 **teaspoon baking soda**
- 1 **teaspoon ground cinnamon**
- ½ **teaspoon salt**
- 1 **cup (6 ounces) semisweet chocolate chips**

1. In a large bowl, cream shortening and sugar until light and fluffy. Beat in the molasses, egg and vanilla. Combine the flour, oats, baking soda, cinnamon and salt; gradually add to creamed mixture and mix well. Stir in chocolate chips.

2. Roll into 1½-in. balls. Place 2 in. apart on greased baking sheets. Bake at 350° for 8-10 minutes or until golden brown. Cool for 5 minutes before removing from pans to wire racks.

PER SERVING *1 cookie equals 140 cal., 7 g fat (2 g sat. fat), 9 mg chol., 106 mg sodium, 20 g carb., 1 g fiber, 2 g pro.*

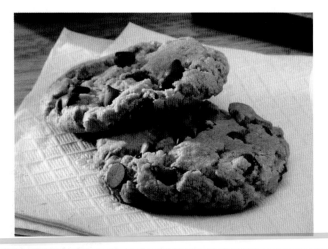

139 CALORIES Caramelized Pear Strudel

This easy, stylish dessert is sure to please everyone. Best served warm, it's delicious with a scoop of light vanilla ice cream or reduced-fat whipped topping.

—**LEAH BEATTY** COBOURG, ON

PREP: 35 MIN. + COOLING • **BAKE:** 20 MIN. + COOLING
MAKES: 10 SERVINGS

- ½ **cup sugar**
- 1 **tablespoon cornstarch**
- 3 **large pears, peeled and finely chopped**
- ½ **cup fresh or frozen cranberries, thawed**
- 2 **tablespoons butter**
- ½ **cup dried cranberries**
- 1 **teaspoon ground ginger**
- 1 **teaspoon grated orange peel**
- ½ **teaspoon ground cinnamon**
- 6 **sheets phyllo dough (14 inches x 9 inches)**
  Cooking spray
- 1 **teaspoon confectioners' sugar**

1. In a large bowl, combine sugar and cornstarch. Add pears and cranberries; toss gently to coat. In a large nonstick skillet, melt butter over medium-high heat. Add fruit mixture; cook and stir for 7-8 minutes or until cranberries pop. Stir in the dried cranberries, ginger, orange peel and cinnamon. Cool.

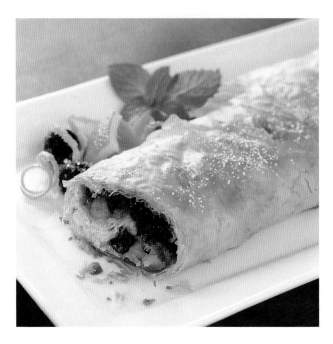

2. Line a baking sheet with foil and coat the foil with cooking spray; set aside. Place one sheet of phyllo dough on a work surface; coat with cooking spray. Repeat the layers five times. (Keep remaining phyllo dough covered with plastic wrap and a damp towel until ready to use each sheet.)

3. Spread cranberry mixture over dough to within 1 in. of edges. Fold in sides. Roll up, starting at a long side. Place seam side down on prepared baking sheet.

4. Bake at 400° for 20-23 minutes or until golden brown. Remove from pan to a wire rack to cool. Dust with confectioners' sugar before serving.

PER SERVING *1 slice equals 139 cal., 3 g fat (1 g sat. fat), 6 mg chol., 50 mg sodium, 30 g carb., 2 g fiber, 1 g pro.* **Diabetic Exchanges:** *1 starch, 1 fruit, ½ fat.*

149 CALORIES
Chocolate Mint Crisps
If you like chocolate and mint, you can't help but love these delicious crispy cookies with their creamy icing! We always make them for the holidays and our guests can never seem to eat just one!
—**KAREN ANN BLAND** GOVE, KS

PREP: 20 MIN. + CHILLING
BAKE: 15 MIN./BATCH + STANDING • **MAKES:** 6½ DOZEN

- 1½ cups packed brown sugar
- ¾ cup butter, cubed
- 2 tablespoons plus 1½ teaspoons water
- 2 cups (12 ounces) semisweet chocolate chips
- 2 eggs
- 2½ cups all-purpose flour
- 1¼ teaspoons baking soda
- ½ teaspoon salt
- 3 packages (4.67 ounces each) mint Andes candies

1. In a heavy saucepan, combine the brown sugar, butter and water. Cook and stir over low heat until butter is melted and mixture is smooth. Remove from the heat; stir in chocolate chips until melted.

2. Transfer to a bowl. Let stand for 10 minutes. With mixer on high speed, add eggs one at a time, beating well after each addition. Combine the flour, baking soda and salt; add to chocolate mixture, beating on low until blended. Cover and refrigerate for 8 hours or overnight.

3. Roll dough into 1-in. balls. Place 3 in. apart on lightly greased baking sheets. Bake at 350° for 11-13 minutes or until edges are set and tops are puffed and cracked (cookies will become crisp after cooling).

4. Immediately top each cookie with a mint. Let stand for 1-2 minutes; spread over cookie. Remove to wire racks; let stand until chocolate is set and cookies are completely cooled.

PER SERVING *2 cookies equals 149 cal., 7 g fat (4 g sat. fat), 20 mg chol., 114 mg sodium, 22 g carb., 1 g fiber, 2 g pro.*

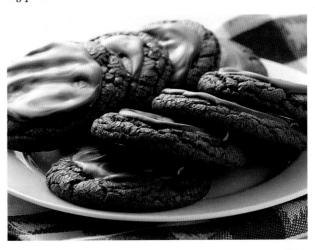

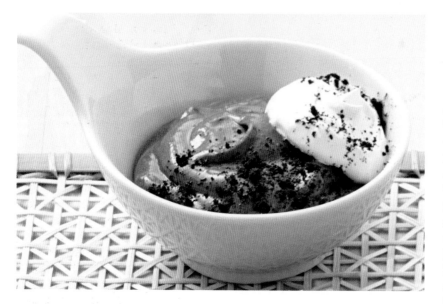

105 CALORIES

Cappuccino Pudding

With a fun combination of chocolate, coffee and cinnamon, this pudding is one of my favorites.

—**CINDY BERTRAND** FLOYDADA, TX

START TO FINISH: 20 MIN.
MAKES: 4 SERVINGS

- 4 teaspoons instant coffee granules
- 1 tablespoon boiling water
- 1½ cups cold fat-free milk
- 1 package (1.4 ounces) sugar-free instant chocolate pudding mix
- ½ teaspoon ground cinnamon
- 1 cup reduced-fat whipped topping
  Additional whipped topping and chocolate wafer crumbs, optional

1. Dissolve coffee in boiling water; set aside. In a large bowl, combine milk, pudding mix and cinnamon. Beat on low speed for 2 minutes. Let stand for 2 minutes or until set.
2. Stir in the coffee; fold in the whipped topping. Spoon into serving dishes. Garnish with additional whipped topping and wafer crumbs if desired.

PER SERVING *½ cup (calculated without optional ingredients) equals 105 cal., 2 g fat (0 sat. fat), 2 mg chol., 48 mg sodium, 17 g carb., 0 fiber, 3 g pro. **Diabetic Exchanges:** ½ starch, ½ fat-free milk.*

131 CALORIES

Warm Chocolate Melting Cups

Our guests often request these lovely cake cups, and they're always surprised that the desserts are so light.

—**KISSA VAUGHN** TROY, TX

PREP: 20 MIN. • **BAKE:** 20 MIN.
MAKES: 10 SERVINGS

- 1¼ cups sugar, divided
- ½ cup baking cocoa
- 2 tablespoons all-purpose flour
- ⅛ teaspoon salt
- ¾ cup water
- ¾ cup plus 1 tablespoon semisweet chocolate chips
- 1 tablespoon brewed coffee
- 1 teaspoon vanilla extract
- 2 eggs
- 1 egg white
- 10 fresh strawberry halves, optional

1. In a small saucepan, combine ¾ cup sugar, cocoa, flour and salt. Gradually stir in water. Bring to a boil; cook and stir for 2 minutes or until thickened. Remove from the heat; stir in the chocolate chips, coffee and vanilla until smooth. Transfer to a large bowl.
2. In another bowl, beat eggs and egg white until slightly thickened. Gradually add remaining sugar, beating until mixture is thick and lemon-colored. Fold into the chocolate mixture.
3. Transfer to ten 4-oz. ramekins coated with cooking spray. Place ramekins in a baking pan; add 1 in. of boiling water to pan. Bake, uncovered, at 350° for 20-25 minutes or just until centers are set. Garnish with strawberry halves if desired. Serve immediately.

PER SERVING *1 serving equals 131 cal., 1 g fat (trace sat. fat), 42 mg chol., 49 mg sodium, 29 g carb., 1 g fiber, 3 g pro. **Diabetic Exchange:** 2 starch.*

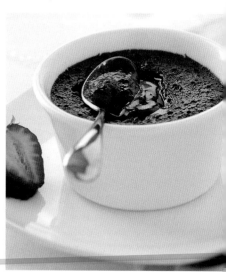

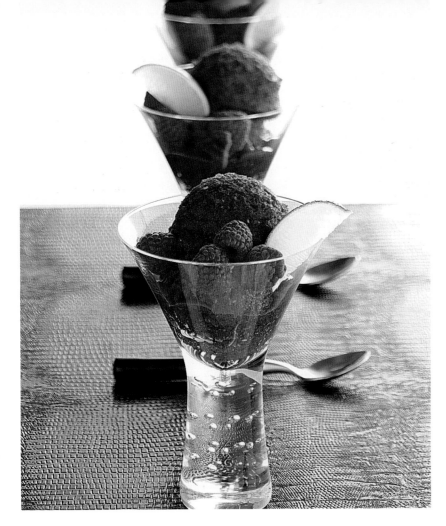

Garnish each serving with raspberries and lime wedges if desired.

PER SERVING *½ cup equals 118 cal., trace fat (trace sat. fat), 0 chol., 3 mg sodium, 31 g carb., 2 g fiber, 1 g pro.* **Diabetic Exchanges:** *1 starch, ½ fruit.*

127 CALORIES ## Makeover Oatmeal Bars

Here's a delicious bar that is even more moist and chewy than the original recipe, but with all the old-fashioned oatmeal flavor and only half the fat!
—**CLYDE WILLIAMS** CHAMBERSBURG, PA

PREP: 10 MIN. • **BAKE:** 15 MIN. + COOLING
MAKES: 20 SERVINGS

- ⅔ **cup sugar**
- ½ **cup unsweetened applesauce**
- ⅓ **cup canola oil**
- 1 **tablespoon maple syrup**
- 2 **cups quick-cooking oats**
- 1 **cup all-purpose flour**
- 1 **teaspoon baking soda**
- ½ **teaspoon salt**
- ½ **teaspoon ground allspice**
- ½ **cup raisins**

1. In a bowl, beat sugar, applesauce, oil and syrup until well blended.
2. In a small bowl, combine the oats, flour, baking soda, salt and allspice; gradually beat into applesauce mixture until blended. Stir in raisins.
3. Spread batter into a 13-in. x 9-in. baking pan coated with cooking spray. Bake at 350° for 15-20 minutes or until edges begin to brown. Cool completely on a wire rack. Cut into bars.

PER SERVING *1 bar equals 127 cal., 4 g fat (trace sat. fat), 0 chol., 123 mg sodium, 21 g carb., 1 g fiber, 2 g pro.* **Diabetic Exchanges:** *1 starch, 1 fat.*

118 CALORIES
Strawberry-Raspberry Ice

I reach for this refreshing snack on hot days. The bright color and summery flavor lure everyone to it! You can use any canned fruit in place of the berries—just be sure to freeze the can first.
—**SANDRA SAKAITIS** ST. LOUIS, MO

PREP: 10 MIN. + FREEZING
MAKES: 3½ CUPS

- 2 **packages (10 ounces each) frozen sweetened sliced strawberries, partially thawed**
- 2 **cups frozen unsweetened raspberries, partially thawed**
- ⅓ **cup sugar**
- 3 **tablespoons lime juice**
- 2 **tablespoons orange juice**
  Fresh raspberries and lime wedges, optional

1. Place strawberries, raspberries, sugar and juices in a blender. Cover and process for 2-3 minutes or until smooth. Transfer to a 13-in. x 9-in. dish. Freeze for 1 hour or until edges begin to firm.
2. Stir and return to freezer. Freeze 2 hours longer or until firm.
3. Just before serving, transfer to a food processor; cover and process for 2-3 minutes or until smooth.

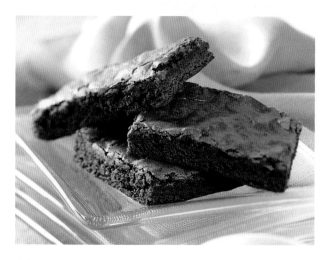

124 CALORIES ## Chewy Chocolate Brownies

Cap off lunch with this sweet treat. The fudgy brownies are so yummy, it's hard to believe they're just 124 calories each!
—**MICHELE DOUCETTE** STEPHENVILLE, NL

PREP: 15 MIN. • **BAKE:** 15 MIN. + COOLING • **MAKES:** 1½ DOZEN

- 3 ounces semisweet chocolate, chopped
- 1 cup packed brown sugar
- 3 tablespoons unsweetened applesauce
- 1 egg
- 1 egg white
- 2 tablespoons canola oil
- 4½ teaspoons light corn syrup
- 2 teaspoons vanilla extract
- 1 cup all-purpose flour
- ¼ cup baking cocoa
- ½ teaspoon baking soda
- ⅛ teaspoon salt

1. In a microwave, melt chocolate; stir until smooth. Cool slightly. Meanwhile, in a large bowl, beat the brown sugar, applesauce, egg, egg white, oil, corn syrup and vanilla. Beat in chocolate until blended. Combine the flour, cocoa, baking soda and salt; beat into brown sugar mixture just until blended.
2. Pour into a 13-in. x 9-in. baking pan coated with cooking spray. Bake at 350° for 15-18 minutes or until a toothpick inserted near the center comes out clean. Cool on a wire rack. Cut into bars.
PER SERVING *1 brownie equals 124 cal., 4 g fat (1 g sat. fat), 12 mg chol., 65 mg sodium, 22 g carb., 1 g fiber, 2 g pro.* **Diabetic Exchanges:** *1½ starch, ½ fat.*

148 CALORIES
Old-Fashioned Molasses Cake

This old-time spice cake is low in fat but big on flavor. Serve it warm for breakfast on a frosty morning or have a square with hot cider on a snowy afternoon. It's a great cold-weather snack.
—**DEANNE BAGLEY** BATH, NY

PREP: 15 MIN. • **BAKE:** 25 MIN. + COOLING • **MAKES:** 9 SERVINGS

- 2 tablespoons reduced-fat butter, softened
- ¼ cup sugar
- 1 egg
- ½ cup molasses
- 1 cup all-purpose flour
- 1 teaspoon baking soda
- ¼ teaspoon ground ginger
- ¼ teaspoon ground cinnamon
- ⅛ teaspoon salt
- ½ cup hot water
- 9 tablespoons fat-free whipped topping

1. In a small bowl, beat butter and sugar until crumbly, about 2 minutes. Beat in egg. Beat in the molasses. Combine the flour, baking soda, ginger, cinnamon and salt; add to butter mixture alternately with water, mixing well after each addition.
2. Transfer to a 9-in. square baking pan coated with cooking spray. Bake at 350° for 25-30 minutes or until a toothpick inserted near the center comes out clean.

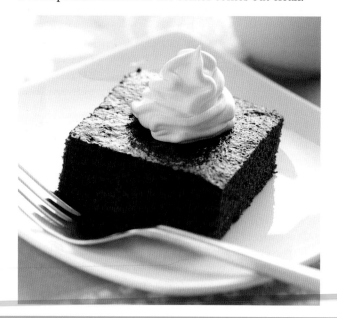

Cool on a wire rack. Cut into squares; garnish with whipped topping.

NOTE *This recipe was tested with Land O'Lakes light stick butter.*

PER SERVING *1 piece with 1 tablespoon whipped topping equals 148 cal., 2 g fat (1 g sat. fat), 28 mg chol., 205 mg sodium, 30 g carb., trace fiber, 2 g pro.* **Diabetic Exchanges:** *2 starch, ½ fat.*

141 CALORIES

Chippy Blond Brownies

If you love chocolate and butterscotch, you won't be able to resist my sweet and chewy brownies. I often include the recipe inside a baking dish as a special wedding present.

—ANNA ALLEN OWINGS MILLS, MD

PREP: 15 MIN. • **BAKE:** 25 MIN.
MAKES: 2 DOZEN

- 6 tablespoons butter, softened
- 1 cup packed brown sugar
- 2 eggs
- 1 teaspoon vanilla extract
- 1¼ cups all-purpose flour
- 1 teaspoon baking powder
- ½ teaspoon salt
- 1 cup (6 ounces) semisweet chocolate chips
- ½ cup chopped pecans

1. In a large bowl, cream butter and brown sugar until light and fluffy. Add the eggs, one at a time, beating well after each addition. Beat in vanilla. Combine the flour, baking powder and salt; gradually add to creamed mixture. Stir in chocolate chips and pecans.

2. Spread into a greased 11-in. x 7-in. baking pan. Bake at 350° for 25-30 minutes or until a toothpick inserted near the center comes out clean. Cool on a wire rack.

PER SERVING *1 brownie equals 141 cal., 7 g fat (3 g sat. fat), 25 mg chol., 104 mg sodium, 19 g carb., 1 g fiber, 2 g pro.*

110 CALORIES ## Dark Chocolate Butterscotch Brownies

My daughters and I love to have homemade brownies. We experimented with many recipes and finally came up with what we think is the best-ever brownie. The rich, satiny frosting and the butterscotch chips are irresistible.

—KIT CONCILUS MEADVILLE, PA

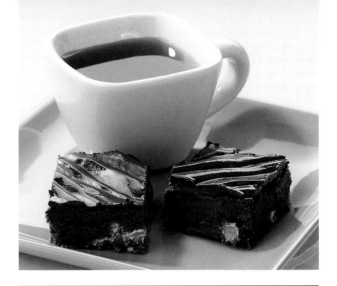

PREP: 25 MIN. • **BAKE:** 25 MIN. + COOLING
MAKES: ABOUT 5 DOZEN

- 4 ounces unsweetened chocolate, chopped
- ¾ cup butter, cubed
- 2 cups sugar
- 3 egg whites
- 1½ teaspoons vanilla extract
- 1 cup all-purpose flour
- 1 cup 60% cocoa bittersweet chocolate baking chips
- 1 cup butterscotch chips

GLAZE
- 1 cup 60% cocoa bittersweet chocolate baking chips
- ¼ cup butter, cubed

1. In a microwave, melt unsweetened chocolate and butter; stir until smooth. Cool slightly. In a large bowl, combine sugar and chocolate mixture. Stir in egg whites and vanilla. Gradually add flour to chocolate mixture. Stir in chips.

2. Spread into a greased 13-in. x 9-in. baking pan. Bake at 350° for 25-30 minutes or until a toothpick inserted near the center comes out clean (do not overbake). Cool on a wire rack.

3. For glaze, in a microwave, melt chips and butter; stir until smooth. Immediately spread over brownies. Cool before cutting.

NOTE *This recipe was tested using Ghirardelli 60% cocoa bittersweet chocolate baking chips. Semisweet chocolate chips may be substituted.*

PER SERVING *1 brownie equals 110 cal., 6 g fat (4 g sat. fat), 9 mg chol., 39 mg sodium, 14 g carb., 1 g fiber, 1 g pro.*

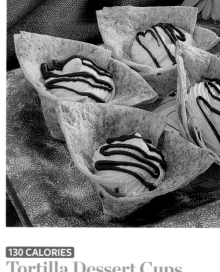

114 CALORIES

Mother Lode Pretzels

I brought these savory-sweet pretzels to a family gathering, and they disappeared from the dessert tray before dessert was even served! My family raves about how awesome they are.

—**CARRIE BENNETT** MADISON, WI

PREP: 35 MIN. + STANDING
MAKES: 4½ DOZEN

- 1 package (10 ounces) pretzel rods
- 1 package (14 ounces) caramels
- 1 tablespoon evaporated milk
- 1¼ cups miniature semisweet chocolate chips
- 1 cup plus 2 tablespoons butterscotch chips
- ⅔ cup milk chocolate toffee bits
- ¼ cup chopped walnuts, toasted

1. With a sharp knife, cut pretzel rods in half; set aside. In a large saucepan over low heat, melt caramels with milk. In a large shallow bowl, combine the chips, toffee bits and walnuts.

2. Pour caramel mixture into a 2-cup glass measuring cup. Dip the cut end of each pretzel piece two-thirds of the way into caramel mixture (reheat in microwave if mixture becomes too thick for dipping). Allow excess caramel to drip off, then roll pretzels in the chip mixture. Place on waxed paper until set. Store in an airtight container.

PER SERVING *1 pretzel equals 114 cal., 5 g fat (3 g sat. fat), 3 mg chol., 104 mg sodium, 17 g carb., 1 g fiber, 1 g pro.*

130 CALORIES

Tortilla Dessert Cups

Diabetics and dessert lovers alike are wowed by these creamy treats. After finding out my mother had diabetes, I went on a search for some good treat recipes that she could still enjoy. No one will guess these are light!

—**SUSAN MILLER** WAKEMAN, OH

PREP: 30 MIN. + CHILLING
MAKES: 20 SERVINGS

- 3 tablespoons sugar
- 2 teaspoons ground cinnamon
- 10 flour tortillas (6 inches)
- 1 package (8 ounces) reduced-fat cream cheese
- 1 cup cold fat-free milk
- 1 package (1 ounce) sugar-free instant white chocolate or vanilla pudding mix
- 2 cups reduced-fat whipped topping
- ¼ cup milk chocolate chips, melted

1. In a small bowl, combine sugar and cinnamon. Coat one side of each tortilla with cooking spray; sprinkle with cinnamon-sugar. Turn tortillas over; repeat on the other side. Cut each tortilla into four wedges.

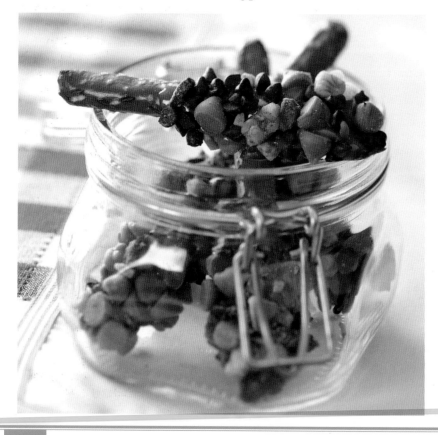

2. For each dessert cup, place round edge of one tortilla wedge in the bottom of a muffin cup, shaping sides to fit cup. Place a second tortilla wedge in the muffin cup, allowing bottom and sides to overlap. Bake at 350° for 10 minutes or until crisp and lightly browned. Cool completely in pan.

3. Meanwhile, for filling, in a small bowl, beat the cream cheese until smooth. In another bowl, whisk the milk and pudding mix for 2 minutes. Let stand for 2 minutes or until soft-set. Beat in cream cheese on low until smooth. Fold in whipped topping. Cover and chill for 1 hour.

4. Carefully remove cups from pan. Pipe or spoon about 3 tablespoons filling into each cup. Drizzle or pipe with melted chocolate. Refrigerate for 5 minutes or until chocolate is set. Store in the refrigerator.

PER SERVING *1 dessert cup equals 130 cal., 4 g fat (2 g sat. fat), 5 mg chol., 178 mg sodium, 19 g carb., trace fiber, 4 g pro.* **Diabetic Exchanges:** *1 starch, 1 fat.*

145 CALORIES

Tropical Meringue Tarts

How special are these tarts! As pretty as an Easter basket, the meringue shells are filled with pudding, then topped with fruit and coconut. The perfect showstopper dessert for company.
—TASTE OF HOME TEST KITCHEN

PREP: 30 MIN. • **BAKE:** 50 MIN. + COOLING
MAKES: 10 SERVINGS

- 4 **egg whites**
- 1 **teaspoon white vinegar**
- 1 **teaspoon vanilla extract**
- 1 **teaspoon cornstarch**
- 1 **cup sugar**
- 1¼ **cups cold fat-free milk**
- 1 **package (1 ounce) sugar-free instant vanilla pudding mix**
- 1 **cup reduced-fat whipped topping**
- 1 **cup cubed fresh pineapple**
- 2 **medium kiwifruit, peeled and sliced**
- 2 **tablespoons flaked coconut, toasted**

1. Place egg whites in a large bowl; let stand at room temperature for 30 minutes. Meanwhile, line a baking sheet with parchment paper or foil. Draw ten 3-in. circles on paper; set aside.

2. Add vinegar and vanilla to egg whites; beat on medium speed until soft peaks form. Beat in cornstarch. Gradually beat in sugar, 2 tablespoons at a time, on high until stiff glossy peaks form and sugar is dissolved.

3. Cut a small hole in the corner of pastry or plastic bag; insert a large star pastry tip (#6B). Fill the bag with meringue.

4. Pipe the meringue in a spiral fashion to fill in circles on prepared pan. Pipe twice around the base of each shell in a spiral fashion to make the sides.

5. Bake at 275° for 50-60 minutes or until set and dry. Turn oven off and leave door closed; leave meringues in oven for 1 hour.

6. For filling, in a large bowl, whisk milk and pudding mix for 2 minutes. Fold in whipped topping. Spoon into the meringue shells. Top with pineapple, kiwi and coconut.

PER SERVING *1 tart equals 145 cal., 2 g fat (1 g sat. fat), 1 mg chol., 157 mg sodium, 30 g carb., 1 g fiber, 3 g pro.* **Diabetic Exchange:** *2 starch.*

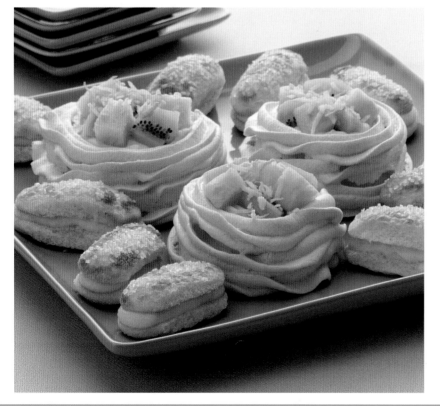

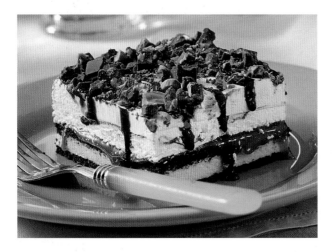

244 CALORIES

Ice Cream Sandwich Dessert

This chocolaty treat is perfect for warm summer days—and so easy to make! With store-bought ice cream sandwiches, you can whip up this dessert in no time.

—CATHIE VALENTINE GRANITEVILLE, SC

PREP: 10 MIN. + FREEZING • **MAKES:** 15-18 SERVINGS

- 17 **miniature ice cream sandwiches, divided**
- 1 **jar (12 ounces) caramel ice cream topping**
- 1 **carton (12 ounces) frozen reduced-fat whipped topping, thawed**
- ¼ **cup chocolate syrup**
- 2 **Symphony candy bars with almonds and toffee (4¼ ounces each), chopped**

Arrange 14 ice cream sandwiches in an ungreased 13-in. x 9-in. dish. Cut remaining sandwiches in half lengthwise; fill in the spaces in the dish. Spread with caramel and whipped toppings. Drizzle with chocolate syrup. Sprinkle with chopped candy bars. Cover and freeze for at least 45 minutes. Cut into squares.
PER SERVING *1 piece equals 244 cal., 10 g fat (6 g sat. fat), 13 mg chol., 105 mg sodium, 39 g carb., 1 g fiber, 3 g pro.*

200 CALORIES Peanut Butter S'mores Bars

I originally made these bars to add something new and colorful to my Christmas cookie trays. When I send them to school with my kids, they disappear in a flash! You can use M&Ms in different colors for all the holidays year-round.
—JULIE WISCHMEIER BROWNSTOWN, IN

PREP: 10 MIN. • **BAKE:** 20 MIN. + CHILLING • **MAKES:** 2 DOZEN

- 1 **tube (16½ ounces) refrigerated peanut butter cookie dough**
- 3½ **cups miniature marshmallows**
- ¾ **cup milk chocolate chips**
- 2 **teaspoons shortening**
- 1½ **cups milk chocolate M&M's**

1. Preheat oven to 350°. Let dough stand at room temperature 5-10 minutes to soften. With floured hands, press dough into an ungreased 13x9-in. baking pan. Bake 18-20 minutes or until lightly browned and edges are firm.
2. Sprinkle with marshmallows; bake 2-3 minutes longer or until marshmallows are puffy.
3. In a microwave, melt chocolate chips and shortening; stir until smooth. Sprinkle M&M's over marshmallows; drizzle with chocolate mixture. Refrigerate until set before cutting.
PER SERVING *1 bar equals 200 cal., 9 g fat (4 g sat. fat), 5 mg chol., 105 mg sodium, 29 g carb., 1 g fiber, 2 g pro.*

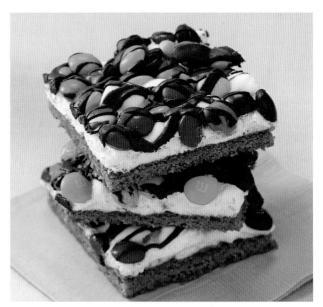

174 CALORIES Tart Cherry Pie

My aunt and I are diabetic, and we both enjoy this yummy fruit pie. Our friends often request it for dessert whenever they come to visit us.
—**BONNIE JOHNSON** DEKALB, IL

PREP: 15 MIN. + COOLING • **MAKES:** 8 SERVINGS

- 2 **cans (14½ ounces each) pitted tart cherries**
- 1 **package (3 ounces) cook-and-serve vanilla pudding mix**
- 1 **package (.3 ounce) sugar-free cherry gelatin**
  Sugar substitute equivalent to 4 teaspoons sugar
- 1 **pastry shell (9 inches), baked**

Drain cherries, reserving juice; set cherries aside. In a large saucepan, combine cherry juice and dry pudding mix. Cook and stir until mixture comes to a boil and is thickened and bubbly. Remove from the heat; stir in gelatin powder and sweetener until dissolved. Stir in cherries; transfer to pastry shell. Cool completely. Store in the refrigerator.

PER SERVING *1 piece equals 174 cal., 7 g fat (3 g sat. fat), 5 mg chol., 162 mg sodium, 25 g carb., 1 g fiber, 2 g pro.* **Diabetic Exchanges:** *1 starch, 1 fat, ½ fruit.*

238 CALORIES Caramel Apple Pizza

I made a favorite recipe lighter by preparing my own cookie crust with less fat and sugar. I also use a combination of fat-free and low-fat cream cheese, as well as fat-free caramel sauce. My family doesn't even notice the difference!
—**TARI AMBLER** SHOREWOOD, IL

PREP: 40 MIN. + COOLING • **MAKES:** 12 SLICES

- ¼ **cup butter, softened**
- ¼ **cup sugar**
- ¼ **cup packed brown sugar**
- 1 **egg**
- 2 **tablespoons canola oil**
- 1 **tablespoon light corn syrup**
- 1 **teaspoon vanilla extract**
- 1 **cup whole wheat pastry flour**
- ¾ **cup all-purpose flour**
- ½ **teaspoon baking powder**
- ¼ **teaspoon salt**
- ¼ **teaspoon ground cinnamon**

TOPPING

- 1 **package (8 ounces) fat-free cream cheese**

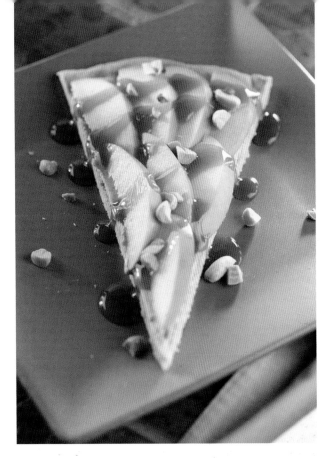

- ¼ **cup packed brown sugar**
- ½ **teaspoon ground cinnamon**
- ½ **teaspoon vanilla extract**
- 3 **medium tart apples, thinly sliced**
- ¼ **cup fat-free caramel ice cream topping**
- ¼ **cup chopped unsalted dry roasted peanuts**

1. In a large bowl, cream butter and sugars until light and fluffy. Beat in the egg, oil, corn syrup and vanilla. Combine the flours, baking powder, salt and cinnamon; gradually add to creamed mixture and mix well.
2. Press dough onto a 14-in. pizza pan coated with cooking spray. Bake at 350° for 12-15 minutes or until lightly browned. Cool on a wire rack.
3. In a small bowl, beat the cream cheese, brown sugar, cinnamon and vanilla until smooth. Spread over crust. Arrange apples over the top. Drizzle with caramel topping; sprinkle with peanuts. Serve immediately.

PER SERVING *1 slice equals 238 cal., 9 g fat (3 g sat. fat), 29 mg chol., 228 mg sodium, 36 g carb., 2 g fiber, 6 g pro.*

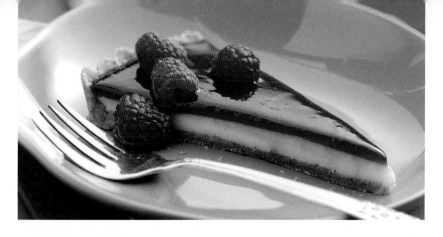

198 CALORIES

Raspberry Custard Tart

With a yummy raspberry layer and nutty homemade crust, our pretty creation will wow your guests! It's hard to believe that a slice isn't an invitation to stray from healthy eating goals.

—TASTE OF HOME TEST KITCHEN

PREP: 25 MIN. • **COOK:** 15 MIN. + CHILLING
MAKES: 12 SERVINGS

- 3 **tablespoons reduced-fat butter**
- ⅓ **cup sugar**
- ¾ **cup all-purpose flour**
- ¼ **cup finely chopped pecans, toasted**

FILLING
- ⅓ **cup sugar**
- ¼ **cup all-purpose flour**
- 2¼ **cups fat-free milk**
- 1 **egg yolk, beaten**
- ¼ **teaspoon almond extract**
- 1 **jar (12 ounces) seedless raspberry spreadable fruit**
- 1½ **cups fresh raspberries**

1. In a small bowl, beat butter and sugar for 2 minutes or until crumbly. Beat in flour and nuts. Coat a 9-in. fluted tart pan with removable bottom with cooking spray. Press crumb mixture onto the bottom and up the sides of pan. Bake at 425° for 8-10 minutes or until lightly browned. Cool on a wire rack.

2. In a small saucepan, combine sugar and flour. Stir in milk until smooth. Cook and stir over medium-high heat until thickened and bubbly. Reduce heat; cook and stir 2 minutes longer. Remove from the heat. Stir a small amount of hot filling into egg yolk; return all to the pan, stirring constantly. Bring to a gentle boil; cook and stir 2 minutes longer. Remove from the heat; gently stir in extract. Pour over crust. Refrigerate until set.

3. In a small bowl, whisk fruit spread until smooth; spread over filling. Garnish with raspberries.

NOTE *This recipe was tested with Land O'Lakes light stick butter.*

PER SERVING *1 piece equals 198 cal., 4 g fat (1 g sat. fat), 22 mg chol., 44 mg sodium, 39 g carb., 2 g fiber, 3 g pro.* **Diabetic Exchanges:** *1½ starch, 1 fruit, ½ fat.*

187 CALORIES Caramel Apple Bread Pudding

Watching your waistline? Relax! This rich, sweet pudding with its luscious caramel topping is pure comfort food--without all the fat. Yum!

—MICHELLE BORLAND PEORIA, IL

PREP: 15 MIN. • **BAKE:** 35 MIN.
MAKES: 8 SERVINGS

- 1 **cup unsweetened applesauce**
- 1 **cup fat-free milk**
- ½ **cup packed brown sugar**
- ½ **cup egg substitute**
- 1 **teaspoon vanilla extract**
- ½ **teaspoon ground cinnamon**
- 5 **cups cubed day-old bread**
- ½ **cup chopped peeled apple**
- ½ **cup fat-free whipped topping**
- ½ **cup fat-free caramel ice cream topping**

1. In a large bowl, combine the applesauce, milk, brown sugar, egg substitute, vanilla and cinnamon. Fold in bread cubes and apple; let stand for 15 minutes or until bread is softened.

2. Pour into an 8-in. square baking dish coated with cooking spray. Bake, uncovered, at 325° for 35-40 minutes or until a knife inserted near the center comes out clean. Serve warm with whipped topping and caramel topping. Refrigerate leftovers.

PER SERVING *1 serving equals 187 cal., 1 g fat (trace sat. fat), 1 mg chol., 201 mg sodium, 40 g carb., 1 g fiber, 4 g pro.*

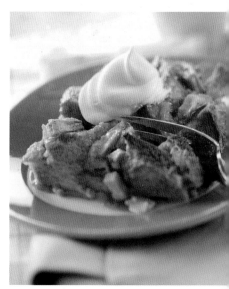

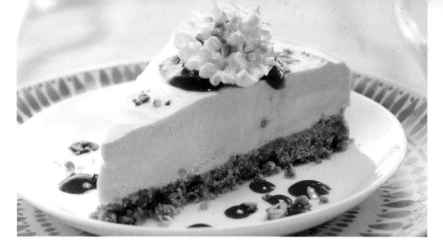

227 CALORIES Mocha Pudding Cakes

Mouthwatering mini cakes are the perfect treat for two. My mom used to make these when I was a little girl. Now I whip them up for a speedy dessert.

—**DEBORA SIMMONS** EGLON, WV

START TO FINISH: 30 MIN.
MAKES: 2 SERVINGS

- ¼ cup all-purpose flour
- 3 tablespoons sugar
- 1½ teaspoons baking cocoa
- ½ teaspoon baking powder
- ⅛ teaspoon salt
- 3 tablespoons 2% milk
- 1½ teaspoons butter, melted
- ¼ teaspoon vanilla extract

TOPPING

- 2 tablespoons brown sugar
- 1½ teaspoons baking cocoa
- 3 tablespoons hot brewed coffee
- 1 tablespoon hot water
  Whipped topping, optional

1. In a small bowl, combine the flour, sugar, cocoa, baking powder and salt. Stir in the milk, butter and vanilla until smooth. Spoon into two 4-oz. ramekins coated with cooking spray.

2. Combine brown sugar and cocoa; sprinkle over batter. Combine coffee and water; pour over topping. Bake at 350° for 15-20 minutes or until a knife inserted near the center comes out clean. Serve warm or at room temperature with whipped topping if desired.

PER SERVING *1 serving (calculated without whipped topping) equals 227 cal., 4 g fat (2 g sat. fat), 9 mg chol., 294 mg sodium, 47 g carb., 1 g fiber, 3 g pro.*

214 CALORIES Frozen Pistachio Dessert with Raspberry Sauce

Raspberry sauce brings bright flavor and a touch of holiday color to my cool and creamy pistachio treat. It'll melt any resistance to dessert!

—**SUZETTE JURY** KEENE, CA

PREP: 35 MIN. + FREEZING
MAKES: 12 SERVINGS

- 1½ cups crushed vanilla wafers (about 45 wafers)
- ¼ cup finely chopped pistachios
- ¼ cup reduced-fat butter, melted
- 1¼ cups fat-free milk
- 1 package (1 ounce) sugar-free instant pistachio pudding mix
- 6 ounces reduced-fat cream cheese
- 1 carton (8 ounces) frozen fat-free whipped topping, thawed, divided
- 1 package (12 ounces) frozen unsweetened raspberries, thawed
- 2 tablespoons sugar
- 2 tablespoons orange liqueur or orange juice
- 2 tablespoons chopped pistachios

1. In a small bowl, combine the wafers, finely chopped pistachios and butter. Press onto the bottom of a 9-in. springform pan coated with cooking spray. Place the pan on a baking sheet. Bake at 350° for 10 minutes or until lightly browned. Cool on a wire rack.

2. Meanwhile, in a small bowl, whisk milk and pudding mix for 2 minutes. Let stand for 2 minutes or until soft-set. In a large bowl, beat cream cheese until smooth. Beat in the pudding.

3. Set aside ¾ cup whipped topping for garnish; fold remaining whipped topping into cream cheese mixture. Pour filling over crust. Freeze for 5 hours or overnight. Cover and refrigerate remaining whipped topping.

4. For sauce, place the raspberries, sugar and liqueur in a food processor. Cover and process for 1-2 minutes or until smooth. Strain and discard seeds and pulp. Refrigerate until serving.

5. Remove dessert from the freezer 15 minutes before serving. Remove sides of pan. Garnish with chopped pistachios and remaining whipped topping. Serve with sauce.

NOTE *This recipe was tested with Land O'Lakes light stick butter.*
PER SERVING *1 slice with 4 teaspoons sauce equals 214 cal., 9 g fat (4 g sat. fat), 18 mg chol., 268 mg sodium, 28 g carb., 2 g fiber, 4 g pro.*
Diabetic Exchanges: *2 starch, 2 fat.*

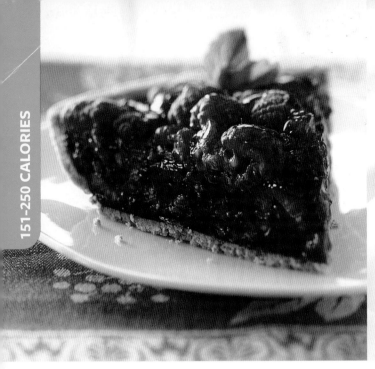

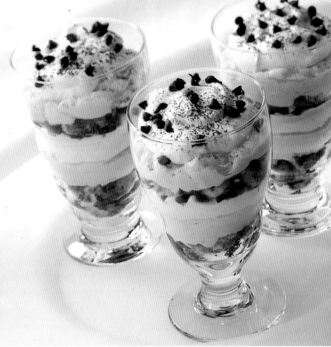

163 CALORIES

Fresh Raspberry Pie

This bright and flavorful raspberry pie is the perfect light ending to a hearty meal. The fruitiness of the filling combines perfectly with the flaky crust for a scrumptious dessert.

—PATRICIA STAUDT MARBLE ROCK, IA

PREP: 20 MIN. + CHILLING
MAKES: 8 SERVINGS

- ¼ **cup sugar**
- 1 **tablespoon cornstarch**
- 1 **cup water**
- 1 **package (.3 ounce) sugar-free raspberry gelatin**
- 4 **cups fresh raspberries**
- 1 **reduced-fat graham cracker crust (8 inches)**
  Reduced-fat whipped topping, optional

1. In a small saucepan, combine the sugar, cornstarch and water until smooth. Bring to a boil, stirring constantly. Cook and stir for 2 minutes or until thickened. Remove from the heat; stir in gelatin until dissolved. Cool for 15 minutes.

2. Place raspberries in the crust; slowly pour gelatin mixture over berries. Chill until set, about 3 hours. Garnish with whipped topping if desired.

PER SERVING *1 piece (calculated without whipped topping) equals 163 cal., 3 g fat (1 g sat. fat), 0 chol., 124 mg sodium, 30 g carb., 4 g fiber, 2 g pro.* **Diabetic Exchanges:** *1½ starch, ½ fruit.*

189 CALORIES

Tiramisu Parfaits

These are a long-time favorite dessert with our family. I think they look so pretty with a drizzle of chocolate or cocoa on top.

—NANCY GRANAMAN
BURLINGTON, IA

PREP: 40 MIN. + CHILLING
MAKES: 6 SERVINGS

- 4½ **teaspoons instant coffee granules**
- ⅓ **cup boiling water**
- 2 **cups cold fat-free milk**
- 2 **packages (1 ounce each) sugar-free instant vanilla pudding mix**
- 4 **ounces fat-free cream cheese**
- 1 **package (3 ounces) ladyfingers, split and cubed**
- 2 **cups fat-free whipped topping**
- 2 **tablespoons miniature chocolate chips**
- 1 **teaspoon baking cocoa**

1. Dissolve coffee in boiling water; cool to room temperature. In a large bowl, whisk milk and pudding mixes for 2 minutes. Let stand for 2 minutes or until soft-set.

2. In another large bowl, beat cream cheese until smooth. Gradually fold in the pudding.

3. Place ladyfinger cubes in a bowl; add coffee and toss to coat. Let stand for 5 minutes.

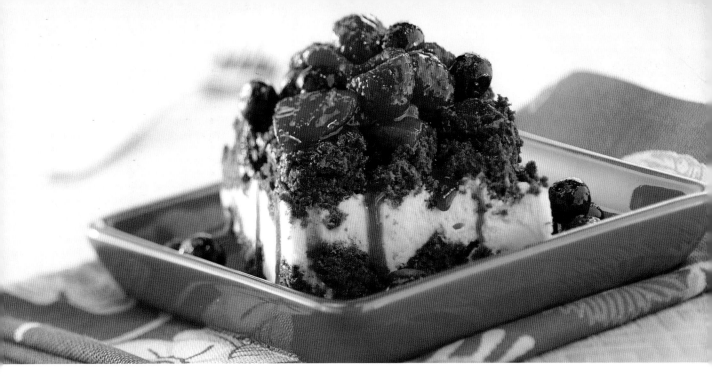

4. Divide half of the ladyfinger cubes among six parfait glasses or serving dishes. Top with half of the pudding mixture, 1 cup whipped topping and 1 tablespoon chocolate chips. Repeat layers.

5. Cover and refrigerate for 8 hours or overnight. Just before serving, dust with cocoa.

PER SERVING *1 parfait equals 189 cal., 3 g fat (1 g sat. fat), 55 mg chol., 573 mg sodium, 32 g carb., 1 g fiber, 7 g pro.* **Diabetic Exchange:** *2 starch.*

233 CALORIES Hot Berries 'n' Brownie Ice Cream Cake

This decadent dessert is like a little taste of heaven. The hot three-berry topping seeps through the chocolate brownie layer and into the cool vanilla ice cream.

—ALLENE BARY-COOPER
WICHITA FALLS, TX

PREP: 20 MIN. • **BAKE:** 30 MIN. + FREEZING
MAKES: 24 SERVINGS

1 package fudge brownie mix (13-inch x 9-inch pan size)
¼ cup water
¼ cup unsweetened applesauce
¼ cup canola oil
2 eggs
1 carton (1¾ quarts) reduced-fat no-sugar-added vanilla ice cream, softened

BERRY SAUCE
2 tablespoons butter
⅓ cup sugar
¼ cup honey
2 tablespoons lime juice
1 tablespoon balsamic vinegar
1 teaspoon ground cinnamon
¼ to ½ teaspoon cayenne pepper
1 quart fresh strawberries, hulled and sliced
2 cups fresh blueberries
2 cups fresh raspberries

1. Prepare brownie mix using water, applesauce, oil and eggs. Bake according to package directions; cool completely on a wire rack.

2. Crumble brownies into 1-in. pieces; sprinkle half into a 13-in. x 9-in. dish coated with cooking spray. Spread evenly with ice cream. Press remaining brownie pieces into ice cream. Cover and freeze for 1 hour or until firm.

3. Remove from freezer 5 minutes before serving. For sauce, in a large skillet, melt the butter over medium heat. Stir in the sugar, honey, lime juice, vinegar, cinnamon and cayenne. Add berries; cook for 3-5 minutes or until heated through, stirring occasionally. Cut cake into squares; top with hot berry sauce.

PER SERVING *1 piece with 3 tablespoons berry sauce equals 233 cal., 9 g fat (3 g sat. fat), 27 mg chol., 140 mg sodium, 36 g carb., 2 g fiber, 4 g pro.* **Diabetic Exchanges:** *2 starch, 1½ fat, ½ fruit.*

220 CALORIES Frozen Yogurt Cookie Dessert

We often prepare this scrumptious but simple dessert for company. Only five ingredients are needed for the creamy flavor sensation. It's easy to use just the portion you want and freeze the rest to enjoy at a later time.

—ELLEN THOMPSON SPRINGFIELD, OH

PREP: 20 MIN. + FREEZING
MAKES: 12 SERVINGS

- 12 reduced-fat Oreo cookies, crushed
- 1 quart low-fat vanilla frozen yogurt, softened
- ⅓ cup chocolate syrup
- ½ cup dry roasted peanuts
- 1 carton (8 ounces) frozen fat-free whipped topping, thawed

1. Set aside 1 tablespoon cookie crumbs. Sprinkle the remaining crumbs into an 11-in. x 7-in. dish coated with cooking spray. Freeze for 10 minutes.

2. Gently spread frozen yogurt over crumbs. Drizzle with chocolate syrup and sprinkle with peanuts. Spread with whipped topping; sprinkle with reserved crumbs.

3. Cover and freeze for at least 2 hours. Remove from the freezer 10 minutes before serving.

PER SERVING *1 piece equals 220 cal., 7 g fat (2 g sat. fat), 3 mg chol., 193 mg sodium, 34 g carb., 1 g fiber, 6 g pro.* **Diabetic Exchanges:** *2 starch, 1 fat.*

167 CALORIES Raspberry Pie with Oat Crust

A diabetic for 30 years, I adapted this recipe to fit my needs. When I serve this pie, no one can believe it's sugarless. I love how tender the oatmeal crust turns out.

—GINNY ARANDAS GREENSBURG, PA

PREP: 25 MIN. + CHILLING
MAKES: 8 SERVINGS

- ¾ cup all-purpose flour
- ½ cup quick-cooking oats
- ½ teaspoon salt
- ¼ cup canola oil
- 3 to 4 tablespoons cold water
- FILLING
- 2 cups water
- 1 package (.8 ounces) sugar-free cook-and-serve vanilla pudding mix
- 1 package (.3 ounce) sugar-free raspberry gelatin
- 4 cups fresh raspberries

1. In a food processor, combine the flour, oats and salt. While processing, slowly drizzle in oil. Gradually add water until a ball forms. Roll out dough between two sheets of waxed paper. Remove top sheet of waxed paper; invert dough into a 9-in. pie plate. Remove remaining waxed paper.

2. Trim and flute edges. Line unpricked pastry with a double thickness of heavy-duty foil. Bake at 450° for 8 minutes. Remove foil; bake 5-7 minutes longer or until golden brown. Cool on a wire rack.

3. In a large saucepan, heat water over medium heat. Whisk in pudding mix. Cook and stir for 5 minutes or until thickened and bubbly. Whisk in gelatin until completely dissolved. Remove from the heat; cool slightly. Fold in raspberries. Spoon into crust. Chill for at least 3 hours or overnight. Refrigerate leftovers.

PER SERVING *1 piece equals 167 cal., 8 g fat (1 g sat. fat), 0 chol., 238 mg sodium, 22 g carb., 5 g fiber, 3 g pro.* **Diabetic Exchanges:** *1½ fat, 1 starch, ½ fruit.*

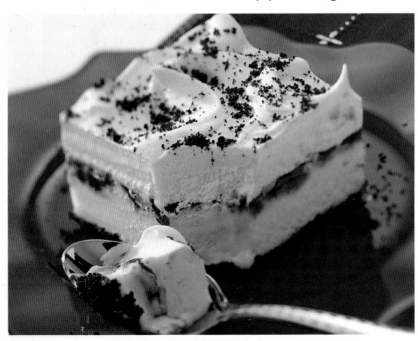

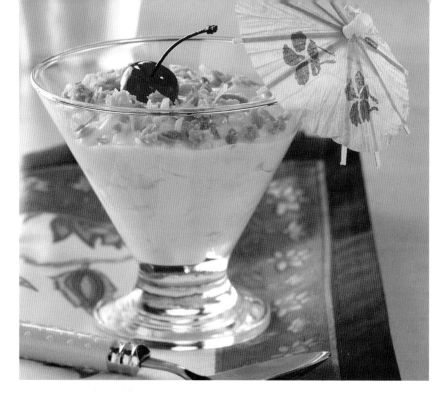

171 CALORIES Pina Colada Pudding Cups

Here's a dessert that is so simple but just chock-full of refreshing pineapple and coconut flavor! A nice light treat after a big meal, it also offers make-ahead convenience for busy hostesses.

—BETTY MAY TOPEKA, KS

PREP: 15 MIN. + CHILLING
MAKES: 8 SERVINGS

- 3 cups fat-free milk
- 2 envelopes whipped topping mix (Dream Whip)
- 2 packages (1 ounce each) sugar-free instant vanilla pudding mix
- 2 cans (8 ounces each) unsweetened crushed pineapple, undrained
- ½ teaspoon coconut extract
- ¼ cup flaked coconut, toasted
- 8 maraschino cherries

1. In a large bowl, whisk the milk, whipped topping and pudding mixes for 2 minutes. Stir in the pineapple and extract.
2. Spoon ¾ cup pudding mixture into eight dessert dishes. Cover and refrigerate for 30 minutes or until chilled.
3. Sprinkle each serving with 1½ teaspoons coconut and top each with a cherry.
PER SERVING *1 pudding cup equals 171 cal., 3 g fat (3 g sat. fat), 2 mg chol., 350 mg sodium, 31 g carb., 1 g fiber, 4 g pro.* **Diabetic Exchanges:** *1½ starch, ½ fruit.*

177 CALORIES Makeover Toffee Crunch Dessert

This is a lightened-up version of one of my favorite desserts. It cuts 90% of the fat and nearly half the calories from the original recipe. Try it for yourself. Guests will never suspect the fluffy layered specialty is on the light side.

—KIM BELCHER KINGSTON MINES, IL

PREP: 20 MIN. + CHILLING
MAKES: 15 SERVINGS

- 1½ cups cold fat-free milk
- 1 package (1 ounce) sugar-free instant vanilla pudding mix
- 2 cartons (8 ounces each) frozen fat-free whipped topping, thawed
- 1 prepared angel food cake (8 to 10 ounces), cut into 1-inch cubes
- 4 Butterfinger candy bars (2.1 ounces each), crushed

1. In a large bowl, whisk milk and pudding mix for 2 minutes. Let stand for 2 minutes or until soft-set. Stir in 2 cups whipped topping. Fold in the remaining whipped topping.
2. In a 13-in. x 9-in. dish coated with cooking spray, layer half of the cake cubes, pudding mixture and crushed candy bars. Repeat layers. Cover and refrigerate for at least 2 hours before serving.
PER SERVING *¾ cup equals 177 cal., 3 g fat (2 g sat. fat), trace chol., 255 mg sodium, 33 g carb., 1 g fiber, 3 g pro.* **Diabetic Exchanges:** *2 starch, ½ fat.*

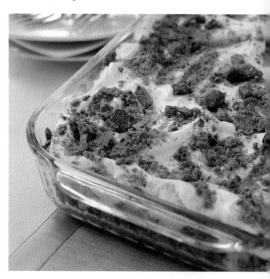

233 CALORIES Tres Leches Cake

Finish off a fiesta with a piece of this classic tender cake. Although it's been lightened, the sweet flavors of the traditional Mexican dessert aren't lost, making it the perfect end to almost any meal.
—**ANNA YEATTS** PINEHURST, NC

PREP: 35 MIN. • **BAKE:** 20 MIN. + CHILLING • **MAKES:** 15 SERVINGS

- 5 eggs, separated
- 1 cup sugar, divided
- 1 tablespoon butter, softened
- ⅓ cup fat-free milk
- 1 teaspoon vanilla extract
- 1 cup all-purpose flour
- 1 teaspoon baking powder

MILK SYRUP

- 1 can (14 ounces) fat-free sweetened condensed milk
- 1 can (12 ounces) fat-free evaporated milk
- 1 cup fat-free half-and-half
- 3 teaspoons vanilla extract
- 15 tablespoons frozen reduced-fat whipped topping
- 15 fresh strawberries

1. Place egg whites in a large bowl; let stand at room temperature for 30 minutes. Coat a 13-in. x 9-in. baking dish with cooking spray and dust with flour; set aside.
2. In a large bowl, beat egg yolks on high speed for 5 minutes or until thick and lemon-colored. Gradually beat in ¾ cup sugar and butter. Stir in milk and vanilla.

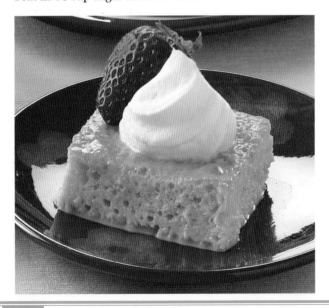

Sift flour and baking powder; gradually add to yolk mixture and mix well (batter will be thick).
3. With clean beaters, beat egg whites on medium speed until soft peaks form. Gradually beat in remaining sugar, 1 tablespoon at a time, on high until stiff peaks form. Gradually fold into batter.
4. Spread evenly into prepared dish. Bake at 350° for 18-22 minutes or until cake springs back when lightly touched. Place on a wire rack.
5. In a large saucepan, combine the condensed milk, evaporated milk and half-and-half. Bring to a boil over medium heat, stirring constantly; cook and stir for 2 minutes. Remove from the heat; stir in vanilla. Cool slightly.
6. Cut cake into 15 pieces, leaving cake in the baking dish. Poke holes in cake with a skewer. Slowly pour a third of the milk syrup over cake, allowing syrup to absorb into the cake. Repeat twice. Let stand for 30 minutes.
7. Cover and refrigerate for 2 hours before serving. Top each piece with whipped topping and a strawberry.
PER SERVING *1 piece equals 233 cal., 3 g fat (2 g sat. fat), 76 mg chol., 126 mg sodium, 42 g carb., 1 g fiber, 8 g pro.*

177 CALORIES Berry Nectarine Buckle

I found this recipe in a magazine quite a long time ago, but have changed it over the years to suit our tastes. We enjoy the combination of three berries plus nectarines, especially with a scoop of low-fat frozen yogurt!
—**LISA SJURSEN-DARLING** SCOTTSVILLE, NY

PREP: 25 MIN. • **BAKE:** 35 MIN. • **MAKES:** 20 SERVINGS

- ⅓ cup all-purpose flour
- ⅓ cup packed brown sugar
- 1 teaspoon ground cinnamon
- 3 tablespoons cold butter

BATTER

- 6 tablespoons butter, softened
- ¾ cup plus 1 tablespoon sugar, divided
- 2 eggs
- 1½ teaspoons vanilla extract
- 2¼ cups all-purpose flour
- 2½ teaspoons baking powder
- ½ teaspoon salt
- ½ cup fat-free milk
- 1 cup fresh blueberries

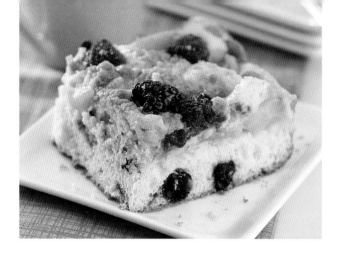

1 **pound medium nectarines, peeled, sliced and patted dry** or 1 **package (16 ounces) frozen unsweetened sliced peaches, thawed and patted dry**
½ **cup fresh raspberries**
½ **cup fresh blackberries**

1. For topping, in a small bowl, combine the flour, brown sugar and cinnamon; cut in butter until crumbly. Set aside.
2. In a large bowl, cream the butter and ¾ cup sugar until light and fluffy. Add eggs, one at a time, beating well after each addition. Beat in vanilla. Combine the flour, baking powder and salt; add to creamed mixture alternately with milk, beating well after each addition. Set aside ¾ cup batter. Fold blueberries into the remaining batter.
3. Spoon into a 13-in. x 9-in. baking dish coated with cooking spray. Arrange nectarines on top; sprinkle with remaining sugar. Drop reserved batter by teaspoonfuls over nectarines. Sprinkle with raspberries, blackberries and reserved topping.
4. Bake at 350° for 35-40 minutes or until a toothpick inserted near the center comes out clean. Serve warm.

PER SERVING *1 piece equals 177 cal., 6 g fat (3 g sat. fat), 35 mg chol., 172 mg sodium, 28 g carb., 1 g fiber, 3 g pro.* **Diabetic Exchanges:** *2 starch, 1 fat.*

197 CALORIES Yummy Chocolate Cake

My husband and I are trying to eat lighter, but we still crave sweets. This moist chocolate cake really helps with that. With the rich frosting, it makes a decadent treat!
—**LADONNA REED** PONCA CITY, OK

PREP: 20 MIN. • **BAKE:** 15 MIN. + COOLING • **MAKES:** 16 SERVINGS

1 **package chocolate cake mix (regular size)**
1 **package (2.1 ounces) sugar-free instant chocolate pudding mix**
1¾ **cups water**
3 **egg whites**
FROSTING
1¼ **cups cold fat-free milk**
¼ **teaspoon almond extract**
1 **package (1.4 ounces) sugar-free instant chocolate pudding mix**
1 **carton (8 ounces) frozen reduced-fat whipped topping, thawed**
Chocolate curls, optional

1. In a large bowl, combine the cake mix, pudding mix, water and egg whites. Beat on low speed for 1 minute; beat on medium for 2 minutes.
2. Pour into a 15-in. x 10-in. x 1-in. baking pan coated with cooking spray. Bake at 350° for 12-18 minutes or until a toothpick inserted near the center comes out clean. Cool on a wire rack.
3. For frosting, place milk and extract in a large bowl. Sprinkle with a third of the pudding mix; let stand for 1 minute. Whisk pudding into milk. Repeat twice with remaining pudding mix. Whisk pudding 2 minutes longer. Let stand for 15 minutes. Fold in whipped topping. Frost cake. Garnish with chocolate curls if desired.

PER SERVING *1 piece (calculated without chocolate curls) equals 197 cal., 5 g fat (3 g sat. fat), trace chol., 409 mg sodium, 35 g carb., 1 g fiber, 3 g pro.* **Diabetic Exchanges:** *2 starch, ½ fat.*

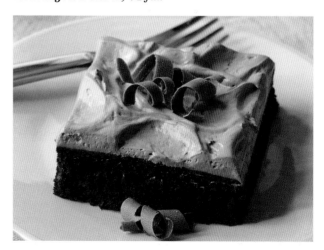

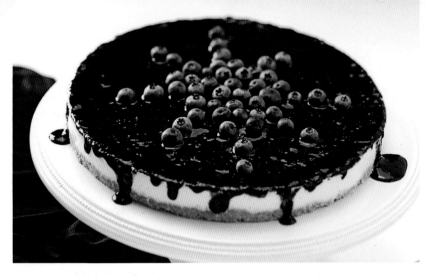

171 CALORIES Lemon Blueberry Cheesecake

For a refreshing alternative to traditional cheesecake, try my no-bake specialty!

—JULIA KLEE BONAIRE, GA

PREP: 30 MIN. + CHILLING
MAKES: 12 SERVINGS

- 1 package (3 ounces) lemon gelatin
- 1 cup boiling water
- 1 cup graham cracker crumbs
- 2 tablespoons butter, melted
- 1 tablespoon canola oil
- 3 cups (24 ounces) fat-free cottage cheese
- ¼ cup sugar

TOPPING

- 2 tablespoons sugar
- 1½ teaspoons cornstarch
- ¼ cup water
- 1⅓ cups fresh or frozen blueberries, divided
- 1 teaspoon lemon juice

1. In a large bowl, dissolve gelatin in boiling water. Cool. In a small bowl, combine the crumbs, butter and oil. Press onto the bottom of a 9-in. springform pan. Chill.
2. In a blender, cover and process cottage cheese and sugar until smooth. While processing, slowly add the cooled gelatin. Pour into crust; cover the cheesecake and refrigerate overnight.
3. For topping, in a small saucepan, combine sugar and cornstarch; gradually stir in water until smooth. Add 1 cup blueberries. Bring to a boil; cook and stir for 2 minutes or until thickened. Stir in lemon juice; cool slightly.
4. Transfer to a blender; cover and process until smooth. Refrigerate until chilled.
5. Run a knife around edge of pan to loosen cheesecake; remove sides of pan. Spread blueberry mixture over the top. Sprinkle with the remaining blueberries.

PER SERVING *1 slice equals 171 cal., 4 g fat (1 g sat. fat), 8 mg chol., 352 mg sodium, 27 g carb., 1 g fiber, 8 g pro.* **Diabetic Exchanges:** *1½ starch, ½ fruit, ½ fat.*

153 CALORIES Best Strawberry Ice Cream

I've made this ice cream often, and it comes out smooth and creamy every time. Our state produces of lot of strawberries, and they are so good!

—LEONE MAYNE FROSTPROOF, FL

PREP: 30 MIN. + CHILLING
PROCESS: 20 MIN. + FREEZING
MAKES: ABOUT 2 QUARTS

- 2 eggs
- 2 cups milk
- 1¼ cups sugar
- 1 cup miniature marshmallows
- 2 cups pureed unsweetened strawberries
- 1 cup half-and-half cream
- ½ cup heavy whipping cream
- 1 teaspoon vanilla extract

1. In a large heavy saucepan, combine eggs and milk; stir in sugar. Cook and stir over medium-low heat until mixture is thickened and coats the back of a spoon, about 14 minutes. Remove from heat; stir in the marshmallows until melted.
2. Set saucepan in ice and stir the mixture for 5-10 minutes or until cool. Stir in remaining ingredients. Cover and refrigerate overnight.
3. When ready to freeze, pour into the cylinder of an ice cream freezer and freeze according to the manufacturer's directions.

PER SERVING *½ cup equals 153 cal., 6 g fat (4 g sat. fat), 48 mg chol., 35 mg sodium, 22 g carb., 1 g fiber, 3 g pro.*

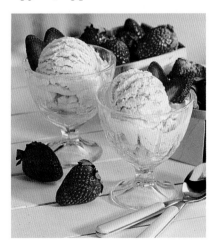

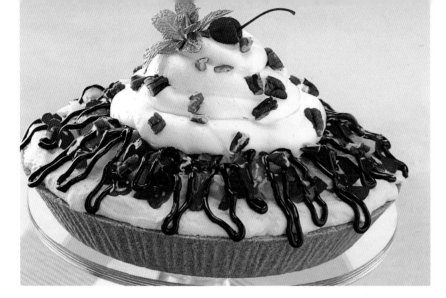

235 CALORIES
Plum Dumplings

Special meals call for elegant desserts, and this one really fills the bill. Sweet plums are halved, then tucked into tender homemade pastry.

—**MARTHA VOSS** DICKINSON, ND

PREP: 30 MIN. • **COOK:** 25 MIN.
MAKES: 6 SERVINGS

- 1½ cups all-purpose flour
- ¼ cup sugar
- 1 teaspoon baking powder
- ⅛ teaspoon salt
- 6 tablespoons 2% milk
- 1 egg, lightly beaten
- 3 medium black plums, halved and pitted
- 1 cup water
- 3 tablespoons butter
  Melted butter and cinnamon-sugar

1. In a large bowl, combine the flour, sugar, baking powder and salt. Stir in milk and egg just until blended. Divide into six portions.
2. On a lightly floured surface, pat each portion of dough into a 5-in. circle. Place a plum half on each circle. Gently bring up corners of dough to center; pinch edges to seal.
3. In a Dutch oven, bring water and butter to a boil. Carefully add dumplings. Reduce heat; cover and simmer for 20-25 minutes or until a toothpick inserted into a dumpling comes out clean. Serve warm with pan juices, melted butter and cinnamon-sugar.
PER SERVING *1 dumpling (calculated without butter and cinnamon-sugar) equals 235 cal., 8 g fat (4 g sat. fat), 52 mg chol., 175 mg sodium, 37 g carb., 1 g fiber, 5 g pro.*

247 CALORIES Banana
Split Cheesecake

Here's a light and festive treat that's sure to dazzle friends and family at the end of any meal. I like to top it with syrup, caramel and pecans for a fantastic look and mouthwatering taste.

—**CHERIE SWEET** EVANSVILLE, IN

PREP: 35 MIN. + FREEZING
MAKES: 10 SERVINGS

- 1 can (8 ounces) unsweetened crushed pineapple, divided
- 2 medium firm bananas, sliced
- 1 reduced-fat graham cracker crust (8 inches)
- 1 package (8 ounces) fat-free cream cheese
- 1½ cups pineapple sherbet, softened
- 1 package (1 ounce) sugar-free instant vanilla pudding mix
- 1 carton (8 ounces) frozen reduced-fat whipped topping, thawed, divided
- 4 maraschino cherries, divided
- 1 tablespoon chocolate syrup
- 1 tablespoon caramel ice cream topping
- 1 tablespoon chopped pecans

1. Drain pineapple, reserving juice. In a small bowl, combine bananas and 2 tablespoons reserved juice; let stand for 5 minutes. Drain bananas, discarding juice. Arrange bananas over bottom of crust; set aside.
2. In a large bowl, beat cream cheese and 2 tablespoons reserved pineapple juice. Gradually beat in sherbet. Gradually add pudding mix; beat 2 minutes longer. Refrigerate ⅓ cup pineapple until serving; fold remaining pineapple into cream cheese mixture. Fold in 2 cups whipped topping; spread evenly over banana slices. Freeze until firm.
3. Remove from the freezer 10-15 minutes before serving. Chop three maraschino cherries and pat dry; arrange cherries and reserved pineapple around edge of pie. Drizzle with chocolate syrup and caramel topping. Dollop remaining whipped topping onto center of pie. Sprinkle with pecans; top with remaining cherry.
PER SERVING *1 piece equals 247 cal., 6 g fat (4 g sat. fat), 3 mg chol., 336 mg sodium, 41 g carb., 1 g fiber, 5 g pro.*

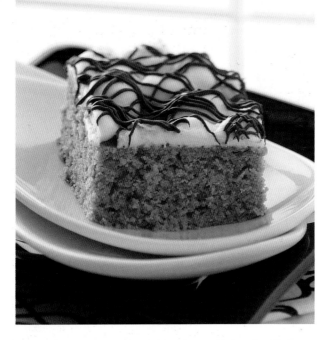

inserted near the center comes out clean. Sprinkle with marshmallows. Bake 4-6 minutes longer or until marshmallows are softened. Cool on a wire rack for 10 minutes.

3. In a microwave, melt chocolate chips; stir until smooth. Drizzle over top of cake. Cool completely on a wire rack.

PER SERVING *1 piece equals 168 cal., 6 g fat (2 g sat. fat), 0 chol., 159 mg sodium, 28 g carb., 2 g fiber, 3 g pro.* ***Diabetic Exchanges:*** *2 starch, 1 fat.*

179 CALORIES Chocolate Ganache Cake

Though our elegant cake looks like something you'd only serve on special occasions, it's actually quite easy to make. So you can enjoy it any time!

—TASTE OF HOME TEST KITCHEN

PREP: 20 MIN. • **BAKE:** 20 MIN. + COOLING • **MAKES:** 12 SERVINGS

- 2 **ounces 53% cacao dark baking chocolate, coarsely chopped**
- 2 **tablespoons butter**
- ¾ **cup boiling water**

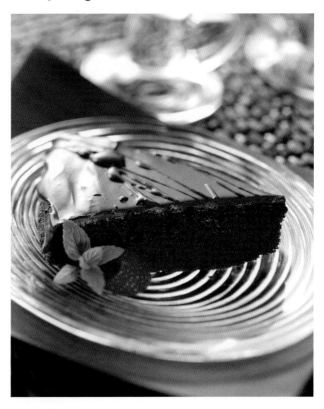

168 CALORIES Yummy S'more Snack Cake

This simple cake comes in a close second to s'mores by the campfire. You can adjust the amount of marshmallows and chocolate chips to your liking.

—DEB WILLIAMS PEORIA, AZ

PREP: 20 MIN. • **BAKE:** 20 MIN. + COOLING • **MAKES:** 20 SERVINGS

- 2½ **cups reduced-fat graham cracker crumbs (about 15 whole crackers)**
- ½ **cup sugar**
- ⅓ **cup cake flour**
- ⅓ **cup whole wheat flour**
- 2 **teaspoons baking powder**
- ¼ **teaspoon salt**
- 3 **egg whites**
- 1 **cup light soy milk**
- ¼ **cup unsweetened applesauce**
- ¼ **cup canola oil**
- 2 **cups miniature marshmallows**
- 1 **cup (6 ounces) semisweet chocolate chips**

1. In a large bowl, combine the first six ingredients. In a small bowl, whisk the egg whites, soy milk, applesauce and oil. Stir into dry ingredients just until moistened. Transfer to a 13-in. x 9-in. baking pan coated with cooking spray.

2. Bake at 350° for 12-15 minutes or until a toothpick

- ¾ cup sugar
- ¼ cup buttermilk
- 1 egg
- 1 teaspoon vanilla extract
- ½ teaspoon orange extract
- 1 cup all-purpose flour
- 1 teaspoon baking soda
- ½ teaspoon salt

GANACHE
- 3 ounces 53% cacao dark baking chocolate, coarsely chopped
- ¼ cup half-and-half cream

1. Place chocolate and butter in a large bowl; add boiling water and stir until smooth. Stir in the sugar, buttermilk, egg and extracts. Combine the flour, baking soda and salt; beat into chocolate mixture just until blended.

2. Transfer to a 9-in. round baking pan coated with cooking spray. Bake at 350° for 18-22 minutes or until a toothpick inserted near the center comes out clean. Cool for 10 minutes before removing from pan to a wire rack to cool completely. Place rack on a waxed paper-lined baking sheet.

3. For ganache, place chocolate in a small bowl. In a small saucepan, bring cream just to a boil. Pour over chocolate; whisk until smooth. Cool for 10 minutes or until slightly thickened.

4. Slowly pour ganache over cake, allowing some ganache to drape over the sides. Refrigerate until serving. Cut into wedges.

PER SERVING *1 slice equals 179 cal., 7 g fat (4 g sat. fat), 26 mg chol., 236 mg sodium, 28 g carb., 1 g fiber, 3 g pro.* **Diabetic Exchanges:** *2 starch, 1 fat.*

199 CALORIES Blackberry Cobbler

This tasty treat has helped my family stay healthy, lose weight and still be able to enjoy dessert! Other kinds of berries or even fresh peaches are just as delicious as substitutes in the cobbler.
—**LESLIE BROWNING** LEBANON, KY

PREP: 15 MIN. + STANDING • **BAKE:** 45 MIN. • **MAKES:** 10 SERVINGS
- ½ cup sugar
- 4½ teaspoons quick-cooking tapioca
- ¼ teaspoon ground allspice
- 5 cups fresh or frozen blackberries, thawed
- 2 tablespoons orange juice

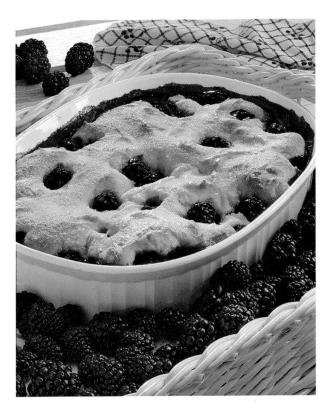

DOUGH
- 1 cup all-purpose flour
- ⅓ cup plus 1 tablespoon sugar, divided
- ¼ teaspoon baking soda
- ¼ teaspoon salt
- ⅓ cup vanilla yogurt
- ⅓ cup fat-free milk
- 3 tablespoons butter, melted

1. In a large bowl, combine the sugar, tapioca and allspice. Add blackberries and orange juice; toss to coat. Let stand for 15 minutes. Spoon into a 2-qt. baking dish coated with cooking spray.

2. In a large bowl, combine the flour, ⅓ cup sugar, baking soda and salt. Combine the yogurt, milk and butter; stir into dry ingredients until smooth. Spread over the berry mixture.

3. Bake at 350° for 20 minutes. Sprinkle with remaining sugar. Bake 25-30 minutes longer or until golden brown. Serve warm.

PER SERVING *1 serving equals 199 cal., 4 g fat (2 g sat. fat), 10 mg chol., 135 mg sodium, 40 g carb., 4 g fiber, 3 g pro.* **Diabetic Exchanges:** *1½ starch, 1 fruit, ½ fat.*

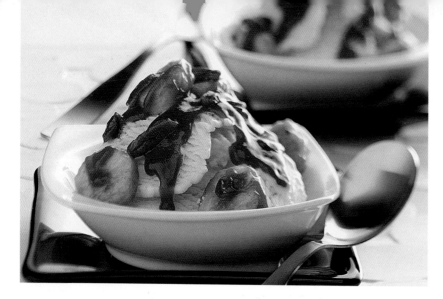

233 CALORIES Bananas Foster Sundaes

I have wonderful memories of eating Bananas Foster in New Orleans, and as a dietitian, I wanted to find a healthier version. I combined the best of two recipes and made some adjustments to create this Southern treat.
—**LISA VARNER** EL PASO, TX

START TO FINISH: 15 MIN.
MAKES: 6 SERVINGS

- 1 **tablespoon butter**
- 3 **tablespoons brown sugar**
- 1 **tablespoon orange juice**
- ¼ **teaspoon ground cinnamon**
- ¼ **teaspoon ground nutmeg**
- 3 **large firm bananas, sliced**
- 2 **tablespoons chopped pecans, toasted**
- ½ **teaspoon rum extract**
- 3 **cups reduced-fat vanilla ice cream**

In a large nonstick skillet, melt butter over medium-low heat. Stir in the brown sugar, orange juice, cinnamon and nutmeg until blended. Add bananas and pecans; cook, stirring gently, for 2-3 minutes or until bananas are glazed and slightly softened. Remove from the heat; stir in extract. Serve with ice cream.

PER SERVING *⅓ cup banana mixture with ½ cup ice cream equals 233 cal., 7 g fat (3 g sat. fat), 23 mg chol., 66 mg sodium, 40 g carb., 2 g fiber, 4 g pro.*

200 CALORIES Fudgy Chocolate Dessert

With a cakelike brownie bottom and layers of chocolate and hot fudge, this scrumptious treat is a chocolate lover's dream. It's my most-requested recipe.
—**BONNIE BOWEN** ADRIAN, MI

PREP: 25 MIN. • **BAKE:** 20 MIN. + CHILLING
MAKES: 20 SERVINGS

- 1 **package chocolate cake mix (regular size)**
- 1 **can (15 ounces) solid-pack pumpkin**
- 3 **cups cold fat-free milk**
- 2 **packages (1.4 ounces each) sugar-free instant chocolate pudding mix**
- 1 **package (8 ounces) fat-free cream cheese**
- 1 **carton (8 ounces) frozen reduced-fat whipped topping, thawed**
- ¼ **cup fat-free hot fudge ice cream topping**
- ¼ **cup fat-free caramel ice cream topping**
- ¼ **cup sliced almonds, toasted**

1. In a large bowl, combine cake mix and pumpkin (mixture will be thick). Spread evenly into a 13-in. x 9-in. baking dish coated with cooking spray.
2. Bake at 375° for 20-25 minutes or until a toothpick inserted near the center comes out clean. Cool completely on a wire rack.
3. In a large bowl, whisk milk and pudding mixes for 2 minutes. Let stand for 2 minutes or until soft-set.
4. In a small bowl, beat cream cheese until smooth. Add pudding; beat until well blended. Spread over cake. Cover and refrigerate for at least 2 hours.
5. Just before serving, spread whipped topping over dessert. Drizzle with fudge and caramel toppings; sprinkle with almonds.

PER SERVING *1 piece equals 200 cal., 5 g fat (2 g sat. fat), 2 mg chol., 376 mg sodium, 35 g carb., 2 g fiber, 5 g pro.* **Diabetic Exchanges:** *2 starch, ½ fat.*

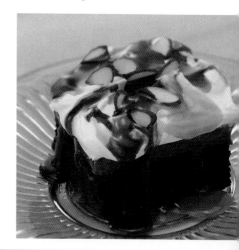

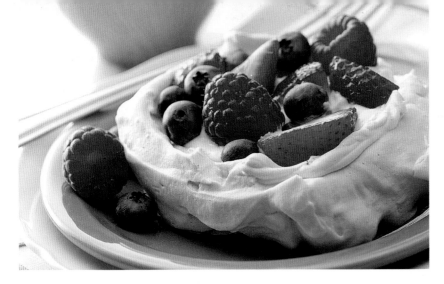

222 CALORIES Meringues with Fresh Berries

Juicy berries and a dollop of light cream fill these puffy meringue desserts. Friends always rave about them.
—AGNES WARD STRATFORD, ON

PREP: 20 MIN. • **BAKE:** 1 HOUR + COOLING
MAKES: 2 SERVINGS

- 2 **egg whites**
- ⅛ **teaspoon cream of tartar**
  Dash salt
- ¼ **cup sugar**
- ¼ **teaspoon vanilla extract**
- 1 **cup mixed fresh berries**
- ½ **teaspoon sugar, optional**
- ⅓ **cup sour cream**
- ⅛ to ¼ **teaspoon rum extract**

1. Place egg whites in a small bowl; let stand at room temperature for 30 minutes. Add cream of tartar and salt; beat on medium speed until soft peaks form. Gradually beat in sugar, 1 tablespoon at a time, on high until stiff peaks form. Beat in vanilla.
2. Drop meringue into two mounds on a parchment paper-lined baking sheet. Shape into 3½-in. cups with the back of a spoon.
3. Bake at 225° for 1 to 1¼ hours or until set and dry. Turn oven off; leave meringues in oven for 1 hour. Remove to wire racks to cool.
4. In a small bowl, combine berries and sugar if desired; let stand for 5 minutes. Combine sour cream and extract; spoon into meringue shells. Top with berries.
PER SERVING *1 serving (calculated without optional sugar) equals 222 cal., 7 g fat (5 g sat. fat), 27 mg chol., 149 mg sodium, 33 g carb., 2 g fiber, 5 g pro.* **Diabetic Exchanges:** *2 starch, 1½ fat, ½ fruit.*

214 CALORIES Coconut Custard Pie

My husband and I are both diabetic. We really appreciate desserts like this creamy custard pie. Coconut extract in the filling and a toasted coconut topping give it a wonderfully sweet flavor.
—EVA WRIGHT GRANT, AL

PREP: 25 MIN.
BAKE: 40 MIN. + CHILLING
MAKES: 8 SERVINGS

- ½ **cup flaked coconut**
- 1 **refrigerated pastry shell (9 inches)**
- 4 **eggs**
- ½ **teaspoon salt**
- 1¾ **cups fat-free milk**
  Sugar substitute equivalent to ½ cup sugar
- 1½ **teaspoons coconut extract**
- ½ **teaspoon vanilla extract**

1. Place coconut in an ungreased 9-in. pie plate. Bake at 350° for 4 minutes, stirring several times; set aside. (Coconut will not be fully toasted.)
2. Line unpricked pastry shell with a double thickness of heavy-duty foil. Bake at 450° for 8 minutes. Remove foil; bake 4-6 minutes longer. Cool.
3. In a bowl, beat the eggs and salt for 5 minutes. (Mixture will be lemon-colored and slightly thickened.) Add the milk, sugar substitute, coconut extract and vanilla. Transfer to crust. (Crust will be full.)
4. Bake at 350° for 30 minutes. Sprinkle with coconut. Bake for 8-10 minutes longer or until a knife inserted near the center comes out clean and coconut is lightly browned. Cool on a wire rack for 1 hour. Refrigerate until chilled.
NOTE *This recipe was tested with Splenda no-calorie sweetener.*
PER SERVING *1 piece equals 214 cal., 12 g fat (6 g sat. fat), 112 mg chol., 320 mg sodium, 20 g carb., trace fiber, 6 g pro.*

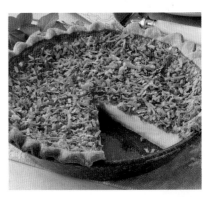

Slow Cooker

Your **slow cooker will be your new best friend** on the Comfort Food Diet. Prepare your meal in the morning or at noon, pop it into the slow cooker and come home to a **delicious hot entree, side or dessert** that will help you meet your **1,400 calorie goal** and satisfy your family!

When you know that **a healthy dinner** is waiting for you at home, you'll be less tempted to grab an unhealthy snack or to hit the drive-thru after work. And **the ease of a slow-cooked meal** means you'll have more time in your day for working out or pursuing other interests.

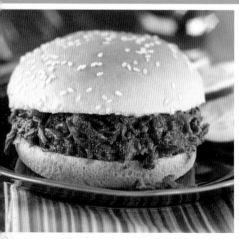

BBQ BEEF SANDWICHES *PAGE 448*

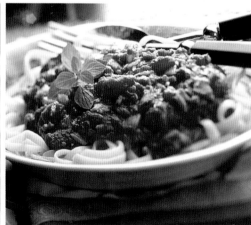

RED CLAM SAUCE *PAGE 466*

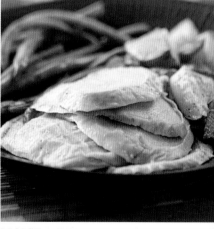

MOIST & TENDER TURKEY BREAST
PAGE 461

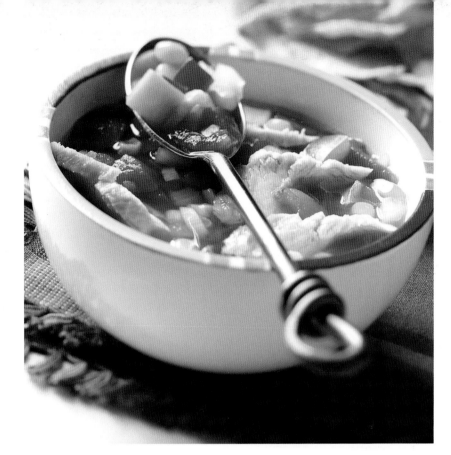

273 CALORIES Beef Burgundy

For this dish, I trim the meat and cut up the veggies the night before. Next day, I toss all the ingredients into the slow cooker. Shortly before dinnertime, I cook the noodles to complete the meal.

—**MARY JO MILLER** MANSFIELD, OH

PREP: 10 MIN. • **COOK:** 5 HOURS
MAKES: 6 SERVINGS

- 1½ pounds beef stew meat, cut into 1-inch cubes
- ½ pound whole fresh mushrooms, halved
- 4 medium carrots, chopped
- 1 can (10¾ ounces) condensed golden mushroom soup, undiluted
- 1 large onion, cut into thin wedges
- ½ cup Burgundy wine or beef broth
- ¼ cup quick-cooking tapioca
- ½ teaspoon salt
- ¼ teaspoon dried thyme
- ¼ teaspoon pepper
  Hot cooked egg noodles

1. In a 5-qt. slow cooker, combine the first 10 ingredients.
2. Cover and cook on low for 5-6 hours or until meat is tender. Serve with noodles.
PER SERVING *1 cup equals 273 cal., 9 g fat (3 g sat. fat), 73 mg chol., 642 mg sodium, 19 g carb., 3 g fiber, 24 g pro.*

143 CALORIES Southwestern Chicken Soup

Here's the perfect recipe for a busy day—because the slow cooker does most of the work for you!

—**HAROLD TARTAR**
WEST PALM BEACH, FL

PREP: 10 MIN. • **COOK:** 7 HOURS
MAKES: 10 SERVINGS (2½ QUARTS)

- 1¼ pounds boneless skinless chicken breasts, cut into thin strips
- 1 tablespoon canola oil
- 2 cans (14½ ounces each) reduced-sodium chicken broth
- 1 package (16 ounces) frozen corn, thawed
- 1 can (14½ ounces) diced tomatoes, undrained
- 1 medium onion, chopped
- 1 medium green pepper, chopped
- 1 medium sweet red pepper, chopped
- 1 can (4 ounces) chopped green chilies
- 1½ teaspoons seasoned salt, optional
- 1 teaspoon ground cumin
- ½ teaspoon garlic powder

1. In a large skillet, saute chicken in oil until lightly browned. Transfer to a 5-qt. slow cooker. Stir in the remaining ingredients.
2. Cover and cook on low for 7-8 hours or until chicken and vegetables are tender. Stir before serving.
PER SERVING *1 cup equals 143 cal., 3 g fat (1 g sat. fat), 31 mg chol., 364 mg sodium, 15 g carb., 3 g fiber, 15 g pro.* **Diabetic Exchanges:** *2 lean meat, 1 starch.*

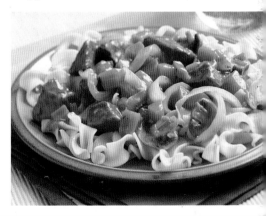

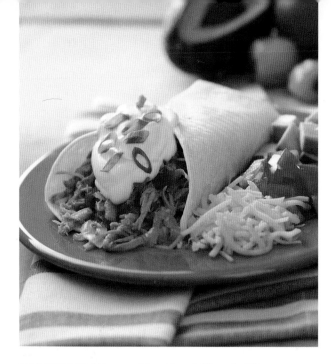

301 CALORIES Slow-Cooked Pork Tacos

Sometimes I'll substitute Bibb lettuce leaves for the tortillas to make crunchy lettuce wraps instead of tacos. Let each person customize these tacos with their own favorite toppings.
—**KATHLEEN WOLF** NAPERVILLE, IL

PREP: 20 MIN. • **COOK:** 4 HOURS • **MAKES:** 10 SERVINGS

- 1 boneless pork sirloin roast (2 pounds), cut into 1-inch pieces
- 1½ cups salsa verde
- 1 medium sweet red pepper, chopped
- 1 medium onion, chopped
- ¼ cup chopped dried apricots
- 2 tablespoons lime juice
- 2 garlic cloves, minced
- 1 teaspoon ground cumin
- ½ teaspoon salt
- ¼ teaspoon white pepper
  Dash hot pepper sauce
- 10 flour tortillas (8 inches), warmed
  Reduced-fat sour cream, thinly sliced green onions, cubed avocado, shredded reduced-fat cheddar cheese and chopped tomato, optional

1. In a 3-qt. slow cooker, combine the first 11 ingredients. Cover and cook on high for 4-5 hours or until meat is tender.

2. Shred pork with two forks. Place about ½ cup pork mixture down the center of each tortilla. Serve with toppings if desired.
PER SERVING *1 taco (calculated without optional toppings) equals 301 cal., 8 g fat (2 g sat. fat), 54 mg chol., 616 mg sodium, 32 g carb., 1 g fiber, 24 g pro.* **Diabetic Exchanges:** *3 lean meat, 2 starch.*

254 CALORIES Spicy Two-Bean Chili

Chili fans will get a kick out of this nontraditional recipe. Tomatoes with green chilies, kidney and black beans and a splash of lime juice lend an original twist. It's wonderful ladled over steaming rice.
—**LESLEY PEW** LYNN, MA

PREP: 20 MIN. • **COOK:** 8 HOURS • **MAKES:** 11 SERVINGS

- 2 pounds ground beef
- 3 large onions, chopped
- 6 garlic cloves, minced
- 2 cans (16 ounces each) kidney beans, rinsed and drained
- 2 cans (15 ounces each) black beans, rinsed and drained
- 2 cans (10 ounces each) diced tomatoes and green chilies, undrained
- 1 can (14½ ounces) chicken broth
- ½ cup lime juice
- 6 tablespoons cornmeal
- ¼ cup chili powder

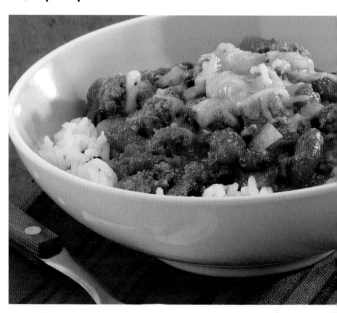

4 teaspoons dried oregano
3 teaspoons ground cumin
2 teaspoons salt
2 teaspoons rubbed sage
½ teaspoon white pepper
½ teaspoon paprika
½ teaspoon pepper
  Hot cooked rice
  Shredded cheddar cheese

1. In a Dutch oven, cook beef and onions over medium heat until meat is no longer pink. Add garlic; cook 1 minute longer. Drain.
2. Transfer to a 5-qt. slow cooker. Stir in the beans, tomatoes, broth, lime juice, cornmeal and seasonings.
3. Cover and cook on low for 8 hours or until heated through. Serve with rice; sprinkle with cheese.
PER SERVING *1 cup (calculated without rice and cheese) equals 254 cal., 8 g fat (3 g sat. fat), 40 mg chol., 906 mg sodium, 24 g carb., 6 g fiber, 21 g pro.*

380 CALORIES Hearty Beef Vegetable Stew

I received this wonderful recipe from a co-worker. It's awesome! A hit with everyone—including our two young children—this stew is as nutritious as it is tasty.
—ANGELA NELSON RUTHER GLEN, VA

PREP: 20 MIN. • **COOK:** 5 HOURS • **MAKES:** 6 SERVINGS

1½ pounds boneless beef chuck roast, cut into 1-inch cubes
2 teaspoons canola oil
1½ pounds red potatoes, cut into 1-inch cubes
3 medium carrots, cut into 1-inch lengths
1 medium onion, chopped
½ cup chopped celery
1 can (28 ounces) crushed tomatoes, undrained
3 tablespoons quick-cooking tapioca
2 tablespoons dried basil

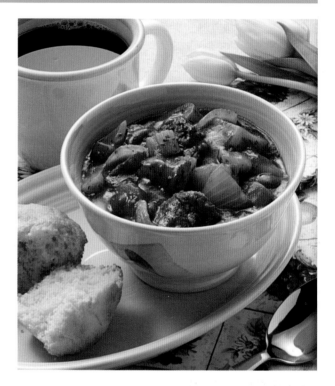

1 tablespoon sugar
½ teaspoon salt
⅛ teaspoon pepper

1. In a large nonstick skillet, brown meat in oil over medium heat. Meanwhile, place the potatoes, carrots, onion and celery in a 5-qt. slow cooker.
2. Drain meat; add to slow cooker. Combine tomatoes, tapioca, basil, sugar, salt and pepper; pour over the top.
3. Cover and cook on high for 5-6 hours or until meat and vegetables are tender.
PER SERVING *1⅓ cups equals 380 cal., 8 g fat (3 g sat. fat), 78 mg chol., 458 mg sodium, 46 g carb., 7 g fiber, 31 g pro.* **Diabetic Exchanges:** *3 lean meat, 2 starch, 2 vegetable.*

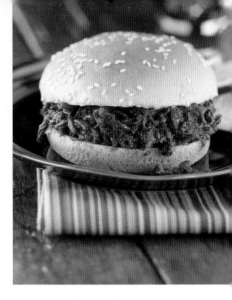

225 CALORIES Brisket with Cranberry Gravy

With just 15 minutes of hands-on work, this tender beef brisket simmers into a delectable entree.

—NOELLE LABRECQUE
ROUND ROCK, TX

PREP: 15 MIN. • **COOK:** 5½ HOURS
MAKES: 12 SERVINGS

- 1 medium onion, sliced
- 1 fresh beef brisket (3 pounds), halved
- 1 can (14 ounces) jellied cranberry sauce
- ½ cup thawed cranberry juice concentrate
- 2 tablespoons cornstarch
- ¼ cup cold water

1. Place onion in a 5-qt. slow cooker; top with brisket. Combine cranberry sauce and juice concentrate; pour over beef. Cover and cook on low for 5½ to 6 hours or until meat is tender.
2. Remove brisket and keep warm. Strain cooking juices, discarding onion; skim fat. Place in a small saucepan and bring to a boil. Combine cornstarch and cold water until smooth; gradually stir into the pan. Cook and stir for 2 minutes or until thickened. Thinly slice brisket across the grain; serve with gravy.

NOTE *This is a fresh beef brisket, not corned beef.*

PER SERVING *3 ounces cooked beef with 3 tablespoons gravy equals 225 cal., 5 g fat (2 g sat. fat), 48 mg chol., 46 mg sodium, 21 g carb., 1 g fiber, 23 g pro.* **Diabetic Exchanges:** *3 lean meat, 1½ starch.*

354 CALORIES BBQ Beef Sandwiches

After years of searching, I found a recipe for shredded barbecue beef that's a hit with all my family and friends. If there's any left over, it freezes well, too.

—REBECCA ROHLAND MEDFORD, WI

PREP: 15 MIN. • **COOK:** 8 HOURS
MAKES: 14 SERVINGS

- 2 cups ketchup
- 1 medium onion, chopped
- ¼ cup cider vinegar
- ¼ cup molasses
- 2 tablespoons Worcestershire sauce
- 2 garlic cloves, minced
- ½ teaspoon salt
- ½ teaspoon ground mustard
- ½ teaspoon pepper
- ¼ teaspoon garlic powder
- ¼ teaspoon crushed red pepper flakes
- 1 boneless beef chuck roast (3 pounds)
- 14 sesame seed hamburger buns, split

1. In a large bowl, combine the first 11 ingredients. Cut roast in half; place in a 5-qt. slow cooker. Pour ketchup mixture over roast. Cover and cook on low for 8-10 hours or until meat is tender.
2. Remove meat and shred with two forks. Skim fat from cooking juices. Return meat to slow cooker; heat through. Using a slotted spoon, serve beef on buns.

PER SERVING *1 sandwich equals 354 cal., 12 g fat (5 g sat. fat), 63 mg chol., 805 mg sodium, 37 g carb., 1 g fiber, 24 g pro.*

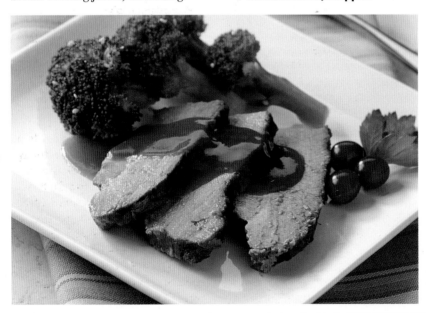

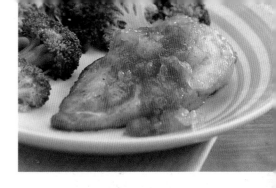

Corn and Broccoli in Cheese Sauce

This popular dish is a standby at our house. My daughter likes to add leftover ham to it. No one will ever guess it's lightened up!

—**JOYCE JOHNSON** UNIONTOWN, OH

PREP: 10 MIN. • **COOK:** 3 HOURS
MAKES: 8 SERVINGS

- 1 package (16 ounces) frozen corn, thawed
- 1 package (16 ounces) frozen broccoli florets, thawed
- 4 ounces reduced-fat process cheese (Velveeta), cubed
- ½ cup shredded cheddar cheese
- 1 can (10¼ ounces) reduced-fat reduced-sodium condensed cream of chicken soup, undiluted
- ¼ cup fat-free milk

1. In a 4-qt. slow cooker, combine the corn, broccoli and cheeses. In a small bowl, combine soup and milk; pour over vegetable mixture.
2. Cover and cook on low for 3-4 hours or until heated through. Stir before serving.

PER SERVING *¾ cup equals 148 cal., 5 g fat (3 g sat. fat), 16 mg chol., 409 mg sodium, 21 g carb., 3 g fiber, 8 g pro.* **Diabetic Exchanges:** *1 starch, 1 medium-fat meat.*

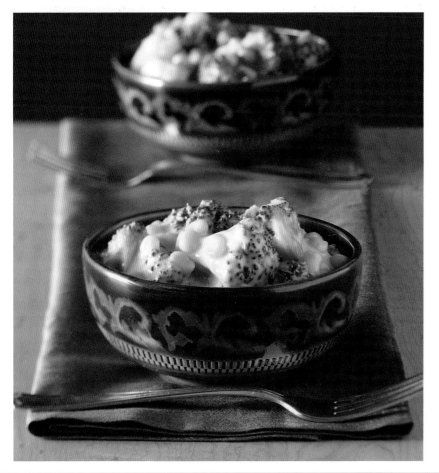

Honey Pineapple Chicken

I adapted a dinnertime favorite for my slow cooker because it's so much easier to do the preparation in advance, then let the chicken cook on its own while I do other things. Your family will love the combination of sweet and savory flavors.

—**CAROL GILLESPIE** CHAMBERSBURG, PA

PREP: 15 MIN. • **COOK:** 3 HOURS
MAKES: 12 SERVINGS

- 3 pounds boneless skinless chicken breast halves
- 2 tablespoons canola oil
- 1 can (8 ounces) unsweetened crushed pineapple, undrained
- 1 cup packed brown sugar
- ½ cup honey
- ⅓ cup lemon juice
- ¼ cup butter, melted
- 2 tablespoons prepared mustard
- 2 teaspoons reduced-sodium soy sauce

1. In a large skillet, brown chicken in oil in batches on both sides; transfer to a 5-qt. slow cooker. In a small bowl, combine the remaining ingredients; pour over chicken.
2. Cover and cook on low for 3-4 hours or until meat is tender. Strain cooking liquid, reserving pineapple. Serve pineapple with the chicken.

PER SERVING *1 serving equals 302 cal., 9 g fat (3 g sat. fat), 73 mg chol., 180 mg sodium, 33 g carb., trace fiber, 23 g pro.*

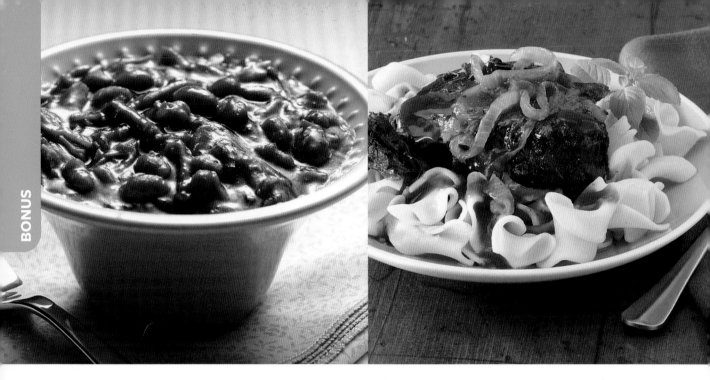

217 CALORIES Slow-Cooked Pork and Beans

I like to get this dish started before leaving for work in the morning. When I get home, my supper's ready! It's a hearty slow cooker meal that is also good for a potluck. A generous helping of tender pork and beans is perfect alongside a slice of warm corn bread.

—PATRICIA HAGER NICHOLASVILLE, KY

PREP: 15 MIN. • **COOK:** 6 HOURS
MAKES: 12 SERVINGS

- 1 **boneless pork loin roast (3 pounds)**
- 1 **medium onion, sliced**
- 3 **cans (15 ounces each) pork and beans**
- 1½ **cups barbecue sauce**
- ¼ **cup packed brown sugar**
- 1 **teaspoon garlic powder**

1. Cut roast in half; place in a 5-qt. slow cooker. Top with onion. In a large bowl, combine the beans, barbecue sauce, brown sugar and garlic powder; pour over meat. Cover and cook on low for 6-8 hours or until meat is tender.

2. Remove roast; shred with two forks. Return meat to slow cooker; heat through.

PER SERVING *1 cup equals 217 cal., 6 g fat (2 g sat. fat), 56 mg chol., 404 mg sodium, 16 g carb., 2 g fiber, 24 g pro.*

302 CALORIES German-Style Short Ribs

Our whole family is excited when I plug in the slow cooker to make these ribs that are fall-off-the-bone tender. We like them served over rice or egg noodles.

—BREGITTE RUGMAN
SHANTY BAY, ON

PREP: 15 MIN. • **COOK:** 8 HOURS
MAKES: 8 SERVINGS

- ¾ **cup dry red wine or beef broth**
- ½ **cup mango chutney**
- 3 **tablespoons quick-cooking tapioca**
- ¼ **cup water**
- 3 **tablespoons brown sugar**
- 3 **tablespoons cider vinegar**
- 1 **tablespoon Worcestershire sauce**
- ½ **teaspoon salt**
- ½ **teaspoon ground mustard**
- ½ **teaspoon chili powder**
- ½ **teaspoon pepper**
- 4 **pounds bone-in beef short ribs**
- 2 **medium onions, sliced**
  Hot cooked egg noodles

1. In a 5-qt. slow cooker, combine the first 11 ingredients. Add ribs and turn to coat. Top with onions.
2. Cover and cook on low for 8-10 hours or until meat is tender. Remove ribs from slow cooker. Skim fat from cooking juices; serve with ribs and noodles.

PER SERVING *1 serving (calculated without noodles) equals 302 cal., 11 g fat (5 g sat. fat), 55 mg chol., 378 mg sodium, 28 g carb., 1 g fiber, 19 g pro.*

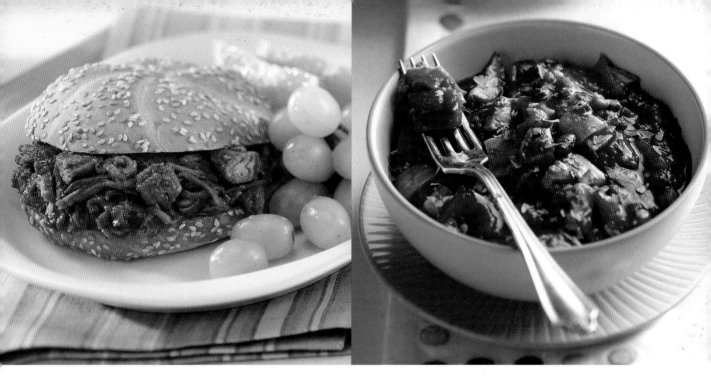

Tangy Pulled Pork Sandwiches

My slow cooker not only makes this one simple meal to fix, but it also keeps the pork moist and tender.

—**BEKI KOSYDAR-KRANTZ** MAYFIELD, PA

PREP: 10 MIN. • **COOK:** 4 HOURS
MAKES: 4 SERVINGS

- 1 **pork tenderloin (1 pound)**
- 1 **cup ketchup**
- 2 **tablespoons plus 1½ teaspoons brown sugar**
- 2 **tablespoons plus 1½ teaspoons cider vinegar**
- 1 **tablespoon plus 1½ teaspoons Worcestershire sauce**
- 1 **tablespoon spicy brown mustard**
- ¼ **teaspoon pepper**
- 4 **kaiser rolls, split**

1. Cut the tenderloin in half; place in a 3-qt. slow cooker. Combine the ketchup, brown sugar, vinegar, Worcestershire sauce, mustard and pepper; pour over pork.

2. Cover and cook on low for 4-5 hours or until meat is tender. Remove meat; shred with two forks. Return to the slow cooker; heat through. Serve on rolls.

PER SERVING *1 sandwich equals 402 cal., 7 g fat (2 g sat. fat), 63 mg chol., 1,181 mg sodium, 56 g carb., 2 g fiber, 29 g pro.*

238 CALORIES
Southwest Turkey Stew

I prefer main dishes that let our whole family eat right. This stew is a hit with both my husband and young children.

—**STEPHANIE HUTCHINSON** HELIX, OR

PREP: 15 MIN. • **COOK:** 5 HOURS
MAKES: 6 SERVINGS

- 1½ **pounds turkey breast tenderloins, cubed**
- 2 **teaspoons canola oil**
- 1 **can (15 ounces) turkey chili with beans, undrained**
- 1 **can (14½ ounces) diced tomatoes, undrained**
- 1 **medium sweet red pepper, chopped**
- 1 **medium green pepper, chopped**
- ¾ **cup chopped onion**
- ¾ **cup salsa**
- 3 **garlic cloves, minced**
- 1½ **teaspoons chili powder**
- ½ **teaspoon salt**
- ½ **teaspoon ground cumin**
- 1 **tablespoon minced fresh cilantro, optional**

In a nonstick skillet, brown turkey in oil; transfer to a 3-qt. slow cooker. Stir in the chili, tomatoes, peppers, onion, salsa, garlic, chili powder, salt and cumin. Cover and cook on low for 5-6 hours or until turkey is no longer pink and vegetables are tender. Garnish with cilantro if desired.

PER SERVING *1¼ cups equals 238 cal., 4 g fat (1 g sat. fat), 65 mg chol., 837 mg sodium, 17 g carb., 5 g fiber, 33 g pro.* **Diabetic Exchanges:** *4 lean meat, 1 vegetable, ½ starch.*

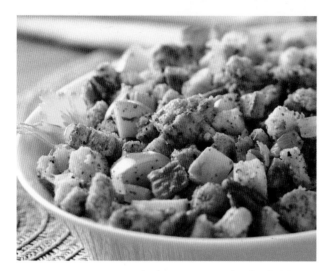

201 CALORIES

Slow-Cooked Sausage Dressing

Here's a holiday dressing that's so delicious, no one will know it's lower in fat. Best of all, it cooks effortlessly in the slow cooker, so the stove and oven are freed up for other dishes!
—RAQUEL HAGGARD EDMOND, OK

PREP: 20 MIN. • **COOK:** 3 HOURS • **MAKES:** 8 CUPS

- ½ pound reduced-fat bulk pork sausage
- 2 celery ribs, chopped
- 1 large onion, chopped
- 7 cups seasoned stuffing cubes
- 1 can (14½ ounces) reduced-sodium chicken broth
- 1 medium tart apple, chopped
- ⅓ cup chopped pecans
- 2 tablespoons reduced-fat butter, melted
- 1½ teaspoons rubbed sage
- ½ teaspoon pepper

1. In a large nonstick skillet, cook the sausage, celery and onion over medium heat until meat is no longer pink; drain. Transfer to a large bowl; stir in the remaining ingredients.
2. Place in a 5-qt. slow cooker coated with cooking spray. Cover and cook on low for 3-4 hours or until heated through and apple is tender, stirring once.
NOTE *This recipe was tested with Land O'Lakes light stick butter.*
PER SERVING ⅔ *cup equals 201 cal., 8 g fat (2 g sat. fat), 17 mg chol., 640 mg sodium, 26 g carb., 3 g fiber, 7 g pro.*

294 CALORIES Tex-Mex Beef Barbecues

I took this dish to a potluck recently, and guests loved it! The sandwiches are just as good made with ground beef instead of brisket. The wonderful recipe came from my mom.
—LYNDA ZUNIGA CRYSTAL CITY, TX

PREP: 20 MIN. • **COOK:** 5 HOURS • **MAKES:** 14 SERVINGS

- 1 fresh beef brisket (3½ pounds)
- 1 jar (18 ounces) hickory smoke-flavored barbecue sauce
- ½ cup finely chopped onion
- 1 envelope chili seasoning
- 1 tablespoon Worcestershire sauce
- 1 teaspoon minced garlic
- 1 teaspoon lemon juice
- 14 hamburger buns, split

1. Cut brisket in half; place in a 5-qt. slow cooker.
2. In a small bowl, combine the barbecue sauce, onion, chili seasoning, Worcestershire sauce, garlic and lemon juice. Pour over beef. Cover and cook on high for 5-6 hours or until meat is tender.
3. Remove beef; cool slightly. Shred and return to the slow cooker; heat through. Serve on buns.
NOTE *This is a fresh beef brisket, not corned beef.*
PER SERVING *1 sandwich equals 294 cal., 7 g fat (2 g sat. fat), 47 mg chol., 732 mg sodium, 28 g carb., 2 g fiber, 28 g pro.* **Diabetic Exchanges:** *3 lean meat, 2 starch.*

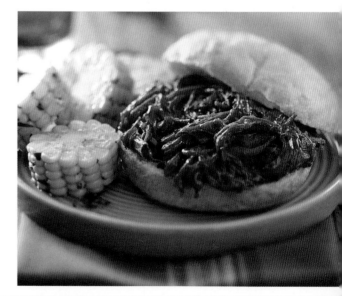

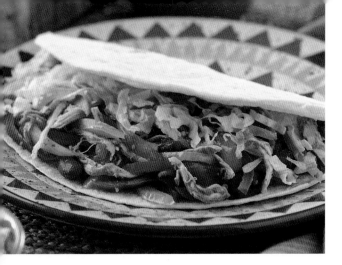

243 CALORIES Creamy Swiss Steak

When I was working, I'd put this Swiss steak in the slow cooker before I left for the day. A creamy mushroom sauce made with canned soup nicely flavors the tender round steak. It's delicious and so nice to come home to!

—**GLORIA CARPENTER** BANCROFT, MI

PREP: 15 MIN. • **COOK:** 8 HOURS • **MAKES:** 8 SERVINGS

- ¾ cup all-purpose flour
- 1 teaspoon salt
- ½ teaspoon pepper
- 2 pounds boneless beef round steak, cut into serving-size portions
- 2 tablespoons butter
- ½ cup chopped onion
- 2 cans (10¾ ounces each) condensed cream of mushroom soup, undiluted
- 1 cup water
  Hot cooked noodles

1. In a large resealable plastic bag, combine the flour, salt and pepper. Add beef, a few pieces at a time, and shake to coat.

2. In a large skillet, brown beef in butter on both sides. Transfer to a 3-qt. slow cooker; top with onion. Combine soup and water; pour over onion. Cover and cook on low for 8-10 hours or until meat is tender. Serve with noodles.

PER SERVING *1 serving (calculated without noodles) equals 243 cal., 8 g fat (4 g sat. fat), 73 mg chol., 624 mg sodium, 13 g carb., 1 g fiber, 28 g pro.*

347 CALORIES
Busy Mom's Chicken Fajitas

Staying at home with a young child makes preparing dinner a challenge, but my slow cooker provides an easy way to fix a low-fat meal. The tender meat in these fajitas is a hit, and the veggies and beans provide a healthy dose of fiber!

—**SARAH NEWMAN** MAHTOMEDI, MN

PREP: 15 MIN. • **COOK:** 5 HOURS • **MAKES:** 6 SERVINGS

- 1 pound boneless skinless chicken breast halves
- 1 can (16 ounces) kidney beans, rinsed and drained
- 1 can (14½ ounces) diced tomatoes with mild green chilies, drained
- 1 each medium green, sweet red and yellow peppers, julienned
- 1 medium onion, halved and sliced
- 2 teaspoons ground cumin
- 2 teaspoons chili powder
- 1 garlic clove, minced
- ¼ teaspoon salt
- 6 flour tortillas (8 inches), warmed
  Shredded lettuce and chopped tomatoes, optional

1. In a 3-qt. slow cooker, combine the chicken, beans, tomatoes, peppers, onion and seasonings. Cover and cook on low for 5-6 hours or until chicken is tender.

2. Remove chicken; cool slightly. Shred chicken and return to the slow cooker; heat through.

3. Spoon about ¾ cup chicken mixture down the center of each tortilla. Top with lettuce and tomatoes if desired.

PER SERVING *1 fajita (calculated without optional toppings) equals 347 cal., 5 g fat (1 g sat. fat), 42 mg chol., 778 mg sodium, 49 g carb., 7 g fiber, 26 g pro.*

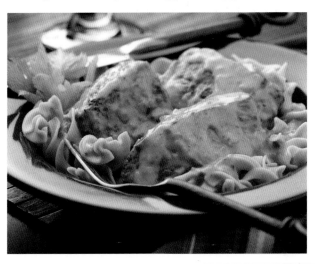

235 CALORIES
Bavarian Pork Loin

My aunt, who often prepared this tender pork roast, shared her cherished recipe with me. What a taste sensation with sauerkraut, carrots, onions and apples!
—**EDIE DESPAIN** LOGAN, UTAH

PREP: 25 MIN.
COOK: 6 HOURS + STANDING
MAKES: 10 SERVINGS

- 1 boneless pork loin roast (3 to 4 pounds)
- 1 can (14 ounces) Bavarian sauerkraut, rinsed and drained
- 1¾ cups chopped carrots
- 1 large onion, finely chopped
- ½ cup unsweetened apple juice
- 2 teaspoons dried parsley flakes
- 3 large tart apples, peeled and quartered

1. Cut roast in half; place in a 5-qt. slow cooker. In a small bowl, combine the sauerkraut, carrots, onion, apple juice and parsley; spoon over roast. Cover and cook on low for 4 hours.
2. Add apples to slow cooker. Cover and cook 2-3 hours longer or until meat is tender. Remove roast; let stand for 10 minutes before slicing. Serve with sauerkraut mixture.

STOVETOP OPTION *Cut roast in half. In a Dutch oven coated with cooking spray, brown roast on all sides. Combine the sauerkraut, carrots, onion, ¾ cup apple juice and parsley; spoon over roast. Bring to a boil. Reduce heat; cover and simmer for 1 hour. Stir in the apples. Cover and simmer for 20-25 minutes longer or until apples are tender and a thermometer reads 160°. Serve as directed.*

PER SERVING *1 serving equals 235 cal., 6 g fat (2 g sat. fat), 68 mg chol., 294 mg sodium, 17 g carb., 2 g fiber, 27 g pro.*

185 CALORIES
Sirloin Roast with Gravy

This recipe is perfect for my husband, who's a meat-and-potatoes kind of guy. The peppery, fork-tender roast combined with the rich gravy creates a tasty centerpiece for any meal.
—**RITA CLARK** MONUMENT, CO

PREP: 15 MIN. • **COOK:** 5½ HOURS
MAKES: 10 SERVINGS

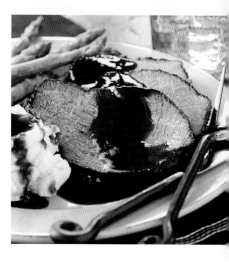

- 1 beef sirloin tip roast (3 pounds)
- 1 to 2 tablespoons coarsely ground pepper
- 1½ teaspoons minced garlic
- ¼ cup reduced-sodium soy sauce
- 3 tablespoons balsamic vinegar
- 1 tablespoon Worcestershire sauce
- 2 teaspoons ground mustard
- 2 tablespoons cornstarch
- ¼ cup cold water

1. Rub roast with pepper and garlic; cut in half and place in a 3-qt. slow cooker. Combine the soy sauce, vinegar, Worcestershire sauce and mustard; pour over beef. Cover and cook on low for 5½ to 6 hours or until the meat is tender.
2. Remove roast and keep warm. Strain cooking juices into a small saucepan; skim fat. Combine cornstarch and water until smooth; gradually stir into cooking juices. Bring to a boil; cook and stir for 2 minutes or until thickened. Serve with beef.

PER SERVING *4 ounces cooked beef with 3 tablespoons gravy equals 185 cal., 6 g fat (2 g sat. fat), 72 mg chol., 318 mg sodium, 4 g carb., trace fiber, 26 g pro.* **Diabetic Exchange:** *4 lean meat.*

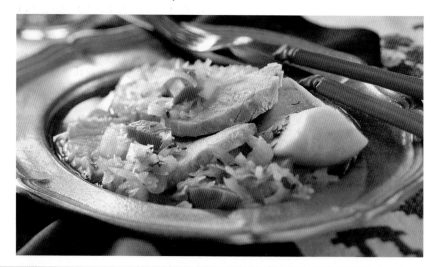

206 CALORIES Makeover Hash Brown Soup

Here's a lightened-up soup with all the rich and creamy goodness you'd expect, but with less fat, sodium and calories. It's just the thing to chase away chills!

—JUDITH WEBB BLUE SPRINGS, MO

PREP: 15 MIN. • **COOK:** 6 HOURS
MAKES: 8 SERVINGS

- 2 green onions, chopped
- 2 teaspoons canola oil
- 1 package (28 ounces) frozen O'Brien potatoes, thawed
- 2 cups 2% milk
- 1 can (10¾ ounces) reduced-fat reduced-sodium condensed cream of chicken soup, undiluted
- 6 turkey bacon strips, diced and cooked
- ½ cup shredded cheddar cheese

1. In a small skillet, saute onions in oil until tender. In a 5-qt. slow cooker, combine the potatoes, milk, soup and onions.

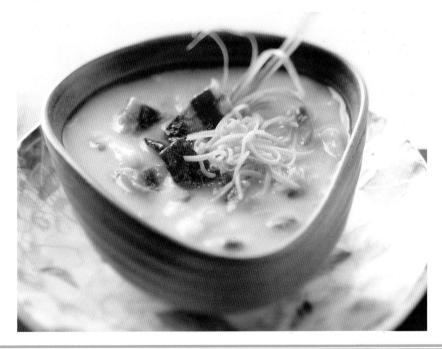

2. Cover and cook on low for 6-7 hours or until heated through. Top each serving with 2 tablespoons bacon and 1 tablespoon cheese.
PER SERVING *¾ cup equals 206 cal., 9 g fat (4 g sat. fat), 26 mg chol., 520 mg sodium, 24 g carb., 2 g fiber, 8 g pro.*

250 CALORIES Slow-Cooker Berry Cobbler

Even during warm weather, you can enjoy the comforting flavors of a homemade cobbler without heating up your kitchen!

—KAREN JAROCKI YUMA, AZ

PREP: 15 MIN. • **COOK:** 2 HOURS
MAKES: 8 SERVINGS

- 1¼ cups all-purpose flour, divided
- 2 tablespoons plus 1 cup sugar, divided
- 1 teaspoon baking powder
- ¼ teaspoon ground cinnamon
- 1 egg, lightly beaten
- ¼ cup fat-free milk

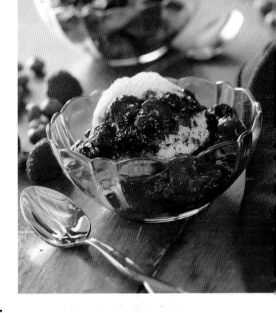

- 2 tablespoons canola oil
- ⅛ teaspoon salt
- 2 cups fresh or frozen raspberries, thawed
- 2 cups fresh or frozen blueberries, thawed
  Low-fat vanilla frozen yogurt, optional

1. In a large bowl, combine 1 cup flour, 2 tablespoons sugar, baking powder and cinnamon. Combine the egg, milk and oil; stir into dry ingredients just until moistened (batter will be thick). Spread batter evenly into a 5-qt. slow cooker coated with cooking spray.
2. In another large bowl, combine the salt and remaining flour and sugar; add berries and toss to coat. Spread over batter.
3. Cover and cook on high for 2 to 2½ hours or until a toothpick inserted in cobbler comes out clean. Serve with frozen yogurt if desired.
PER SERVING *1 piece (calculated without frozen yogurt) equals 250 cal., 4 g fat (trace sat. fat), 27 mg chol., 142 mg sodium, 51 g carb., 4 g fiber, 3 g pro.*

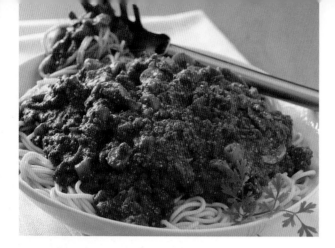

PER SERVING *1 cup equals 220 cal., 9 g fat (3 g sat. fat), 49 mg chol., 729 mg sodium, 15 g carb., 3 g fiber, 20 g pro.* **Diabetic Exchanges:** *2 lean meat, 1 starch, ½ fat.*

245 CALORIES Beef Roast Dinner

Since this healthy dish is slow cooked, you can use less-costly roasts and have the same mouthwatering results you'd get with more expensive cuts. Change up the veggies for variety, nutrition or to suit your tastes!

—**SANDRA DUDLEY** BEMIDJI, MN

PREP: 20 MIN. • **COOK:** 8 HOURS • **MAKES:** 10 SERVINGS

- 1 pound red potatoes (about 4 medium), cubed
- ¼ pound small fresh mushrooms
- 1½ cups fresh baby carrots
- 1 medium green pepper, chopped
- 1 medium parsnip, chopped
- 1 small red onion, chopped
- 1 beef rump roast or bottom round roast (3 pounds)
- 1 can (14½ ounces) beef broth
- ¾ teaspoon salt
- ¾ teaspoon dried oregano
- ¼ teaspoon pepper
- 3 tablespoons cornstarch
- ¼ cup cold water

220 CALORIES Zippy Spaghetti Sauce

This thick and hearty sauce goes a long way to satisfy a hungry family. To make sure I have the ingredients on hand, I always keep a bag of chopped green pepper in my freezer and minced garlic in my fridge.

—**ELAINE PRIEST** DOVER, PA

PREP: 20 MIN. • **COOK:** 6 HOURS • **MAKES:** ABOUT 3 QUARTS

- 2 pounds lean ground beef (90% lean)
- 1 cup chopped onion
- ½ cup chopped green pepper
- 2 cans (15 ounces each) tomato sauce
- 1 can (28 ounces) diced tomatoes, undrained
- 1 can (12 ounces) tomato paste
- ½ pound sliced fresh mushrooms
- 1 cup grated Parmesan cheese
- ½ to ¾ cup dry red wine or beef broth
- ½ cup sliced pimiento-stuffed olives
- ¼ cup dried parsley flakes
- 1 to 2 tablespoons dried oregano
- 2 teaspoons Italian seasoning
- 2 teaspoons minced garlic
- ½ teaspoon salt
- 1 teaspoon pepper
  Hot cooked spaghetti

1. In a large skillet, cook the beef, onion and green pepper over medium heat until meat is no longer pink; drain. Transfer to a 5-qt. slow cooker.

2. Stir in tomato sauce, tomatoes, tomato paste, mushrooms, cheese, wine, olives, parsley, oregano, Italian seasoning, garlic, salt and pepper.

3. Cover and cook on low for 6-8 hours. Serve sauce with spaghetti.

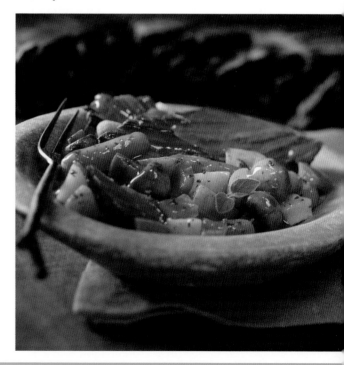

BONUS

1. Place vegetables in a 5-qt. slow cooker. Cut roast in half; place in slow cooker. Combine the broth, salt, oregano and pepper; pour over meat.Cover and cook on low for 8 hours or until meat is tender.

2. Remove meat and vegetables to a serving platter; keep warm. Skim fat from cooking juices; transfer to a small saucepan. Bring liquid to a boil.

3. Combine cornstarch and water until smooth. Gradually stir into the pan. Bring to a boil; cook and stir for 2 minutes or until thickened. Serve with meat and vegetables.

PER SERVING *4 ounces cooked beef with ⅔ cup vegetables and ¼ cup gravy equals 245 cal., 7 g fat (2 g sat. fat), 82 mg chol., 427 mg sodium, 16 g carb., 2 g fiber, 29 g pro.*
***Diabetic Exchanges:** 4 lean meat, 1 starch.*

229 CALORIES Chunky Chicken Soup

I am a stay-at-home mom who relies on my slow cooker for fast, nutritious meals with minimal cleanup and prep time. I knew this recipe was a hit when I didn't have any leftovers and my husband asked me to make it again.
—**NANCY CLOW** MALLORYTOWN, ON

PREP: 15 MIN. • **COOK:** 4½ HOURS • **MAKES:** 7 SERVINGS

- 1½ pounds boneless skinless chicken breasts, cut into 2-inch strips
- 2 teaspoons canola oil
- ⅔ cup finely chopped onion
- 2 medium carrots, chopped
- 2 celery ribs, chopped
- 1 cup frozen corn
- 2 cans (10¾ ounces each) condensed cream of potato soup, undiluted
- 1½ cups chicken broth
- 1 teaspoon dill weed
- 1 cup frozen peas
- ½ cup half-and-half cream

1. In a large skillet over medium-high heat, brown chicken in oil. Transfer to a 5-qt. slow cooker; add the onion, carrots, celery and corn.

2. In a large bowl, whisk the soup, broth and dill until blended; stir into slow cooker. Cover and cook on low for 4 hours or until chicken and vegetables are tender.

3. Stir in peas and cream. Cover and cook 30 minutes longer or until heated through.

PER SERVING *1 cup equals 229 cal., 7 g fat (3 g sat. fat), 66 mg chol., 629 mg sodium, 17 g carb., 3 g fiber, 24 g pro.*

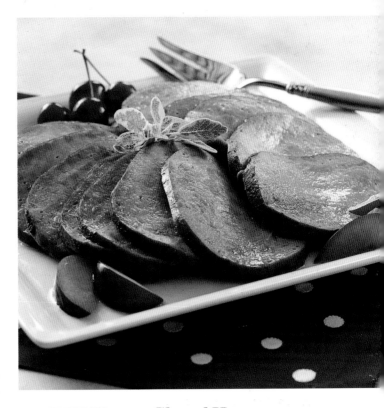

166 CALORIES Honey-Glazed Ham

Here's an easy solution for feeding a large group. The simple ham is perfect for family dinners where time spent out of the kitchen is as valuable as space in the oven.
—**JACQUIE STOLZ** LITTLE SIOUX, IA

PREP: 10 MIN. • **COOK:** 4½ HOURS • **MAKES:** 14 SERVINGS

- 1 boneless fully cooked ham (4 pounds)
- 1½ cups ginger ale
- ¼ cup honey
- ½ teaspoon ground mustard
- ½ teaspoon ground cloves
- ¼ teaspoon ground cinnamon

1. Cut ham in half; place in a 5-qt. slow cooker. Pour ginger ale over ham. Cover and cook on low for 4-5 hours or until heated through.

2. Combine the honey, mustard, cloves and cinnamon; stir until smooth. Spread over the ham; cook for 30 minutes longer.

PER SERVING *4 ounces ham equals 166 cal., 5 g fat (2 g sat. fat), 66 mg chol., 1,347 mg sodium, 8 g carb., trace fiber, 24 g pro.*

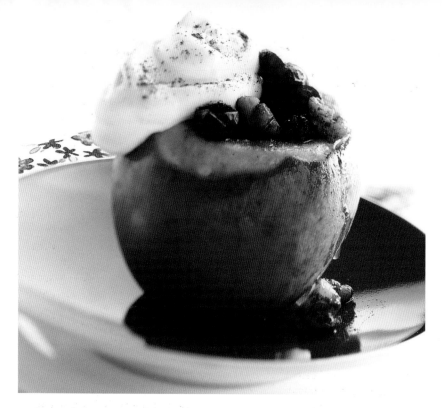

1 small onion, finely chopped
1 boneless pork shoulder butt roast (2½ pounds)
1 bottle (18 ounces) barbecue sauce
½ cup water
¼ cup honey
6 garlic cloves, minced
1 teaspoon seasoned salt
1 teaspoon ground ginger
8 submarine buns, split

1. Place onion and roast in a 5-qt. slow cooker. In a small bowl, combine the barbecue sauce, water, honey, garlic, seasoned salt and ginger; pour over meat. Cover and cook on high for 5-6 hours or until meat is tender.
2. Remove meat; cool slightly. Shred meat with two forks and return to the slow cooker; heat through. Serve on buns. Cut sandwiches in half.

PER SERVING *½ sub sandwich equals 417 cal., 13 g fat (4 g sat. fat), 81 mg chol., 867 mg sodium, 44 g carb., 2 g fiber, 29 g pro.*

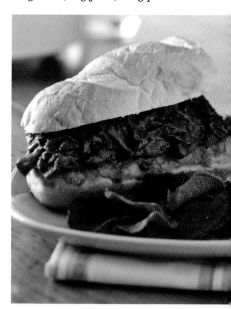

136 CALORIES Cranberry-Stuffed Apples

Cinnamon, nutmeg and walnuts add a homey autumn flavor to these stuffed apples. The slow cooker does most of the work for me!

—GRACIELA SANDVIGEN
ROCHESTER, NY

PREP: 10 MIN. • **COOK:** 4 HOURS
MAKES: 5 SERVINGS

5 medium apples
⅓ cup fresh or frozen cranberries, thawed and chopped
¼ cup packed brown sugar
2 tablespoons chopped walnuts
¼ teaspoon ground cinnamon
⅛ teaspoon ground nutmeg
Whipped cream or vanilla ice cream, optional

1. Core apples, leaving bottoms intact. Peel top third of each apple; place in a 5-qt. slow cooker.

Combine the cranberries, brown sugar, walnuts, cinnamon and nutmeg; spoon into apples.
2. Cover and cook on low for 4-5 hours or until apples are tender. Serve with whipped cream or ice cream if desired.
PER SERVING *1 apple (calculated without whipped cream or ice cream) equals 136 cal., 2 g fat (trace sat. fat), 0 chol., 6 mg sodium, 31 g carb., 4 g fiber, 1 g pro.* **Diabetic Exchanges:** *1 starch, 1 fruit.*

417 CALORIES
Pulled Pork Subs

Honey and ground ginger are the flavor boosters behind my no-stress sandwiches. A bottle of barbecue sauce quickly ties it all together.

—DENISE DAVIS PORTER, ME

PREP: 15 MIN. • **COOK:** 5 HOURS
MAKES: 16 SERVINGS

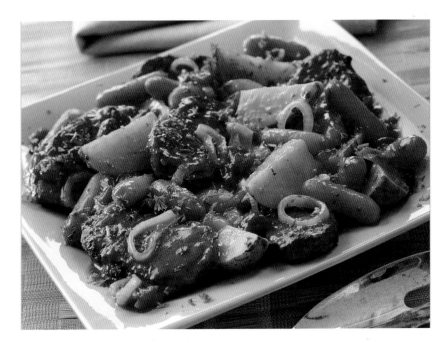

402 CALORIES
Swiss Steak Supper

Here's a satisfying slow-cooked dinner that's loaded with veggies. To save a step, I like to season the steak with peppered seasoned salt instead of using both seasoned salt and pepper.

—KATHLEEN ROMANIUK
CHOMEDEY, QC

PREP: 20 MIN. • **COOK:** 5 HOURS
MAKES: 6 SERVINGS

- 1½ **pounds beef top round steak**
- ½ **teaspoon seasoned salt**
- ¼ **teaspoon coarsely ground pepper**
- 1 **tablespoon canola oil**
- 3 **medium potatoes**
- 1½ **cups fresh baby carrots**
- 1 **medium onion, sliced**
- 1 **can (14½ ounces) Italian diced tomatoes**
- 1 **jar (12 ounces) home-style beef gravy**
- 1 **tablespoon minced fresh parsley**

1. Cut steak into six serving-size pieces; flatten to ¼-in. thickness.

Rub with seasoned salt and pepper. In a large skillet, brown beef in oil on both sides; drain.

2. Cut each potato into eight wedges. In a 5-qt. slow cooker, layer the potatoes, carrots, beef and onion. Combine tomatoes and gravy; pour over the top.

3. Cover and cook on low for 5-6 hours or until meat and vegetables are tender. Sprinkle with parsley.

PER SERVING *1 serving equals 402 cal., 6 g fat (2 g sat. fat), 67 mg chol., 822 mg sodium, 53 g carb., 5 g fiber, 33 g pro.*

255 CALORIES
Cranberry-Mustard Pork Loin

This dressed-up pork loin is so easy that you only have to spend a few minutes preparing it. The roast is a family favorite because it's so tasty, and a favorite of mine because it's so fast to get started!

—LAURA COOK WILDWOOD, MO

PREP: 15 MIN. • **COOK:** 4 HOURS
MAKES: 8 SERVINGS

- 1 **boneless pork loin roast (2 pounds)**
- 1 **can (14 ounces) whole-berry cranberry sauce**
- ¼ **cup Dijon mustard**
- 3 **tablespoons brown sugar**
- 3 **tablespoons lemon juice**
- 1 **tablespoon cornstarch**
- ¼ **cup cold water**

1. Place roast in a 3-qt. slow cooker. Combine the cranberry sauce, mustard, brown sugar and lemon juice; pour over roast. Cover and cook on low for 4 to 5 hours or until meat is tender. Remove roast and keep warm.

2. Strain cooking juices into a 2-cup measuring cup; add enough water to measure 2 cups. In a small saucepan, combine cornstarch and cold water until smooth; stir in cooking juices. Bring to a boil; cook and stir for 2 minutes or until thickened. Serve with pork.

PER SERVING *3 ounces cooked pork equals 255 cal., 6 g fat (2 g sat. fat), 56 mg chol., 236 mg sodium, 28 g carb., 1 g fiber, 22 g pro.*

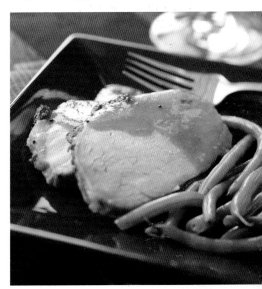

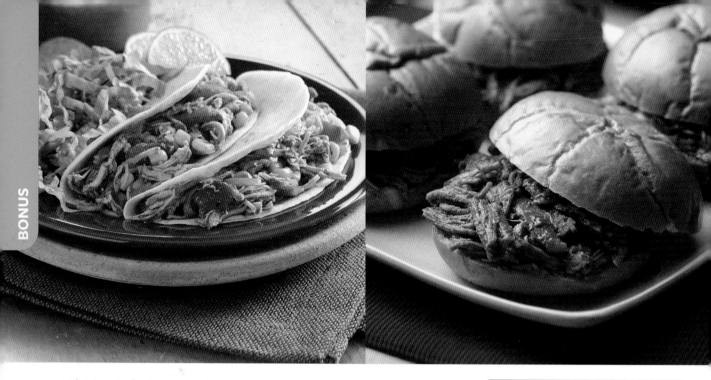

148 CALORIES

Lime Chicken Tacos

Fresh lime adds zest to an easy filling for tortillas, and leftovers would be a refreshing topping for any taco salad. This fun recipe is great for a casual dinner with friends or family.
—**TRACY GUNTER** BOISE, ID

PREP: 10 MIN. • **COOK:** 5½ HOURS
MAKES: 12 TACOS

- 1½ **pounds boneless skinless chicken breasts**
- 3 **tablespoons lime juice**
- 1 **tablespoon chili powder**
- 1 **cup frozen corn**
- 1 **cup chunky salsa**
- 12 **fat-free flour tortillas (6 inches), warmed**
  Sour cream, shredded cheddar cheese and shredded lettuce, optional

1. Place the chicken in a 3-qt. slow cooker. Combine lime juice and chili powder; pour over chicken. Cover and cook on low 5-6 hours or until chicken is tender.
2. Remove chicken; cool slightly. Shred meat with two forks and return to the slow cooker. Stir in corn and salsa.
3. Cover and cook on low for 30 minutes or until heated through. Serve in tortillas with sour cream, cheese and lettuce if desired.

PER SERVING *1 taco (calculated without sour cream and cheese) equals 148 cal., 2 g fat (trace sat. fat), 31 mg chol., 338 mg sodium, 18 g carb., 1 g fiber, 14 g pro.* ***Diabetic Exchanges:*** *2 lean meat, 1 starch.*

410 CALORIES ## Slow-Cooked Pork Barbecue

I need only five ingredients to make sweet and tender pulled pork for sandwiches. You can easily adjust or add seasonings to suit your family's tastes.
—**CONNIE JOHNSON** SPRINGFIELD, MO

PREP: 15 MIN. • **COOK:** 5 HOURS
MAKES: 10 SERVINGS

- 1 **boneless pork loin roast (3 to 4 pounds)**
- 1½ **teaspoons seasoned salt**
- 1 **teaspoon garlic powder**
- 1 **cup cola, divided**
- 1 **cup barbecue sauce**
- 10 **sandwich buns, split**

1. Cut roast in half; place in a 5-qt. slow cooker. Sprinkle with seasoned salt and garlic powder. Pour ¼ cup cola over roast. Cover and cook on low for 4-5 hours or until meat is tender.
2. Remove roast; cool slightly. Shred meat with two forks and return to slow cooker. Combine barbecue sauce and remaining cola; pour over meat. Cover and cook on high for 1-2 hours or until sauce is thickened. Serve on buns.

PER SERVING *1 sandwich equals 410 cal., 11 g fat (3 g sat. fat), 68 mg chol., 886 mg sodium, 41 g carb., 1 g fiber, 35 g pro.*

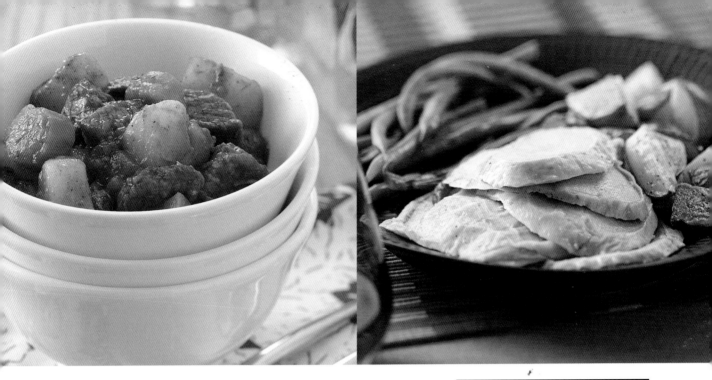

266 CALORIES Southwestern
Beef Stew

A zippy stew seasoned with picante sauce is ideal on cold winter evenings. It's ready in minutes after you come home from a long day at work.
—**REGINA STOCK** TOPEKA, KS

PREP: 30 MIN. • **COOK:** 8¼ HOURS
MAKES: 7 SERVINGS

- 2 **pounds beef stew meat, cut into 1-inch cubes**
- 1 **jar (16 ounces) picante sauce**
- 2 **medium potatoes, peeled and cut into ½-inch cubes**
- 4 **medium carrots, cut into ½-inch slices**
- 1 **large onion, chopped**
- 1 **teaspoon chili powder**
- ¼ **teaspoon salt**
- ¼ **teaspoon ground cumin**
- 1 **tablespoon cornstarch**
- ¼ **cup cold water**

1. In a large nonstick skillet coated with cooking spray, brown beef on all sides; drain. Transfer to a 3-qt. slow cooker. Stir in the picante sauce, potatoes, carrots, onion, chili powder, salt and cumin.
2. Cover and cook on low 8-9 hours or until the meat and vegetables are tender.
3. In a small bowl, combine cornstarch and water until smooth; stir into stew. Cover and cook on high for 15 minutes or until thickened.
PER SERVING *1 cup equals 266 cal., 9 g fat (3 g sat. fat), 81 mg chol., 436 mg sodium, 18 g carb., 2 g fiber, 26 g pro.* ***Diabetic Exchanges:*** *3 lean meat, 2 vegetable, ½ starch.*

318 CALORIES Moist &
Tender Turkey Breast

This easy entree is sure to be popular in your home. Everyone will love the irresistible taste, and you'll appreciate how quickly it comes together.
—**HEIDI VAWDREY** RIVERTON, UTAH

PREP: 10 MIN. • **COOK:** 4 HOURS
MAKES: 12 SERVINGS

- 1 **bone-in turkey breast (6 to 7 pounds)**
- ½ **cup water**
- 4 **fresh rosemary sprigs**
- 4 **garlic cloves, peeled**
- 1 **tablespoon brown sugar**
- ½ **teaspoon coarsely ground pepper**
- ¼ **teaspoon salt**

Place turkey breast and water in a 6-qt. slow cooker. Place rosemary and garlic around turkey. Combine the brown sugar, pepper and salt; sprinkle over turkey. Cover and cook on low for 4-6 hours or until turkey is tender.
PER SERVING *6 ounces cooked turkey equals 318 cal., 12 g fat (3 g sat. fat), 122 mg chol., 154 mg sodium, 2 g carb., trace fiber, 47 g pro.*

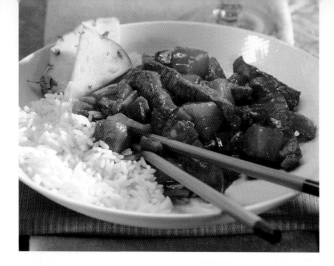

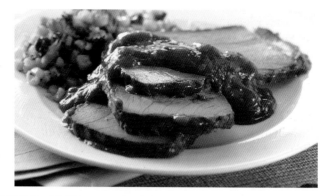

312 CALORIES

Slow-Cooked Sweet 'n' Sour Pork

Even though a co-worker gave me this recipe more than 20 years ago, my family still enjoys it today.
—MARTHA NICKERSON HANCOCK, ME

PREP: 20 MIN. • **COOK:** 6½ HOURS • **MAKES:** 6 SERVINGS

 2 **tablespoons plus 1½ teaspoons paprika**
 1½ **pounds boneless pork loin roast, cut into 1-inch strips**
 1 **tablespoon canola oil**
 1 **can (20 ounces) unsweetened pineapple chunks**
 1 **medium onion, chopped**
 1 **medium green pepper, chopped**
 ¼ **cup cider vinegar**
 3 **tablespoons brown sugar**
 3 **tablespoons reduced-sodium soy sauce**
 1 **tablespoon Worcestershire sauce**
 ½ **teaspoon salt**
 2 **tablespoons cornstarch**
 ¼ **cup cold water**
    Hot cooked rice, optional

1. Place paprika in a large resealable plastic bag. Add pork, a few pieces at a time, and shake to coat. In a nonstick skillet, brown pork in oil in batches over medium-high heat. Transfer to a 3-qt. slow cooker.
2. Drain pineapple, reserving juice; refrigerate the pineapple. Add the pineapple juice, onion, green pepper, vinegar, brown sugar, soy sauce, Worcestershire sauce and salt to slow cooker. Cover and cook on low for 6-8 hours or until meat is tender.
3. Combine cornstarch and water until smooth; stir into pork mixture. Add pineapple. Cover and cook for

30 minutes longer or until sauce is thickened. Serve over rice if desired.
PER SERVING *1 cup pork mixture (calculated without rice) equals 312 cal., 10 g fat (3 g sat. fat), 73 mg chol., 592 mg sodium, 28 g carb., 2 g fiber, 27 g pro.* **Diabetic Exchanges:** *3 lean meat, 1 fruit, ½ starch, ½ fat.*

267 CALORIES Picante Beef Roast

I created Picante Beef Roast because I love the flavor of taco seasoning and think it shouldn't be reserved just for tacos! My recipe couldn't be easier, and it works great with a pork roast, too.
—MARGARET THIEL LEVITTOWN, PA

PREP: 15 MIN. • **COOK:** 8 HOURS • **MAKES:** 8 SERVINGS

 1 **beef rump roast or bottom round roast (3 pounds), trimmed**
 1 **jar (16 ounces) picante sauce**
 1 **can (15 ounces) tomato sauce**
 1 **envelope taco seasoning**
 3 **tablespoons cornstarch**
 ¼ **cup cold water**

1. Cut roast in half; place in a 5-qt. slow cooker. In a large bowl, combine the picante sauce, tomato sauce and taco seasoning; pour over roast. Cover and cook on low for 8-9 hours or until meat is tender.
2. Remove meat to a serving platter; keep warm. Skim fat from cooking juices; transfer 3 cups to a small saucepan. Bring liquid to a boil. Combine cornstarch and water until smooth. Gradually stir into the pan. Bring to a boil; cook and stir for 2 minutes or until thickened. Serve with roast.
PER SERVING *5 ounces cooked beef with ⅓ cup gravy equals 267 cal., 8 g fat (3 g sat. fat), 102 mg chol., 983 mg sodium, 11 g carb., trace fiber, 34 g pro.*

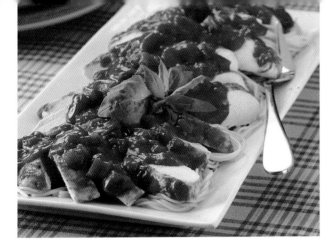

231 CALORIES Slow-Cooked Italian Chicken

With its nicely seasoned tomato sauce, this enticing chicken is especially good over pasta or rice. My father always loved to have me make this.

—DEANNA D'AURIA BANNING, CA

PREP: 20 MIN. • **COOK:** 4 HOURS • **MAKES:** 4 SERVINGS

- 4 boneless skinless chicken breast halves (4 ounces each)
- 1 can (14½ ounces) reduced-sodium chicken broth
- 1 can (14½ ounces) stewed tomatoes, cut up
- 1 can (8 ounces) tomato sauce
- 1 medium green pepper, chopped
- 1 green onion, chopped
- 1 garlic clove, minced
- 3 teaspoons chili powder
- 1 teaspoon ground mustard
- ½ teaspoon pepper
- ¼ teaspoon garlic powder
- ¼ teaspoon onion powder
- ⅓ cup all-purpose flour
- ½ cup cold water
  Hot cooked pasta

1. Place chicken in a 3-qt. slow cooker. In a bowl, combine the broth, tomatoes, tomato sauce, green pepper, onion, garlic and seasonings; pour over chicken. Cover and cook on low for 4-5 hours or until meat is tender. Remove chicken and keep warm.

2. Pour cooking juices into a large saucepan; skim fat. Combine flour and cold water until smooth; stir into juices. Bring to a boil; cook and stir for 2 minutes or until thickened. Serve with chicken and pasta.

PER SERVING *1 chicken breast half with ½ cup sauce (calculated without pasta) equals 231 cal., 3 g fat (1 g sat. fat), 63 mg chol., 818 mg sodium, 22 g carb., 3 g fiber, 28 g pro.* **Diabetic Exchanges:** *3 lean meat, 1 starch, 1 vegetable.*

211 CALORIES Coconut-Pecan Sweet Potatoes

These delicious sweet potatoes cook effortlessly in the slow cooker so you can tend to other things. Coconut adds new mouthwatering flavor to this classic side dish.

—RAQUEL HAGGARD EDMOND, OK

PREP: 15 MIN. • **COOK:** 4 HOURS • **MAKES:** 12 SERVINGS

- 4 pounds sweet potatoes, peeled and cut into chunks
- ½ cup chopped pecans
- ½ cup flaked coconut
- ⅓ cup sugar
- ⅓ cup packed brown sugar
- ¼ cup reduced-fat butter, melted
- ½ teaspoon ground cinnamon
- ¼ teaspoon salt
- ½ teaspoon coconut extract
- ½ teaspoon vanilla extract

1. Place sweet potatoes in a 5-qt. slow cooker coated with cooking spray. Combine the pecans, coconut, sugar, brown sugar, butter, cinnamon and salt; sprinkle over potatoes.

2. Cover and cook on low for 4 hours or until potatoes are tender. Stir in extracts.

NOTE *This recipe was tested with Land O'Lakes light stick butter.*

PER SERVING *⅔ cup equals 211 cal., 7 g fat (3 g sat. fat), 5 mg chol., 103 mg sodium, 37 g carb., 3 g fiber, 2 g pro.*

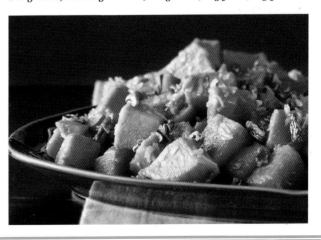

> "I pre-pay for evening Zumba classes. It's an incentive to make sure I go each week. Grab a friend and try it. It's so much fun. Twenty pounds down this year!"

—SONYA TOEWS

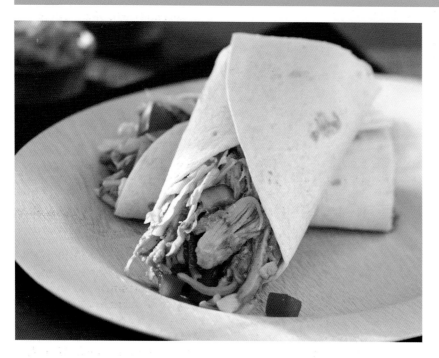

320 CALORIES

Pork Burritos

I've been making this recipe for 20 years, changing it here and there until I created the perfect version. It's a favorite of friends and family alike.

—SHARON BELMONT LINCOLN, NE

PREP: 20 MIN. • **COOK:** 8 HOURS
MAKES: 14 SERVINGS

- 1 boneless pork sirloin roast (3 pounds)
- ¼ cup reduced-sodium chicken broth
- 1 envelope reduced-sodium taco seasoning
- 1 tablespoon dried parsley flakes
- 2 garlic cloves, minced
- ½ teaspoon pepper
- ¼ teaspoon salt
- 1 can (16 ounces) refried beans
- 1 can (4 ounces) chopped green chilies
- 14 flour tortillas (8 inches), warmed
  Optional toppings: shredded lettuce, chopped tomatoes, chopped green pepper, guacamole, reduced-fat sour cream and shredded reduced-fat cheddar cheese

1. Cut roast in half; place in a 4- or 5-qt. slow cooker. In a small bowl, combine the broth, taco seasoning, parsley, garlic, pepper and salt. Pour over roast. Cover and cook on low for 8-10 hours or until meat is very tender.

2. Remove pork from the slow cooker; cool slightly. Shred with two forks; set aside. Skim fat from cooking liquid; stir in beans and chilies. Return pork to the slow cooker; heat through.

3. Spoon ½ cup pork mixture down the center of each tortilla; add toppings of your choice. Fold sides and ends over filling and roll up.

TO FREEZE BURRITOS *Roll up burritos without toppings. Wrap individually in paper towels, then foil. Transfer to a resealable plastic bag. May be frozen for up to 2 months. To use frozen burritos, unwrap foil. Place paper towel-wrapped burritos on a microwave-safe plate. Microwave on high for 3-4 minutes or until heated through. Serve with toppings of your choice.*

PER SERVING *1 burrito (calculated without optional toppings) equals 320 cal., 9 g fat (3 g sat. fat), 61 mg chol., 606 mg sodium, 33 g carb., 2 g fiber, 26 g pro. Diabetic Exchanges: 2 starch, 2 lean meat, 1 fat.*

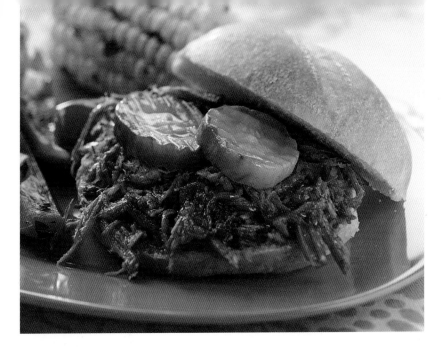

Shredded Barbecue Beef Sandwiches

I like to serve these scrumptious sandwiches with coleslaw either on the side—or right on the sandwich. You can freeze any leftover meat for a quick meal later on.

—BUNNY PALMERTREE
CARROLLTON, MS

PREP: 10 MIN. • **COOK:** 10 HOURS
MAKES: 16 SERVINGS

- 1 can (10½ ounces) condensed beef broth, undiluted
- 1 cup ketchup
- ½ cup packed brown sugar
- ½ cup lemon juice
- 3 tablespoons steak sauce
- 2 garlic cloves, minced
- 1 teaspoon pepper
- 1 teaspoon Worcestershire sauce
- 1 beef eye round roast (3½ pounds), cut in half
- 1 teaspoon salt
- 16 sandwich buns, split
  Dill pickle slices, optional

1. In a small bowl, whisk the first eight ingredients. Pour half of mixture into a 5-qt. slow cooker. Sprinkle beef with salt; add to slow cooker and top with remaining broth mixture.

2. Cover and cook on low for 10-12 hours or until meat is tender. Shred meat with two forks and return to slow cooker. Using a slotted spoon, place ½ cup beef mixture on each bun. Top with pickles if desired.

PER SERVING *1 sandwich (calculated without pickles) equals 370 cal., 8 g fat (2 g sat. fat), 46 mg chol., 963 mg sodium, 47 g carb., 1 g fiber, 28 g pro.*

Round Steak Sauerbraten

My easy version of an Old World classic takes just minutes to prepare for the slow cooker. The flavorful beef is also delicious with white rice or dirty rice.

—LINDA BLOOM MCHENRY, IL

PREP: 20 MIN. • **COOK:** 6½ HOURS
MAKES: 10 SERVINGS

- 1 envelope brown gravy mix
- 2 tablespoons plus 1½ teaspoons brown sugar
- 2½ cups cold water, divided
- 1 cup chopped onion
- 2 tablespoons white vinegar
- 2 teaspoons Worcestershire sauce
- 2 bay leaves
- 2½ pounds beef top round steak, cut into 3-inch x ½-inch strips
- 2 teaspoons salt
- 1 teaspoon pepper
- ¼ cup cornstarch
- 10 cups hot cooked egg noodles

1. In a 5-qt. slow cooker, combine the gravy mix, brown sugar, 2 cups water, onion, vinegar, Worcestershire sauce and bay leaves.

2. Sprinkle beef with salt and pepper; stir into gravy mixture. Cover and cook on low 6-8 hours or until meat is tender.

3. Combine cornstarch and remaining water until smooth; stir into beef mixture. Cover and cook on high for 30 minutes or until thickened. Discard bay leaves. Serve with noodles.

PER SERVING *¾ cup beef mixture with 1 cup noodles equals 331 cal., 6 g fat (2 g sat. fat), 96 mg chol., 741 mg sodium, 37 g carb., 2 g fiber, 32 g pro.* **Diabetic Exchanges:** *3 lean meat, 2½ starch.*

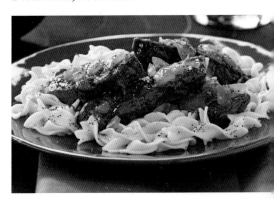

`199 CALORIES` Slow-Cooked Sirloin

My family of five likes to eat beef, and this recipe is a favorite.
I usually serve it with homemade bread or rolls to soak up every
last drop of the tasty gravy.
—**VICKI TORMASCHY** DICKINSON, ND

PREP: 20 MIN. • **COOK:** 3½ HOURS • **MAKES:** 6 SERVINGS

- 1 **beef top sirloin steak (1½ pounds)**
- 1 **medium onion, cut into 1-inch chunks**
- 1 **medium green pepper, cut into 1-inch chunks**
- 1 **can (14½ ounces) reduced-sodium beef broth**
- ¼ **cup Worcestershire sauce**
- ¼ **teaspoon dill weed**
- ¼ **teaspoon dried thyme**
- ¼ **teaspoon pepper**
  Dash crushed red pepper flakes
- 2 **tablespoons cornstarch**
- 2 **tablespoons water**

1. In a large nonstick skillet coated with cooking spray,
brown beef on both sides. Place onion and green pepper
in a 3-qt. slow cooker. Top with beef. Combine the
broth, Worcestershire sauce, dill, thyme, pepper and
pepper flakes; pour over beef. Cover and cook on high
for 3-4 hours or until meat reaches desired doneness
and vegetables are crisp-tender.

2. Remove beef and keep warm. Combine cornstarch and
water until smooth; gradually stir into cooking juices.
Cover and cook on high for 30 minutes or until slightly
thickened. Return beef to the slow cooker; heat through.
PER SERVING *1 serving equals 199 cal., 6 g fat (2 g sat.
fat), 68 mg chol., 305 mg sodium, 8 g carb., 1 g fiber,
26 g pro.* **Diabetic Exchanges:** *3 lean meat, 1 vegetable.*

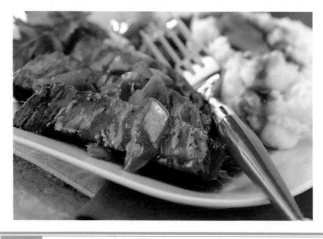

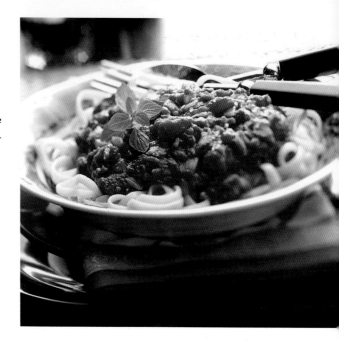

`305 CALORIES` Red Clam Sauce

This luscious sauce tastes like you've worked on it all day.
Instead, it simmers hands-free while you do other things.
What a great way to jazz up pasta!
—**JOANN BROWN** LATROBE, PA

PREP: 25 MIN. • **COOK:** 3 HOURS • **MAKES:** 4 SERVINGS

- 1 **medium onion, chopped**
- 1 **tablespoon canola oil**
- 2 **garlic cloves, minced**
- 2 **cans (6½ ounces each) chopped clams, undrained**
- 1 **can (14½ ounces) diced tomatoes, undrained**
- 1 **can (6 ounces) tomato paste**
- ¼ **cup minced fresh parsley**
- 1 **bay leaf**
- 1 **teaspoon sugar**
- 1 **teaspoon dried basil**
- ½ **teaspoon dried thyme**
- 6 **ounces linguine, cooked and drained**

1. In a small skillet, saute onion in oil until tender. Add
garlic; cook 1 minute longer.

2. Transfer to a 1½- or 2-qt. slow cooker. Stir in the
clams, tomatoes, tomato paste, parsley, bay leaf, sugar,
basil and thyme.

3. Cover and cook on low for 3-4 hours or until heated
through. Discard bay leaf. Serve with linguine.

BONUS

STOVETOP OPTION *Saute onion and garlic as directed in a large saucepan. Add the diced tomatoes, tomato paste, parsley, bay leaf, sugar, basil and thyme. Bring to a boil. Reduce heat; cover and simmer for 45 minutes, stirring occasionally. Stir in clams; heat through. Serve as directed.*

PER SERVING *1 cup sauce with ¾ cup cooked linguine equals 305 cal., 5 g fat (trace sat. fat), 15 mg chol., 553 mg sodium, 53 g carb., 7 g fiber, 15 g pro.*

278 CALORIES Vegetable Beef Stew

Here is a variation on traditional beef stew that I came across. With sweet flavor from apricots and squash, we think it has South American or Cuban flair. The addition of corn makes it even more filling and hearty.
—**RUTH RODRIGUEZ** FORT MYERS BEACH, FL

PREP: 10 MIN. • **COOK:** 5½ HOURS • **MAKES:** 4 SERVINGS

- ¾ pound beef stew meat, cut into ½-inch cubes
- 2 teaspoons canola oil
- 1 can (14½ ounces) beef broth
- 1 can (14½ ounces) stewed tomatoes, cut up
- 1½ cups cubed peeled butternut squash
- 1 cup frozen corn, thawed
- 6 dried apricot or peach halves, quartered
- ½ cup chopped carrot
- 1 teaspoon dried oregano
- ¼ teaspoon salt
- ¼ teaspoon pepper
- 2 tablespoons cornstarch
- ¼ cup water
- 2 tablespoons minced fresh parsley

1. In a nonstick skillet, cook beef over medium heat in oil until no longer pink; drain. Transfer to a 3-qt. slow cooker. Add the broth, tomatoes, squash, corn, apricots, carrot, oregano, salt and pepper.
2. Cover and cook on high for 5-6 hours or until vegetables and meat are tender.
3. Combine cornstarch and water until smooth; gradually stir into stew. Cover and cook on high for 30 minutes or until thickened. Stir in parsley.
PER SERVING *1½ cups equals 278 cal., 9 g fat (3 g sat. fat), 53 mg chol., 717 mg sodium, 32 g carb., 5 g fiber, 21 g pro.* **Diabetic Exchanges:** *2 lean meat, 2 vegetable, 1½ starch, ½ fat.*

300 CALORIES Slow-Cooked Mac 'n' Cheese

The name of this recipe alone is enough to make mouths water. This is comfort food at its finest: rich, hearty and extra-cheesy. It serves nine as a side dish, though you might just want to make it your main course!
—**SHELBY MOLINA** WHITEWATER, WI

PREP: 25 MIN. • **COOK:** 2 HOURS • **MAKES:** 9 SERVINGS

- 2 cups uncooked elbow macaroni
- 1 can (12 ounces) reduced-fat evaporated milk
- 1½ cups fat-free milk
- ⅓ cup egg substitute
- 1 tablespoon butter, melted
- 8 ounces reduced-fat process cheese (Velveeta), cubed
- 2 cups (8 ounces) shredded sharp cheddar cheese, divided

1. Cook macaroni according to package directions; drain and rinse in cold water. In a large bowl, combine the evaporated milk, milk, egg substitute and butter. Stir in the process cheese, 1/2 cups sharp cheddar cheese and macaroni.
2. Transfer to a 3-qt. slow cooker coated with cooking spray. Cover and cook on low for 2-3 hours or until center is set, stirring once. Sprinkle with remaining sharp cheddar cheese.
PER SERVING *¾ cup equals 300 cal., 12 g fat (9 g sat. fat), 45 mg chol., 647 mg sodium, 29 g carb., 1 g fiber, 19 g pro.* **Diabetic Exchanges:** *2 starch, 2 medium-fat meat.*

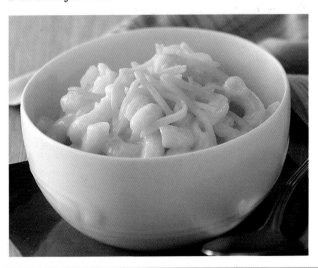

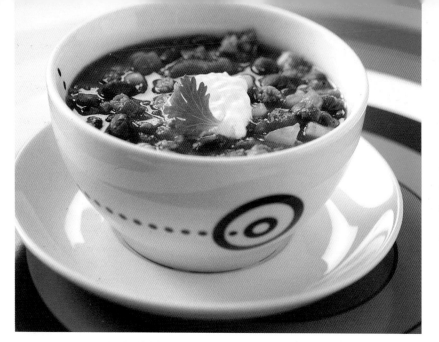

349 CALORIES
Family-Pleasing Turkey Chili

My children really love this recipe, and it's become one of their favorite comfort foods. It's relatively inexpensive, and the leftovers are wonderful!

—SHEILA CHRISTENSEN
SAN MARCOS, CA

PREP: 25 MIN. • **COOK:** 4 HOURS
MAKES: 6 SERVINGS (2¼ QUARTS)

- 1 pound lean ground turkey
- 1 medium green pepper, finely chopped
- 1 small red onion, finely chopped
- 2 garlic cloves, minced
- 1 can (28 ounces) diced tomatoes, undrained
- 1 can (16 ounces) kidney beans, rinsed and drained
- 1 can (15 ounces) black beans, rinsed and drained
- 1 can (14½ ounces) reduced-sodium chicken broth
- 1¾ cups frozen corn, thawed
- 1 can (6 ounces) tomato paste
- 1 tablespoon chili powder
- ½ teaspoon pepper
- ¼ teaspoon ground cumin
- ¼ teaspoon garlic powder
  Optional toppings: reduced-fat sour cream and minced fresh cilantro

1. In a large nonstick skillet, cook the turkey, green pepper and onion over medium heat until meat is no longer pink. Add garlic; cook for 1 minute longer. Drain.

2. Transfer to a 4-qt. slow cooker. Stir in the tomatoes, kidney beans, black beans, broth, corn, tomato paste, chili powder, pepper, cumin and garlic powder.

3. Cover and cook on low for 4-5 hours or until chili is heated through. Serve with optional toppings if desired.

PER SERVING *1½ cups (calculated without optional toppings) equals 349 cal., 7 g fat (2 g sat. fat), 60 mg chol., 725 mg sodium, 47 g carb., 12 g fiber, 27 g pro.* **Diabetic Exchanges:** *3 lean meat, 2 starch, 2 vegetable.*

357 CALORIES
Spicy French Dip

If I'm cooking for a party or family get-together, I can put this beef in the slow cooker in the morning, then concentrate on other preparations. It's a great time-saver and never fails to get rave reviews.

—GINNY KOEPPEN WINNFIELD, LA

PREP: 5 MIN. • **COOK:** 8 HOURS
MAKES: 12 SERVINGS

- 1 beef sirloin tip roast (3 pounds), cut in half
- ½ cup water
- 1 can (4 ounces) diced jalapeno peppers, drained
- 1 envelope Italian salad dressing mix
- 12 crusty rolls (5 inches)

1. Place beef in a 5-qt. slow cooker. In a small bowl, combine the water, jalapenos and dressing mix; pour over beef. Cover and cook on low for 8-10 hours or until meat is tender.

2. Remove beef and shred using two forks. Skim fat from cooking juices. Serve beef on rolls with juice.

PER SERVING *1 sandwich with 3 tablespoons juice equals 357 cal., 9 g fat (4 g sat. fat), 68 mg chol., 877 mg sodium, 37 g carb., 2 g fiber, 31 g pro.* **Diabetic Exchanges:** *3 lean meat, 2 starch.*

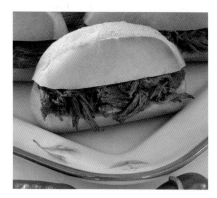

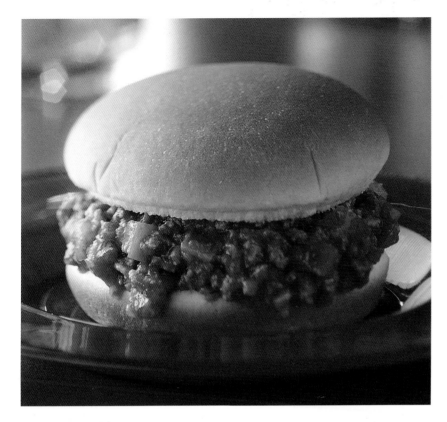

- 1 pound smoked kielbasa or Polish sausage, sliced
- ½ pound boneless skinless chicken breasts, cut into 1-inch cubes
- 1 can (14½ ounces) beef broth
- 1 can (14½ ounces) diced tomatoes, undrained
- 2 celery ribs, chopped
- ⅓ cup tomato paste
- 4 garlic cloves, minced
- 1 tablespoon dried parsley flakes
- 1½ teaspoons dried basil
- 1 teaspoon cayenne pepper
- ½ teaspoon salt
- ½ teaspoon dried oregano
- 1 pound cooked medium shrimp, peeled and deveined
- 2 cups cooked rice

1. In a 4-qt. slow cooker, combine the first 12 ingredients. Cover and cook on low for 6-7 hours or until chicken is no longer pink.
2. Stir in shrimp and rice. Cover and cook 15 minutes longer or until heated through.
PER SERVING *1 cup equals 228 cal., 11 g fat (4 g sat. fat), 95 mg chol., 692 mg sodium, 12 g carb., 1 g fiber, 18 g pro.* **Diabetic Exchanges:** *2 lean meat, 1 starch, 1 fat.*

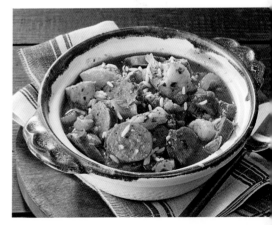

---

247 CALORIES

Turkey Sloppy Joes

These tangy sandwiches go over well at gatherings large and small. I frequently take them to potlucks, and I'm always asked what my secret ingredient is!
—**MARYLOU LARUE** FREELAND, MI

PREP: 15 MIN. • **COOK:** 4 HOURS
MAKES: 8 SERVINGS

- 1 pound lean ground turkey
- 1 small onion, chopped
- ½ cup chopped celery
- ¼ cup chopped green pepper
- 1 can (10¾ ounces) reduced-sodium condensed tomato soup, undiluted
- ½ cup ketchup
- 2 tablespoons prepared mustard
- 1 tablespoon brown sugar
- ¼ teaspoon pepper
- 8 hamburger buns, split

1. In a large skillet coated with cooking spray, cook the turkey, onion, celery and green pepper over medium heat until meat is no longer pink; drain. Stir in the soup, ketchup, mustard, brown sugar and pepper.
2. Transfer to a 3-qt. slow cooker. Cover and cook on low for 4 hours. Serve on buns.
PER SERVING *1 sandwich equals 247 cal., 7 g fat (2 g sat. fat), 45 mg chol., 553 mg sodium, 32 g carb., 2 g fiber, 14 g pro.* **Diabetic Exchanges:** *2 starch, 1½ lean meat.*

228 CALORIES Jambalaya

Sausage, chicken and shrimp keep this dish hearty and satisfying. Made easy with canned items, it's perfect for casual family get-togethers.
—**SHERRY HUNTWORK** GRETNA, NE

DO-IT-YOURSELF
Meal Planning Worksheet

DATE: _____

FOOD	CALORIES	FOOD	CALORIES
planned breakfast		actual breakfast	
_____	_____	_____	_____
_____	_____	_____	_____
_____	_____	_____	_____
_____		_____	

PLANNED BREAKFAST TOTAL CALORIES: | **ACTUAL BREAKFAST TOTAL CALORIES:**

FOOD	CALORIES	FOOD	CALORIES
planned lunch		actual lunch	
_____	_____	_____	_____
_____	_____	_____	_____
_____	_____	_____	_____

PLANNED LUNCH TOTAL CALORIES: | **ACTUAL LUNCH TOTAL CALORIES:**

FOOD	CALORIES	FOOD	CALORIES
planned dinner		actual dinner	
_____	_____	_____	_____
_____	_____	_____	_____
_____	_____	_____	_____

PLANNED DINNER TOTAL CALORIES: | **ACTUAL DINNER TOTAL CALORIES:**

FOOD	CALORIES	FOOD	CALORIES
planned snacks		actual snacks	
_____	_____	_____	_____

PLANNED SNACKS TOTAL CALORIES: | **ACTUAL SNACKS TOTAL CALORIES:**

PLANNED TOTAL CALORIES: | **ACTUAL TOTAL CALORIES:**

exercise _____

_____

DO-IT-YOURSELF
Meal Planning Worksheet

DATE: _____

FOOD	CALORIES	FOOD	CALORIES
planned breakfast		actual breakfast	

PLANNED BREAKFAST TOTAL CALORIES:

planned lunch		actual lunch	

PLANNED LUNCH TOTAL CALORIES:

planned dinner		actual dinner	

PLANNED DINNER TOTAL CALORIES:

planned snacks		actual snacks	

PLANNED SNACKS TOTAL CALORIES:

ACTUAL BREAKFAST TOTAL CALORIES:

ACTUAL LUNCH TOTAL CALORIES:

ACTUAL DINNER TOTAL CALORIES:

ACTUAL SNACKS TOTAL CALORIES:

PLANNED TOTAL CALORIES:

ACTUAL TOTAL CALORIES:

exercise _____

index by food category

To help you find the perfect dish for your family, we've created three different indexes.

This first one is divided into food and meal categories as well as major ingredients. Use this index to find recipes that call for a specific item or when you want to find a perfect sandwich, snack or salad.

You'll also notice that major categories are broken down a bit. If you look up "Chicken," for instance, you'll notice that there are subcategories for lunch dishes and dinner options.

Best of all, every entry in every index offers the calorie count per serving of that item. Planning a healthy meal for your family has never been easier!

Fudgy Chocolate Dessert
(200 CALORIES), 442

Granola Fudge Clusters
(114 CALORIES), 410

Ice Cream Sandwich Dessert
(244 CALORIES), 428

Marbled Chocolate Cheesecake Bars
(95 CALORIES), 406

Mocha Pudding Cakes
(227 CALORIES), 431

Mother Lode Pretzels
(114 CALORIES), 426

Oatmeal Chip Cookies
(140 CALORIES), 420

Peanut Butter S'mores Bars
(200 CALORIES), 428

Rocky Road Treat (145 CALORIES), 415

Tiramisu Parfaits (189 CALORIES), 431

Tortilla Dessert Cups
(130 CALORIES), 426

Trail Mix Clusters (79 CALORIES), 82

Warm Chocolate Melting Cups
(131 CALORIES), 422

White Chocolate Cranberry Cookies
(113 CALORIES), 413

White Chocolate Pretzel Snack
(63 CALORIES), 72

Wonton Sundaes (83 CALORIES), 402

Yummy Chocolate Cake
(197 CALORIES), 437

Yummy S'more Snack Cake
(168 CALORIES), 440

CINNAMON

Apple-Cinnamon Oatmeal Mix
(176 CALORIES), 115

Caramel Apple Bread Pudding
(187 CALORIES), 430

Chewy Granola Bars
(160 CALORIES), 98

Cinnamon-Honey Grapefruit
(63 CALORIES), 90

Cinnamon-Raisin Bites
(82 CALORIES), 88

Cranberry-Stuffed Apples
(136 CALORIES), 458

Hot Berries 'n' Brownie Ice Cream Cake
(233 CALORIES), 433

Nutmeg Waffles (196 CALORIES), 99

Old-Fashioned Molasses Cake
(148 CALORIES), 424

Raisin Oatmeal Mix
(186 CALORIES), 104

Slow-Cooker Berry Cobbler
(250 CALORIES), 455

Spiced Butternut Squash Soup
(131 CALORIES), 150

Spiced Oatmeal Mix (210 CALORIES), 139

COCONUT

Coconut-Cherry Cream Squares
(142 CALORIES), 419

Coconut Custard Pie
(214 CALORIES), 443

Coconut-Pecan Sweet Potatoes
(211 CALORIES), 463

Pina Colada Pudding Cups
(171 CALORIES), 435

Tropical Meringue Tarts
(145 CALORIES), 427

COFFEE

Cafe Mocha Mini Muffins
(81 CALORIES), 91

Cappuccino Mousse
(125 CALORIES), 418

Cappuccino Pudding
(105 CALORIES), 422

Frappe Mocha (80 CALORIES), 80

Mocha Pudding Cakes
(227 CALORIES), 431

Spiced Coffee with Cream
(55 CALORIES), 70

Tiramisu Parfaits (189 CALORIES), 431

Warm Chocolate Melting Cups
(131 CALORIES), 422

CORN & GRITS

Alfresco Bean Salad
(146 CALORIES), 372

Baked Corn Pudding
(186 CALORIES), 381

Baked Southern Grits
(158 CALORIES), 118

Black Bean Taco Pizza
(264 CALORIES), 249

Cajun Buttered Corn
(105 CALORIES), 377

Chive 'n' Garlic Corn
(159 CALORIES), 378

Chunky Chicken Soup
(229 CALORIES), 457

Confetti Scrambled Egg Pockets
(207 CALORIES), 134

Corn and Broccoli in Cheese Sauce
(148 CALORIES), 449

Corn 'n' Red Pepper Medley
(130 CALORIES), 382

Corn Potato Pancakes
(180 CALORIES), 384

Corny Chicken Wraps
(363 CALORIES), 340

Crab Cakes with Fresh Lemon
(311 CALORIES), 304

Family-Pleasing Turkey Chili
(349 CALORIES), 468

Fast Refried Bean Soup
(117 CALORIES), 148

Garlic Cheese Grits (186 CALORIES), 121

Hominy Taco Chili (274 CALORIES), 184

Marvelous Chicken Enchiladas
(336 CALORIES), 289

Mexican Veggies (70 CALORIES), 347

Sauteed Corn with Tomatoes & Basil
(85 CALORIES), 346

Southwestern Beef Strips
(304 CALORIES), 291

Southwestern Chicken Soup
(143 CALORIES), 445

Southwestern Goulash
(224 CALORIES), 241

Tomato Corn Salad (84 CALORIES), 348

Turkey Burritos with Fresh Fruit Salsa
(371 CALORIES), 335

Zippy Corn Chowder
(190 CALORIES), 145

CORN BREAD & CORNMEAL

Cornmeal Oven-Fried Chicken
(244 CALORIES), 209

Cranberry Cornmeal Dressing
(205 CALORIES), 388

Hamburger Corn Bread Casserole
(339 CALORIES), 280

CRANBERRIES

Apple Cranberry Delight
(70 CALORIES), 404

Berry Barbecued Pork Roast
(262 CALORIES), 287

Brisket with Cranberry Gravy
(225 CALORIES), 448

Caramelized Pear Strudel
(139 CALORIES), 420

Cran-Orange Pork Medallions
(339 CALORIES), 284

Cranberry Almond Macaroons
(91 CALORIES), 396

Cranberry Cornmeal Dressing
(205 CALORIES), 388

Cranberry-Mustard Pork Loin
(255 CALORIES), 459

Cranberry-Stuffed Apples
(136 CALORIES), 458

White Chocolate Cranberry Cookies
(113 CALORIES), 413

Slow-Cooker Berry Cobbler
(250 CALORIES), 455
Wonton Sundaes (83 CALORIES), 402
PIES & TARTS
Coconut Custard Pie
(214 CALORIES), 443
Fresh Raspberry Pie
(163 CALORIES), 432
No-Bake Cheesecake Pie
(141 CALORIES), 419
Raspberry Custard Tart
(198 CALORIES), 430
Raspberry Pie with Oat Crust
(167 CALORIES), 434
Tart Cherry Pie (174 CALORIES), 429
Tropical Meringue Tarts
(145 CALORIES), 427

DRESSING
Cranberry Cornmeal Dressing
(205 CALORIES), 388
Slow-Cooked Sausage Dressing
(201 CALORIES), 452

EGGS (ALSO SEE BREAKFASTS)
Baked Corn Pudding
(186 CALORIES), 381
Herbed Potato Salad
(142 CALORIES), 368
Herbed Tuna Sandwiches
(332 CALORIES), 177
Special Egg Salad (259 CALORIES), 160

FISH SEE SEAFOOD.

FRUIT (ALSO SEE SPECIFIC KINDS)
Berry & Yogurt Phyllo Nests
(72 CALORIES), 92
Berry Nectarine Buckle
(177 CALORIES), 436
Berry Turkey Sandwiches
(356 CALORIES), 189
Berry Yogurt Cups (98 CALORIES), 97
Breakfast Crepes with Berries
(182 CALORIES), 102
Breakfast Sundaes (266 CALORIES), 127
Broiled Fruit Dessert
(80 CALORIES), 395
Chocolate Fruit Dip (88 CALORIES), 81
Chunky Fruit 'n' Nut Fudge
(92 CALORIES), 401
Citrus Fish Tacos (411 CALORIES), 325
Creamy Chicken Salad
(261 CALORIES), 181
Custard Berry Parfaits
(119 CALORIES), 119
Dried Fruit Muesli (228 CALORIES), 126

Fruit Cup with Citrus Sauce
(63 CALORIES), 93
Fruit Juice Pops (149 CALORIES), 417
Fruit Smoothies (97 CALORIES), 92
Fruited Dutch Baby
(203 CALORIES), 127
Fruited Turkey Salad Pitas
(393 CALORIES), 204
Fruited Turkey Wraps
(332 CALORIES), 162
Fruity Cereal Bars (105 CALORIES), 411
Fruity Crab Pasta Salad
(322 CALORIES), 168
Granola-to-Go Bars
(130 CALORIES), 101
Hot Berries 'n' Brownie Ice Cream Cake
(233 CALORIES), 433
Icy Fruit Pops (66 CALORIES), 69
Mahi Mahi with Nectarine Salsa
(247 CALORIES), 236
Melon 'n' Grape Medley
(74 CALORIES), 354
Meringues with Fresh Berries
(222 CALORIES), 443
Mint Berry Blast (65 CALORIES), 95
Mixed Berry French Toast Bake
(297 CALORIES), 140
Polynesian Stir-Fry
(339 CALORIES), 274
Sangria Gelatin Ring
(80 CALORIES), 409
Slow-Cooker Berry Cobbler
(250 CALORIES), 455
Spinach & Citrus Salad
(52 CALORIES), 351
Sun-Kissed Smoothies
(100 CALORIES), 91
Sunrise Slushies (73 CALORIES), 95
Sweet Berry Bruschetta
(92 CALORIES), 89
Teriyaki Chicken Salad with Poppy
    Seed Dressing (361 CALORIES), 198
Trail Mix Clusters (79 CALORIES), 82
Turkey Burritos with Fresh Fruit Salsa
(371 CALORIES), 335
Yogurt Fruit Smoothies
(225 CALORIES), 129

GROUND BEEF
LUNCHES
Barbecue Beef Sandwiches
(348 CALORIES), 179
Barley Beef Skillet (400 CALORIES), 195
Best Sloppy Joes (274 CALORIES), 163
Chili Beef Quesadillas
(353 CALORIES), 190

Easy Beef Barley Soup
(317 CALORIES), 173
Family-Favorite Cheeseburger Pasta
(391 CALORIES), 196
Fully Loaded Chili (351 CALORIES), 191
Grilled Italian Meatball Burgers
(399 CALORIES), 203
Hominy Taco Chili (274 CALORIES), 184
Italian Beef and Shells
(396 CALORIES), 204
Lasagna Soup (280 CALORIES), 185
Makeover Gourmet Enchiladas
(358 CALORIES), 192
Pumpkin Sloppy Joes for 2
(350 CALORIES), 171
Spicy Two-Bean Chili
(254 CALORIES), 446
Taco Salad Wraps (345 CALORIES), 175
Zesty Hamburger Soup
(222 CALORIES), 177
Zippy Spaghetti Sauce
(220 CALORIES), 456
DINNERS
Chili Mac Casserole
(358 CALORIES), 316
Enchilada Casser-Ole!
(357 CALORIES), 327
French Cheeseburger Loaf
(277 CALORIES), 306
Hamburger Corn Bread Casserole
(339 CALORIES), 280
Hamburger Noodle Casserole
(319 CALORIES), 262
"Little Kick" Jalapeno Burgers
(254 CALORIES), 260
Makeover Tater-Topped Casserole
(340 CALORIES), 256

HAM & PROSCIUTTO
Asparagus Ham Roll-Ups
(69 CALORIES), 88
Baked Deli Focaccia Sandwich
(240 CALORIES), 143
Brunch Enchiladas (258 CALORIES), 130
Cordon Bleu Appetizers
(86 CALORIES), 65
Ham and Apricot Crepes
(258 CALORIES), 137
Ham 'n' Cheese Squares
(141 CALORIES), 101
Ham 'n' Chickpea Soup
(312 CALORIES), 174
Ham Asparagus Spirals
(49 CALORIES), 73
Ham Potato Puffs
(165 CALORIES), 122

INDEX

Veggie Cheese Ravioli
(322 CALORIES), 292
Veggie-Cheese Stuffed Shells
(326 CALORIES), 295
Weekday Lasagna (280 CALORIES), 296
Weeknight Beef Skillet
(319 CALORIES), 314
Zippy Spaghetti Sauce
(220 CALORIES), 456

SIDE DISHES
Couscous with Mushrooms
(230 CALORIES), 391
Creamy Macaroni 'n' Cheese
(312 CALORIES), 387
Garden Primavera Fettuccine
(373 CALORIES), 382
Garlic-Herb Orzo Pilaf
(361 CALORIES), 390
Savory Skillet Noodles
(160 CALORIES), 374
Slow-Cooked Mac 'n' Cheese
(300 CALORIES), 467
Southwestern Pasta & Cheese
(389 CALORIES), 393
Zucchini Pasta (219 CALORIES), 390

PEACHES
Baked Blueberry & Peach Oatmeal
(277 CALORIES), 124
Dijon-Peach Pork Chops
(360 CALORIES), 324
Peach Smoothie (68 CALORIES), 66
Peach-Stuffed French Toast
(267 CALORIES), 128
Spicy Chicken Breasts with Pepper Peach Relish (263 CALORIES), 263
Waffles with Peach-Berry Compote
(251 CALORIES), 133

PEAS
Chicken Fettuccine Alfredo
(425 CALORIES), 329
Creamed Peas and Carrots
(191 CALORIES), 368
Favorite Irish Stew (271 CALORIES), 253
Garlic Chicken Penne
(429 CALORIES), 329
Holiday Peas (87 CALORIES), 353
Orange-Glazed Pork Stir-Fry
(277 CALORIES), 302
Peas a la Francaise (112 CALORIES), 379
Peas in Cheese Sauce
(114 CALORIES), 370
Skillet Arroz con Pollo
(373 CALORIES), 318
Texas Caviar (77 CALORIES), 78
Turkey a la King (350 CALORIES), 170

PEPPERS
SEE BELL PEPPERS; HOT PEPPERS.

PINEAPPLE
Broiled Pineapple Dessert
(98 CALORIES), 399
Hawaiian Breakfast Cups
(131 CALORIES), 123
Honey Pineapple Chicken
(302 CALORIES), 449
Malibu Chicken Bundles
(400 CALORIES), 331
Pina Colada Pudding Cups
(171 CALORIES), 435
Pineapple Beef Kabobs
(412 CALORIES), 314
Pineapple Cabbage Saute
(85 CALORIES), 363
Pineapple Chicken Fajitas
(402 CALORIES), 201
Pineapple Pudding Cake
(131 CALORIES), 412
Slow-Cooked Sweet 'n' Sour Pork
(312 CALORIES), 462
Snapper with Spicy Pineapple Glaze
(304 CALORIES), 251
Sweet and Sour Chicken
(428 CALORIES), 336
Tropical Meringue Tarts
(145 CALORIES), 427

PIZZA
Baked Potato Pizza (359 CALORIES), 313
Black Bean Taco Pizza
(264 CALORIES), 249
Greek Pizzas (320 CALORIES), 256
Grilled Artichoke-Mushroom Pizza
(283 CALORIES), 300
Pizza Lover's Pie (305 CALORIES), 277
Pizza Roll-Up (316 CALORIES), 287

POLENTA
Mini Polenta Pizzas (57 CALORIES), 77
Ratatouille with Polenta
(195 CALORIES), 156
Spiced Polenta Steak Fries
(121 CALORIES), 385

POPCORN
Cajun Popcorn (77 CALORIES), 71
Parmesan Popcorn (49 CALORIES), 75
Sunflower Popcorn Bars
(96 CALORIES), 81
Sweet 'n' Salty Popcorn
(91 CALORIES), 83
Tex-Mex Popcorn (44 CALORIES), 66

PORK (ALSO SEE BACON & CANADIAN BACON; HAM & PROSCIUTTO; SAUSAGE & PEPPERONI)

LUNCHES
Pork Burritos (320 CALORIES), 464
Pulled Pork Subs (417 CALORIES), 458
Slow-Cooked Pork Tacos
(301 CALORIES), 446
Tangy Pulled Pork Sandwiches
(402 CALORIES), 451

DINNERS
Apple-Cherry Pork Chops
(350 CALORIES), 247
Apple Pork Stir-Fry
(370 CALORIES), 312
Bavarian Pork Loin
(235 CALORIES), 454
Berry Barbecued Pork Roast
(262 CALORIES), 287
Braised Pork Chops
(180 CALORIES), 241
Chinese Pork 'n' Noodles
(398 CALORIES), 316
Chops 'n' Kraut (311 CALORIES), 290
Cran-Orange Pork Medallions
(339 CALORIES), 284
Cranberry-Mustard Pork Loin
(255 CALORIES), 459
Dijon-Peach Pork Chops
(360 CALORIES), 324
Easy Barbecued Pork Chops
(312 CALORIES), 307
Gingered Pork Tenderloin
(214 CALORIES), 207
Glazed Pork Chops
(246 CALORIES), 244
Glazed Pork Medallions
(200 CALORIES), 221
Glazed Pork Tenderloin
(263 CALORIES), 270
Grilled Pork Chops with Cilantro Salsa
(240 CALORIES), 230
Grilled Pork Tenderloin
(171 CALORIES), 238
Grilled Stuffed Pork Tenderloin
(296 CALORIES), 281
Herbed Pork and Potatoes
(358 CALORIES), 334
Honey Lemon Schnitzel
(298 CALORIES), 257
Jalapeno-Apricot Pork Tenderloin
(378 CALORIES), 323
Onion-Dijon Pork Chops
(261 CALORIES), 295

Quick Creamed Spinach
(131 CALORIES), 385
Skillet Pasta Florentine
(383 CALORIES), 330
Southwest Pasta Bake
(328 CALORIES), 265
Spinach & Citrus Salad
(52 CALORIES), 351
Spinach and Mushroom Smothered
Chicken (203 CALORIES), 238
Spinach-Feta Chicken Rolls
(272 CALORIES), 272
Spinach Omelet Brunch Roll
(160 CALORIES), 103
Spinach-Tomato Phyllo Bake
(216 CALORIES), 219
Tofu Spinach Lasagna
(227 CALORIES), 226
Tortellini Primavera
(341 CALORIES), 286
Turkey Roulades (184 CALORIES), 214
Wilted Garlic Spinach
(66 CALORIES), 357

SQUASH
Brown Sugar Squash
(216 CALORIES), 386
Grandma's Stuffed Yellow Squash
(103 CALORIES), 378
Greek-Style Squash
(80 CALORIES), 360
Italian Squash Casserole
(99 CALORIES), 344
Mediterranean Summer Squash
(69 CALORIES), 365
Rice with Summer Squash
(123 CALORIES), 375
Sizzling Beef Kabobs
(227 CALORIES), 218
Turkey 'n' Squash Lasagna
(311 CALORIES), 285

STEWS (ALSO SEE CHILI; SOUPS)
Hearty Beef Vegetable Stew
(380 CALORIES), 447
Jamaican-Style Beef Stew
(285 CALORIES), 184
Jambalaya (228 CALORIES), 469
Old-Fashioned Lamb Stew
(273 CALORIES), 176
Potato-Lentil Stew
(295 CALORIES), 180
Southwest Turkey Stew
(238 CALORIES), 451
Southwestern Beef Stew
(266 CALORIES), 461
Vegetable Beef Stew
(278 CALORIES), 467

STRAWBERRIES
Best Strawberry Ice Cream
(153 CALORIES), 438
Jellied Champagne Dessert
(96 CALORIES), 397
Mixed Berry Pizza (110 CALORIES), 415
Orange Strawberry Smoothies
(120 CALORIES), 108
Strawberry Banana Delight
(78 CALORIES), 405
Strawberry Mango Smoothies
(100 CALORIES), 83
Strawberry-Raspberry Ice
(118 CALORIES), 423
Strawberry Tofu Smoothies
(136 CALORIES), 111
Strawberry Watermelon Slush
(89 CALORIES), 67
Tres Leches Cake (233 CALORIES), 436
Waffles with Peach-Berry Compote
(251 CALORIES), 133
Warm Chocolate Melting Cups
(131 CALORIES), 422
Watermelon Berry Sorbet
(95 CALORIES), 404

STUFFING SEE DRESSING.

SWEET POTATOES
Chipotle Sweet Potato and Spiced
Apple Purees (224 CALORIES), 388
Coconut-Pecan Sweet Potatoes
(211 CALORIES), 463
Sweet Potato & Black Bean Chili
(252 CALORIES), 168
Sweet Potato Banana Bake
(189 CALORIES), 366
Sweet Potato Casserole
(186 CALORIES), 371

TOFU
Orange Strawberry Smoothies
(120 CALORIES), 108
Raspberry Key Lime Crepes
(222 CALORIES), 138
Strawberry Tofu Smoothies
(136 CALORIES), 111
Tofu Spinach Lasagna
(227 CALORIES), 226

TOMATOES
Alfresco Bean Salad
(146 CALORIES), 372
Anytime Frittata (138 CALORIES), 106
Asparagus Tomato Salad
(81 CALORIES), 351
Baked Mostaccioli
(278 CALORIES), 258

Basil Cherry Tomatoes
(42 CALORIES), 347
Bow Ties with Chicken & Shrimp
(399 CALORIES), 324
Cacciatore Chicken Breasts
(272 CALORIES), 266
Caprese Tomato Bites
(63 CALORIES), 72
Cheese Tomato Egg Bake
(110 CALORIES), 102
Chops 'n' Kraut (311 CALORIES), 290
Colorful Beef Wraps
(325 CALORIES), 307
Creole Chicken (320 CALORIES), 305
Fantastic Fish Tacos
(314 CALORIES), 252
Grape Tomato Mozzarella Salad
(85 CALORIES), 358
Greek Pizzas (320 CALORIES), 256
Grilled Pork Chops with Cilantro Salsa
(240 CALORIES), 230
Hearty Spaghetti Sauce
(163 CALORIES), 246
Hominy Taco Chili (274 CALORIES), 184
Italian Cabbage Casserole
(223 CALORIES), 212
Italian Hot Dish (391 CALORIES), 322
Italian Pasta Casserole
(335 CALORIES), 306
Jamaican-Style Beef Stew
(285 CALORIES), 184
Jambalaya (228 CALORIES), 469
Lasagna Soup (280 CALORIES), 185
Meatless Chili Mac (214 CALORIES), 237
Meatless Zucchini Lasagna
(272 CALORIES), 303
Mediterranean Breakfast Pitas
(267 CALORIES), 141
Mediterranean Shrimp 'n' Pasta
(368 CALORIES), 330
Mexican-Inspired Turkey Burgers
(312 CALORIES), 288
Parmesan Tomato (54 CALORIES), 344
Pork 'n' Penne Skillet
(264 CALORIES), 291
Presto Chicken Tacos
(215 CALORIES), 147
Ranch Chicken Salad Sandwiches
(257 CALORIES), 172
Red Clam Sauce (305 CALORIES), 466
Sauteed Corn with Tomatoes & Basil
(85 CALORIES), 346
Skillet Tacos (267 CALORIES), 305
Slow-Cooked Italian Chicken
(231 CALORIES), 463

alphabetical index

With *Best of Comfort Food Diet Cookbook*, serving your family healthy and tasty meals is a breeze. This index (organized by recipe title) also offers the per-serving calorie count of every dish.

If you have a hard time recalling the names of all the favorites you've prepared from this book, simply begin to highlight those dishes that get thumbs-up approval from your family. You could also put a blank sticky note on the back of this book and write down the titles of the recipes your family enjoys most.

INDEX

index by calories

The Taste of Home Comfort Food Diet's success rests on the calories you consume each day. To help you plan your caloric intake and daily menus, this index categorizes recipes by type (snacks, breakfast, dinner, etc.). The items are then broken down into their applicable calorie ranges.

When looking for a dinner that's on the lighter side, see the 86 dishes listed under "Dinners: 250 Calories or Less." If you saved a few more calories for the end of the day, consider the recipes found under "Dinners: 251 to 350 Calories." There you'll find 128 recipes.

With a little help from this index, you'll be amazed at how easy it is to meet your goals and make the Taste of Home Comfort Food Diet a healthy and delicious part of your life.

DINNERS

251-350 CALORIES

Photography Credits

boxed lunch, page 5
matka_Wariatka/Shutterstock.com

notebook, page 6
Galushko Sergey/Shutterstock.com

yoga posture, page 7
Deklofenak/Shutterstock.com

stacked apples, page 10
Ultrashock/Shutterstock.com

roasted salmon, page 11
Yuri Arcurs/Shutterstock.com

dairy products, page 11
matka_Wariatka/Shutterstock.com

rice with beans & peppers, page 4, page 11
Tobik/Shutterstock.com

MyPlate, page 12
Basheera Designs/Shutterstock.com

nutrition label, page 15
XAOC/Shutterstock.com

fruit bowl, page 17
Ildi Papp/Shutterstock.com

popcorn, page 17
Jiri Hera/Shutterstock.com

shopping basket, page 18
Yelena Panyukova/Shutterstock.com

cherry tomatoes, page 19
Larina Natalia/Shutterstock.com

fresh blueberries, page 19
Kati Molin/Shutterstock.com

grilled chicken breast, page 19
barbaradudzinska/Shutterstock.com

healthy dip, page 20
Wiktory/Shutterstock.com

shopping list, page 20
Gina Sanders/Shutterstock.com

cupcakes in pan, page 21
Monkey Business Images/Shutterstock.com

woman shopping for corn, page 22 Yuri Arcurs/Shutterstock.com

chopping veggies, page 25
auremar/Shutterstock.com

salmon with lemon, page 26
DUSAN ZIDAR/Shutterstock.com

peppermint candy, page 26
J. Broadwater/Shutterstock.com

veggies with hummus, page 27
keko64/Shutterstock.com

lunch snack, page 27
Juriah Mosin/Shutterstock.com

eating on couch, page 30
Luis Camargo/Shutterstock.com

walking on grass, page 34
Rafal Olechowski/Shutterstock.com

walking family, page 35
Dmitriy Shironosov/Shutterstock.com

woman walking, page 35
Christopher Edwin Nuzzaco/Shutterstock.com

woman stretching, page 36
Monalyn Gracia/Corbis

woman hiking, page 37
Jordan Siemens/Getty Images

mixed nuts, page 37
Nadja Antonova/Shutterstock.com

compass, page 37
STILLFX/Shutterstock.com

couple hiking, page 37
Tyler Olson/Shutterstock.com

couple resting by tree, page 37
Tyler Olson/Shutterstock.com

plate of veggies, page 39
picamaniac/Shutterstock.com

chili peppers, page 40
Cogipix/Shutterstock.com

cucumbers, page 40
Teresa Kasprzycka/Shutterstock.com

arugula in bowl, page 40
Cogipix/Shutterstock.com

summer drink, page 41
Tamara Kulikova/Shutterstock.com

blackberries, page 84
ninette_luz/Shutterstock.com

peanut butter, page 85
Simone van den Berg/Shutterstock.com